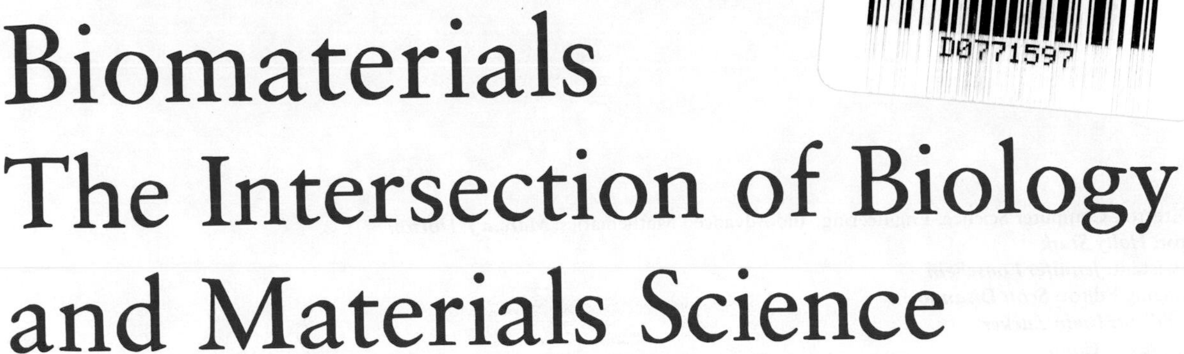

Biomaterials
The Intersection of Biology and Materials Science

J. S. Temenoff

Wallace H. Coulter Department of Biomedical Engineering
Georgia Tech and Emory University, Atlanta, GA

A. G. Mikos

Departments of Bioengineering and Chemical and Biomolecular Engineering
Rice University, Houston, TX

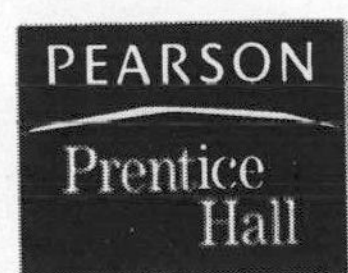

Pearson Education International

Editorial Director, Computer Science, Engineering, and Advanced Mathematics: ***Marcia J. Horton***
Senior Editor: ***Holly Stark***
Editorial Assistant: ***Jennifer Lonschein***
Senior Managing Editor: ***Scott Disanno***
Production Editor: ***Irwin Zucker***
Art Director: ***Jayne Conte***
Cover Designer: ***Bruce Kenselaar***
Art Editor: ***Thomas Benfatti***
Manufacturing Manager: ***Alexis Heydt-Long***
Manufacturing Buyer: ***Lisa McDowell***
Senior Marketing Manager: ***Tim Galligan***

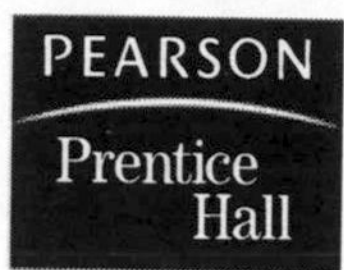

Pearson Prentice Hall
Pearson Education, Inc.
Upper Saddle River, New Jersey 07458

Printed in the United States of America

10 9 8 7 6 5 4 3

ISBN 0-13-235044-0
978-0-13-235044-0

Pearson Education LTD., *London*
Pearson Education Australia Pty, Limited, *Sydney*
Pearson Education Singapore, Pte. Ltd
Pearson Education North Asia Ltd., *Hong Kong*
Pearson Education Canada, Ltd., *Toronto*
Pearson Education de Mexico, S.A. de C.V.
Pearson Education Japan, *Tokyo*
Pearson Education Malaysia, Pte. Ltd.
Pearson Education, Inc., *Upper Saddle River, New Jersey*

Dedications

To my mother, who encouraged me to ask "Why?"
and my father, who encouraged me to ask "How?"
(JST)

To Mary, Georgios, and Lydia
(AGM)

Contents

2

Chemical Structure of Biomaterials 32

3

Physical Properties of Biomaterials 101

5

Biomaterial Degradation 177

6

Biomaterial Processing 205

9

Cell Interactions with Biomaterials 314

10

13

Biomaterials and Thrombosis 428

Foreword

Biomaterials have received considerable attention over the last thirty years as a means of treating diseases and easing suffering. The focus of treatment is no longer in conventional passive devices but rather a combination of device-integrated biomaterials and the necessary therapeutic treatment. Biomaterials have found applications in approximately 8,000 various kinds of medical devices that have been used in repairing skeletal systems, returning cardiovascular functionality, replacing organs, and repairing or returning senses. Even though biomaterials have had a pronounced impact in medical treatment, a need still exists to be able to design and develop better polymer, ceramic, and metal systems along with the ability to characterize and test their properties. This book is the first in a long time to point out such need and to give students a clear picture of how to approach such subjects.

The two authors take a fresh approach to the problem. They focus on a thorough materials analysis that does not take shortcomings on mechanical properties, structure or molecular analysis, but at the same time offers a thorough presentation of biological considerations in a succinct way.

Polymeric biomaterials originated as off-the-shelf materials that clinicians were able to use in solving a problem—dialysis tubing was originally made of cellulose acetate, vascular grafts were fabricated from Dacron, and artificial hearts were molded from polyurethanes. However, these materials did not possess the chemical, physical, and biological properties necessary to prevent further complications. Thus, recent advances in synthetic techniques have allowed these properties to be imparted on biomaterials that help to alleviate the accompanying biocompatibility issues. This becomes so clear in this book!

Much consideration is given to the design of a material for a specific application. Certain properties of the material must be controlled so as to perform the necessary function and elicit the appropriate response. These properties can be tailored to the specific need by carefully controlling the structural characteristics, modifying the surface properties, and employing biomimetic characteristics in the material design. Biomimetic principles are gaining widespread acceptance in the development of biomaterials, especially for drug delivery, regenerative medicine, and nanotechnology. The use of protein moieties and protein-like components on the surface or in the bulk of synthetic materials contacting biological systems has certain advantage over traditional systems. The authors are to be congratulated for pointing this out.

This book will be a successful text because it recognizes that biomaterials are first and foremost *materials!* The authors provide a refreshing approach to the medical aspects of biomaterials. It has exceptionally lucid chapters on Cell/Materials and Protein/Materials interactions. The students will finally understand immunology when they read Chapter 12. And thrombosis, one of the most important problems of biomaterials, is simply expertly presented in Chapter 13.

This textbook is a comprehensive fundamental text that will undoubtedly become a staple in biomaterials education. It addresses the right amount of knowledge and will fill a major gap in the field of biomaterials science. Professors Temenoff and Mikos have made a great service to the field.

Nicholas A. Peppas, Sc.D.
Fletcher S. Pratt Chair of Chemical Engineering,
Biomedical Engineering, and Pharmacy
University of Texas at Austin

Preface

Intersect: to share a common area (*Merriam-Webster Dictionary*)

Although this book is entitled *Biomaterials: The Intersection of Biology and Materials Science*, we believe that this field has evolved over approximately the past fifty years from the intersection of multiple disparate viewpoints, including materials science, biology, engineering, and clinical, business, and regulatory perspectives. With this history, the multidisciplinary nature of biomaterials is inescapable. As educators in this field, we have taken on the particular challenge of preparing students with a broad range of backgrounds to address the complex issues associated with designing and implementing new biomedical devices.

With this in mind, we set out to write a balanced and cohesive textbook that would introduce fundamental concepts of biomaterials to undergraduate engineering majors in their second year of study or later. Given this target audience, the text assumes basic knowledge of chemistry and physics, but does not require in-depth exposure to more complex mathematical concepts such as partial differential equations, or any knowledge of cell biology or biochemistry.

After an overview of the scope of the biomaterials field, Chapter 1 reviews basic chemical principles required to understand the forces underlying the material structures introduced in Chapter 2. Chapters 3 and 4 provide more information about physical and mechanical properties of the main classes of biomaterials (metals, ceramics, and polymers). Throughout these sections, material classes are compared and contrasted to further student knowledge of how each may be optimal for different applications. After discussion of how materials are "built up" from their subunits, in Chapters 5 and 6, we turn to how these materials are "torn down" (degraded) in the body and how processing parameters affect key material properties, such as degradation and mechanical strength.

Chapters 7 and 8 are both the physical and intellectual centers of this text as they represent contact between the materials science and the biological concepts in the book. Topics covered in these chapters include surface modification techniques and their effects on protein adsorption. Chapter 9 relates how cells react to these adsorbed proteins in general, before leading into a discussion of particular cell responses (acute inflammation and wound healing) in Chapters 10 and 11. No depiction of biological response to implanted materials would be complete without a discussion of immune response and hypersensitivity (Chapter 12), thrombosis (Chapter 13) and infection, tumorigenesis, and pathologic calcification (Chapter 14).

To maintain a balanced discussion, the fourteen chapters in this book were purposefully divided into seven chapters on materials science, and seven chapters on the biological response. Continuing the spirit of "intersection," characterization methods and regulatory issues were not written as insular sections, but rather included throughout book as appropriate.

The twenty-first century will surely present even greater challenges to the biomaterialist in integrating ever more complex biological knowledge into the design of improved materials. We believe that exploration of overlap between these disparate fields is essential and hope that this book provides a first step for many future biomaterialists in discovering vital intersections of their own.

Acknowledgments

The development and production of a textbook such as this is an ambitious undertaking that requires the contributions of a myriad of talented and dedicated individuals. Accordingly, we would like to acknowledge the several individuals and institutions whose assistance and perseverance made the completion of this text possible. Two individuals were indispensable in the preparation of this work. Kurt Kasper, Ph.D. (Rice University) provided summaries for each of the chapters, authored the example problems that occur throughout the text, contributed to writing select sections of the text, and worked diligently in editing the various drafts of this book. Mark Sweigart, Ph.D. (Rice University) wrote the end-of-chapter problems, industriously assembled all of the figures for this textbook, formatted all of the equations, and patiently edited the text for stylistic consistency. Elizabeth Christensen, Ph.D. (Rice University) and Michael Hacker, Ph.D. (Rice University) contributed select figures and kindly compiled literature reports that were integrated into the material in this text. Additionally, we thank the entire biomaterials faculty at Georgia Tech and Emory University for their feedback during the preparation of the text, particularly Julia Babensee, Ph.D. and Andrés García, Ph.D., who contributed to the end-of-chapter problems.

Further, we are indebted to the various pioneers in biomaterials research who thoroughly reviewed the first draft of this book. Specifically, we extend our deep appreciation to James M. Anderson, M.D., Ph.D. (Case Western Reserve University), Joel D. Bumgardner, Ph.D. (University of Memphis), Arnold I. Caplan, Ph.D. (Case Western Reserve University), M. Cindy Farach-Carson, Ph.D. (University of Delaware), Paul S. Engel, Ph.D. (Rice University), John A. Jansen, D.D.S., Ph.D. (Radboud University Nijmegen Medical Center), Robert Langer, Sc.D. (Massachusetts Institute of Technology), Nicholas A. Peppas, Sc.D. (University of Texas at Austin), Alan J. Russell, Ph.D. (University of Pittsburgh), and Frederick J Schoen, M.D., Ph.D. (Brigham and Women's Hospital) for their meticulous reviews and constructive comments.

We would also like to acknowledge several individuals who played vital roles in the evaluation and development of the text. Particularly, we thank Valeria Milam, Ph.D. (Georgia Tech) for helping to test this book in the classroom and for providing valuable alterations to the various drafts of the text. We also thank Larry McIntire, Ph.D. and Robert Nerem, Ph.D. for their comments on this book, as well as for providing a dynamic and supportive environment in which to test this text. We appreciate the teaching assistants and students in the Georgia Tech Introduction to Biomaterials classes (BMED 4823/MSE 4803 and BMED/MSE 4751) in the Spring and Fall Semesters of 2006 and the Spring Semester of 2007 for their patience during the classroom testing of this textbook. We also thank Simon Young, D.D.S. (Rice University) and the graduate students in the laboratory of Johnna Temenoff, Ph.D. at Georgia Tech/Emory University (namely, Kelly Brink, Derek Doroski, Jeremy Lim, and Peter Yang) for their perseverance and diligence in helping edit the final drafts of this book.

We extend also our gratitude to several other individuals who were essential in attending to the details surrounding the production of this book. Carol D. Lofton (Rice University) worked tirelessly to secure the copyright permissions needed for publication. Also, the staff in the Coulter Department of Biomedical Engineering at Georgia Tech/Emory University kindly assisted in the preparations of the various drafts of the text and in obtaining the required copyright permissions. Finally, we acknowledge the artistic talent of Karen Ku, who drew the inspirational art work appearing on the cover of this book.

J. S. Temenoff
A. G. Mikos

Materials for Biomedical Applications

CHAPTER 1

Main Objective

To understand what the field of biomaterials encompasses, to appreciate the general concerns of a biomaterialist, and to review principles from general chemistry as needed.

Specific Objectives

1. To understand the breadth of the field and important consensus definitions relating to biomaterials.
2. To be able to compare/contrast natural and synthetic materials.
3. To be able to compare/contrast surface and bulk properties and understand that design criteria depend on the final application.
4. To understand that the material induces a biological response which can, in turn, affect the material performance.
5. To understand that the form of the material can influence its properties and the biological response to its implantation.
6. To understand how electron structure contributes to various types of bonding.

1.1 Introduction to Biomaterials

This chapter is designed to provide a general overview of the breadth of the field of biomaterials and discuss briefly all the aspects of this discipline that will be explored more fully in later chapters. In addition, it provides important basic definitions and background information for the remainder of the book. The chapter begins with a discussion of the scope and history of biomaterials science and the role of the biomaterialist. In later sections, degradative, surface and bulk properties of materials are related to the choices incumbent upon biomaterialists as they design/select the optimal material for particular applications. Finally, a review of basic chemical principles underlying important material properties is presented.

1.1.1 Important Definitions

Biomaterials is a wide-ranging field, encompassing aspects of basic biology, medicine, engineering, and materials science, that has developed to its current form primarily since World War II. Because of the breadth of the field, confusion often exists about what a biomaterial is, and, in particular, the role of the biomaterialist in modern medicine. Therefore, we begin our discussion of biomaterials science with key definitions to better characterize the discipline.

According to a consensus decision by a panel of experts, a **biomaterial** is

> A material intended to interface with biological systems to evaluate, treat, augment, or replace any tissue, organ or function of the body [1].

Therefore, **biomaterials science** is the study of biomaterials and their interactions with the biological environment [2]. This includes subjects relating to materials science, such as mechanical properties of materials or surface modification of implants, as well as biological topics such as immunology, toxicology, and wound healing processes.

Regardless of which aspect of biomaterials science is addressed, the "bio" of "biomaterial" cannot be forgotten. Because the overall goal of the field is the development of materials that will be implanted in humans, one of the most important concepts in biomaterials science is that of *biocompatibility*. According to another consensus definition, **biocompatibility** is

> The ability of a material to perform with an appropriate host response in a specific application [1].

Thus, a **biomaterialist**, as a practitioner of biomaterials science, is responsible for alterations to the composition of a biomaterial and/or its fabrication process in order to control the biological response and produce an implant with maximal biocompatibility. As the above definitions indicate, a biomaterialist must consider both the material properties and the biological reaction to ensure that the chosen material is appropriate for the given application. Therefore, this book will address both the materials science (Chapters 1-7) and the biological (Chapters 8-14) aspects of biomaterials, with the goal of introducing principles to guide future biomaterialists in the selection and development of optimal materials for a wide variety of applications and implantation sites.

EXAMPLE PROBLEM 1.1

Are the following items biomaterials? Why or why not?

(a) contact lens
(b) splinter
(c) vascular graft
(d) crutches

Solution: "A biomaterial is a material intended to interface with biological systems to evaluate, treat, augment, or replace any tissue, organ or function of the body [1]." (a) and (c) are biomaterials according to this definition. (a) interfaces with the ocular environment to augment the light-focusing function of the eye for vision. Similarly, (c) interfaces with the vascular environment to replace vascular (venous/arterial) function. (b) is not intended to interface with the biological environment or to serve a biological function. (d) could be viewed either as a biomaterial or not by the given definition. It depends upon the justification of the terms "augment," "replace," and "interface." ■

1.1.2 History and Current Status of the Field

Although we consider biomaterials a relatively young field, its origins date back thousands of years. Archaeologists have uncovered remains of humans containing metal dental implants from as early as 200 A.D., and it is known that linen was used as a suture material by the Egyptians. However, the development of the biomaterials field significantly increased after World War II with the widespread availability of synthetic materials that were originally designed for use in the war. [3]

For example, implantation of plastics (synthetic polymers) in humans was first reported in the 1940s. Many of these first attempts centered around poly(methyl methacrylate), which had been previously employed as a material for aircraft, and nylon, a common parachute material. However, the field progressed quickly from these first materials to encompass a wide range of material types. The two decades after World War II saw the advent, among others, of the first successful artificial hip (metallic biomaterials), kidney dialysis machines (originally using a natural polymer derivative, cellulose), and vascular grafts (another naturally derived polymer, silk). [3]

The long-term success of these devices was due, in addition to the advancement in materials, to better surgical techniques, including proper sterilization, and patient monitoring. Also, a greater knowledge of biology, particularly as it related to biocompatibility, had a significant impact on the field of biomaterials. Although in the first few decades after World War II any material could be placed in a patient in an emergency situation, the need for biomaterial regulation was soon recognized, and national and international standards requiring rigorous testing before implantation were developed. [3]

Today, biomaterials represent a significant portion of the healthcare industry, with an estimated market size of over $9 billion per year in the United States (see Table 1.1). Some of the most common medical devices that possess a large biomaterial component include replacement heart valves, synthetic vascular grafts, hip and knee replacements, heart-lung machines, and renal dialysis equipment.

In the cardiovascular area, approximately 100,000 replacement heart valves [2] and 300,000 vascular grafts are implanted each year in the United States. Figure 1.1 depicts one typical design of a heart valve, while synthetic vascular grafts are shown in Figure 1.2. After insertion, both of these devices can restore proper blood flow and thus greatly improve the patient's ability to function normally. However, a number of problems can occur. For replacement heart valves, the most common complications include blood clotting, mechanical failure, and infection (see Fig. 1.3). In vascular grafts, blood clotting or overgrowth of tissue that blocks the interior of the vessel and prevents blood flow can be causes for device failure.

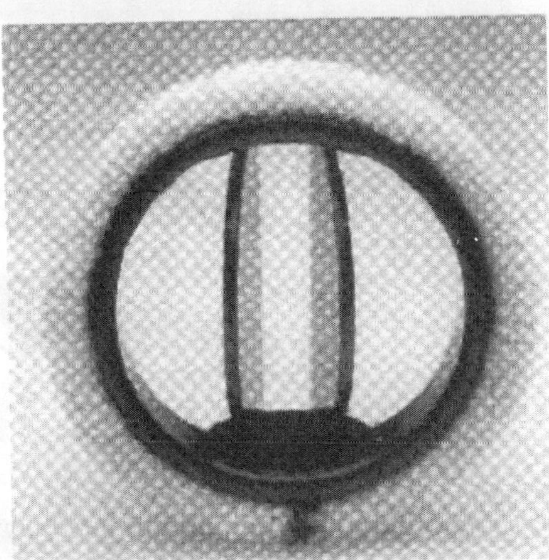

Figure 1.1
Image of a bileaflet heart valve prosthesis. (Reprinted with permission from [2])

TABLE 1.1

Biomaterials in the U.S. Healthcare Market

Total U.S. health care expenditures (2000)	$1,400,000,000,000
Total U.S. health research and development (2001)	$82,000,000,000
Number of employees in the medical device industry (2003)	300,000
Registered U.S. medical device manufacturers (2003)	13,000
Total U.S. medical device market (2002)	$77,000,000,000
U.S. market for disposable medical supplies (2003)	$48,600,000,000
U.S. market for biomaterials (2000)	$9,000,000,000
Individual medical device sales:	
Diabetes management products (1999)	$4,000,000,000
Cardiovascular devices (2002)	$6,000,000,000
Orthopedic-musculoskeletal surgery U.S. market (1998)	$4,700,000,000
Wound care U.S. market (1998)	$3,700,000,000
In vitro diagnostics (1998)	$10,000,000,000
Numbers of devices (U.S.):	
Intraocular lenses (2003)	2,500,000
Contact lenses (2000)	30,000,000
Vascular grafts	300,000
Heart valves	100,000
Pacemakers	400,000
Blood bags	40,000,000
Breast prostheses	250,000
Catheters	200,000,000
Heart-lung (Oxygenators)	300,000
Coronary stents	1,500,000
Renal dialysis (number of patients, 2001)	320,000
Hip prostheses (2002)	250,000
Knee prostheses (2002)	250,000
Dental implants (2000)	910,000

(Reprinted with permission from [2])

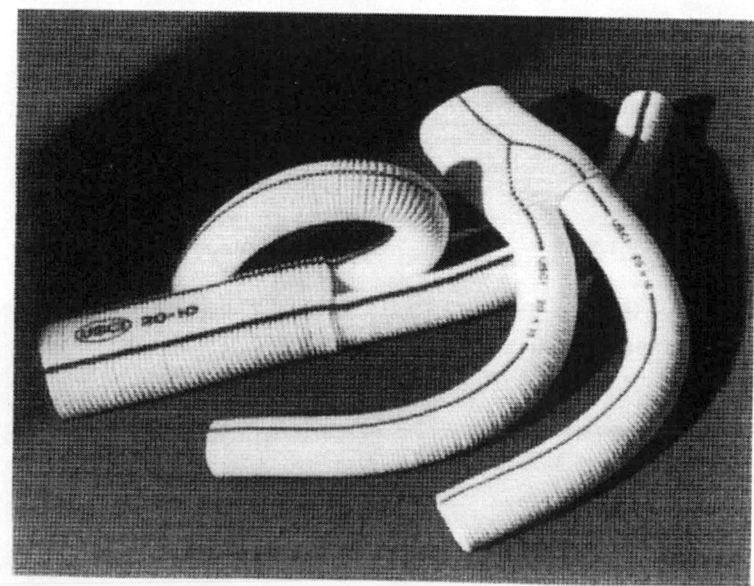

Figure 1.2
Image of vascular grafts constructed of expanded poly (tetrafluoroethylene). (Reprinted with permission from [4])

Over 500,000 artificial joint replacements, such as the knee or hip, are implanted yearly in the United States [2]. An example of an artificial hip is shown in Figure 1.4. Such replacements restore the ability to walk, or even engage in moderate athletic activity, and thus greatly improve the patient's quality of life. Over time, however, these prostheses can loosen, leading to tissue damage and creating the need for a second surgery to repair or replace the implant.

Heart-lung machines, like that seen in Figure 1.5, are used daily in operating rooms worldwide to recirculate blood externally, allowing a patient's heart to be stopped so that surgery can be performed on it. Although the development of such devices was crucial to the field of cardiac surgery and saves the lives of many patients each year, certain problems remain. Due in part to the limitations of the current biomaterial filters, the heart-lung machine is unable to attain the efficiency of the native lung for blood oxygenation. This, in turn, requires higher pumping pressures than are normally exerted by the heart, which can lead to blood cell lysis (breakage). In addition, anticoagulants are required to prevent blood clotting, thereby increasing the risk of uncontrolled bleeding after surgery.

Approximately 300,000 patients in the United States with compromised kidney function must receive renal dialysis three times per week [5] to remove waste from the blood in order to maintain life. In this procedure, the blood is pumped across a dialysis membrane, which allows waste products of certain size to flow out of the blood (see Fig. 1.6). However, this device suffers from problems similar to those described for the heart-lung machine, including blood cell lysis, and the potential for infection or undesired activation of a portion of the body's immune response (the complement system, discussed in Chapter 12).

1.1.3 Future Directions

Over the course of the past 50 years, several stages in biomaterials development can be identified. Starting in the 1960s–1970s, the first generation of biomaterials was designed to be **inert**, or not reactive with the body, thereby decreasing the potential for negative immune response to the implant. In the 1990s, this concept was gradually replaced with a second generation of materials designed to be **bioactive**, interacting in a positive manner with the body to promote localized healing.

Because biomaterials science occupies a unique niche at the corner of several disciplines, advances in disparate subjects have propelled the field to its current status. Experiments providing detailed knowledge of cell and molecular biology and genetics have led to the development of these "smart" or "instructive" materials, which can help guide the biological response in the implant area. Advances in surgical

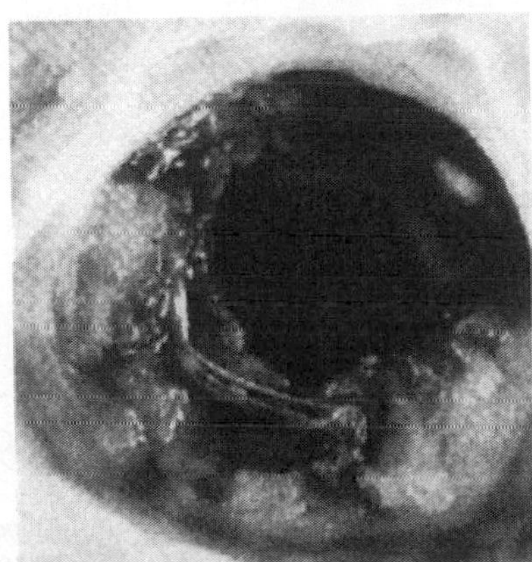

Figure 1.3
Image of blood clots on a bileaflet heart valve. (Reprinted with permission from [6])

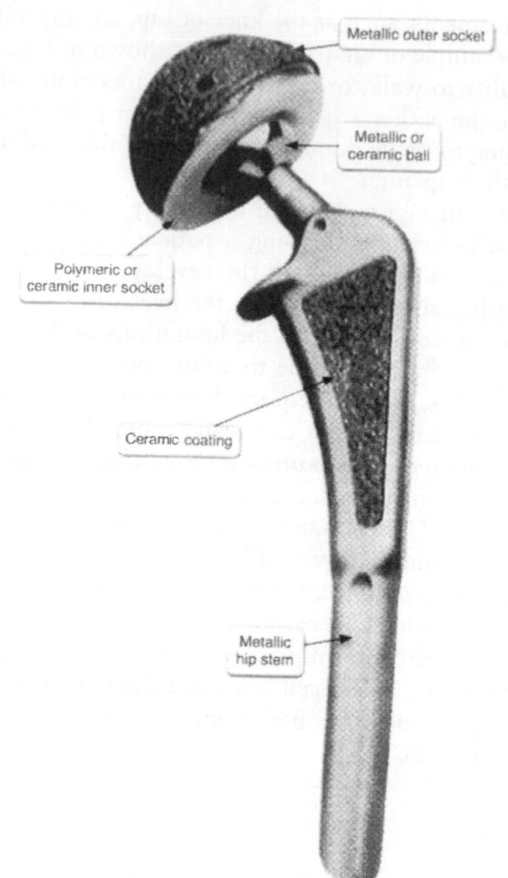

Figure 1.4
An orthopedic hip implant, exhibiting the use of all three classes of biomaterials: metals, ceramics and polymers. In this case, the stem, which is implanted in the femur (upper bone of the leg), is made with a metallic biomaterial. The implant may be coated with a ceramic to improve attachment to the bone, or a polymeric cement (not shown) can be used to hold the stem in place. At the top of the hip stem is a ball (metal or ceramic) that works in conjunction with the corresponding socket to facilitate motion in the joint. The corresponding inner socket is made out of either a polymer (for a metallic ball) or ceramic (for a ceramic ball), and attached to the pelvis by a metallic socket. (Adapted with permission from [7])

techniques like minimally invasive surgery have promoted the design of injectable materials that can be applied locally and with minimal pain to the patient. New developments in materials science, such as composites involving nano-scale objects as reinforcing agents, have inspired the creation of a new set of nano-structured biomaterials.

Further advances in all of these fields are expected to have a great impact on the future of biomaterials. Thus, as we move forward in the new millennium, we stand on the edge of another generation—biomaterials that are designed to become completely integrated and cause the full reproduction of damaged tissue, as exemplified

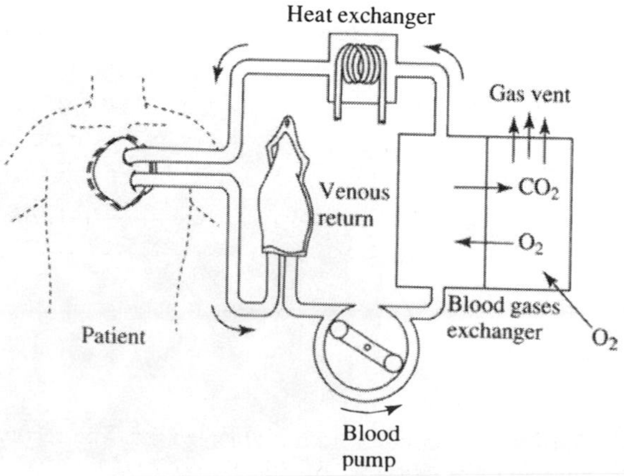

Figure 1.5
Schematic of a heart-lung machine setup. (Reprinted with permission from [5].)

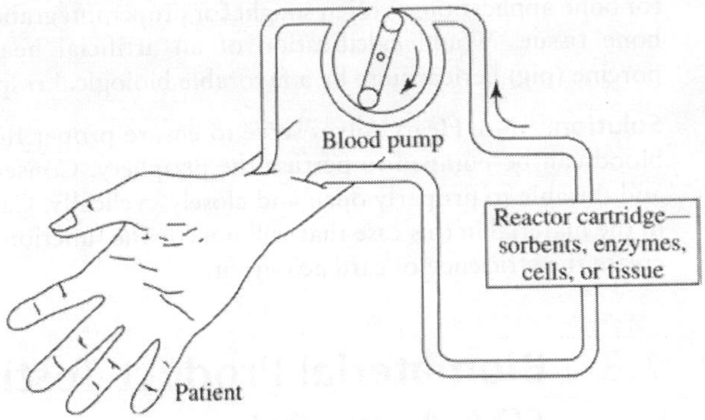

Figure 1.6
Schematic of kidney dialysis setup. (Reprinted with permission from [5])

in current research in biomaterials for tissue engineering applications. The perpetual evolution of new processes and materials makes the field of biomaterials very dynamic. This book is therefore designed to relate basic principles in biology and materials science to both currently used materials as well as potential design parameters for the next generation of biomaterials.

1.2 Biological Response to Biomaterials

One of the major concerns of the biomaterialist is the biological response to the chosen material, which determines its biocompatibility. Immediately after implantation, inflammation usually occurs. Clinically, this is characterized by redness, swelling, warmth, and pain around the implant site. However, this is usually temporary, and may be resolved in a number of ways, including complete integration of the material into the surrounding tissue or isolation of the implant with fibrous encapsulation.

Depending on the implant site and the nature of the material, other reactions may also ensue, such as activation of the immune system, localized blood clotting, infection, tumor formation, or implant calcification. Although many of these responses are not desirable, certain reactions may be acceptable, depending on the application. For example, calcification of an implant used to support bone tissue may be necessary to ensure good integration between the biomaterial and the surrounding bone.

Factors such as the type of material, the shape of the implant, material degradation characteristics, surface chemical properties, and bulk chemical and mechanical properties have been identified as important to the overall biocompatibility of a biomaterial and to its suitability for specific applications. Therefore, the biomaterialist must select the material type and processing method to obtain optimal degradative, surface, and bulk characteristics, keeping in mind the final location and application of the implant.

At the most basic level, it is the protein and cellular response to the material that determines the overall success of the implant. Therefore, characterization of these responses is necessary. Experiments assessing both cell/protein interactions with biomaterials and overall biocompatibility can be carried out either *in vitro* or *in vivo*. *In vitro* (literally "in glass" [1]) tests take place in a well-controlled laboratory environment, while *in vivo* experiments require biomaterial implantation in a living system, such as an animal model [1].

EXAMPLE PROBLEM 1.2

The biological response to a material is of utmost concern to a biomaterialist. The response must be appropriate for the desired application. For example, calcification of implant materials for bone applications is often sought for proper integration of the implant with the surrounding bone tissue. Would calcification of an artificial heart valve composed of decellularized porcine (pig) pericardium be a favorable biological response? Why or why not?

Solution: No. Heart valves serve to ensure proper fluid flow patterns in the heart, so that blood can be pumped to perfuse the periphery. Consequently, heart valves must be flexible and durable to properly open and closely cyclically. Calcification leads to undesired stiffness of the material in this case that will impede the function of the valve (opening/closing) and decrease the efficiency of cardiac output. ■

1.3 Biomaterial Product Testing and FDA Approval

The ultimate *in vivo* event takes place upon final device implantation in humans. However, due to ethical concerns, before this can occur, many *in vitro* and *in vivo* biocompatibility tests must be performed. These are dictated by and analyzed in accordance with standards compiled by agencies such as the *ASTM International (ASTM)* and the *International Organization for Standardization (ISO)*.[1] These agencies are responsible for the development of technical standards for materials, products, systems, and services. More specifics on these guidelines are found in later sections of this book.

The steps to producing a product involving a biomaterial are outlined by regulatory agencies such as the U.S. Food and Drug Administration (FDA). Approval by this agency is required in order to sell a biomedical product in the United States. Biomedical product development generally includes the following stages (adapted from [8]):

1. *In vitro* testing
2. *In vivo* studies with healthy experimental animals
3. *In vivo* studies with animal models of disease (if applicable)
4. Controlled clinical trials

Results from all of these tests are reported to the FDA to prove that the new device is both safe and effective. The amount of testing and whether or not clinical trials are required depends on the perceived danger of the proposed product. Based on their intended use, products are classified as Class I, II, or III [9]. Class III devices are more complicated and perform tasks more directly related to saving or sustaining life. Thus, they are subject to the most rigorous standards, including, usually, the requirement of clinical trials. It is also important to note here that the FDA approves devices, not materials, so currently, specific biomaterials can only be used in the context of approved final devices.

1.4 Types of Biomaterials

One of the primary roles of the biomaterialist is to choose the appropriate source of material for a specific application. In general, materials are classified as **organic** if they contain carbon or **inorganic** if they do not. More specifically, biomaterials fall into one of three categories of materials: metals, ceramics, or polymers.

---

[1] *ASTM International* was originally the *American Society for Testing and Materials*. Also, *ISO* is derived from the Greek word "isos" due to variations in the translation of *International Organization for Standardization*.

TABLE 1.2

Metals Commonly Used in Biomedical Applications

Metal	Applications
Cobalt-chromium alloys	Artificial heart valves, dental prostheses, orthopedic fixation plates, artificial joint components, vascular stents
Gold and platinum	Dental fillings, electrodes for cochlear implants
Silver-tin-copper alloys	Dental amalgams
Stainless steel	Dental prostheses, orthopedic fixation plates, vascular stents
Titanium alloys	Artificial heart valves, dental implants, artificial joint components, orthopedic screws, pacemaker cases, vascular stents

1.4.1 Metals

Metals are inorganic materials possessing non-directional metallic bonds with highly mobile electrons (see Section 1.7 for more on bond types). A list of metals and alloys (combinations of multiple elemental metals) commonly used in biomedical applications is found in Table 1.2. In addition to their ability to conduct electricity, metals are strong and relatively easily formed into complex shapes. This makes metals a suitable material for orthopedic (hip and knee) replacements (Fig. 1.4), for dental fillings and implants for craniofacial restoration, and for cardiovascular applications such as stents and pacemaker leads.

1.4.2 Ceramics

Ceramics are inorganic materials composed of non-directional ionic bonds between electron-donating and electron-accepting elements. Ceramic materials most often employed as biomaterials are listed in Table 1.3. Ceramics may contain crystals, like metals, or may be non-crystalline (amorphous) **glasses**. Ceramics are very hard and more resistant to degradation in many environments than metals. However, they are quite brittle because of the nature of ionic bonds. Due to the similarity between the chemistry of ceramics and that of native bone, ceramics are most often used as a part of orthopedic implants or as dental materials (Fig. 1.4). Because of their brittle nature, they are commonly employed in applications requiring small loads.

TABLE 1.3

Ceramics Commonly Used in Biomedical Applications

Ceramic	Applications
Aluminum oxides	Orthopedic joint replacement components, orthopedic load-bearing implants, implant coatings, dental implants
Bioactive glasses	Orthopedic and dental implant coatings, dental implants, facial reconstruction components, bone graft substitute materials
Calcium phosphates	Orthopedic and dental implant coatings, dental implant materials, bone graft substitute materials, bone cements

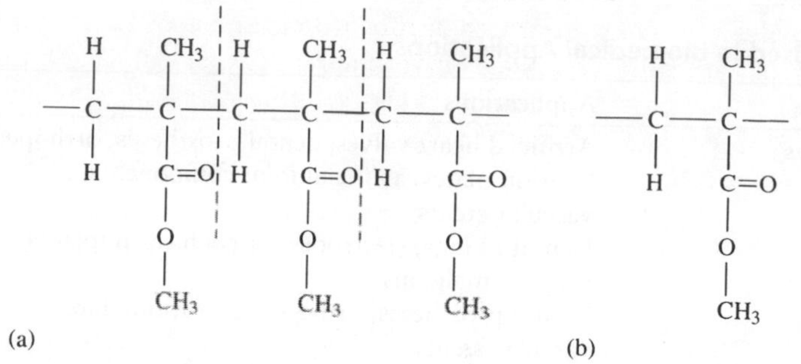

Figure 1.7
Chemical structure of poly (methyl methacrylate), a polymer commonly used as a bone cement. (a) shows a section of the polymer chain, with the dotted lines indicating the repeating unit, which is also shown in (b).

1.4.3 Polymers

Unlike the other two classes of biomaterials, **polymers** are organic materials possessing long chains that are held together by directional covalent bonds (Fig. 1.7). Polymers are widely used in biomedical applications (Fig. 1.4) due to the range of physical and chemical properties possible with these materials [10]. Examples of some of the synthetic (man-made) polymers that are often used as biomaterials are found in Table 1.4. Alternatively, polymers that are derived from natural sources, such as proteins commonly found in the body, have been widely explored as biomaterials. Common uses for these types of polymers are also listed in Table 1.4.

Regardless of the origin of the polymer, there are several polymer sub-classes that are useful to the biomaterialist in that each may be particularly suited to certain

TABLE 1.4

Synthetic and Naturally Derived Polymers Commonly Used in Biomedical Applications

Polymer	Applications
Synthetic	
Poly(2-hydroxyethyl methacrylate)	Contact lenses
Poly(dimethyl siloxane)	Breast implants, contact lenses, knuckle replacements
Poly(ethylene)	Orthopedic joint implants
Poly(ethylene glycol)	Pharmaceutical fillers, wound dressings
Poly(ethylene terephthalate)	Vascular grafts, sutures
Poly(ε-caprolactone)	Drug delivery devices, sutures
Poly(lactic-co-glycolic acid)	Resorbable meshes and sutures
Poly(methyl methacrylate)	Bone cements, diagnostic contact lenses
Poly(tetrafluoroethylene)	Vascular grafts, sutures
Poly(isoprene)	Gloves
Poly(propylene)	Sutures
Naturally derived	
Alginate	Wound dressings
Chitosan	Wound dressings
Collagen	Orthopedic repair matrices, nerve repair matrices, tissue engineering matrices
Elastin	Skin repair matrices
Fibrin	Hemostatic products, tissue sealants
Glycosaminoglycan	Orthopedic repair matrices
Hyaluronic acid	Orthopedic repair matrices

tissue types. For example, **elastomers** can sustain substantial deformation at low stresses and return rapidly to their initial dimensions upon release of the stress [1], suggesting that they may be suitable for cardiovascular applications, where tissue elasticity is an important property. Another category of polymers called **hydrogels** exhibit the ability to swell in water and to retain a significant fraction of water within their structures without completely dissolving [1]. Due to their high water content, hydrogels have been explored for a variety of soft tissue applications.

It is also possible to form **composite** materials to improve bulk or surface properties of biomaterials. Composites are materials consisting of two or more chemically distinct components, one of which is often a polymer [11]. Composites are often created to optimize mechanical properties. In this case, a fiber-reinforcing material (usually carbon) is dispersed throughout a polymer. Although a detailed discussion of composite materials is beyond the scope of this text, it is interesting to note that many consider the structure of human tissues to resemble a fiber-reinforced composite.

1.4.4 Naturally Derived vs. Synthetic Polymers

Naturally based polymers can be derived from sources within the body (collagen, fibrin, or hyaluronic acid) or outside the body (chitosan, alginate). One of the most common natural biomaterials found in the human body is the protein **collagen.** Many different types of collagen exist in various tissues, and several of these, particularly types I and II, have been explored as biomaterials. Another protein-based material, **fibrin,** results from the combination of the blood clotting factors fibrinogen and thrombin. Both collagen and fibrin have been used in tissue engineering attempts to repair cartilage defects and in other orthopedic applications.

In addition to proteins, naturally based polymers may be derived from sugars (carbohydrates). **Hyaluronic acid** is an example of a carbohydrate molecule occurring in human tissues that is often employed as a biomaterial. However, the source of other carbohydrate-derived materials may be non-human. Chitosan, a sugar-based substance found in arthropod exoskeletons; agarose, which is formed by algae; and alginate, derived from seaweed, are all currently being investigated as biomaterials for a variety of applications. For example, a combination of chitosan and alginate has been examined for wound dressings.

There are advantages and disadvantages to both natural and synthetic polymers, and particular materials may lend themselves to certain applications over others. In many cases, naturally derived polymers have chemical compositions similar to the tissues they are replacing. Therefore, they may be more fully integrated into the surrounding tissue over time or more easily altered (remodeled) in response to changes in tissue needs. However, concerns exist about the feasibility of finding large amounts of some of these materials for clinical applications, their relatively low mechanical properties, and the assurance of pathogen removal. In addition, regions of these molecules may be recognized as "foreign" by the body's immune system, leading to a type of material "rejection." Further potential problems arise when the biomaterial is based on not a single naturally occurring polymer, but decellularized tissue. Here, unwanted calcification leading to device failure (discussed in Chapter 14) is a particular concern.

In contrast, synthetic polymers can be easily mass-produced and sterilized, so supply issues are not a problem. Additionally, their physical, chemical, mechanical and degradative properties can be tailored for specific applications. However, unless specifically treated, most synthetic materials do not interact with tissues in an active manner and therefore cannot direct or aid in healing around the implant site. Also, few synthetic polymers have been approved by regulatory agencies for use in humans in specific applications.

Regardless of source, all of the materials described in this section are polymeric, so they have a number of key properties in common and can all be modified or processed using similar techniques. Therefore, in the following chapters, the term "polymer" will be used to refer, for the most part, to both naturally derived and synthetic materials.

EXAMPLE PROBLEM 1.3

Which of the following classes of biomaterials would be most appropriate for use to fabricate an artificial tendon, a tissue that must sustain substantial deformation at low forces and return rapidly to its original dimensions upon release of the stress? Why?

(a) metals
(b) ceramics
(c) polymers

Solution: (c) Because of the wide range of mechanical properties attainable with polymeric materials, elastomeric polymers are easily found. Metals and ceramics, however, typically allow for little tensile deformation before failure, and they typically require large stresses for small elongations in tension.

■

1.5 Processing of Biomaterials

In addition to the material type, the processing method is another important choice for the biomaterialist. Processing can affect bulk properties such as strength, as well as surface properties of materials. In fact, many processing techniques have been developed to alter only the surface physical or chemical properties without affecting the rest of the material. These include spraying a ceramic coating on a metal hip implant to improve integration with the surrounding bone or coating a catheter with antibiotics to prevent infection (see Chapter 7 for more on these methods).

Processing is also necessary to form materials into specified shapes. The shape of the material alters the surface area available, which, in turn, can affect the degradative properties and the biological response. Implant geometry is often dictated by the characteristics of the tissue to be replaced. For instance, biomaterials may be fabricated into sheets for skin applications, cylinders for vascular grafts, or a ball-and-cup combination for hip replacement.

1.6 Important Properties of Biomaterials

The selection of the biomaterial and appropriate processing techniques for a given application is determined primarily by the degradative, surface, and bulk properties of the material. As explained below, each of these characteristics directly affects the biological response; thus, these are the most important aspects to consider when designing an optimal biomaterial for a given implant type.

1.6.1 Degradative Properties of Biomaterials

The shape and size of the implant, its location in the body, and the chemical, physical, and mechanical bulk and surface properties of the biomaterial affect its degradation *in vivo*. Although the temperature and pH of body fluids are relatively mild, during inflammation cells may be recruited to the area and produce active substances to transform the region into a harsh environment, thus promoting material degradation.

Degradation can be an undesired side effect of implantation, or it may be designed into the chemical nature of the biomaterial. Such biodegradable materials are currently under investigation as carriers for cells and bioactive factors for tissue engineering applications. For both desired and undesired degradation, the time before failure (environmental stability) is crucial to implant design. In addition, the biocompatibility of degradation by-products must be examined along with the biocompatibility of the intact material. Because the nature and amount of degradation depends strongly on the chemistry and mechanical demands of the implant site, *in vivo* testing is often required to accurately assess biomaterial degradation time and any possible inflammatory response.

1.6.2 Surface Properties of Biomaterials

On a mechanistic level, the biological response to a material is highly affected by the proteins that attach (adsorb) to its surface. Biomaterial surface properties determine protein adsorption, and thus are a key consideration for the biomaterialist. The **surface** of a material is defined to be the few atomic layers on the exterior of the object. Surface properties can be different than those in the rest of the material (the **bulk**) due to special processing schemes that alter only the outermost layers of the material, or as a result of interactions with cells and proteins in the body.

Surface properties include both chemical and physical characteristics. An example of a surface chemical property is hydrophobicity. A **hydrophobic** material (literally, "water-fearing") contains many chemical moieties that do not interact favorably with water [1]. In contrast, **hydrophilic** ("water-loving") materials have an affinity for water [1]. Hydrophobicity is one of the most important parameters affecting the adsorption of proteins to a biomaterial in an aqueous environment, such as that found *in vivo*.

Surface physical properties, such as surface roughness, also impact the protein and cellular response to a biomaterial. A rough topography, which may be caused by a combination of chemistry and processing techniques, can act to physically trap biological constituents at the implant surface, thereby altering the interactions between the biomaterial and the surrounding tissue.

EXAMPLE PROBLEM 1.4

Would a hydrophobic or hydrophilic polymer be a more appropriate choice for a contact lens application? Why? Would a melting temperature (T_m) of the polymer above 37°C or below 37°C be more appropriate for this application? Why?

Solution: A hydrophilic polymer would be more appropriate to interface with the aqueous environment of the eye. Additionally, a melting temperature above 37°C would be more appropriate, as one would not want the polymer to be molten at body temperature (37°C) in this application. ■

EXAMPLE PROBLEM 1.5

A 1 ml droplet of distilled water is dropped onto each material A and B as shown. Which material is more hydrophilic? Justify your answer.

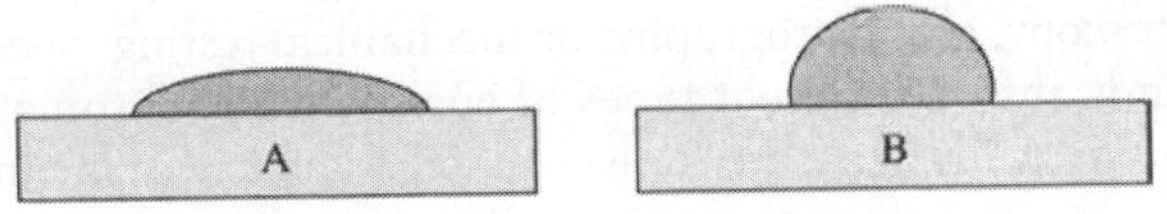

Solution: Material A is more hydrophilic. For a given volume of water, the surface area of interaction is greatest for A. Thus, it is more hydrophilic—that is, it has a greater affinity for water than B. ■

1.6.3 Bulk Properties of Biomaterials

Overall biocompatibility depends also in part on the properties of the bulk material. In addition, this is often the most important parameter in determining the suitability of certain materials for specific applications. Bulk properties may play a smaller role than surface characteristics in determining the initial inflammatory response. However, they have a large long-term impact, since a biomaterial with inappropriate bulk properties will very likely lead to device failure.

Bulk characteristics of biomaterials include mechanical properties, physical properties and chemical composition. **Mechanical properties**, such as strength and stiffness, are extremely important in that they should match, as much as possible, the properties of the tissue to be replaced. Specifically, tissues may exhibit distinctly different mechanical properties in different directions (**anisotropy**). This is due to the unique function of many tissues. For example, a long bone in the leg can support more load along its length than in other directions, since this is where most of the force is exerted during walking or standing. Therefore, although mechanical requirements in a given location can be complex, they must be taken into consideration when selecting a suitable replacement. Additionally, fatigue properties are crucial because many implants will need to withstand repeated loading to reproduce the desired function in the body. For example, heart valves open over 40 million times per year in the average human, making material fatigue properties a key selection parameter when designing artificial heart valves.

Mechanical properties of materials are highly affected by their physical and chemical characteristics. Bulk **physical properties** include crystallinity and thermal transitions, such as melting point. Crystallinity is important because, in addition to mechanical properties, it alters water uptake, which can impact the degradative properties of the biomaterial, as well as its interactions with surrounding cells and proteins. Transition points, such as melting temperature, are also crucial, since the biomaterial must be stable over a long period of time at body temperature.

The **chemical composition** of a biomaterial dictates the other bulk properties, just as the chemistry at the surface determines many of the surface properties. As with the surface, one of the major chemical characteristics of the bulk material is its degree of hydrophobicity. Many chemical properties are, at the most basic level, a result of the type of bonds present in the material (discussed in Section 1.7).

1.6.4 Characterization Techniques

In order to better understand how degradative, surface, and bulk properties affect the biological response to a biomaterial, it is important first to measure them. A plethora of techniques, both quantitative and qualitative, have been developed to examine material properties and are discussed in more detail throughout the text. **Quantitative** procedures produce a numerical measure of a property (in absolute or relative units), whereas **qualitative** experiments give a general overview of the property of interest, without supplying a numerical value. For example, the act of observing a material under a microscope is qualitative, while the techniques discussed below are more quantitative.

Quantitative characterization of degradative and bulk properties often involves a form of spectroscopy, chromatography, or mechanical testing. **Spectroscopy** measures how compounds absorb different types of energy, while **chromatography** uses various means to physically separate molecules on the basis of chemical characteristics such as charge or size. Mechanical assessment of materials is performed with a mechanical testing frame that allows for controlled loading of the sample by pulling, pushing, or bending it at a preset rate.

Because surfaces are chemically active, many surface analysis techniques require special preparation procedures or equipment to prevent contamination. However, despite these limitations, a wide range of surface characterization methods has been developed. Many methods involve modifications of techniques for bulk properties, such as spectroscopy. In addition, more qualitative methods, like various types of microscopy, can provide valuable information on the structure and topography of the biomaterial surface.

EXAMPLE PROBLEM 1.6

For each of the following methods for the determination of the degradation profile of a hydrogel, indicate whether it is quantitative or qualitative:

(a) visual inspection at each time point
(b) hydrogel mass measurements at each time point

Solution:

(a) is a qualitative measure, whereas **(b)** is a quantitative measure. ■

1.7 Principles of Chemistry

Generally, when designing or selecting a biomaterial that is most appropriate for a specific application, one is, in essence, considering the chemical constitution of the material, since this dictates all the other important characteristics. Therefore, in this section, we review basic chemical principles as an introduction to understanding why each class of materials exhibits certain distinctive properties. The relation of chemical structure to macroscopic properties, a key aspect of materials science, will be revisited in later chapters.

1.7.1 Atomic Structure

Although many subatomic species have been discovered, in this text we will use the simplified model that divides an atom into a nucleus and orbiting electrons (Fig. 1.8). The nucleus contains protons and neutrons, which are much larger than the orbiting electrons. The number of protons (each having a positive charge of 1.67×10^{-19} Coulombs (C)) is the atom's **atomic number** (Z). In an electrically neutral atom, this positive charge is balanced by an equal number of electrons, each of which has a negative charge equal in magnitude to that of a proton. Neutrons are electrically neutral but do contribute significantly to the **atomic mass**.

Atomic mass is usually measured in **atomic mass units** (amu). One amu is roughly equivalent to the mass of a proton or neutron (1.66×10^{-24} g). For example, carbon has six protons and six neutrons, giving an atomic mass of 12 amu.[2] Atomic weight of an element can be reported in amu, or in mass per mole. One **mole** of material contains 6.023×10^{23} (Avogadro's number) molecules. 1 amu/molecule = 1 g/mol of that element.

[2]Atomic weights reported on the periodic table (Fig. 1.14), are actually weighted averages of the masses of different isotopes of an element. **Isotopes** have the same number of protons and electrons, but differ in the number of neutrons in the nucleus.

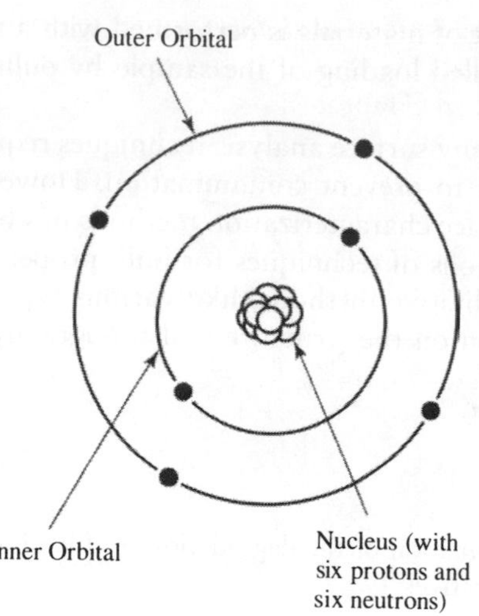

Figure 1.8
The Bohr atomic model, which separates the atom into a nucleus (containing protons and neutrons) and orbiting electrons. For an electrically neutral atom, the positive charge of the nucleus is balanced by an equal number of electrons. In this model, electrons are depicted as orbiting the nucleus in discrete energy states, or orbitals, which are separated by a finite amount of energy. (Reprinted with permission from [12])

1.7.2 Atomic Models

Over the past century, a detailed theory based on **quantum mechanics** has been developed that explains that electrons moving around a nucleus have both wave-like and particle-like qualities. Although an in-depth treatment of this subject is beyond the scope of this book, an examination of simple models depicting both of these qualities is presented. Both models are correct, and both will be used to describe material phenomena in later chapters, depending on which provides the clearest explanation.

1.7.2.1 Bohr Model One of the first (and simplest) models developed based on quantum mechanical principles was the **Bohr model** of the atom (Fig. 1.8). Here, electrons are thought to orbit the nucleus in discrete energy states, or orbitals. Orbitals are separated by a finite amount of energy, so to move from one orbital to another, an electron would have to gain or lose a set amount of energy. If an atom is exposed to energy of a certain frequency, it may gain a discrete amount of this energy and promote one of its electrons to a higher orbital (see Figure 1.9). After this occurs, the electron will often return to its normal orbital (ground state), emitting a

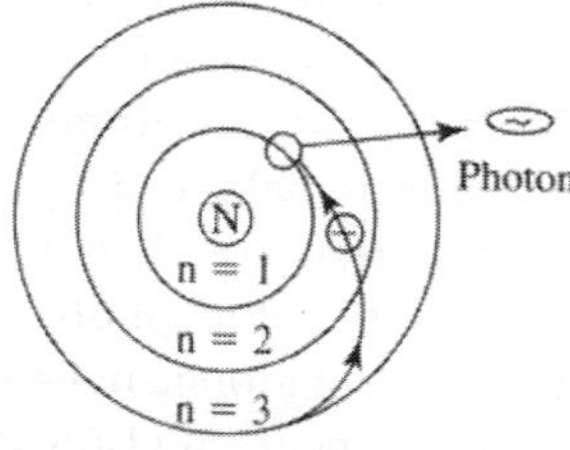

Figure 1.9
If exposed to energy of a certain frequency, atoms may enter an excited state and promote one or more electrons to a higher orbital. After this occurs, the electron will often return to its normal orbital (ground state), emitting a photon of energy equal to the difference in energy between the original orbital and the excited-state orbital. (Adapted with permission from [13])

photon of energy equal to the difference in energy between the original orbital and the excited-state orbital. These photon emissions are the basis of a number of materials characterization techniques, as discussed in Chapter 2.

1.7.2.2 Wave-Mechanical Model The Bohr model failed to explain several phenomena involving electrons, which led to the development of the **wave-mechanical model** of the atom. In this model, electrons, instead of being small particles, are considered to have wave-like characteristics and are described by equations for wave motion. Here, orbitals are thought of as the probability that an electron will occupy a certain space around the nucleus and are characterized by probability functions (electron clouds). Figure 1.10 compares the probability of finding the hydrogen electron at a given distance from the nucleus as depicted by both the Bohr and wave-mechanical atomic models.

1.7.3 Atomic Orbitals

1.7.3.1 Shapes of Subshells (Orbitals) Per the wave-mechanical model, three of four parameters called **quantum numbers** dictate the size, shape and orientation of the electron probability functions. More specifically, this model terms the discrete Bohr energy states *electron shells*, which can further be divided into *subshells* (often called orbitals). Subshells are designated by lowercase letters *s, p, d* or *f*. Each subshell can have several energy states that are specified by the third quantum number. For example, there are five states for a *d* subshell, three states for a *p* subshell, and only one for an *s* subshell. Plotting the wave functions in three dimensions reveals

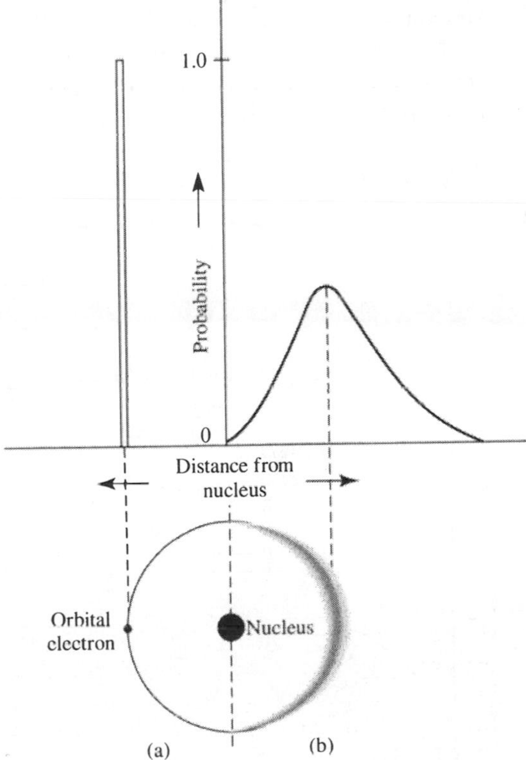

Figure 1.10
The distribution of the hydrogen electron as depicted by both the (a) Bohr and (b) wave-mechanical atomic models. Orbitals have discrete energy levels in both the Bohr and wave-mechanical models. However, in the wave-mechanical model, orbitals are thought of as the probability that an electron will occupy a certain space around the nucleus, and they are characterized by probability functions (electron clouds). (Reprinted with permission from J.D. Jastrzebski, *The Nature and Properties of Engineering Materials,* 3rd ed. as appears in [14].)

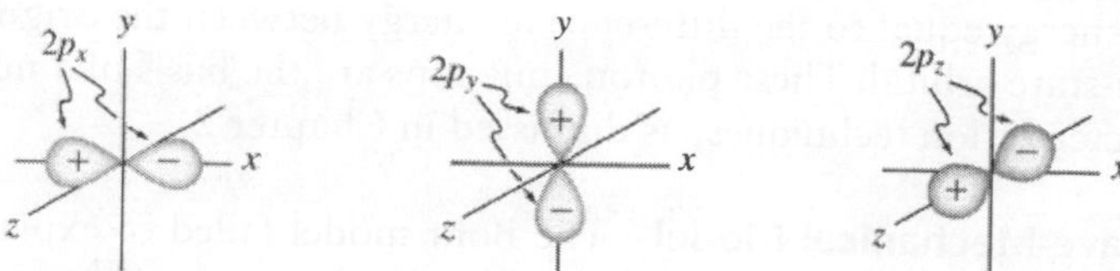

Figure 1.11
Depiction of the energy states for the $2p$ subshell. Because each subshell has a characteristic shape as determined by the electron probability functions (dumbbell-shaped for p subshells), the different energy states are represented by identical subshells oriented along different axes (x, y, and z). (Reprinted with permission from [15].)

that each subshell has only one characteristic shape. The different energy states are then depicted by identical subshells oriented in different directions (usually x, y, and z for the p-subshell; see Fig. 1.11). Thus, the Bohr model was further refined by the wave-mechanical model, which divides the shells into subshells, each of which has its associated energy value.

1.7.3.2 Order of Subshells and the Aufbau Principle Solutions to wave equations using all possible quantum numbers give the set of shells and subshells for all elements (Fig. 1.12). It is important to note that, in this system, the lower the shell number, the lower the energy (energy associated with 1*s* orbital is less than for 2*s*, etc.). Additionally, the energy of the subshells in each shell increases from *s* to *f*. However, energy states can overlap between shells—this is especially true of *d* and *f* subshells. For example, the energy associated with the 3*d* subshell is greater than that for the 4*s*.

Following these general rules of energy states, it would seem logical that electrons would prefer to be in the lowest energy state possible and therefore would fill the shells and subshells in order of increasing energy. This, combined with another

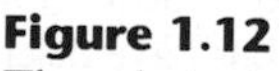

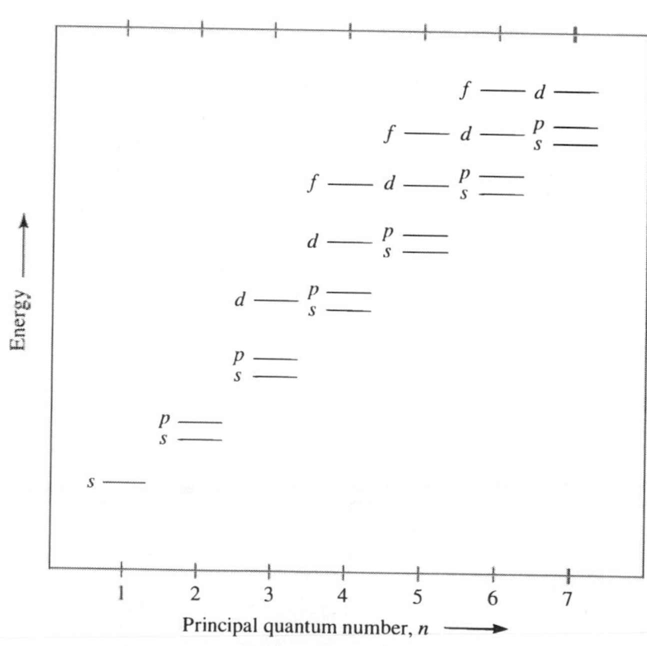

Figure 1.12
The relative energies of shells and subshells for all elements. Note that the lower the shell number, the lower the energy (e.g. energy associated with 1*s* is less than for 2*s*). Additionally, the energy of the subshells in each shell increases from *s* to *f*. However, energy states can overlap between shells (e.g. energy of the 3*d* subshell is greater than that of the 4*s*). (Reprinted with permission from Ralls et al., *Introduction to Materials Science and Engineering* as appears in [14].)

quantum-mechanical theory, the **Pauli exclusion principle**, which requires that each state can hold no more than two electrons (with opposite spin), provides the groundwork to predict the **electron configuration** of an atom. To sequentially add electrons to energy states is called the **Aufbau principle** and is governed by the following set of rules:

1. Lower energy states are filled before higher ones.
2. No energy state may be occupied by more than two electrons (Pauli exclusion principle) and each of these electrons must have a different orientation to their intrinsic angular momentum (spin). An electron's spin has two possible orientations and is designated with an up- or down-facing arrow (Fig. 1.13). The energy state is filled when it contains two electrons with opposite spin. Therefore, *s* subshells contain a maximum of 2 electrons, *p* can contain 6, and *d* can contain 10.
3. **Hund's rule** dictates that in subshells with more than one energy state (such as the three *p* subshells), each subshell will first be filled with one electron. Subsequently, a second electron with opposing spin will be added to each subshell.

Electron configuration is usually noted by a superscript with the number of electrons in that shell-subshell combination. For hydrogen, this would be $1s^1$, while carbon is designated $1s^2 2s^2 2p^2$. Table 1.5 gives the electron configurations for selected common elements. There are actually a variety of electron configurations; the one that can be predicted following the rules described above is considered the **ground state** for that atom. However, through a variety of means, atoms can enter an **excited state** where one or more electrons are found at higher energy levels. Atomic excitation is the basis of a number of spectroscopic techniques discussed later in this text.

1.7.4 Valence Electrons and the Periodic Table

Following the Aufbau principle, some atoms are found to have completely filled orbitals (called a **closed-shell configuration**). These elements are more stable and thus do not participate in most chemical reactions. Other elements have partially filled orbitals (**open-shell configuration**).

Valence electrons are those that occupy the outermost shell (here, we are most concerned with the *s* and *p* subshells). If these subshells of the valence shell are not filled, an element may share or exchange valence electrons with other elements to become more stable. This is the basis of formation of primary bonds, which will be discussed in the following sections.

The **periodic table** organizes elements with increasing atomic number based on number of valence electrons (Fig. 1.14). The elements are placed in the seven

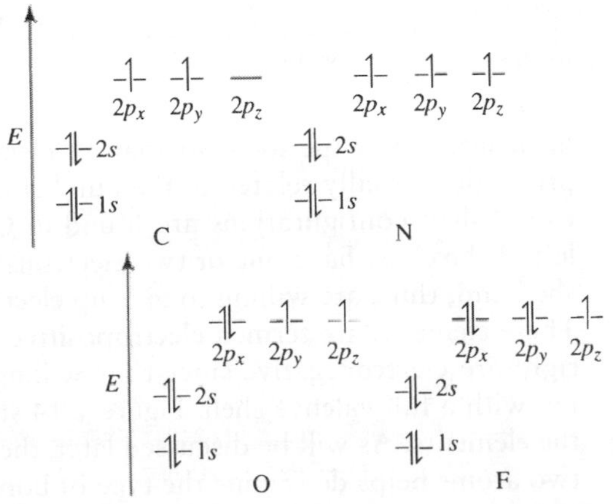

Figure 1.13
Stable electron configurations for carbon (C), nitrogen (N), oxygen (O), and fluorine (F). The Pauli exclusion principle states that each energy state may be occupied by at most two electrons possessing different orientation to their intrinsic angular momentum (indicated by an up- or down-facing arrow). Therefore, *s* subshells contain a maximum of 2 electrons, *p* can contain 6, *d* can contain 10, etc. In these four examples, the *s* subshells are full, whereas the p subshells (which consist of 2 electrons in the *p* subshells for carbon and up to 5 for fluorine) are not. (Reprinted with permission from [15])

TABLE 1.5

Ground State Electron Configurations for Selected Common Elements

Element	Symbol	Atomic Number	Electron Configuration
Hydrogen	H	1	$1s^1$
Helium	He	2	$1s^2$
Lithium	Li	3	$1s^2 2s^1$
Beryllium	Be	4	$1s^2 2s^2$
Boron	B	5	$1s^2 2s^2 2p^1$
Carbon	C	6	$1s^2 2s^2 2p^2$
Nitrogen	N	7	$1s^2 2s^2 2p^3$
Oxygen	O	8	$1s^2 2s^2 2p^4$
Fluorine	F	9	$1s^2 2s^2 2p^5$
Neon	Ne	10	$1s^2 2s^2 2p^6$
Sodium	Na	11	$1s^2 2s^2 2p^6 3s^1$
Magnesium	Mg	12	$1s^2 2s^2 2p^6 3s^2$
Aluminum	Al	13	$1s^2 2s^2 2p^6 3s^2 3p^1$
Silicon	Si	14	$1s^2 2s^2 2p^6 3s^2 3p^2$
Phosphorus	P	15	$1s^2 2s^2 2p^6 3s^2 3p^3$
Sulfur	S	16	$1s^2 2s^2 2p^6 3s^2 3p^4$
Chlorine	Cl	17	$1s^2 2s^2 2p^6 3s^2 3p^5$
Argon	Ar	18	$1s^2 2s^2 2p^6 3s^2 3p^6$
Potassium	K	19	$1s^2 2s^2 2p^6 3s^2 3p^6 4s^1$
Calcium	Ca	20	$1s^2 2s^2 2p^6 3s^2 3p^6 4s^2$
Scandium	Sc	21	$1s^2 2s^2 2p^6 3s^2 3p^6 3d^1 4s^2$
Titanium	Ti	22	$1s^2 2s^2 2p^6 3s^2 3p^6 3d^2 4s^2$
Vanadium	V	23	$1s^2 2s^2 2p^6 3s^2 3p^6 3d^3 4s^2$
Chromium	Cr	24	$1s^2 2s^2 2p^6 3s^2 3p^6 3d^5 4s^1$
Manganese	Mn	25	$1s^2 2s^2 2p^6 3s^2 3p^6 3d^5 4s^2$
Iron	Fe	26	$1s^2 2s^2 2p^6 3s^2 3p^6 3d^6 4s^2$
Cobalt	Co	27	$1s^2 2s^2 2p^6 3s^2 3p^6 3d^7 4s^2$
Nickel	Ni	28	$1s^2 2s^2 2p^6 3s^2 3p^6 3d^8 4s^2$
Copper	Cu	29	$1s^2 2s^2 2p^6 3s^2 3p^6 3d^{10} 4s^1$
Zinc	Zn	30	$1s^2 2s^2 2p^6 3s^2 3p^6 3d^{10} 4s^2$
Gallium	Ga	31	$1s^2 2s^2 2p^6 3s^2 3p^6 3d^{10} 4s^2 4p^1$
Germanium	Ge	32	$1s^2 2s^2 2p^6 3s^2 3p^6 3d^{10} 4s^2 4p^2$
Arsenic	As	33	$1s^2 2s^2 2p^6 3s^2 3p^6 3d^{10} 4s^2 4p^3$
Selenium	Se	34	$1s^2 2s^2 2p^6 3s^2 3p^6 3d^{10} 4s^2 4p^4$
Bromine	Br	35	$1s^2 2s^2 2p^6 3s^2 3p^6 3d^{10} 4s^2 4p^5$
Krypton	Kr	36	$1s^2 2s^2 2p^6 3s^2 3p^6 3d^{10} 4s^2 4p^6$

(Adapted with permission from [14].)

horizontal rows (periods) so that all elements in a column (group) have similar properties, usually related to the number of valence electrons present. Those with closed-shell configurations are found in Group 18. In general, those toward the left of the chart have one or two electrons more than are needed for a full valence shell and, thus, are willing to give up electrons to become positively charged ions. These elements are termed **electropositive**. In contrast, those elements toward the right are **electronegative** since they willingly accept electrons to form a negative ion with a full valence shell. Figure 1.14 shows the electronegativity values for all the elements. As will be discussed later, the difference in electronegativity between two atoms helps determine the type of bond formed between them.

Key: Atomic number / Element / Atomic mass / Electronegativity value (e.g., 22 Ti 47.88 1.5)

1	2	3	4	5	6	7	8	9	10	11	12	13	14	15	16	17	18
1 **H** 1.008 2.1																	2 **He** 4.003 -
3 **Li** 6.941 1.0	4 **Be** 9.012 1.5											5 **B** 10.81 2.0	6 **C** 12.01 2.5	7 **N** 14.01 3.0	8 **O** 16.00 3.5	9 **F** 19.00 4.0	10 **Ne** 20.18 -
11 **Na** 22.99 0.9	12 **Mg** 24.31 1.2											13 **Al** 26.98 1.5	14 **Si** 28.09 1.8	15 **P** 30.97 2.1	16 **S** 32.07 2.5	17 **Cl** 35.45 3.0	18 **Ar** 39.95 -
19 **K** 39.10 0.8	20 **Ca** 40.08 1.0	21 **Sc** 44.96 1.3	22 **Ti** 47.88 1.5	23 **V** 50.94 1.6	24 **Cr** 52.00 1.6	25 **Mn** 54.94 1.5	26 **Fe** 55.85 1.8	27 **Co** 58.93 1.8	28 **Ni** 58.69 1.8	29 **Cu** 63.55 1.9	30 **Zn** 65.38 1.6	31 **Ga** 69.72 1.6	32 **Ge** 72.59 1.8	33 **As** 74.92 2.0	34 **Se** 78.96 2.4	35 **Br** 79.90 2.8	36 **Kr** 83.80 -
37 **Rb** 85.47 0.8	38 **Sr** 87.62 1.0	39 **Y** 88.91 1.2	40 **Zr** 91.22 1.4	41 **Nb** 92.91 1.6	42 **Mo** 95.94 1.8	43 **Tc** 98 1.9	44 **Ru** 101.1 2.2	45 **Rh** 102.9 2.2	46 **Pd** 106.4 2.2	47 **Ag** 107.9 1.9	48 **Cd** 112.4 1.7	49 **In** 114.8 1.7	50 **Sn** 118.7 1.8	51 **Sb** 121.8 1.9	52 **Te** 127.6 2.1	53 **I** 126.9 2.5	54 **Xe** 131.3 -
55 **Cs** 132.9 0.7	56 **Ba** 137.3 0.9	57 **La*** 138.9 1.1	72 **Hf** 178.5 1.3	73 **Ta** 180.9 1.5	74 **W** 183.9 1.7	75 **Re** 186.2 1.9	76 **Os** 190.2 2.2	77 **Ir** 192.2 2.2	78 **Pt** 195.1 2.2	79 **Au** 197.0 2.4	80 **Hg** 200.6 1.9	81 **Tl** 204.4 1.8	82 **Pb** 207.2 1.9	83 **Bi** 209.0 1.9	84 **Po** 209 2.0	85 **At** 210 2.2	86 **Rn** 222 -
87 **Fr** 223 0.7	88 **Ra** 226 0.9	89 **Ac*** 227 1.1															

Figure 1.14
The periodic table of elements organizes elements with increasing atomic number based on number of valence electrons. Elements with closed-shell configurations are found in Group 18. The symbol * indicates the location of the Lanthanoids and Actinoids (not shown) (Adapted with permission from [16], and L. Pauling, *The Nature of The Chemical Bond and the Structure of Molecules and Crystals: An Introduction to Modern Chemistry*, 3rd ed. as appears in [14].)

1.7.5 Ionic Bonding

1.7.5.1 Bonding and Force-Distance Curves **Primary bonds** involve the sharing or transfer of valence electrons and are stronger than secondary bonds, which will be discussed later in this chapter. Equations describing primary bonding can best be visualized by considering what would happen as two atoms are slowly brought together over a large distance (Fig. 1.15). At first, there will be no interaction since the atoms are too far apart. However, as they move closer, they will begin to exert both attractive and repulsive forces on each other. The strength of these forces depends on the distance between the atoms. The cause of the attractive force varies depending on the type of bonding, but this force governs the interaction between the atoms at intermediate distances. At very close distances, there is a strong repulsive force that results from the overlap of the core and valence electron shells from the two atoms.

The total force (F_{total}) between the two atoms at any given separation distance (r) is the sum of the attractive (F_A) and repulsive (F_R) forces:

$$F_{total}(r) = F_A(r) + F_R(r) \tag{1.1}$$

As shown in Fig. 1.15, at a certain separation distance, r_0, an equilibrium is reached where there is no total force:

$$F_A(r_0) + F_R(r_0) = 0 \tag{1.2}$$

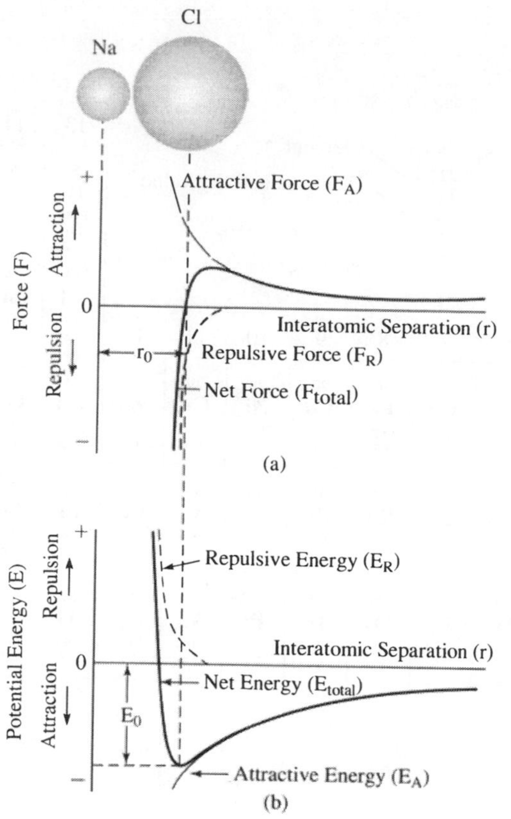

Figure 1.15
(a) Attractive, repulsive and total forces between two atoms as a function of separation distance. The strength of the attractive and repulsive forces depends on the distance, with repulsive forces predominating at small separation lengths due to the overlap of the core and valence electron shells from the two atoms. (b) Attractive, repulsive and total energies between two atoms as a function of separation distance. Note that, at r_0, there is a minimum in the total energy curve—the corresponding energy E_0 is considered the bonding energy for the pair of atoms. (Adapted with permission from [14], and [12].)

Because there is no total force at this distance, atoms prefer to remain at this spacing and will resist attempts to force movement closer or further apart. The distance r_0 is measured from the center of one atom to the center of the other and is considered to be the **bond length** between the two atoms.

Since energy (E) is defined as force (F) over a distance (r), the above equation can be converted from terms of force to terms of energy through integration over an infinite separation distance:

$$E_{total}(r) = \int_{\infty}^{r} F_{total}(r')dr' = \int_{\infty}^{r} F_A(r')dr' + \int_{\infty}^{r} F_R(r')dr' = E_A(r) + E_R(r) \qquad (1.3)$$

Figure 1.15(b) depicts the attractive (E_A), repulsive (E_R), and total energies (E_{total}) based on separation distance (r). Like the force curves [Fig. 1.15(a)], the total energy curve is the sum of the contributions of the attractive and repulsive energies. Also in correspondence to the force curve, at r_0, there is a minimum in the total energy curve. This is the **bonding energy** for the two atoms, and represents the amount of energy that would be required to separate them to an infinite distance.

1.7.5.2 Characteristics of the Ionic Bond There are three types of primary bonds: ionic, covalent, and metallic. The concepts of bond energy and separation distance detailed above are valid for all types of primary bonds, although the magnitude and shape of the energy vs. distance curves may differ. We begin our discussion with ionic bonding, since this type follows the above models for bond force and energy most directly.

Ionic bonds occur between atoms that have large differences in electronegativity, for example, between elements in Group 1 and Group 16 or 17. A common molecule demonstrating ionic bonding is NaCl. In this case, the single electron in the valence shell of Na ($1s^2 2s^2 2p^6 3s^1$) is transferred to the highly electronegative Cl, which is one electron short of a full valence shell ($1s^2 2s^2 2p^6 3s^2 3p^5$). Through this transfer, a positive ion (**cation**) of Na (Na^+) and negative ion (**anion**) of Cl (Cl^-) is formed, with both ions having full valence shells. This generates an electrostatic attraction between the two ions, which is the source of the attractive force in the force-separation distance curves for ionic bonds. The magnitude of this force, the **Coulombic force** (F_C), is a function of both the charge of the ions and their separation distance (r); that is,

$$F_C(r) = \frac{-K_C}{r^2} \tag{1.4}$$

$$K_C = k_0(Z_1 q)(Z_2 q) \tag{1.5}$$

where r is the separation distance between the centers of ions 1 and 2, Z_1 and Z_2 are the valence of the charged ions, k_0 is a proportionality constant ($9 \times 10^9\ \mathrm{VmC^{-1}}$) and q is the charge of a single electron. The corresponding equation for the repulsive force (F_R) reflects the large increase seen as the ions are forced closer together:

$$F_R(r) = \frac{-K_R}{r^n} \tag{1.6}$$

where K_R and n are constants, with $n > 2$. As discussed above, these equations can then be integrated to obtain the corresponding attractive and repulsive energies.

Ionic bonds have the same magnitude in all directions and thus are termed non-directional. To ensure stability, each negative ion must be surrounded in three dimensions by positive ions, and vice versa. This imposes constraints on the structure of ionic crystals. Ionic bonds are most commonly found in ceramic materials. As described previously, ceramics demonstrate characteristic mechanical properties (hardness and brittleness) that can be directly related to this bond type.

1.7.6 Covalent Bonding

Covalent bonds are formed through the sharing of valence electrons, rather than complete electron transfer, as for ionic bonds. In this case, there are electronegative elements but no electropositive ones. Since there is no ion formation with covalent bonds, the attractive force found as a part of the force-separation distance curve is not strictly Coulombic, but attraction does exist between the atomic cores and shared electrons. The corresponding repulsive force is generated when core electrons from the atoms come in proximity to each other. Covalent bonds are found in polymeric biomaterials.

1.7.6.1 Atomic Orbitals and Hybridization The number of covalent bonds that an atom can form depends on the number of valence electrons present. As mentioned previously, atomic subshells (also called orbitals) have specific shapes and orientations. In order to increase the probability of forming covalent bonds, these orbitals can change energy and shape (**hybridize**). For example, typically carbon would have two valence electrons in the $2s$ and two in the $2p$. However, in methane (CH_4), the carbon has gained enough energy to promote one $2s$ electron to the third p orbital and then all of the valence orbitals are altered to form four sp^3 hybrid orbitals. The shape of these hybrid orbitals is depicted in Fig. 1.16. Although energy is required for promotion of an electron between orbitals, the newly formed hybrid

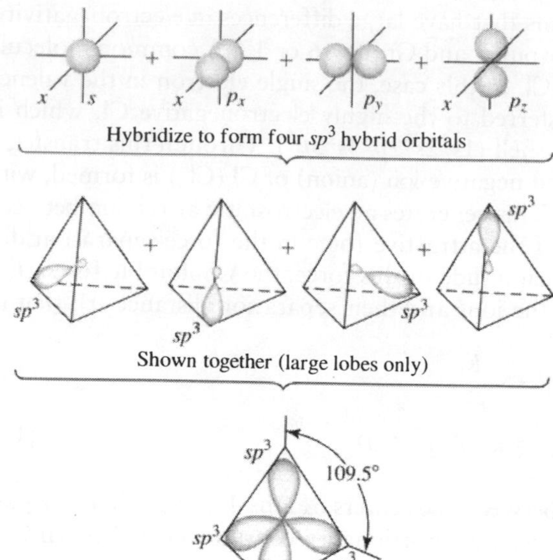

Figure 1.16
Formation of four sp^3 hybrid orbitals from one valence electron in the 2*s* and three in the 2*p*. Each of the newly formed hybrid orbitals have a large lobe that can be directed toward other atoms to promote covalent binding. (Adapted with permission from [17].)

orbitals have a large lobe that can be directed toward other atoms to promote covalent binding. The energy released as the bond is formed more than compensates for the original energy requirement for hybridization.

Depending on the number of valence electrons, *sp*, sp^2 and sp^3 hybrid orbitals are possible. The orientation of the large lobes in each case is somewhat different and is governed by the idea that, due to electrostatic repulsion between the electrons, the most stable atomic structure will place the lobes as far apart as possible. Spatial orientations of the most common hybrid orbital types are found in Fig. 1.17. The spatial orientation of the hybrid orbitals affects where bonding occurs and results in different bond angles for different compounds. These bond angles play an important role in the physical properties of synthetic and naturally derived polymers.

Unlike ionic bonding, covalent bonding is directional because the shared electrons lie in line between the two atoms. This directionality affects the overall properties

Atomic orbital set	Hybrid orbital set	Geometry	Examples
s,p	Two *sp*	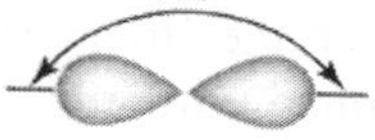 180° Linear	BeF_2, $HgCl_2$
s,p,p	Three sp^2	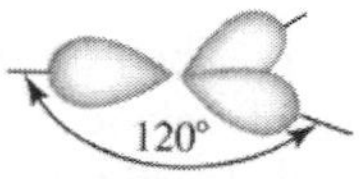 120° Trigonal planar	BF_3, SO_3
s,p,p,p	Four sp^3	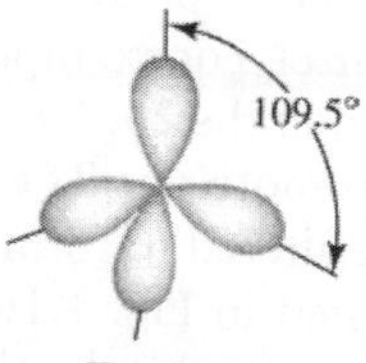 109.5° Tetrahedral	CH_4, NH_3, H_2O, NH_4^+

Figure 1.17
Spatial orientations of the most common hybrid orbital types. The spatial orientation of the hybrid orbitals affects where bonding occurs and results in different bond angles for different compounds. (Adapted with permission from [17].)

(a)

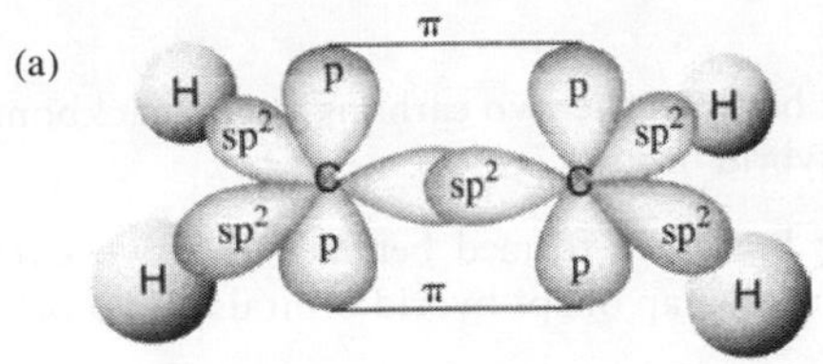

(b)

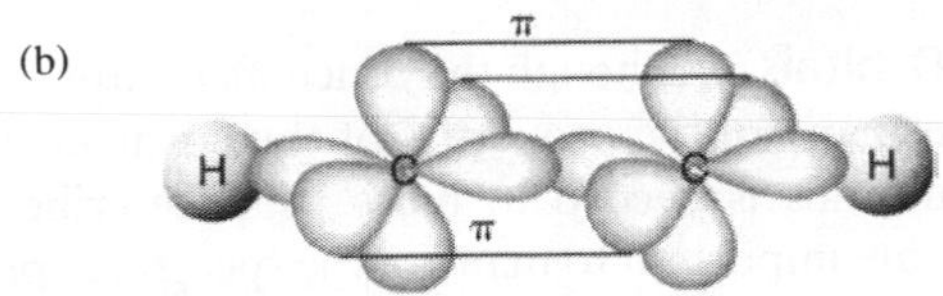

Figure 1.18
π bonds in ethylene and acetylene molecules. (a) Bonds found in the ethylene molecule. σ bonds are formed along the internuclear axis between two atoms, such as the sp^2 orbital between carbon and each hydrogen and the sp^2 orbital between the two carbon atoms. This leaves two electrons in the unhybridized p orbitals, which can then interact in a sideways fashion to complete the valence shell of each carbon, thus forming a π bond parallel to the internuclear axis. (b) Bonds found in the acetylene molecule. A second π bond is formed in a similar manner to ethylene. π bonds are not as strong as σ bonds, but their presence can affect the properties and activity of proteins and synthetic polymers. (Adapted with permission from [17].)

of covalently bonded materials. Bonds formed along the internuclear axis of two atoms are called **sigma (σ) bonds**. These are the type of bonds most often associated with covalent binding. However, in certain cases, such as for double or triple bonds [such as are found in ethylene (C_2H_4) or acetylene (C_2H_2)—see Fig. 1.18], we must consider a second type of bond, the **pi (π) bond**. In ethylene, instead of hybridizing to sp^3 orbitals as happens in CH_4, each carbon has three of the valence electrons in sp^2 hybrid orbitals and one in a regular p orbital. The sp^2 orbitals form σ bonds between one carbon, each hydrogen, and the other carbon [Fig. 1.18(a)]. This leaves two electrons in the unhybridized p orbitals, one associated with each carbon. These p orbitals can then interact in a sideways fashion to complete the valence shell of each carbon, thus forming a π bond perpendicular to the internuclear axis.

A second π bond is formed in a similar manner in the acetylene molecule [C–C triple bond, see Fig. 1.18(b)]. π bonds are not as strong as σ bonds, but can affect rigidity of materials because they constrain certain parts of molecules in planar orientations. Therefore, the presence of such bonds have an impact on the properties and activity of proteins and synthetic polymers.

EXAMPLE PROBLEM 1.7

Determine the orbital structures of the backbones of the following polymers:

(a) $\left[\mathrm{CH_2{-}CH_2} \right]$

(b) $\left[\mathrm{CH{=}CH} \right]$

(c) $\left[\mathrm{C{\equiv}C} \right]$

Solution:

(a) A σ bond is formed between the two carbons in the backbone of poly(ethylene) by the overlap of two sp^3 hybrid orbitals.

(b) A σ bond and a π bond are formed between the two carbons in the backbone of poly(acetylene) by the overlap of sp^2 hybrid orbitals and p orbitals, respectively.

(c) A σ bond and two π bonds are formed between the two carbons in the backbone of poly(yne) by the overlap of sp hybrid orbitals and p orbitals, respectively. ■

1.7.6.2 Molecular Orbitals Although the concepts of atomic orbitals and hybridization serve to explain many of the properties of the covalent bond, another model involving **molecular orbitals** is needed to more fully describe energy absorption and excited states, which are important to many of the spectroscopic techniques that will be discussed later in this text. Molecular orbitals have many of the same properties as atomic orbitals, but they are associated with an entire molecule. Like atomic orbitals, they have definite energy levels and can hold only two electrons, each with different spins. There are two types of molecular orbitals: bonding and antibonding (Fig. 1.19).

In **bonding molecular orbitals**, the wave functions describing the electrons in atomic orbitals from two different atoms overlap in a reinforcing way and enhance each other. Thus, there is a high probability of finding the electrons in the region along the internuclear axis, where there is a strong attraction to the nuclei. This is very stable, and therefore the electrons are at a lower energy than they were in their respective atomic orbitals. The bonding molecular orbital is the basis for covalent bonds between atoms.

On the other hand, in **antibonding molecular orbitals**, the electrons' wave functions overlap in a destructive way and cancel each other in the region between the nuclei, and the greatest electron density is found on the opposite sides of the nuclei (Fig. 1.19). Since this excludes electrons from the very area where a bond should form, this orbital is less stable (has higher energy) than the corresponding atomic orbitals of the individual atoms.

Like atomic orbitals, there are both σ and π molecular orbitals (Fig. 1.20). σ bonding and antibonding molecular orbitals describe the electron density in the line between two nuclei, while π bonding and antibonding molecular orbitals arise from the sideways overlap of atomic orbitals and therefore describe the electron density in spatial orientations other than along the internuclear axis (Fig. 1.20).

1.7.6.3 Mixed Bonds From the above descriptions of the bond types, it can be assumed that ionic bonds are formed primarily when there is a large difference in

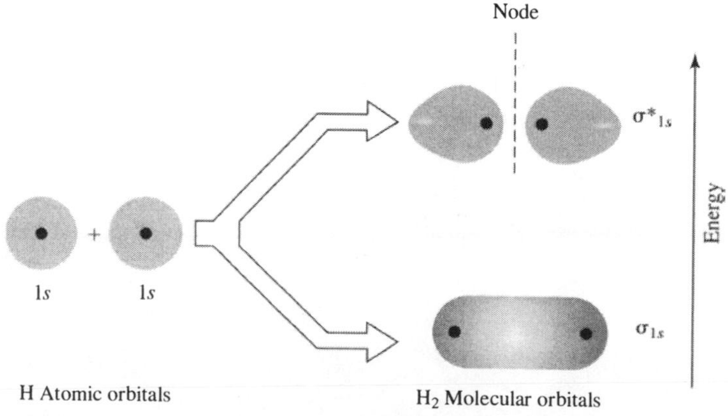

Figure 1.19
The combination of two H 1s atomic orbitals to form bonding (σ) and anti-bonding (σ^*) molecular orbitals in H_2. In bonding molecular orbitals, the wave functions describing the electrons in atomic orbitals from two different atoms overlap in a reinforcing way and enhance each other. This orbital is very stable, and therefore the electrons are at a lower energy than they were in their respective atomic orbitals. On the other hand, in antibonding molecular orbitals, the electrons' wave functions overlap in a destructive way and cancel each other in the region between the nuclei (a node is formed between the nuclei). Since this excludes electrons from the very area where a bond should form, this orbital is less stable (has higher energy) than the corresponding atomic orbitals of the individual atoms. (Adapted with permission from [17].)

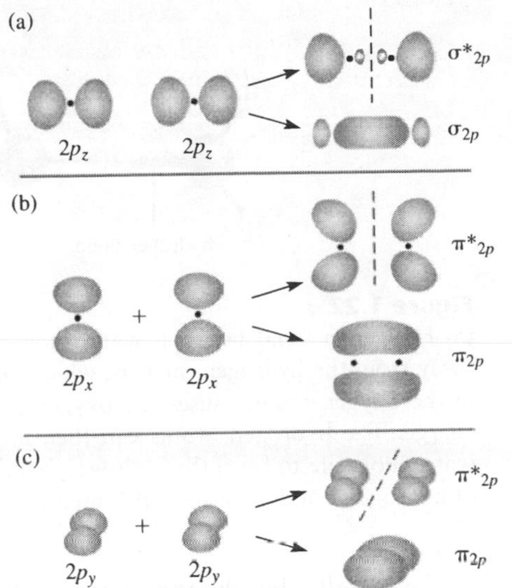

Figure 1.20
(a) σ molecular orbitals. σ bonding and antibonding molecular orbitals describe the electron density in the line between two nuclei. (b–c) π molecular orbitals. π bonding and antibonding molecular orbitals arise from the sideways overlap of atomic orbitals and therefore describe the electron density in spatial orientations other than that along the internuclear axis. (Adapted with permission from [17].)

electronegativity between the elements in a compound, and covalent bonds are formed when there is a smaller difference. However, this is a simplified explanation and, in reality, there is a gradual shift between the bond types. Thus, many bonds have characteristics that are partially ionic and partially covalent. Calculations suggest that a difference in electronegativity of approximately 1.7 results in a bond with half-covalent and half-ionic properties. Many ceramics have bonds that display mixed characteristics. As expected, the extent to which a material's bonds exhibit ionic or covalent characteristics will affect its general physical properties.

1.7.7 Metallic Bonding

Metallic bonds are generally formed in materials containing elements that are electropositive. Because there are no electronegative elements to accept the valence electrons, the electrons are donated to the entire structure. This creates a "cloud" or "sea" of electrons that are mobile and surround a core of cations (Fig. 1.21). Metallic bonds do involve electron sharing, like covalent bonds, but are non-directional, like ionic bonds. Here, the valence electrons are considered to be delocalized and have equal probability of being associated with any of the ion cores. The mobility of electrons in metals is what leads to their high electrical conductivity.

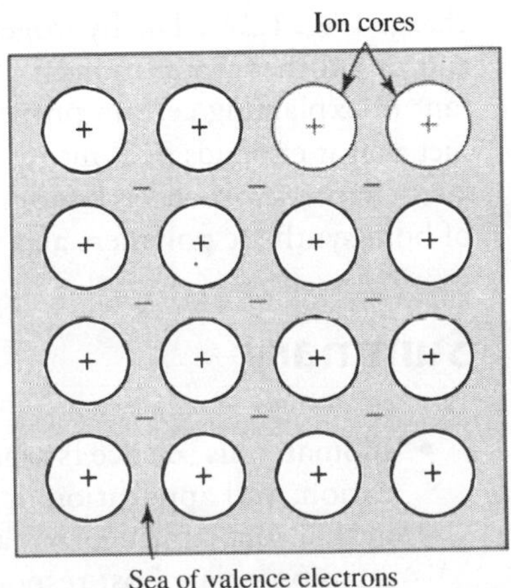

Figure 1.21
Schematic of metallic bonding. Because there are no electronegative elements to accept the valence electrons, the electrons are donated to the entire structure. This creates a "cloud" or "sea" of electrons that are mobile and surround a core of cations. (Reprinted with permission from [14])

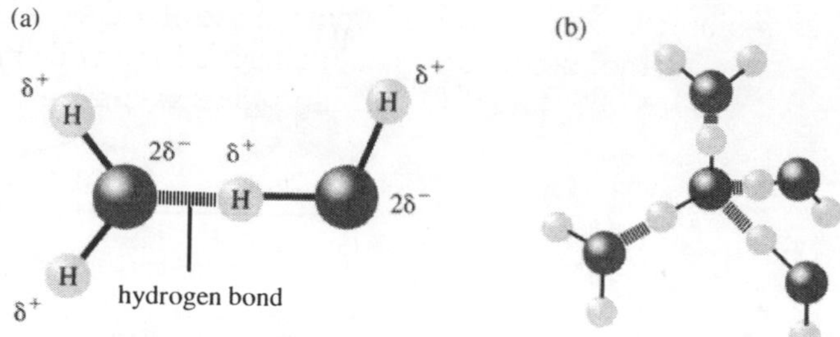

Figure 1.22
(a) Hydrogen bond between water molecules. The electronegative oxygen draws electrons away from the hydrogen nucleus, which, in combination with the extra, unbonded electrons in the oxygen atom, causes the oxygen portion of the molecule to carry a partial negative charge. The hydrogen atoms can then interact with the negative (oxygen) end of another water molecule to form the hydrogen bond. (b) An illustration of a three-dimensional lattice of hydrogen bonds in water. (Adapted with permission from [18])

In metallic bonds, the attractive force seen as part of the force-separation distance curve is caused by the electrostatic attraction between the positively charged ion cores and the negatively charged electron clouds. Similar to the other bond types, a repulsive force is generated when the filled shells of the ion cores start to overlap.

1.7.8 Secondary Forces

Although the type of primary bonds a material possesses dictates many of its properties, **secondary bonds** (or **van der Waals bonds**) can play a large role as well. Secondary bonds involve attraction between atoms that require neither electron transfer nor electron sharing. Thus, they are substantially weaker than primary bonds. In general, this attraction occurs between molecules that, for various reasons, have a portion that is slightly positively charged and a portion that is slightly negatively charged (a **molecular dipole**). The positive end of one molecule then associates with the negative end of another via Coulombic attraction, forming a three-dimensional network.

Although it is possible to have temporary (fluctuating) dipole molecules, which give rise to van der Waals forces, the strongest type of secondary bonding occurs with molecules considered to be permanent dipoles. These are called **polar molecules** and include water (H_2O). In water, the electronegative oxygen draws electrons away from the hydrogen nuclei. This, in combination with the extra, unbonded electrons in the oxygen atom, causes the oxygen portion of the molecule to carry a partial negative charge (Fig. 1.22). The hydrogen atoms can then interact with the negative (oxygen) end of another water molecule, forming a **hydrogen bond**. These bonds are important in explaining certain properties of water, such as its high heat capacity and the fact that it expands as it moves from a liquid to solid state (freezes). As discussed in later chapters, hydrogen bonding is also essential to the structure (and thus function) of both synthetic polymers and naturally formed materials such as proteins.

Summary

- Biomaterials science is a broad field that involves the development, characterization, and application of materials to interface with biological systems in the evaluation, treatment, or augmentation of biological functions while invoking an appropriate host response.

- The field of biomaterials has evolved from the use of industrial materials in the 1940s to the advent of more "designer" materials for a wide range of applications, such as prosthetic heart valves, hip replacements, and kidney dialysis membranes.
- The biological response to a biomaterial is influenced largely by the properties of the material, including the shape, degradation characteristics, surface chemistry, bulk material chemistry, and mechanical properties. In turn, this biological response can have an effect on the material itself.
- The three general categories of biomaterials are metals, ceramics, and polymers.
- Polymeric materials can be either synthetic or naturally derived. Naturally derived polymers originate from biological sources and may closely mimic tissues targeted for replacement and integrate well into the surrounding tissue, but they are often of limited supply, have low mechanical properties, and pose the potential for pathogen transmission. Synthetic polymers, on the other hand, can be produced and sterilized in large quantities with properties tailored for specific applications, but they are usually not capable of interacting with surrounding tissue in an active manner.
- The envisioned final application of a biomaterial dictates the properties and design criteria required of the biomaterial. Surface properties, such as surface roughness and degree of hydrophobicity, are defined by the outermost few atomic layers of the material and highly influence interaction with the surrounding biological environment, especially in the short term. The bulk properties of the material include mechanical properties, physical properties, and chemical composition, which strongly affect the overall performance and long-term stability of the implant.
- The method in which a biomaterial is processed imparts that material with a certain form or geometry. The form of the biomaterial can influence the properties of the material and the biological response to the material. For example, thin sheets are well suited for skin replacements, and flexible, hollow cylinders are appropriate for vascular grafts.
- One of the primary considerations for selection of a biomaterial is the chemical composition of the material. Basic models of molecular chemistry state that an atom is composed of a core nucleus of protons and neutrons orbited by a number of electrons equal to the number of protons. The exact location of the electrons in orbit can be described in terms of discrete energy states (Bohr model) or in terms of space-occupying probabilities (wave-mechanical model). The Aufbau principle, the Pauli exclusion principle, and Hund's rule work in concert to provide a mechanism for predicting the electron configuration of an atom. Atoms with different electron configurations can interact in different ways in various forms of bonding, including ionic bonding (electron transfer), covalent bonding (electron sharing), metallic bonding (nondirectional electron sharing), and bonding through secondary forces, such as hydrogen bonding.

Problems

1.1 One common biomaterial application is the construction of an arterial graft, a device that replaces a section of an artery. An artery is a flexible blood vessel that withstands varying pressures and regulates the flow of blood. Arteries also provide a smooth interior surface to inhibit blood clotting within the vessel.

(a) You need to design an arterial graft. List some advantages and disadvantages of each of the three major types of biomaterials. Which would you choose for this application?
(b) What specific material characteristics need to be considered for the arterial graft application?
(c) Would you use a natural or synthetic material for this application? What are the advantages and disadvantages of each?

1.2 Various biomaterials can be used for joint replacement applications, such as hip implants (see Fig. 1.4). A hip joint replacement must withstand large forces (standing on one leg results in a load of 2.4 times body weight on the femoral head [19]; jumping and running generate higher forces) normally transferred through the hip joint. It must also allow for proper rotation of the joint.
(a) Which of the three major types of biomaterials would you use for the femoral stem? Why?
(b) Would integration of the femoral stem with the surrounding tissue be an acceptable biological response? Why or why not?

References

1. Williams, D.F. *The Williams Dictionary of Biomaterials*. Liverpool: Liverpool University Press, 1999.
2. Ratner, B.D., A.S. Hoffman, F.J. Schoen, and J.E. Lemons. "Biomaterials Science: A Multidisciplinary Endeavor," in *Biomaterials Science: An Introduction to Materials in Medicine*, B.D. Ratner, A.S. Hoffman, F.J. Schoen, and J.E. Lemons, Eds., 2nd ed. San Diego: Elsevier Academic Press, pp. 1–9, 2004.
3. Ratner, B.D. "A History of Biomaterials," in *Biomaterials Science: An Introduction to Materials in Medicine*, B.D. Ratner, A.S. Hoffman, F.J. Schoen, and J.E. Lemons, Eds., 2nd ed. San Diego: Elsevier Academic Press, pp. 10–19, 2004.
4. Park, J.B. and R.S. Lakes, *Biomaterials: An Introduction*, 2nd ed. New York: Plenum Press, 1992.
5. Malchesky, P.S. "Extracorporeal Artificial Organs," in *Biomaterials Science: An Introduction to Materials in Medicine*, B.D. Ratner, A.S. Hoffman, F.J. Schoen, and J.E. Lemons, Eds., 2nd ed. San Diego: Elsevier Academic Press, pp. 514–526, 2004.
6. Padera, Jr., R.F. and F.J. Schoen. "Cardiovascular Medical Devices," in *Biomaterials Science: An Introduction to Materials in Medicine*, B.D. Ratner, A.S. Hoffman, F.J. Schoen, and J.E. Lemons, Eds., 2nd ed. San Diego: Elsevier Academic Press, pp. 470–494, 2004.
7. Guida, G. and D. Hall, "Hip Joint Replacements," in *Integrated Biomaterials Science*, R. Barbucci, Ed. New York: Kluwer, pp. 491–525, 2002.
8. Galletti, P.M. "Prostheses and Artificial Organs," in *The Biomedical Engineering Handbook*, J.D. Bronzino, Ed., 1st ed. Boca Raton: CRC Press, pp. 1828–1837, 1995.
9. http://www.fda.gov. "United States Food and Drug Administration." Washington, DC.
10. Mark, J.E. *Physical Properties of Polymers Handbook*. Woodbury: American Institute of Physics, 1996.
11. Migliaresi, C. and H. Alexander. "Composites," in *Biomaterials Science: An Introduction to Materials in Medicine*, B.D. Ratner, A.S. Hoffman, F.J. Schoen, and J.E. Lemons, Eds., 2nd ed. San Diego: Elsevier Academic Press, pp. 181–197, 2004.
12. Shackelford, J.F., *Introduction to Materials Science for Engineers*, 5th ed. Upper Saddle River: Prentice Hall, 2000.
13. Pollack, Herman W. *Materials Science and Metallurgy*, 4th ed. Englewood Cliffs, NJ: Prentice Hall, 1998.
14. Callister, Jr., W.D. *Materials Science and Engineering: An Introduction*, 3rd ed. New York: John Wiley and Sons, 1994.
15. Vollhardt, K.P.C. and N.E. Schore, *Organic Chemistry*, 2nd ed. New York: W. H. Freeman, 1994.
16. Schaffer, J.P., A. Saxena, S.D. Antolovich, J. Sanders, T. H., and S.B. Warner, *The Science and Design of Engineering Materials*, 2nd ed. Boston: McGraw-Hill, 1998.
17. Brown, T.L., J. LeMay, H.E., and B.E. Bursten, *Chemistry: The Central Science*, 6th ed. Englewood Cliffs: Prentice Hall, 1994.
18. Alberts, B., D. Bray, J. Lewis, M. Raff, K. Roberts, and J. Watson, *Molecular Biology of the Cell*, 3rd ed. New York: Garland Publishing, 1994.
19. Villarraga, M.L. and C.M. Ford. "Applications of Bone Mechanics," in *Bone Mechanics Handbook*, S.C. Cowin, Ed., 2nd ed. Boca Raton: CRC Press, 2001.

Additional Reading

Bhat, S.V. *Biomaterials*, 2nd ed. Harrow: Alpha Science International Ltd., 2005.

Duncan, E. "Development and Regulation of Medical Products Using Biomaterials," in *Biomaterials Science: An Introduction to Materials in Medicine*, B.D. Ratner, A.S. Hoffman, F.J. Schoen, and J.E. Lemons, Eds., 2nd ed. San Diego: Elsevier Academic Press, pp. 788–793, 2004.

Galletti, P.M. and C.K. Colton. "Artificial Lungs and Blood-Gas Exchange Devices," in *The Biomedical Engineering Handbook*, J.D. Bronzino, Ed., 1st ed. Boca Raton: CRC Press, pp. 1879–1897, 1995.

Hallab, N.J., J.J. Jacobs, and J.L. Katz. "Orthopedic Applications," in *Biomaterials Science: An Introduction to Materials in Medicine*, B.D. Ratner, A.S. Hoffman, F.J. Schoen, and J.E. Lemons, Eds., 2nd ed. San Diego: Elsevier Academic Press, pp. 526–555, 2004.

Lemons, J.E. "Voluntary Consensus Standards," in *Biomaterials Science: An Introduction to Materials in Medicine*, B.D. Ratner, A.S. Hoffman, F.J. Schoen, and J.E. Lemons, Eds., 2nd ed. San Diego: Elsevier Academic Press, pp. 783–788, 2004.

Silver, F.H. and D.L. Christiansen. *Biomaterials Science and Biocompatibility*. New York: Springer, 1999.

Temenoff, J.S., E.S. Steinbis, and A.G. Mikos. "Biodegradable Scaffolds," in *Orthopedic Tissue Engineering: Basic Science and Practice*, V.M. Goldberg and A.I. Caplan, Eds. New York: Marcel Dekker, pp. 77–103, 2004.

Voet, D. and J.G. Voet. *Biochemistry*, 3rd ed. New York: John Wiley and Sons, 2004.

Vogler, E.A., "Role of Water in Biomaterials," in *Biomaterials Science: An Introduction to Materials in Medicine*, B.D. Ratner, A.S. Hoffman, F.J. Schoen, and J.E. Lemons, Eds., 2nd ed. San Diego: Elsevier Academic Press, pp. 59–65, 2004.

Yannas, I.V. "Natural Materials," in *Biomaterials Science: An Introduction to Materials in Medicine*, B.D. Ratner, A.S. Hoffman, F.J. Schoen, and J.E. Lemons, Eds., 2nd ed. San Diego: Elsevier Academic Press, pp. 127–137, 2004.

CHAPTER 2 Chemical Structure of Biomaterials

Main Objective

To understand the different types of bonding and how these are organized into material subunits for metals, ceramics and polymers.

Specific Objectives

1. To compare and contrast building blocks of polymers, metals and ceramics.
2. To understand and be able to produce lattice parameters for simple crystal structures in metals and ceramics.
3. To compare and contrast types of defects and impurities in metals and ceramics.
4. To understand and use simple models of diffusion.
5. To understand general methods of polymer synthesis.
6. To understand how the chemical structure of polymers affects their ability to form regular structures (crystals).
7. To understand the theory behind and possible limitations to various chemical composition characterization techniques presented.

2.1 Introduction: Bonding and the Structure of Biomaterials

This chapter will focus on how the types of bonds described in Chapter 1 relate in three dimensions to form different classes of biomaterials. In order to more fully appreciate the differences between these material types, the structures of metals, ceramics and polymers will be compared and contrasted.

For this discussion, it is important to distinguish between crystalline and amorphous materials. In **crystalline** substances, atoms are arranged in a periodic pattern resulting in long-range order. **Amorphous** materials lack this systematic atomic arrangement and can be considered to possess a molecular structure much more like that of a liquid. Although metals are typically crystalline, ceramic and polymeric materials can be either crystalline or amorphous, depending on their chemical constituents and processing method.

2.2 Structure of Metals

We begin our discussion of chemical structures with metallic biomaterials. These materials have been widely explored for a variety of biomedical applications, but are best known as the basis of joint replacements. Metals are crystalline, and because metallic bonding is nondirectional, there are a wide variety of atomic configurations possible to create a number of crystal structures.

2.2.1 Crystal Structures

A number of physical properties depend on the crystal structure of a material. For ease of communication, crystal structures are usually described on the basis of their unit cells. A **unit cell** is the configuration of atoms in a small section of the crystal that is repeated again and again in three dimensions to form the final material. Although the limits of the unit cell are arbitrarily chosen, standard cells are parallelepipeds with corners coinciding with the centers of atoms. Figure 2.1 depicts a diagram of a simple cubic unit cell and its relationship to three-dimensional atomic structure.

When discussing crystal structures, it is convenient to compare them using parameters such as **coordination number** and **atomic packing factor (APF)**. Each atom in a crystal has a coordination number equal to the number of nearest-neighbor atoms. The APF is based on the **atomic hard-sphere model**, which depicts each atom as a sphere requiring a fixed volume (Fig. 2.2). APF is a means of discussing how much unoccupied space there is in a particular structure and is found using:

$$\text{APF} = \frac{\text{volume of atoms in a unit cell}}{\text{total unit cell volume}}$$

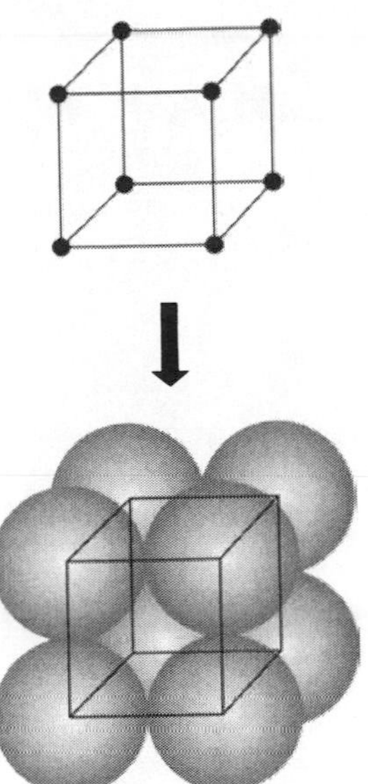

Figure 2.1
Schematic of a simple cubic unit cell and its relationship to three-dimensional atomic structure. The corners of the unit cell coincide with the centers of the atoms in the final structure. (Reprinted with permission from [1])

2.2.1.1 Face-Centered Cubic Structure Although a simple cubic unit cell like that shown in Fig. 2.1 is easy to visualize, in reality, very few materials of interest adopt this crystal structure. In fact, metals have a variety of crystal structures depending on temperature, processing and alloying. For many metals, a common crystal structure is **face-centered cubic** (FCC). Aluminum, copper, lead, silver and gold are

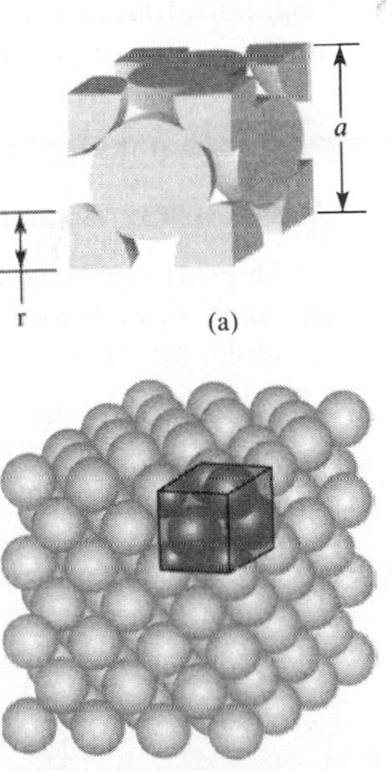

Figure 2.2
(a) The atomic hard-sphere model of a face-centered cubic unit cell. The parameter a is the unit cell edge length and r is the atomic radius. In this geometry, there are atoms located at each of the corners as well as the centers of each face. The atomic packing factor for FCC crystals is 0.74, and the coordination number is 12. (b) Relationship of a unit cell to the larger structure of an FCC crystal. Note how atoms (or lattice points) are shared between multiple unit cells (e.g. each corner lattice point is shared between eight unit cells, whereas face-centered atoms are shared between two unit cells). (Adapted with permission from [2] and [3])

TABLE 2.1

Crystal Structure for Common Metals

Metal	Crystal Structure[a]	Atomic Radius[b] (nm)	Metal	Crystal Structure	Atomic Radius (nm)
Aluminum	FCC	0.1431	Molybdenum	BCC	0.1363
Cadmium	HCP	0.1490	Nickel	FCC	0.1246
Chromium	BCC	0.1249	Platinum	FCC	0.1387
Cobalt	HCP	0.1253	Silver	FCC	0.1445
Copper	FCC	0.1278	Tantalum	BCC	0.1430
Gold	FCC	0.1442	Titanium (α)	HCP	0.1445
Iron (α)	BCC	0.1241	Tungsten	BCC	0.1371
Lead	FCC	0.1750	Zinc	HCP	0.1332

[a] FCC = face-centered cubic; HCP = hexagonal close-packed; BCC = body-centered cubic.

[b] A nanometer (nm) equals 10^{-9} m; to convert from nanometers to angstrom units (Å), multiply the nanometer value by 10.

(Reprinted with permission from [4].)

some of the metals that exhibit this structure at room temperature (see Table 2.1). In this geometry, atoms are located at each of the corners as well as the centers of each face (Fig. 2.2). Examining the hard sphere model in Fig. 2.2, the unit cell edge length (a) and the atomic radius (r) can be related through the formula

$$a = 2r\sqrt{2} \tag{2.1}$$

In a FCC crystal, the corner atoms are shared by eight unit cells and the face atoms are shared by two. Therefore, $\left(8 \times \frac{1}{8}\right) + \left(6 \times \frac{1}{2}\right)$ or the equivalent of four atoms belong to each unit cell. Using the expressions for volume of a sphere and cube, the calculation for APF results in 0.74. This is the largest fraction obtainable using atoms all having the same radius.

Also shown in Fig. 2.2, the coordination number for FCC crystals is 12. As an example, the atom in the center of the front face of the cell has four corner nearest neighbors, four face atoms touching from behind, and another four equivalent neighbor face atoms in the unit cell in front of it, coming out of the page (not shown).

EXAMPLE PROBLEM 2.1

Consider a FCC crystal, as shown in Fig. 2.2.

(a) Show why the relation between r and a is $a = 2r\sqrt{2}$.
(b) Apply this relationship and the knowledge that a FCC crystal has the equivalent of 4 atoms per unit cell to show that the APF for FCC crystals is 0.74.

Solution:

(a) Consider one side of the FCC crystal as shown:

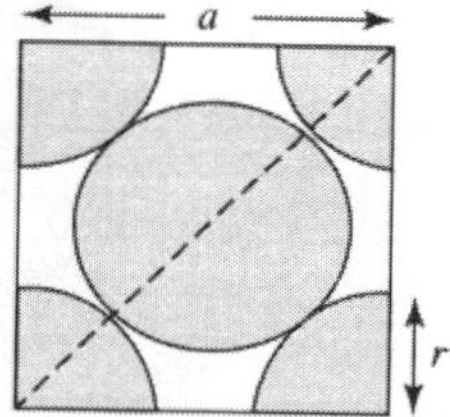

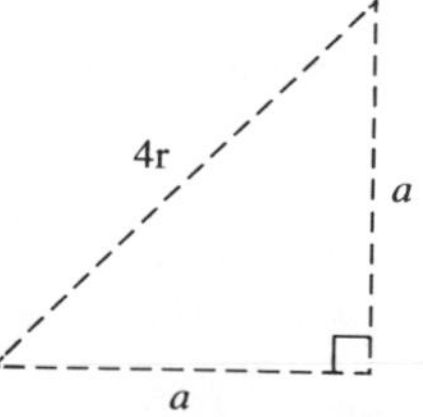

It is apparent that a right triangle can be drawn with two sides equal to a and the hypotenuse equal to $4r$, as the atoms are in contact. Thus, through the use of the Pythagorean Theorem, we obtain

$$a^2 + a^2 = (4r)^2$$
$$2a^2 = 16r^2$$
$$a^2 = 8r^2$$
$$a = 2r\sqrt{2}$$

(b) The volume of a unit cell is as follows: $V_{unit\ cell} = a^3$.

Substituting the relation from part (a) gives $V_{unit\ cell} = (2r\sqrt{2})^3$.
A FCC unit cell contains the equivalent of 4 atoms; thus, the volume occupied by atoms in the unit cell is as follows:

$$V_{atoms} = 4\left(\tfrac{4}{3}\pi r^3\right)$$

The APF is the ratio of the volume of the unit cell occupied by atoms to the volume of the unit cell, and can be expressed as follows:

$$APF = \frac{V_{atoms}}{V_{unit\ cell}} = \frac{(16/3)\pi r^3}{16r^3\sqrt{2}} = \frac{\pi}{3\sqrt{2}} = 0.74$$ ■

2.2.1.2 Body-Centered Cubic Structure Another common crystal structure for metals such as chromium or iron is the **body-centered cubic** (BCC, see Table 2.1). This unit cell is depicted in Fig. 2.3. In this structure, there are atoms at all eight corners and a single atom at the center of the cube. From the figure, the unit cell edge length (a) and the atomic radius (r) are related by the formula

$$a = \frac{4r}{\sqrt{3}} \qquad (2.2)$$

In a BCC crystal, the corner atoms are shared by eight unit cells and the central atom is not shared. Therefore, $\left(8 \times \frac{1}{8}\right) + 1$ or the equivalent of 2 atoms belong to each unit cell. This results in an APF of 0.68, which is less than that for a FCC crystal. Similarly, the coordination number for the BCC structure is lower (8). This can

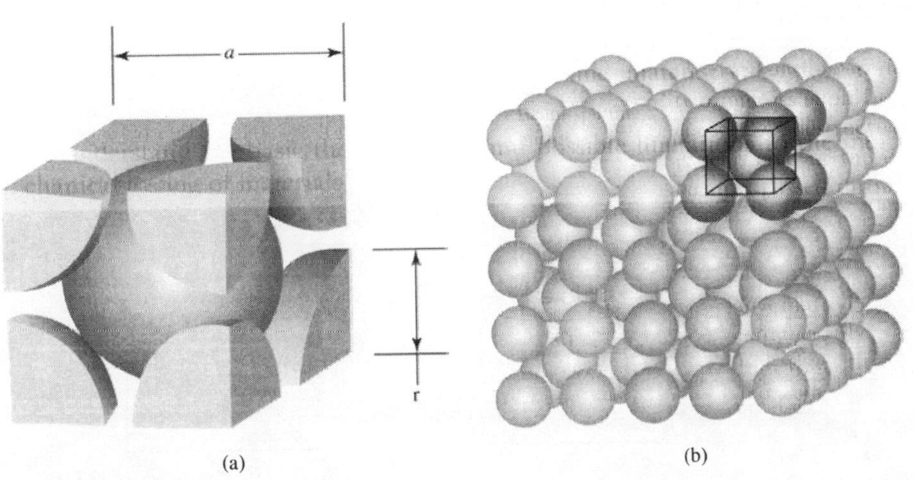

Figure 2.3
(a) The atomic hard-sphere model of a body-centered cubic unit cell. The parameter a is the unit cell edge length and r is the atomic radius. In this geometry, there are atoms at all eight corners and a single atom at the center of the cube. The atomic packing factor for BCC crystals is 0.68, and the coordination number is 8. (b) The relationship of a unit cell to the larger structure of a BCC crystal. Note how only the corner atoms are shared among multiple (eight) unit cells. (Adapted with permission from [2] and [3].)

be seen most easily by taking the atom at the center of the cube, which has the eight corner atoms as nearest neighbors (Fig. 2.3).

Although we have focused on cubic unit cell geometries, metals often have other types of unit cells. Another common type is based on a hexagonal structure. Metals with **hexagonal close-packed** (HCP) unit cells include cobalt and titanium (see Table 2.1). However, detailed descriptions of this and more complicated unit cell geometries are beyond the scope of this text.

2.2.2 Crystal Systems

As mentioned above, since there are many types of crystal structures, it is typically more convenient to represent these geometries as **lattice structures**, as depicted in Fig. 2.4. In this convention, the vertices of the unit cell are called **lattice points.** The unit cell can be completely defined by determining the lengths of the edges of the unit cell (a, b, and c), and the angles between each of the axes (α, β, and γ, see Fig. 2.4). These six values are referred to as **lattice parameters.** (Note that in lattice systems, the exact placement of individual atoms in the unit cell is ignored.)

There exist seven unique combinations of lattice parameters, each of which is a **crystal system.** These include the cubic and hexagonal systems mentioned above, as well as several others shown in Table 2.2. As seen in Fig. 2.5, a given crystal system can produce more than one crystal structure. For example, both FCC and BCC crystals belong to the cubic crystal system.

To further expand the utility of the crystal lattice concept, a coordinate system known as **Miller indices** has been developed to indicate the location of points and the orientation of planes in the lattice structure. Due to the complexity of the geometries involved in some crystal systems, we will confine our discussion of this notation to cubic crystals only. In the following example, a FCC crystal is used to demonstrate how Miller indices expedite naming points in such a unit cell (Fig. 2.6).

As shown in the figure, this notation uses a right-hand Cartesian coordinate system that is aligned with the edges of the unit cell. The coordinates of a certain atom are written as h, k, l, where the three indices represent fractions of the lattice parameters a, b, and c. Following these guidelines, the atom at B would be indicated by 0,1,0. An atom located at point D would be 1,1,1 and an atom in the center of the face, such as H, would be 1/2,1,1/2.

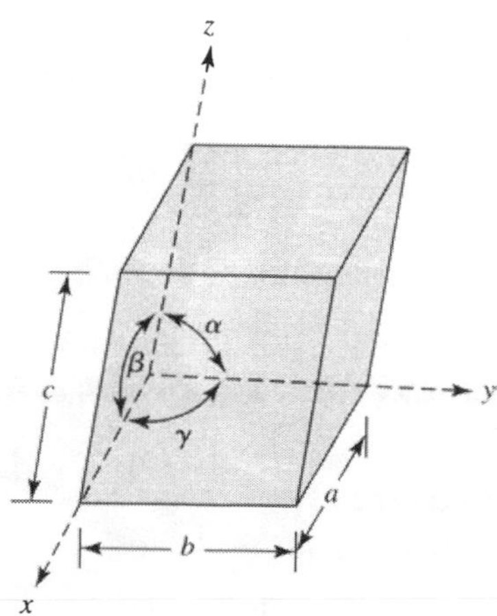

Figure 2.4
Generic lattice structure for a unit cell. The unit cell can be defined by the lengths of the edges of the unit cell (a, b, and c) and the angles between each axis (α, β, and γ). (Reprinted with permission from [4].)

TABLE 2.2

The Seven Main Crystal Systems and their Corresponding Lattice Parameters and Angles

System	Axial lengths and angles[a]	Unit cell geometry
Cubic	$a = b = c, \alpha = \beta = \gamma = 90°$	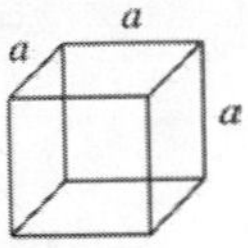
Tetragonal	$a = b \neq c, \alpha = \beta = \gamma = 90°$	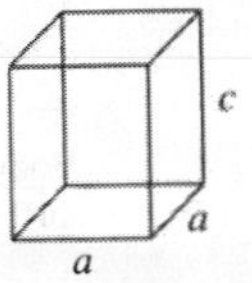
Orthorhombic	$a \neq b \neq c, \alpha = \beta = \gamma = 90°$	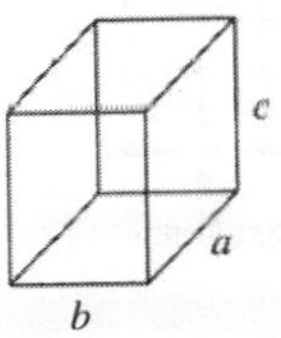
Rhombohedral	$a = b = c, \alpha = \beta = \gamma \neq 90°$	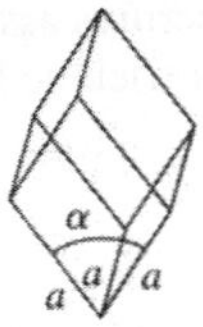
Hexagonal	$a = b \neq c, \alpha = \beta = 90°, \gamma = 120°$	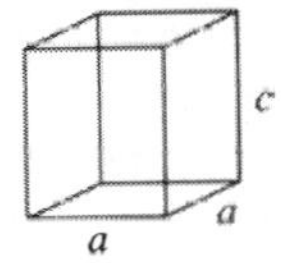
Monoclinic	$a \neq b \neq c, \alpha = \gamma = 90° \neq \beta$	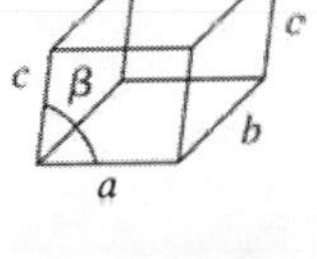
Triclinic	$a \neq b \neq c, \alpha \neq \beta \neq \gamma \neq 90°$	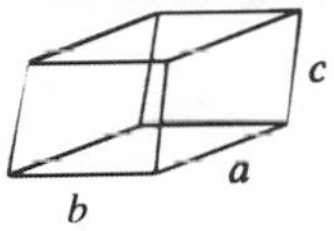

[a] The lattice parameters, a, b, and c are unit cell edge lengths. The lattice parameters α, β, and γ are angles between adjacent unit cell axes where α is the angle viewed *along* the a axis (i.e., the angle *between* the b and c axes). The inequality sign ($\neq$) means that equality is not required. Accidental equality occasionally occurs in some structures.

(Reprinted with permission from [1].)

Planes in crystal structures are designated similarly using Miller indices. Again, the axes are placed along the edges of the unit cell (Fig. 2.7). The following steps are then performed:

1. Determine the points at which the plane intersects the x, y, and z axes. If the plane is parallel to an axis, the intercept for that axis is taken to be ∞.
2. Take the reciprocal of the intercepts.

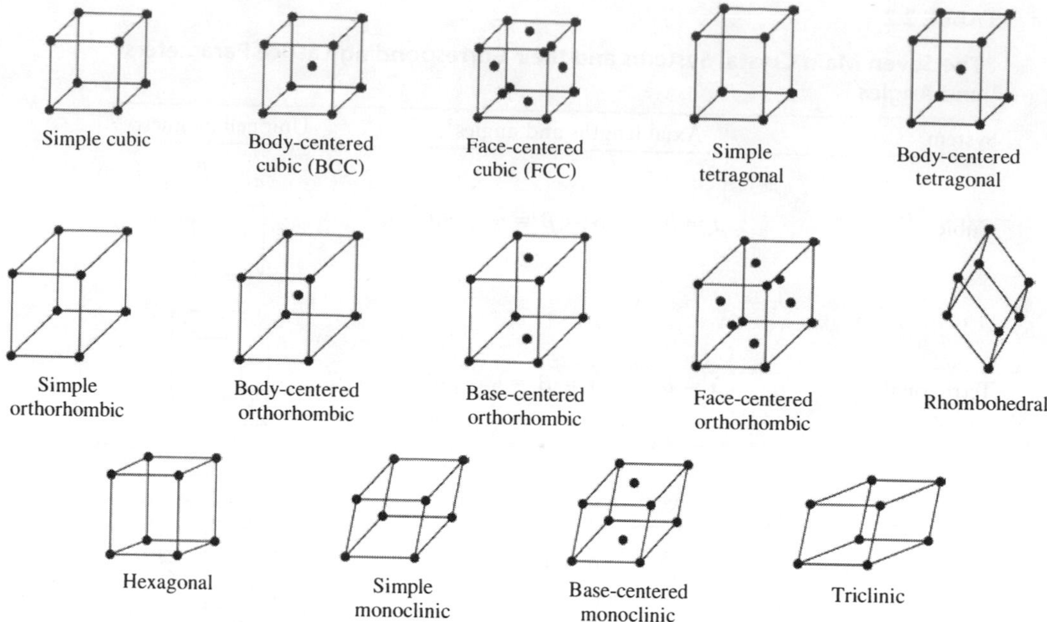

Figure 2.5
The crystal structures associated with the cubic, tetragonal, orthorhombic, rhombohedral, hexagonal, monoclinic, and triclinic lattice systems. (Adapted with permission from [1].)

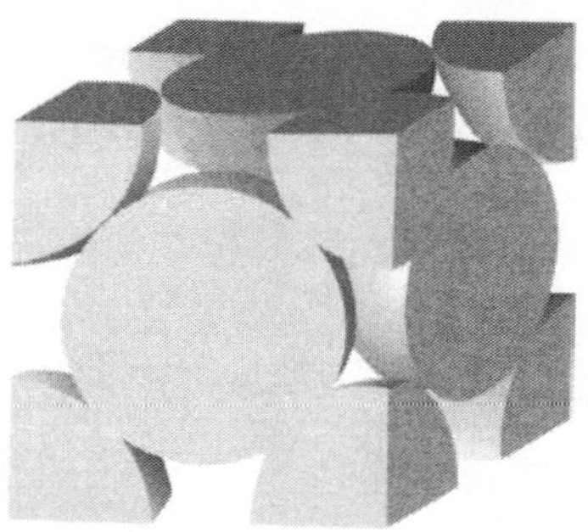

(a)

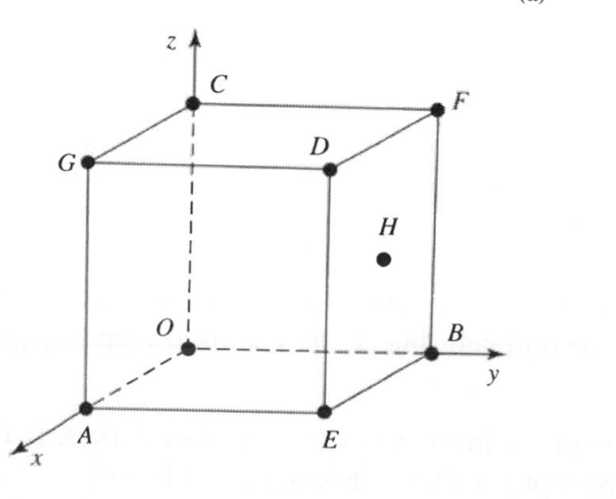

Position	Coordinate
O	0, 0, 0 (Origin)
A	1, 0, 0
B	0, 1, 0
C	0, 0, 1
D	1, 1, 1
E	1, 1, 0
F	0, 1, 1
G	1, 0, 1
H	1/2, 1, 1/2

(b)

Figure 2.6
(a) Hard-sphere model of face-centered cubic unit cell. (b) Corresponding diagram of unit cell with select points depicted using Miller indices. The coordinates of a certain atom are written as h, k, l, where the three indices represent fractions of the lattice parameters a, b, and c. In this figure, the origin has been arbitrarily defined as point O. (Adapted with permission from [2] and [5].)

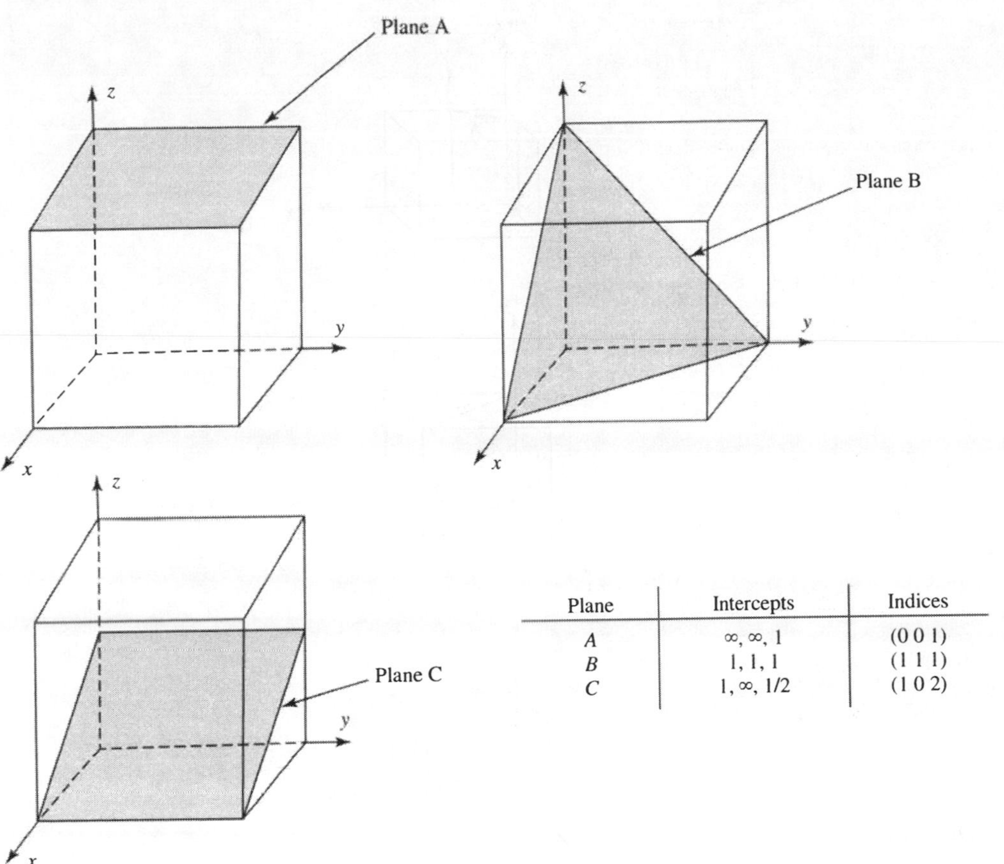

Plane	Intercepts	Indices
A	∞, ∞, 1	(0 0 1)
B	1, 1, 1	(1 1 1)
C	1, ∞, 1/2	(1 0 2)

Figure 2.7
Three planes and their resulting Miller indices, which indicate the orientation of the plane. Indices are based on the reciprocal of the intercepts. (Adapted with permission from [5].)

3. Multiply by an integer to clear fractions.
4. Record integer indices in parentheses with no commas (h k l).
5. Negative numbers are indicated by a bar over the integer.

Using this procedure, plane *A* in Fig. 2.7 has intercepts ∞, ∞, 1 and, thus, its Miller indices are (0 0 1). Similarly, plane *B* has intercepts 1,1,1 and indices (1 1 1), while plane *C* has intercepts 1, ∞, $\frac{1}{2}$ and indices (1 0 2).

EXAMPLE PROBLEM 2.2

Calculate the Miller indices for planes *A*, *B*, and *C*. Note that by convention negative values for indices are denoted with a bar above the number, rather than a negative sign before the number.

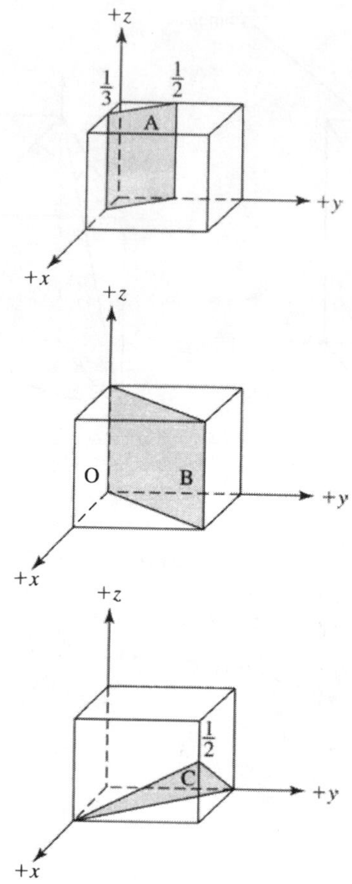

Solution:

For plane A:

	x	y	z
Plane A intercepts	1/3	1/2	∞
reciprocals	3	2	0
indices	(3	2	0)

For plane B:

Since this particular example goes through the origin (O), the origin must be shifted to the edge of the unit cell as follows:

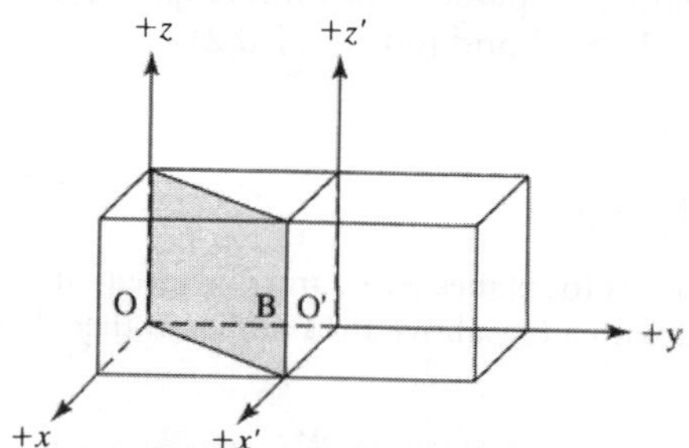

You then use this new origin to determine the intercepts of the plane:

	x	y	z
Plane B intercepts	1	−1	∞
reciprocals	1	−1	0
indices	(1	$\bar{1}$	0)

For plane C:

	x	y	z
Plane C intercepts	1	1	$-1/2$
reciprocals	1	1	-2
indices	(1	1	$\bar{2}$)

■

2.2.3 Defects in Crystal Structures

Our discussion in the previous section assumed a perfect structure for all crystals. However, the formation of a perfect crystal is impossible to achieve under normal conditions. Defects in the crystal structure can be either detrimental or beneficial to the physical and mechanical properties of a material, as we will see in the following chapters. There are several different types of defects, and they are often named according to the number of dimensions affected by the imperfection. We will focus in this chapter on **point defects**, which involve only one or two atoms in a crystal.

2.2.3.1 Point Defects The most common types of point defects are vacancies and self-interstitials, both of which are depicted in Fig. 2.8. A **vacancy** is found at a lattice site where an atom would normally be present, but is currently missing. A **self-interstitial** occurs when an atom from the crystal is crowded into the interstitial space between two adjacent atoms, occupying a space that would otherwise be empty.

Defects occur as a natural result of the thermodynamics of crystal growth. While an in-depth discussion of crystal formation is beyond the scope of this book, a simplified explanation is that the creation of defects is favorable because they increase the entropy of the system. Following these principles, the number of vacancies (N_v) in a crystal can be related to the absolute temperature (T) of the system by the formula

$$N_v = Ne^{\frac{-Q_v}{kT}} \tag{2.3}$$

where N is the total number of atomic sites (atoms + vacancies), Q_v is the activation energy for formation of a vacancy, and k is Boltzmann's constant (1.38×10^{-23} J/atom-K or 8.62×10^{-5} eV/atom-K).

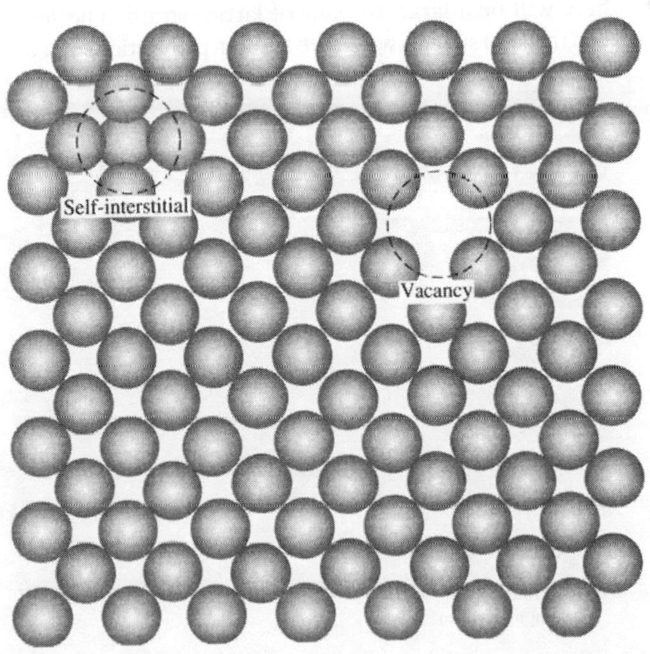

Figure 2.8
Point defects in crystal structures. A vacancy is found at a lattice site where an atom would normally be present, but is currently missing. A self-interstitial occurs when an atom from the crystal is crowded into the interstitial space between surrounding atoms, occupying a space that would otherwise be empty. (Adapted with permission from [2].)

While the formation of defects is thermodynamically favorable, both vacancies and self-interstitials cause strains on the local lattice structure (**lattice strain**). In fact, interstitial defects are uncommon in metals because, in these materials, the atom is so much larger than the interstitial space that it produces large regional distortions in the lattice structure.

2.2.3.2 Impurities In a general sense, the presence of impurities in a material may be considered a type of point defect since they affect the local lattice structure and induce a degree of lattice strain. Impurities can be an artifact of material processing or can be added deliberately to alter the final properties of the material. Like defects, the addition of impurities increases the entropy of the system.

A **solid solution** is formed if the normal crystal structure is maintained upon addition of the impurity atoms. As in a liquid solution, mixing occurs on the atomic level to create a new substance in which each type of atom is homogeneously distributed. In this case, the host material is known as the **solvent**, while the impurity is the **solute**. The solute atoms can either fill spaces between the solvent atoms (**interstitial solution**) or take the place of the solvent atoms (**substitutional solution**) (Fig. 2.9).

While it is not entirely possible to predict when interstitial or substitutional solutions will be formed, interstitial solutions generally occur when the solute atom is smaller than the solvent, allowing for its placement in the interstitial spaces without extreme lattice strain. In the same vein, it has been found that substitutional solutions are favored for a variety of solute/solvent ratios if the following conditions are met:

1. The difference in the size of the atomic radii of the solvent and solute atoms must be less than approximately 15%.
2. The electronegativities of the two atoms must be similar.
3. The valence charges of the two atoms must be similar.
4. The crystal structure of the two atomic species must be identical (important only for solutions in which there is a large fraction of solute).

These are the **Hume-Rothery rules**, named after the person who first suggested them. The first rule is a result of the fact that if the size difference of a solute atom is too great, the solvent atoms will be forced away from their equilibrium bonding positions and there will be a large amount of lattice strain. The second and third conditions assure that the two species will have similar properties such as bond lengths and strengths.

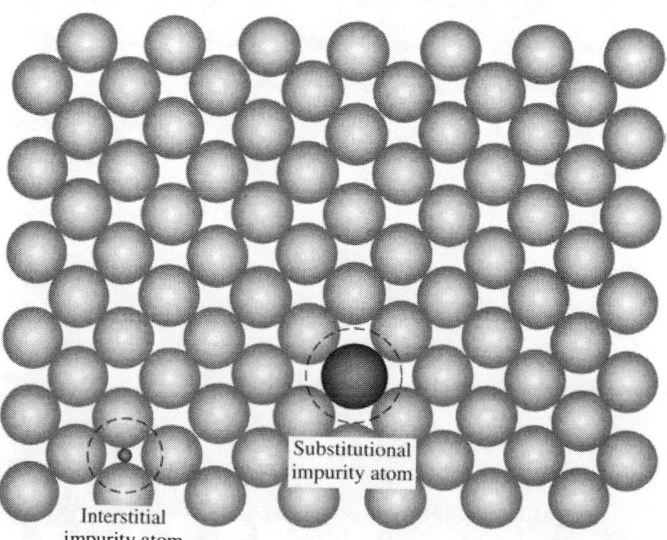

Figure 2.9
Impurities in crystal structures. In this case, the host material is termed the solvent, while the impurity is the solute. The solute atoms can either fill spaces between the solvent atoms (interstitial solution) or take the place of the solvent atoms (substitutional solution). (Adapted with permission from [5])

The best-known solid solutions are metal alloys. In **alloys**, the impurity atom has been added in a particular concentration to improve properties of the host material. Alloys are commonly used to increase strength (see Chapter 4), impart corrosion resistance (see Chapter 5), or improve electrical properties of a pure metal. Common interstitial solid solution alloys include steels (alloys of carbon and iron), which form the basis of stainless steel orthopedic implants. Cobalt-chromium alloys, used for similar applications, are examples of substitutional solid solutions. The concentration of the various species in an alloy can be described in terms of **weight percent composition**, which is the weight of a certain element in relation to the total weight of the alloy. Alternatively, **atom percent composition**, the number of moles of a particular element related to the total moles of all the elements in the alloy, can be used.

EXAMPLE PROBLEM 2.3

The titanium alloy Ti–6Al–4V is a common metal employed in the manufacture of orthopedic implants. This weight percent composition of the alloy is 90 percent Ti, 6 percent Al, and 4 percent V. Determine the following for a Ti–6Al–4V femoral head component of a hip implant (mass of component is 3.0 lbs):

(a) The mass (in grams) of each element in the implant.
(b) The number of moles of each element in the implant.
(c) The atom percent composition of the implant.

Solution:

(a) (3.0 lbs)(0.4536 kg/lb)(1000 g/kg) = 1,361 g (mass of implant)

(0.9)(1,361 g) = 1,225 g Ti in the implant

(0.06)(1,361 g) = 82 g Al in the implant

(0.04)(1,361 g) = 54 gV in the implant

(b) (1,225 g Ti)(1/47.9 g/mole Ti) = 25.6 moles Ti in the implant

(82 g Al)(1/27.0 g/mole Al) = 3.0 moles Al in the implant

(54 g V)(1/50.9 g/mole V) = 1.1 moles V in the implant

(c) Total moles = 25.6 + 3.0 + 1.1 = 29.7 moles

(25.6/29.7) = 86.2% Ti in the implant (atom percent)

(3.0/29.7) = 10.1% Al in the implant (atom percent)

(1.1/29.7) = 3.7% V in the implant (atom percent)

■

2.2.4 Solid State Diffusion

In the preceding section, we have discussed point defects (and impurities) as if they were fixed in the crystal lattice. In reality, this is not the case—motion of defects and impurities can occur throughout the material. This occurs through **diffusion**, which is the movement of material via atomic motion. Since at room temperature most metals are solids, the type of diffusion that occurs through metals is often referred to as **solid state diffusion.** Diffusion can occur in pure metals, with atoms exchanging positions (**self-diffusion**), or atoms of another type can diffuse into the metal (**inter-diffusion or impurity diffusion**). Diffusion of other elements into metals, or diffusion of defects within metals, can have significant effects on their overall physical and mechanical properties.

2.2.4.1 Diffusion Mechanisms Diffusion can be seen as a series of atomic jumps from position to position in a crystal. For an atom to make these jumps, there must be an empty adjacent site and the atom must possess enough energy to change position. Since atoms are always vibrating within their bonds, at any given time a certain fraction possesses enough vibrational energy to overcome both the energy barrier associated with breaking bonds and an increase in lattice strain during atomic movement to diffuse to a neighboring site. The fraction possessing the required amount of energy increases as the temperature of the material increases.

Two main types of diffusion occur in metals. The first kind is **vacancy diffusion.** As the name implies, in this type of diffusion an atom jumps to an adjacent vacancy, thereby exchanging the location of the atom and the vacancy [Fig. 2.10(a)]. Because of this, the direction of atomic diffusion is opposite to that of vacancy diffusion.

The second type of diffusion found in metals is **interstitial diffusion.** In this case, an atom migrates from one interstitial position to a neighboring position [Fig. 2.10(b)]. This usually occurs only with small atoms such as hydrogen, carbon, nitrogen and oxygen that can easily fit into the interstitial spaces. Because of the small size of the diffusing species and their increased mobility, interstitial diffusion generally occurs more rapidly than vacancy diffusion.

2.2.4.2 Modeling of Diffusion Mathematical models involving differential equations have been developed to describe various kinds of diffusion. Many of these are generalized equations that apply to diffusion in gases and liquids as well as solids. We will confine the following discussion to models of **steady-state diffusion,** the case in which the diffusion flux does not change with time.

The amount of diffusion that can occur under a certain set of conditions is dependent on several factors. One of these is the time over which the movement of

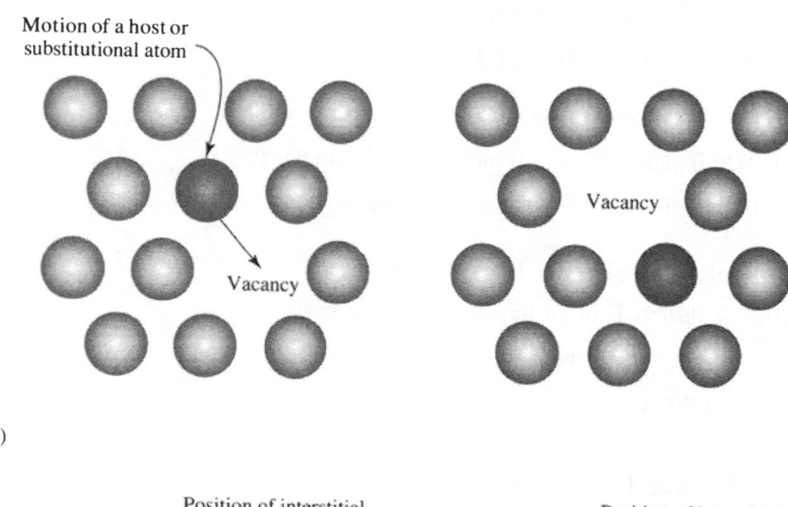

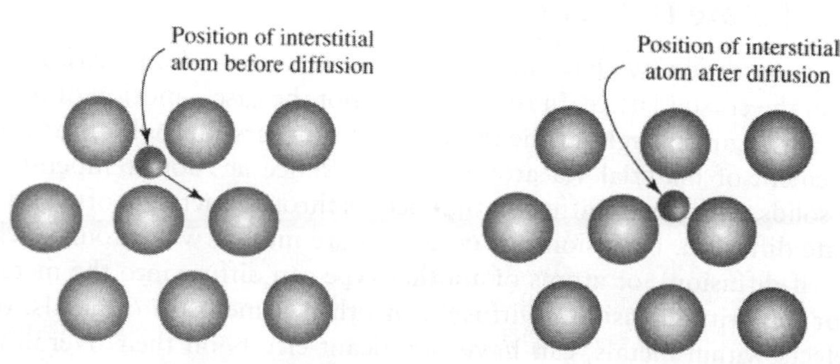

Figure 2.10
(a) Vacancy diffusion in metals. As the name implies, in this type of diffusion an atom jumps to an adjacent vacancy, thereby exchanging the location of the atom and the vacancy. Because of this, the direction of atomic diffusion is opposite to that of vacancy diffusion. (b) Interstitial diffusion in metals. In this case, an atom migrates from one interstitial position to a neighboring position. This usually occurs only with small atoms that can easily fit into the interstitial spaces. (Adapted with permission from [4].)

atoms is allowed to occur. One way to express the rate of atom transfer is the **diffusion flux** (J), which is the mass (or number of atoms) M diffusing through a certain cross-sectional area (A) per unit time (t). This can be written as

$$J = \frac{M}{At} \tag{2.4}$$

Or, as a differential equation,

$$J = \frac{1}{A}\frac{dM}{dt} \tag{2.5}$$

where J typically has units of kg/m^2-s or atoms/m^2-s.

As mentioned above, if J does not change with time, this is steady-state diffusion. One example of steady-state diffusion is the movement of gas atoms across a thin metal plate, given that the concentrations (partial pressures) of the gas on both sides of the plate are held constant [Fig. 2.11(a)].

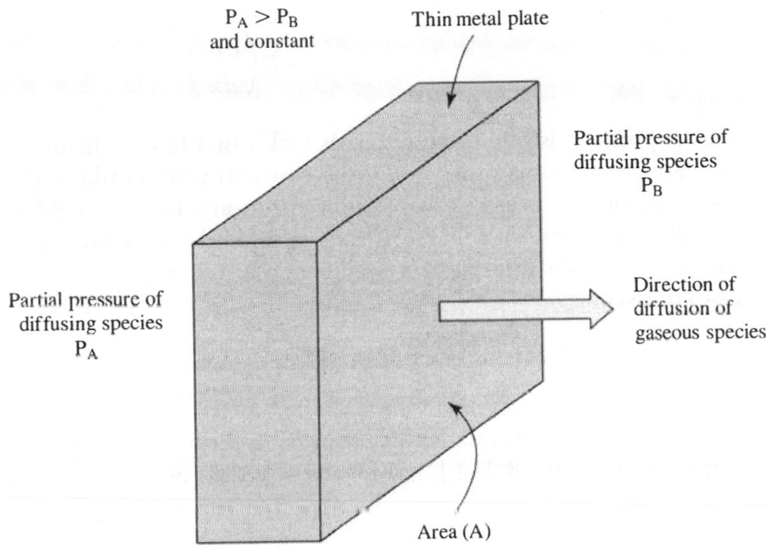

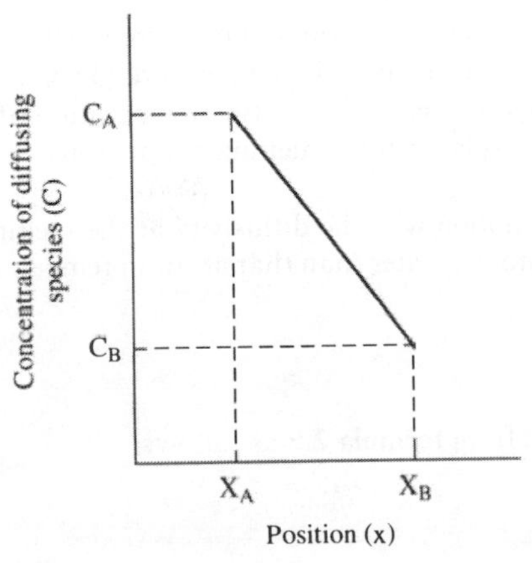

Figure 2.11
(a) Schematic of diffusion across a thin plate, an example of steady-state diffusion. Diffusion flux (J) is the mass (or number of atoms) M diffusing through a certain cross-sectional area (A) per unit time (t). If J does not change with time, this is steady-state diffusion, which occurs here because the partial pressures of gas on each side of the plate are held constant. (b) Concentration profile for situation shown in (a). The slope between two positions (e.g., x_A and x_B) is the concentration gradient between these two points. (Reprinted with permission from [4].)

If the concentration (C) of the gas atoms is plotted against position in the sheet (x) as shown in Fig. 2.11(b), this graph is called the **concentration profile.** The slope between two positions (e.g., x_A and x_B) is the **concentration gradient** between these two points:

$$\text{Concentration gradient} = \frac{dC}{dx} \tag{2.6}$$

As shown in the figure, in this case, the concentration gradient is taken to be linear, so

$$\frac{dC}{dx} = \frac{\Delta C}{\Delta x} = \frac{C_A - C_B}{x_A - x_B} \tag{2.7}$$

For diffusion problems, concentration is usually expressed in terms of mass of diffusing atoms (here, gas atoms) per unit volume of solid (kg/m^3 or g/cm^3).

For the situation depicted in Fig. 2.11(a), the diffusion flux is proportional to the concentration gradient according to

$$J = -D\left(\frac{dC}{dx}\right) \tag{2.8}$$

This expression is often referred to as **Fick's first law** of diffusion. The negative sign indicates that atoms move *down* the concentration gradient (from areas of higher concentration to areas of lower concentration). D (called **diffusivity**) is a proportionality constant with units of m^2/s. It depends on parameters of a given system, such as a crystal's interplanar spacing, and is also dependent on temperature. D can be expressed as

$$D = D_0 e^{\frac{-Q}{RT}} \tag{2.9}$$

where D_0 is a constant with units of m^2/s, Q is the activation energy for diffusion, R is the gas constant (8.314 J/mol-K) and T is the absolute temperature of the system.

EXAMPLE PROBLEM 2.4

Consider the alloy $TiAl_3$, which readily oxidizes to form a layer of Al_2O_3. Assuming that the activation energy of diffusion of oxygen through the Al_2O_3 layer is 337.66 kJ/mole and that the frequency factor (D_0) is 167.2×10^{-4} m^2/s, determine the following:

(a) The diffusivity througth the Al_2O_3 layer at room temperature (25°C).
(b) The diffusivity througth the Al_2O_3 layer at body temperature (37°C).
(c) The diffusivity througth the Al_2O_3 layer at the melting temperature of Al_2O_3 (2045°C).
(d) The diffusivity througth the Al_2O_3 layer at the melting temperature of Ti (1662°C).
(e) The diffusivity at absolute zero.
(f) Explain in terms of molecular motion why the diffusivity at the melting temperature of Al_2O_3 is many orders of magnitude greater than that at room temperature or even body temperature.

Solution:

(a) The diffusivity (D) is calculated from formula 2.9 as follows:

$$D = D_0 e^{\frac{-Q}{RT}}$$

The problem states that $Q = 337.66$ kJ/mole and $D_o = 167.2 \times 10^{-4}$ m^2/s.

The gas constant R = 8.314 J/mole-K. Recall that temperatures in C convert to K by K = °C + 273.

$$D = 167.2 \cdot 10^{-4}\ [\mathrm{m^2/s}]e^{\frac{-337.66 \times 10^3\ \mathrm{J/mole}}{(8.314\ \mathrm{J/mole})(298\ K)}}$$

$$\underline{D = 1.41 \cdot 10^{-61}\ \mathrm{m^2/s}}$$

(b) $$D = 167.2 \cdot 10^{-4}\ [\mathrm{m^2/s}]e^{\frac{-337.66 \times 10^3\ \mathrm{J/mole}}{(8.314\ \mathrm{J/mole})(310\ K)}}$$

$$\underline{D = 2.18 \cdot 10^{-59}\ \mathrm{m^2/s}}$$

(c) $$D = 167.2 \cdot 10^{-4}\ [\mathrm{m^2/s}]e^{\frac{-337.66 \times 10^3\ \mathrm{J/mole}}{(8.314\ \mathrm{J/mole})(2318\ K)}}$$

$$\underline{D = 4.25 \cdot 10^{-10}\ \mathrm{m^2/s}}$$

(d) $$D = 167.2 \cdot 10^{-4}\ [\mathrm{m^2/s}]e^{\frac{-337.66 \times 10^3\ \mathrm{J/mole}}{(8.314\ \mathrm{J/mole})(1935\ K)}}$$

$$\underline{D = 1.34 \cdot 10^{-11}\ \mathrm{m^2/s}}$$

(e) Absolute zero is at 0K and represents a complete absence of molecular motion. Without molecular motion, diffusion can not occur, thus the diffusivity would be zero.

(f) This problem examines the diffusivity of oxygen through the Al_2O_3 layer of $TiAl_3$. As the melting temperature of Al_2O_3 is given to be 2045°C, the aluminum oxide is a solid at the much lower temperatures of 25°C (room temperature) and 37°C (body temperature). In the solid state, molecular motion is very limited due to the lower thermal energy in the material. Thus, diffusion of oxygen through the material is greatly impeded at these temperatures. However, at the melting temperature, the thermal energy has reached a sufficient level to facilitate molecular motion. In this state, diffusion of oxygen can occur much more readily. ■

2.3 Structure of Ceramics

Like metals, ceramic biomaterials have found their primary use in joint replacement applications due to their strength and excellent wear properties. Because the bonds in ceramics are partially to totally ionic in nature, crystal structures in ceramic materials are thought of as being composed of ions rather than atoms. The variety of chemical compositions of ceramic materials results in a wider range of crystal structures than with metals. A few of the most common are discussed in the following sections.

2.3.1 Crystal Structures

Ceramic crystal structure is affected by two parameters that are not concerns in metallic structures: the magnitude of the electrical charge on the constituent ions and the physical size of these ions. The former is important because the crystal must remain electrically neutral. Thus, crystal structure of NaCl should allow the pairing of one Na^+ ion with one Cl^- ion. However, for CaF_2, two F^- ions must be allowed to interact with a single Ca^{2+} ion.

The second characteristic requires the knowledge of the radii of both the cations (r_c) and anions (r_a) composing a ceramic material (see Table 2.3). Cations are generally smaller than anions because electron-electron repulsion decreases with the loss of electrons from the valence shell and the nucleus is able to pull the remaining electrons closer. For an optimally stable structure, cations prefer to contact the maximum allowable number of anions (and vice versa for the anions). In this case, an ion's coordination number refers to the number of nearest neighbors with opposite charge and it depends on the r_c/r_a ratio. One can see in Fig. 2.12 that certain ratios will not allow close contact between cations and anions and thus produce unstable structures.

TABLE 2.3

Radii of both the Cations (r_c) and Anions (r_a) Composing a Ceramic Material (for a Coordination Number of 6)

Cation	Ionic Radius (nm)	Anion	Ionic Radius (nm)
Al^{3+}	0.053	Br^-	0.196
Ba^{2+}	0.136	Cl^-	0.181
Ca^{2+}	0.100	F^-	0.133
Cs^+	0.170	I^-	0.220
Fe^{2+}	0.077	O^{2-}	0.140
Fe^{3+}	0.069	S^{2-}	0.184
K^+	0.138		
Mg^{2+}	0.072		
Mn^{2+}	0.067		
Na^+	0.102		
Ni^{2+}	0.069		
Si^{4+}	0.040		
Ti^{4+}	0.061		

(Reprinted with permission from [4].)

Based on this concept, a minimum r_c/r_a ratio that will allow each coordination number has been determined (see Table 2.4). Each coordination number is associated with a certain nearest-neighbor geometry. For example, for a coordination number of 4, the cation is found at the center of a tetrahedron, with anions at each corner (see Table 2.4). The most common coordination numbers for ceramics are 4, 6, and 8.

2.3.1.1 AX Crystal Structures For ceramics in which both the cation and anion have the same charge, an equal number of each is required for a stable crystal structure. These are called AX crystals, with A representing the cation and X representing the anion. The most common AX structure is the **sodium chloride structure**. The coordination number for both cations (Na^+) and anions (Cl^-) is 6, and the unit cell is depicted in Fig. 2.13. As seen in the figure, the structure can be thought of as two interpenetrating FCC-type crystals, one composed of anions and the other of cations. Compounds such as MgO, MnS, LiF and FeO also follow this structure.

Another prevalent AX crystal has the **cesium chloride structure**. The coordination number in this case is 8 for both the Cs^+ and Cl^- ions and the unit cell is shown in Fig. 2.14. In this unit cell, the anions are located at the vertices of a cube with a single cation at the center. The locations of anions and cations in the unit cell can be interchanged to produce the same crystal structure. Although it looks similar, this is not a BCC crystal since there are two different atoms (ions) involved.

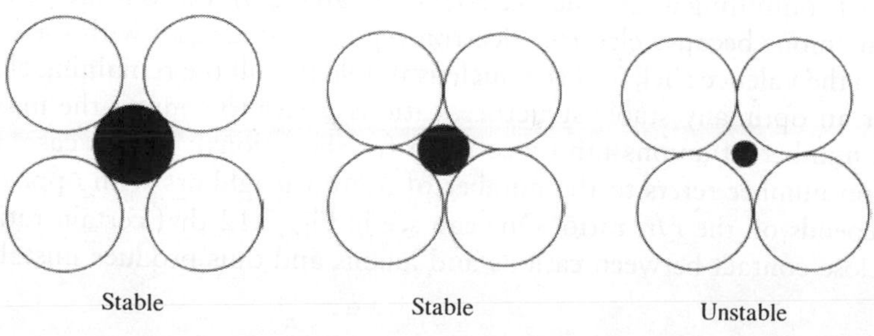

Figure 2.12
Examples of stable and unstable coordination in ionic crystals (black circles are cations). An ion's coordination number refers to the number of nearest neighbors with opposite charge. As shown here, a single coordination number can produce either stable or unstable structures, depending on the relative sizes of the cations and anions. (Reprinted with permission from [4].)

TABLE 2.4

Critical r_c/r_a Ratios and Associated Nearest-Neighbor Geometries for each Coordination Number (r_c = *cation radius length*, r_a = *anion radius length*)

Coordination Number	Lower Critical (r_c/r_a) Value	(r_c/r_a) Stability Range	Geometry*
2	0	$0 < r_c/r_a < 0.155$	Always possible
3	0.155	$0.155 < r_c/r_a < 0.225$	
4	0.225	$0.225 < r_c/r_a < 0.414$	
6	0.414	$0.414 < r_c/r_a < 0.732$	
8	0.732	$0.732 < r_c/r_a < 1$	

*In this column, $r = r_c$ and $R = r_a$

(Adapted with permission from [5].)

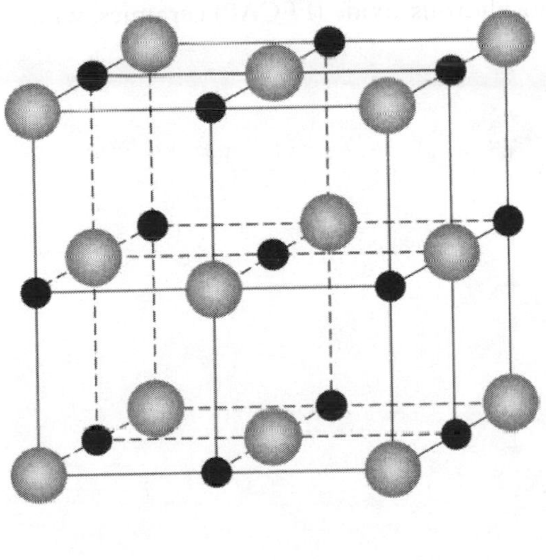

Figure 2.13
The unit cell for an ionic crystal having a sodium chloride structure. The coordination number for both cations (Na^+) and anions (Cl^-) is 6. The structure can be thought of as two interpenetrating FCC-type crystals, one composed of anions and the other of cations. (Adapted with permission from [4].)

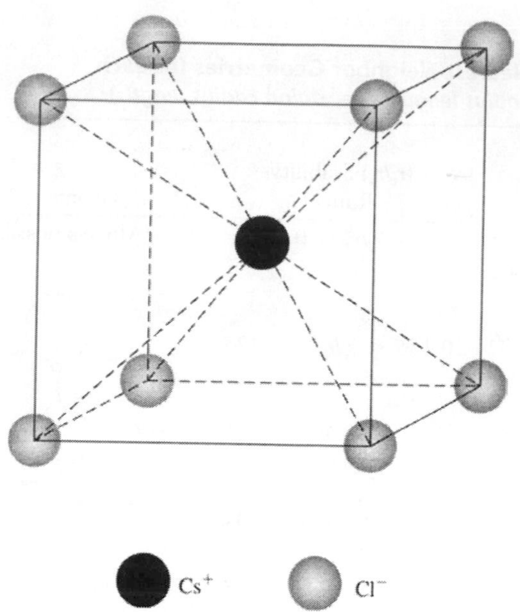

Figure 2.14
The unit cell for an ionic crystal having a cesium chloride structure. The coordination number in this case is 8 for both the Cs^+ and Cl^- ions. In this unit cell, the anions are located at the vertices of a cube with a single cation at the center. Although it looks similar, this is not a BCC crystal since there are two different atoms (ions) involved. (Adapted with permission from [4].)

2.3.1.2 A_mX_p Crystal Structures Ceramic materials are often composed of cations and anions that do not have equal charges, leading to compounds with the formula A_mX_p, where m and/or $p \neq 1$. A common example is found in fluorite (CaF_2). The coordination number for Ca^{2+} is 8, and the system exhibits a cubic coordination geometry (Fig. 2.15). The cations are at the center of the cube, with the anions at the corners. The crystal structure is similar to that of CsCl, (Fig. 2.14) except that only half of the center positions are occupied by Ca^{2+} ions.

It is also possible for compounds to have more than one type of cation, leading to $A_mB_nX_p$ crystal structures, which are more complicated than those presented here. These and even more complex combinations are commonly found in various ceramic biomaterials. This is mainly due to the fact that most ceramics developed for biomedical applications are mixtures of several ionic species, such as zinc-sulfate-calcium-phosphate (ZSCAP) ceramics, which include $ZnSO_4$, ZnO, CaO and P_2O_5, or ferric-calcium-phosphorous-oxide (FECAP) ceramics, which include Fe_2O_3, CaO, and P_2O_5.

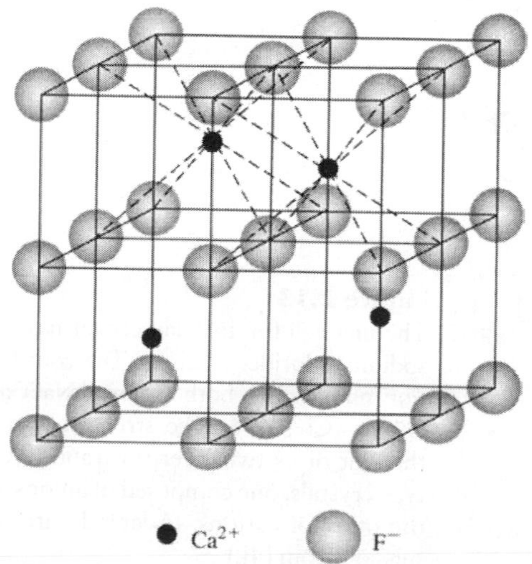

Figure 2.15
The unit cell for an ionic crystal having a fluorite (CaF_2) structure. In this case, the cations and anions do not have equal charges. In this structure, the cations are at the center of the cube with the anions at the corners. The crystal structure is similar to that of CsCl, except that only half of the center positions are occupied by Ca^{2+} ions. (Adapted with permission from [4].)

2.3.1.3 Carbon-Based Materials Although carbon-based materials do not neatly fall into any of the classes of materials (metals, ceramics or polymers), one common form, **graphite,** is sometimes considered a ceramic. Even though it does not possess a standard unit cell, graphite is crystalline. As depicted in Fig. 2.16, the structure consists of planes of hexagonally arranged carbon atoms. Within the planes, each carbon atom is bonded covalently to three neighbors, while the fourth valence electron participates in van der Waals interactions with the plane above it. A property of graphite that is important to the biomaterialist is its ability to adsorb gases. This is used in the formation of **pyrolytic carbon,** in which carbon in the gaseous state is deposited onto another material (in this case, graphite). Pyrolytic carbon has been used in a number of cardiovascular devices, including replacement heart valves.

An additional synthetic form of carbon can be found in **single-walled nanotubes** (SWNT) and **multi-walled nanotubes** (MWNT). A single-walled nanotube can be visualized as a single sheet of graphite rolled to form a tube. Similarly, a multi-walled nanotube can be visualized as a tube rolled from multiple layers of graphite sheets. These carbon nanotubes are generally a few nanometers in diameter and on the order of a micron in length. The SWNT can be characterized by the degree of chirality or "twist" in its structure. A two-dimensional vector, $\mathbf{C}_h$ (Fig. 2.17), can be defined to describe the chirality of the SWNT, such that

$$\mathbf{C}_h = n\mathbf{a}_1 + m\mathbf{a}_2 \equiv (n, m) \tag{2.10}$$

The structure of a SWNT is defined by the indices, n and m, of the two basis vectors $\mathbf{a}_1$ and $\mathbf{a}_2$, where n and m must be integers. Tubes for which $n = m$ are termed "armchair" tubes, and tubes for which $m = 0$ are termed "zigzag" tubes. These terms refer to the pattern of carbon atoms that one would see along the vector $\mathbf{C}_h$. The tubes for all other integer values of n and m are referred to as "chiral" tubes, as the carbon chains appear to spiral around the tubes in these cases. SWNTs have been explored for use in the mechanical reinforcement of biomaterials for several applications, including the reinforcement of synthetic polymers for orthopedic applications.

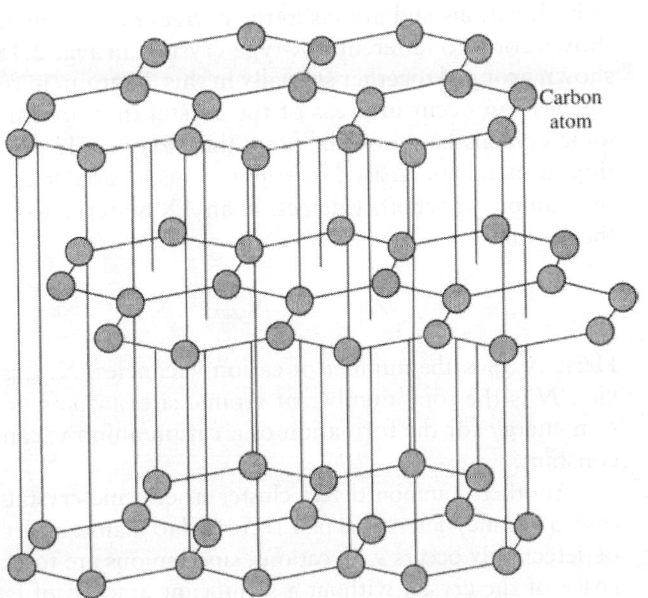

Figure 2.16
Crystal structure of graphite. The structure is composed of planes of hexagonally arranged carbon atoms. Within the planes, each carbon atom is bonded covalently to three neighbors, while the fourth valence electron participates in van der Waals interactions with the plane above it. A biomaterial based on graphite is pyrolytic carbon, in which carbon in the gaseous state is deposited on a graphite surface. (Adapted with permission from [4].)

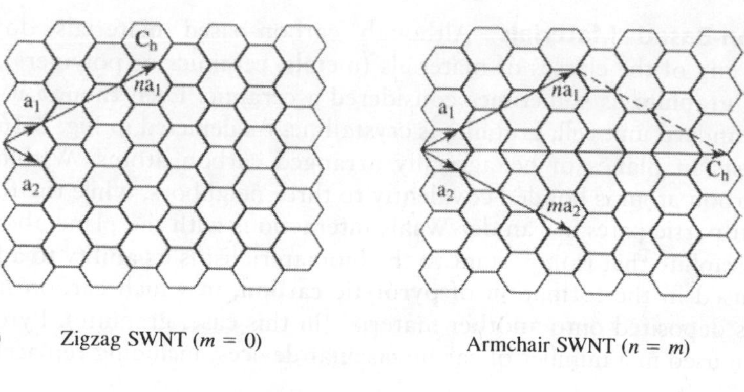

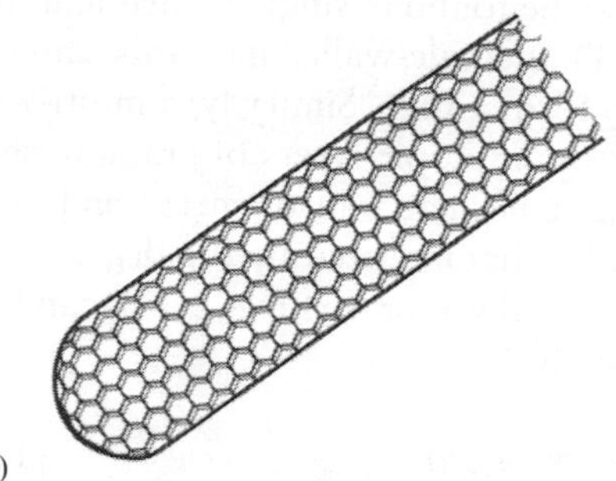

Figure 2.17
The structure of single-walled carbon nanotubes (SWNTs). (a) The sheets of graphite represented in this figure could be visualized to form a SWNT by rolling one side of the sheet in contact with the other. The twist or chirality of the SWNT is defined by a two-dimensional vector, C_h. Two special cases of SWNT are the zigzag ($m = 0$) and armchair ($n = m$) conformations. These terms refer to the pattern of carbon atoms that one would see along the C_h vector. (b) The 3D structure of a carbon nanotube.

2.3.2 Defects in Crystal Structures

2.3.2.1 Point Defects As with metals, a number of defect types have been observed in ceramic crystals. Both interstitial and vacancy point defects can occur for either the cation or anion. It is important to note that an additional constraint exists in the formation of defects in ceramic materials as compared with metals. Because ceramics are ionic in nature, the defect should not affect the electroneutrality of the material. Therefore, individual point defects do not occur since that would leave the crystal with a net charge; instead, groups of defects are formed.

One such defect group is called a **Schottky defect**, in which there are vacancies in both cations and anions in the correct ratio to maintain neutrality. This defect is shown for two different AX-type crystals in Fig. 2.18. Although the vacancies are shown grouped together spatially in this diagram, in reality, the anion and cation vacancies can occur in areas of the crystal that are far apart. Defects are created in ionic crystals based on the same thermodynamic principles that drive their formation in metals (increased entropy). Thus, a similar expression can be used to relate the number of Schottky defects in an AX material to the absolute temperature (T) of the sample:

$$N_{v,cat} = N_{v,an} = Ne^{\frac{-Q_{vp}}{2kT}} \tag{2.11}$$

Here, $N_{v,cat}$ is the number of cation vacancies, $N_{v,an}$ is the number of anion vacancies, N is the total number of atomic sites (atoms + vacancies), Q_{vp} is the activation energy for the formation of a cation/anion vacancy pair, and k is Boltzmann's constant.

Another common defect cluster in ceramic crystals is the **Frenkel defect.** In this case, a vacancy/interstitial pair is created to maintain electroneutrality. Usually this type of defect only occurs with cations, since anions are too large to reside in the interstitial space of the crystal without a significant amount of lattice strain. A typical Frenkel

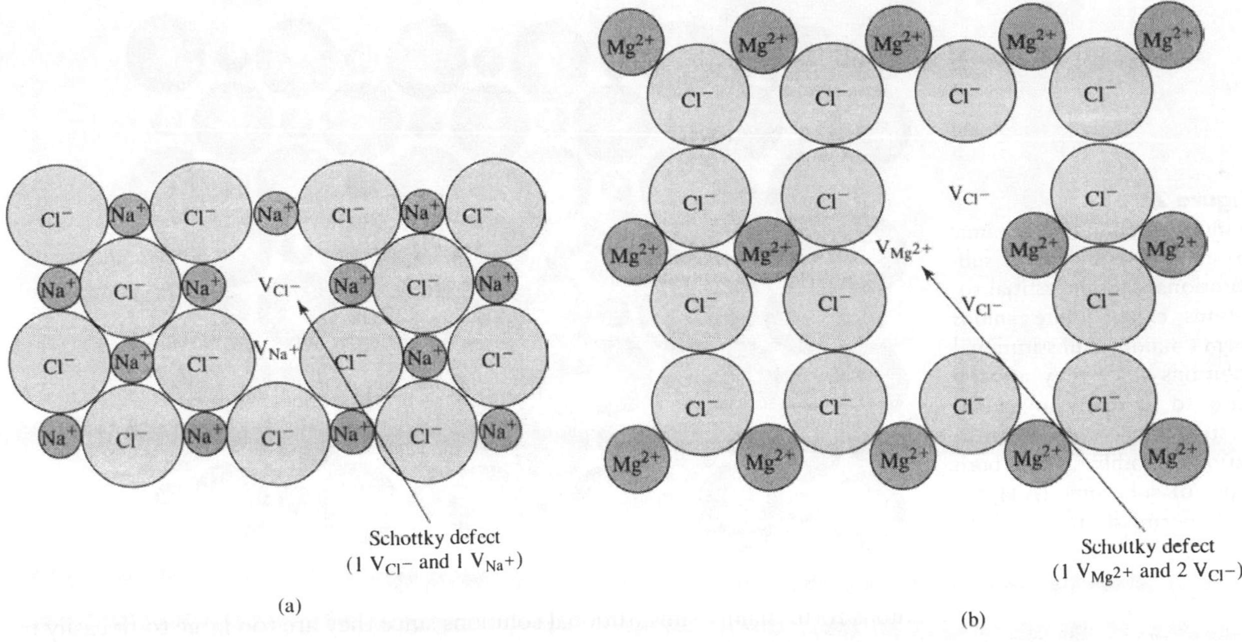

Figure 2.18
(a&b) Schottky defects in ceramic crystals. As shown here for AX (a) and A_mX_p (b) type crystals, there are vacancies in both cations and anions in the correct ratio to maintain electroneutrality. Although the vacancies are shown grouped together spatially in this diagram, in reality, the anion and cation vacancies can occur in areas of the crystal that are quite distant. (Adapted with permission from [5].)

defect is shown in Fig. 2.19. The equation describing the number of Frenkel defects as a function of absolute temperature (T) is

$$N_v = N_i = Ne^{\frac{-Q_{vi}}{2kT}} \quad (2.12)$$

where N_v is the number of vacancies, N_i is the number of interstitials, N is the total number of atomic sites (atoms + vacancies), Q_{vi} is the activation energy for formation of a vacancy and an interstitial, and k is Boltzmann's constant. The extent of both Schottky and Frenkel defects affect the mechanical properties of ceramic biomaterials as they can act as stress concentrators (see section 4.3.3).

2.3.2.2 Impurities Impurities similar to those in metal crystals are often found in ceramic crystals. Solid solutions can be formed and the same terminology (solvent and solute) applies. Although both substitutional and interstitial solutions exist, solute

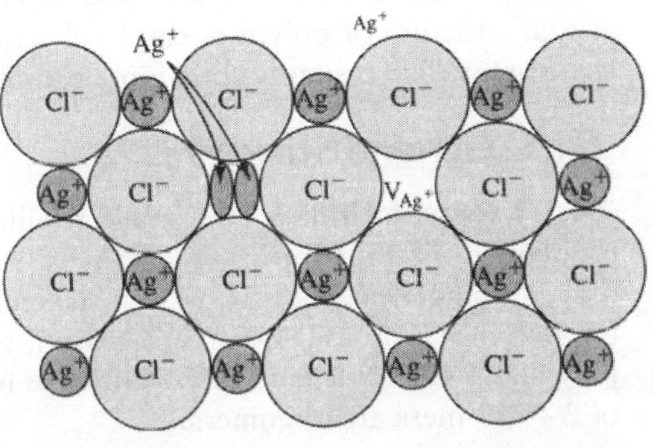

Figure 2.19
Frenkel defects in ceramic crystals. In this case, a vacancy/interstitial pair is created to maintain electroneutrality. Usually this type of defect only occurs with cations, since anions are too large to reside in the interstitial space of the crystal without a significant amount of lattice strain. (Adapted with permission from [5].)

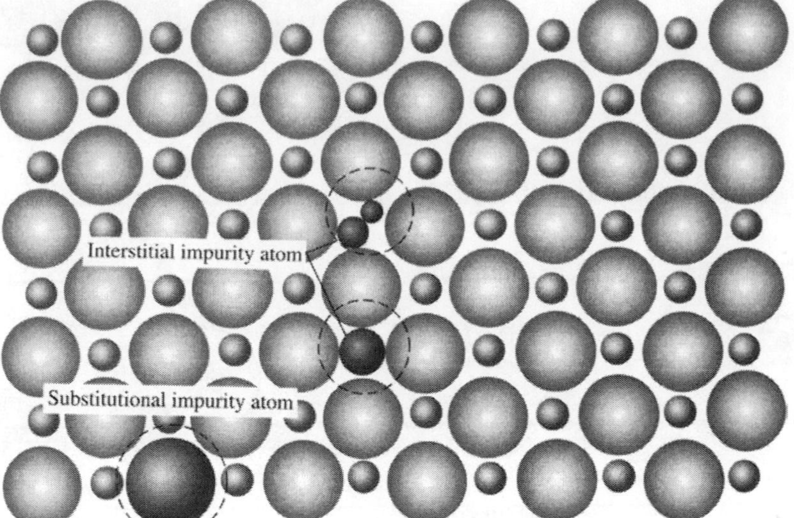

Figure 2.20
Impurities found in ceramic crystals. Although both substitutional and interstitial solutions exist, solute anions form mainly substitutional solutions since they are too large to fit easily in the interstitial space. In contrast, cations readily form both types of solutions. (Adapted with permission from [6].)

anions form mainly substitutional solutions since they are too large to fit easily in the interstitial space. Cations, in contrast, readily form both types of solutions (Fig. 2.20).

As with the point defect clusters discussed above, the addition of the impurity must not affect the electroneutrality of the host material. For stability, the solute ion must be similar in size and charge to the solvent ion. If this is not the case (for example, if a Ca^{2+} ion substitutes for a Na^+ ion in NaCl), the lattice compensates, often through forcing vacancies of host ions (ejection of additional Na^+ ion to restore neutrality). These are additional vacancies from the normal thermal vacancies described by the equations above.

As in metals, diffusion of point defects and impurities can occur within ionic crystals. The rate of diffusion depends on temperature and can be modeled with the same equations as discussed above for diffusion in metals. A main difference is that there must be simultaneous diffusion of at least two species (ions and vacancies) to maintain electroneutrality within the material.

2.4 Structure of Polymers

The third major type of biomaterials is polymeric materials. Polymers are also called **macromolecules** because of their size, which can be on the order of 10^5–10^6 g/mol. Many polymers, both naturally derived and synthetic, have hydrogen-carbon covalent bonds as a main constituent. The variety of possible polymers and their corresponding range of physical and mechanical properties have led to their use in applications as diverse as vascular graft replacements and bone cements. Both amorphous and crystalline polymeric materials are used in clinical applications. However, before the crystal structure of polymers can be described, we must first explain their chemical structure, which is significantly more complex than that of metals or ceramics.

2.4.1 General Structure

2.4.1.1 Repeat Units The smallest building block of a polymer is called a **mer** ("polymer" literally means "many mers"). A mer is a structural entity composed of a fixed number of atoms in a given structure that is repeated over and over to form the polymer (Fig. 2.21). For this reason, a mer is often called the **repeat unit** of a polymer. A molecule containing only one mer is a **monomer**, while those composed of 2–~10 mers are **oligomers**.

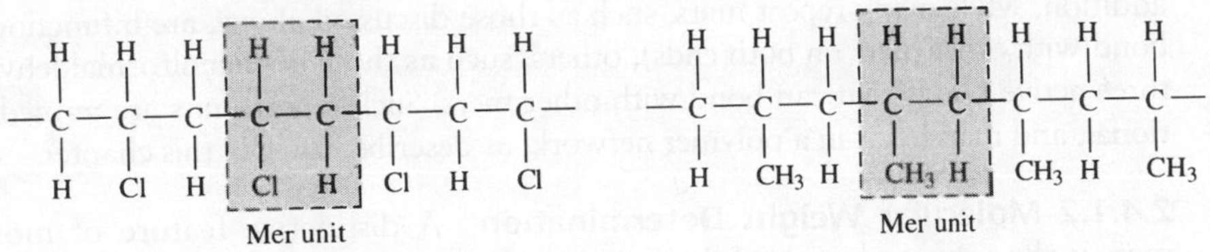

Mer unit   Mer unit

Figure 2.21
Examples of mer units in polymers. A mer is a structural entity composed of a fixed number of atoms in a given structure that is repeated over and over to form the polymer. (Adapted with permission from [4].)

As seen in Table 2.5, repeat units for common polymers can be **saturated**, such as those in poly(ethylene)[1] or poly(vinyl chloride), in which each carbon in the mer is bonded to four other atoms (two carbons and two other types of atoms). Alternatively, they may be unsaturated, such as those for poly(isoprene), see Fig. 2.26 in which two of the carbons in the repeat unit are bonded with double bonds. The presence of unsaturated repeat units can affect the crystallinity and crosslinking of polymers, as discussed in Chapter 3. In

TABLE 2.5
Structure of Common Polymers

Polymer	Structure
Poly(ethylene)(PE)	$\left[CH_2-CH_2 \right]_n$
Poly(ethylene glycol) (PEG)	$\left[CH_2-CH_2-O \right]_n$
Poly(styrene) (PS)	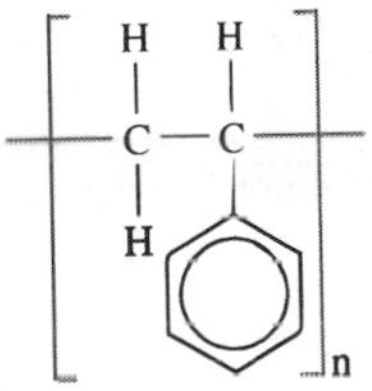 $\left[CH(H)-CH(C_6H_5) \right]_n$
Poly(methyl methacrylate) (PMMA)	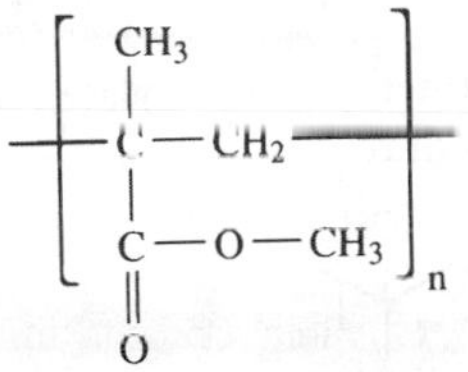 $\left[C(CH_3)(C(=O)-O-CH_3)-CH_2 \right]_n$
Poly(glycolic acid) (PGA)	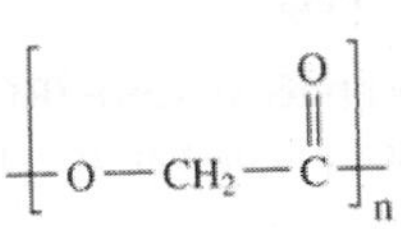 $\left[O-CH_2-C(=O) \right]_n$
Poly(lactic acid) (PLA)	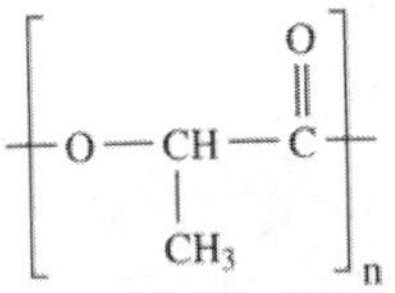 $\left[O-CH(CH_3)-C(=O) \right]_n$
Poly(tetrafluoroethylene) (PTFE)	$\left[CF_2-CF_2 \right]_n$

[1]Standard guidelines for polymer nomenclature generally require that polymers be named by prefixing "poly" to the name, offset in parentheses, of the structural repeating unit of the polymer. If the name of the structural repeating unit of the polymer is only one word, then the parentheses are optional. For example, poly(ethylene) can also be written as polyethylene; whereas, the parentheses are required for poly(vinyl chloride).

addition, while many repeat units, such as those discussed above, are **bifunctional** (may bond with other mers on both ends), others, such as those in phenolformaldehyde, have three active bonds that can bond with other mers. Such repeat units are termed **trifunctional**, and may result in a polymer network, as described later in this chapter.

2.4.1.2 Molecular Weight Determination A distinctive feature of most polymers is the extreme length of their chains. One way to represent this is the **degree of polymerization** (number of repeat units in a polymer), usually indicated by the letter *n* in the chemical formula for the polymer.

For example, the notation

$$\ldots CH_2{-}CH_2{-}CH_2{-}CH_2{-}CH_2{-}CH_2{-}CH_2{-}CH_2\ldots$$

can be abbreviated as

$$-\!\!\left[-CH_2-CH_2-\right]_n\!\!-$$

Alternatively, the polymer's size can be described in terms of the molecular weight of the chain.

EXAMPLE PROBLEM 2.5

Determine the molecular weight of the following polymers:

(a) Poly(ethylene)[2], a material commonly used in the wearing surface of the acetabular cup component of hip prostheses.

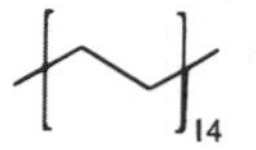

14

(b) Poly(tetrafluoroethylene), a material commonly employed in the fabrication of vascular grafts.

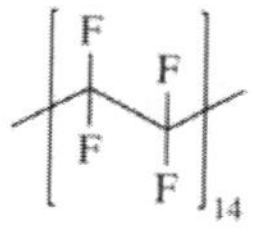

F F F F 14

(c) Poly(methylmethacrylate), a material commonly used as a bone cement in orthopedic procedures.

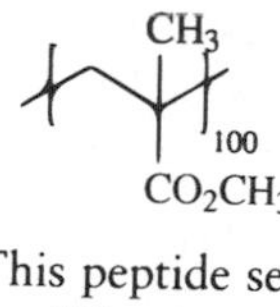

CH_3 100 CO_2CH_3

(d) This peptide sequence (RGD, or arginine, glycine, aspartic acid), commonly used in the modification of materials to increase cell adhesion to the material.

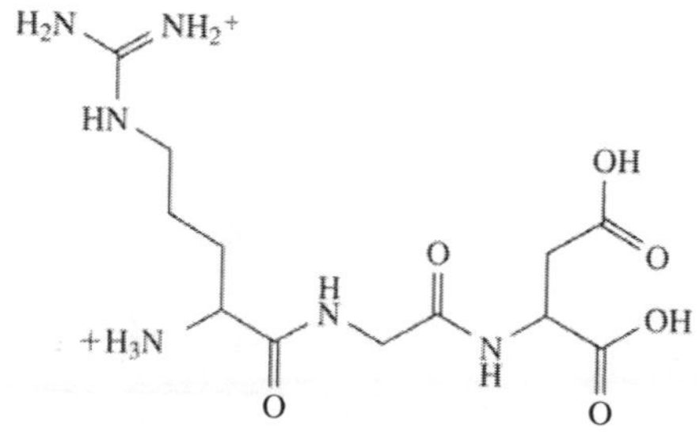

H_2N NH_2^+ HN OH O O H N OH $+H_3N$ N H O O

[2]In many of the problems and figures in the remainder of the book, this condensed structural notation, often used by organic chemists, will be used. In this type of notation, carbon-carbon bonds are represented by dark lines, and the writing of "C" and the appropriate number of "Hs" to fulfill the valence shell of each carbon is omitted. A more detailed structure of poly(ethylene) is found in Table 2.5.

Solution:

(a) Molecular weight of the repeat unit:
2 carbon atoms and 4 hydrogen atoms per repeat unit

$$\text{Atomic mass of carbon} = 12 \text{ g/mole}$$
$$\text{Atomic mass of hydrogen} = 1 \text{ g/mole}$$
$$2(12 \text{ g/mole}) + 4(1 \text{ g/mole}) = 28 \text{ g/mole/repeat unit}$$

Since there are 14 repeat units in this polymer chain, the molecular weight of the polymer equals 14 times the molecular weight of the repeat unit, plus 2 hydrogen atoms, one to terminate each end of the polymer chain:

$$28 \text{ g/mole/repeat unit} \times 14 \text{ repeat units} + 2 \text{ hydrogen atoms} \times (1 \text{ g/mole hydrogen}) = \underline{394 \text{ g/mole}}$$

(b) Molecular weight of the repeat unit:
2 carbon atoms and 4 fluorine atoms per repeat unit

$$\text{Atomic mass of carbon} = 12 \text{ g/mole}$$
$$\text{Atomic mass of fluorine} = 19 \text{ g/mole}$$
$$2(12 \text{ g/mole}) + 4(19 \text{ g/mole}) = 100 \text{ g/mole/repeat unit}$$

Since there are 14 repeat units in this polymer chain, the molecular weight of the polymer equals 14 times the molecular weight of the repeat unit, plus 2 hydrogen atoms, one to terminate each end of the polymer chain:

$$100 \text{ g/mole/repeat unit} \times 14 \text{ repeat units} + 2 \text{ hydrogen atoms} \times (1 \text{ g/mole hydrogen}) = \underline{1{,}402 \text{ g/mole}}$$

(c) Molecular weight of the repeat unit:
5 carbon atoms, 8 hydrogen atoms and 2 oxygen atoms per repeat unit

$$\text{Atomic mass of carbon} = 12 \text{ g/mole}$$
$$\text{Atomic mass of hydrogen} = 1 \text{ g/mole}$$
$$\text{Atomic mass of oxygen} = 16 \text{ g/mole}$$
$$5(12 \text{ g/mole}) + 8(1 \text{ g/mole}) + 2(16 \text{ g/mole}) = 100 \text{ g/mole/repeat unit}$$

Since there are 100 repeat units in this polymer chain, the molecular weight of the polymer equals 100 times the molecular weight of the repeat unit, plus 2 hydrogen atoms, one to terminate each end of the polymer chain:

$$100 \text{ g/mole/repeat unit} \times 100 \text{ repeat units} + 2 \text{ hydrogen atoms} \times (1 \text{ g/mole hydrogen}) = \underline{10{,}002 \text{ g/mole}}$$

(d) This is a peptide (RGD or arginine, glycine, aspartic acid). There is no repeat unit for this peptide. The elemental composition of the peptide is as follows:

Carbon: 12 atoms
Hydrogen: 24 atoms
Nitrogen: 6 atoms
Oxygen: 6 atoms

Thus, the molecular weight of the peptide is as follows:

$$12(12 \text{ g/mole C}) + 24(1 \text{ g/mole H}) + 6(14 \text{ g/mole N}) + 6(16 \text{ g/mole O}) = \underline{348 \text{ g/mole}}$$

■

During synthesis, polymers with a distribution of molecular weights are formed. Therefore, an average molecular weight is generally determined. There are two common definitions for average molecular weight, **number-average molecular weight** ($\overline{M}_n$) and **weight-average molecular weight** ($\overline{M}_w$). The number-average molecular weight is found by dividing the chains into a series of size ranges and computing the fraction of chains with that size. This can be written

$$\overline{M}_n = \sum_i x_i M_i \tag{2.13}$$

where

$$x_i = \frac{N_i}{\sum_i N_i} \tag{2.14}$$

N_i is the number of chains with molecular weight M_i. M_i represents an average molecular weight for the chosen molecular weight range.

The weight-average molecular weight is calculated using the weight fraction of the chains within the selected size ranges; that is,

$$\overline{M}_w = \sum_i w_i M_i \tag{2.15}$$

where

$$w_i = \frac{W_i}{\sum_i W_i} \tag{2.16}$$

and

$$W_i = N_i M_i \tag{2.17}$$

It should be noted that as the size range chosen to define N_i and M_i becomes smaller and smaller, these expressions approach the averaging of each individual chain. The reason that both types of average molecular weight are calculated is that while $\overline{M}_n$ treats all polymer chains equally, for $\overline{M}_w$, the larger chains make a larger contribution to the final value. In some cases, $\overline{M}_w$ can be correlated more directly with the mechanical and physical properties of the material (Table 2.6).

The **polydispersity index** (*PI*) is the ratio of the two molecular weights:

$$PI = \frac{\overline{M}_w}{\overline{M}_n} \tag{2.18}$$

The smallest possible value for the *PI* is 1.00 (all the polymer molecules have the same molecular weight), and it increases as the molecular weight distribution broadens (Fig. 2.22).

TABLE 2.6

Relationship Between Molecular Weight of Poly(Lactic Acid) and Mechanical Properties

Weight average molecular weight	Tensile modulus* (MPa)	Flexural modulus* (MPa)
50,000	1200	1400
100,000	2700	3000
300,000	3000	3250

**Descriptors of different mechanical properties, discussed in Chapter 4*

(Adapted with permission from [7].)

PPF:

PS:

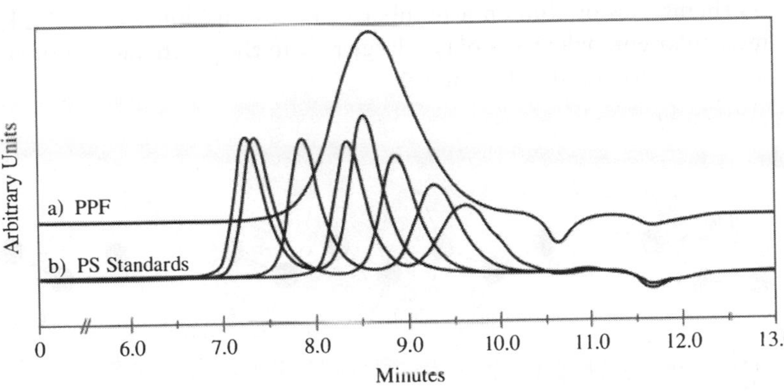

Figure 2.22
Diagram based on results from a type of size-exclusion chromatography (gel permeation chromatography) of poly(propylene fumarate) (PPF) and different poly (styrene) (PS) standards. In this type of chromatography, the larger molecular weight polymer exits first and is detected at an earlier time.

PPF: $\overline{M}_n$: 3,580

PS standards from left to right: $\overline{M}_n$: 26,600, $\overline{M}_n$: 23,300, $\overline{M}_n$: 10,000, $\overline{M}_n$: 4,620, $\overline{M}_n$: 3,260, $\overline{M}_n$: 1,790, $\overline{M}_n$: 869, $\overline{M}_n$: 423.

Note that the PPF peak is much broader than that of the standards. While the polydispersity of the PPF synthesized in the laboratory is near 2, the PS standards are synthesized in such a manner so their PI is near 1. At lower molecular weights, this is more difficult, so the PI of the lowest standard ($\overline{M}_n$ 423) is 1.22.

EXAMPLE PROBLEM 2.6

Consider the following polymer size fractions of a given polymer sample:

Fraction	Molecular Weight	Number of Chains
1	5,000	1,000
2	10,000	1,000
3	1,000,000	3

(a) Calculate the number-average molecular weight of the polymer.
(b) Calculate the weight-average molecular weight of the polymer.
(c) Which average molecular weight determination did the 3 chains of molecular weight 1,000,000 most significantly affect? Why?
(d) Calculate the polydispersity index of the polymer.

Solution:

(a) $\overline{M}_n = \dfrac{\sum_i N_i M_i}{\sum_i N_i}$

In this case,

$\overline{M}_n = [(1{,}000 \times 5{,}000) + (1{,}000 \times 10{,}000) + (3 \times 1{,}000{,}000)]/(1{,}000 + 1{,}000 + 3)$
$= \underline{8{,}987\ Da}$ [Note: 1 Da = 1 g/mole]

(b) $\overline{M}_w = \dfrac{\sum_i N_i M_i^2}{\sum_i N_i M_i}$

In this case, $\overline{M}_w = [1{,}000 \times (5{,}000)^2 + 1{,}000 \times (10{,}000)^2 + 3 \times (1{,}000{,}000)^2]/[(1{,}000 \times 5{,}000) + (1{,}000 \times 10{,}000) + (3 \times 1{,}000{,}000)] = \underline{173{,}611 \text{ Da}}$

(c) The 3 chains of 1,000,000 molecular weight most significantly affected the weight-average molecular weight, as this quantity considers the molecular weight of each species present in a weighted fashion to give greater influence to the fractions with the higher molecular weight than those with simply the highest number of chains.

(d) $PI = \frac{\overline{M}_w}{\overline{M}_n}$

In this case, $PI = (173{,}611 \text{ Da})/(8{,}987 \text{ Da}) = \underline{19}$ (note that PI does not carry units) ■

2.4.1.3 Mer Configuration One of the most striking aspects of polymers (and one that distinguishes them from metals and ceramics) is that single macromolecules can take a variety of shapes. This is primarily caused by the rotation of the carbon atoms in the backbone, the way changing the position of individual links in a chain will change the path of the entire chain (Fig. 2.23). Thus, polymers may fold back on themselves or contain a number of bends and kinks (Fig. 2.24). These types of molecular entanglements play a large role in the mechanical properties of polymers, as will be discussed in Chapter 4.

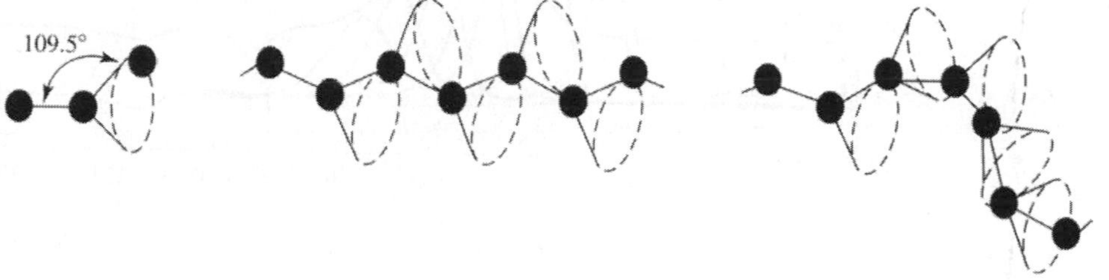

Figure 2.23
Conformations of polymers. Single macromolecules can take a variety of shapes, primarily due to the rotation of the carbon atoms in the backbone. (Adapted with permission from [8].)

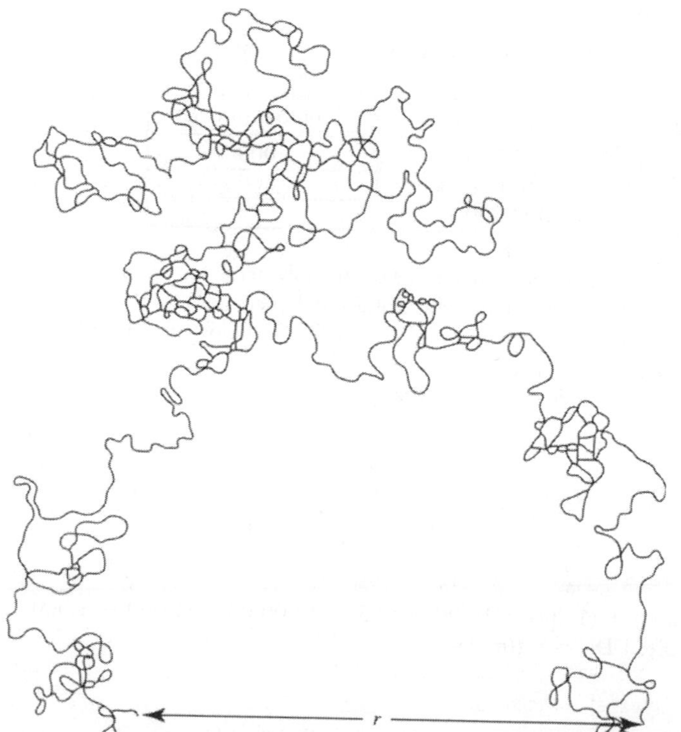

Figure 2.24
Depiction of a typical conformation for a polymer molecule. Note the large number of bends and kinks present. These types of molecular entanglements play a large role in the mechanical properties of polymers. The end-to-end distance of the polymer chain is denoted by r. (Adapted with permission from [9].)

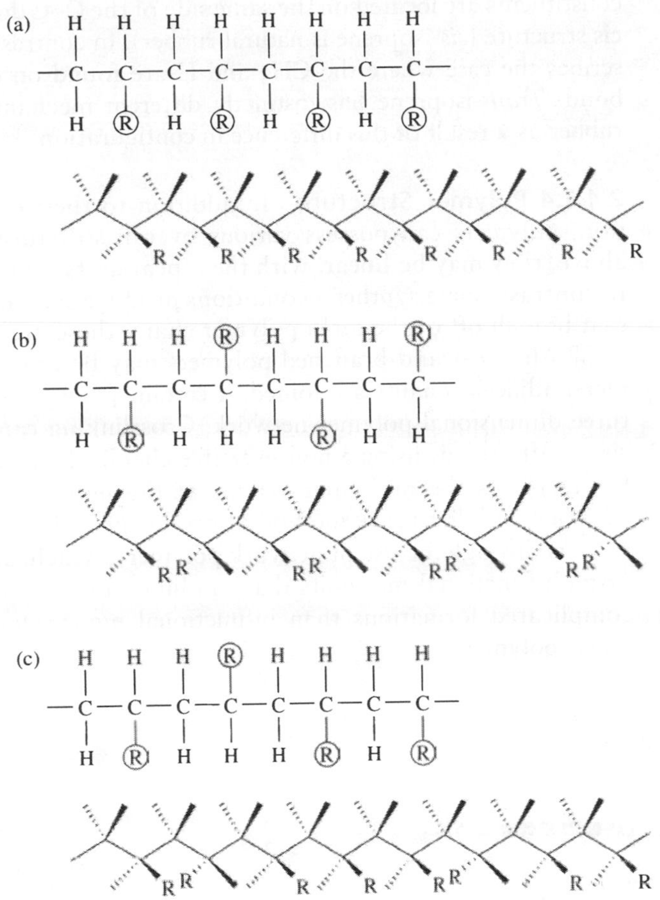

Figure 2.25
Common polymer configurations ("R" represents a generic side group or atom). (a) Isotactic configuration—R groups are arranged on the same side of the chain. (b) Syndiotactic configuration—R groups alternate positions on either side of the chain. (c) Atactic configuration—R groups are situated randomly. In this representation, the solid extensions are oriented out of the page and the dashed are into the page. (Adapted with permission from [4].)

On a molecular level, the bending of polymer molecules is due to the conformation of individual repeat units. The term **conformation** is used to describe the part of the structure of a molecule that can be changed by rotation around single bonds. Repeat unit (and thus polymer) conformation can be highly affected by chemical composition. The presence of bulky side groups [like the benzene ring in poly(styrene)] impairs rotation around the backbone. In a more extreme case, when rigid C–C double bonds are present, no rotation is possible around the backbone and conformation is effectively "frozen."

Polymer conformation is also influenced by the placement of the repeat units. **Configuration** is the part of the structure of a molecule that cannot be changed except by the breaking and reforming of primary bonds. There are several common polymer configurations, as depicted in Fig. 2.25. In this figure, "R" represents a generic side group or atom [such as the benzene ring in poly(styrene) or the Cl atom in poly(vinyl chloride)]. If the R groups are arranged on the same side of the chain, this is an **isotactic configuration.** If they alternate positions on either side of the chain, this is a **syndiotactic configuration.** If the R groups are situated randomly, this is an **atactic configuration.** It is easy to see from these examples that conversion between two configurations requires the breaking of chemical bonds, whereas moving between different polymer conformations involves only bond rotation. In reality, any given polymer chain contains a mixture of configurations. The predominant configuration is determined primarily by the synthesis method.

In the special case where the repeat unit contains a C–C double bond, two configurations are possible (Fig. 2.26). For poly(isoprene), when both the CH_3 and H

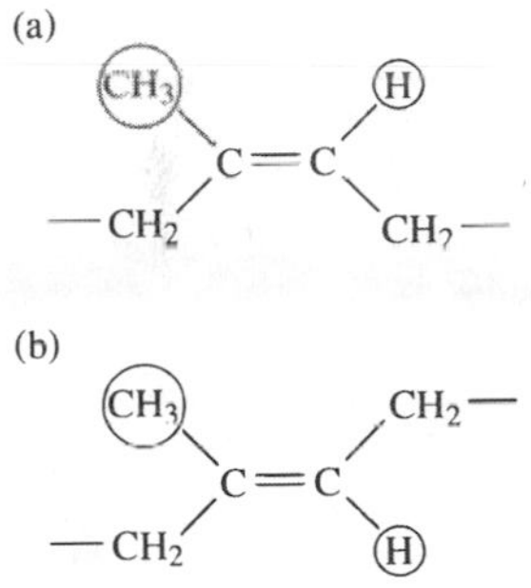

Figure 2.26
Polymer configurations with a C–C double bond [above example: poly(isoprene)]. a) cis configuration—CH_3 and H constituents are found on the same side of the C–C double bond (*cis*-isoprene is natural rubber). b) trans configuration—CH_3 and H are found on opposite sides of the double bond. (Adapted with permission from [4].)

constituents are located on the same side of the C–C double bond, this is termed the **cis** structure (*cis*-isoprene is natural rubber). In contrast, the **trans** configuration describes the case where the CH_3 and H are found on opposite sides of the double bond. *Trans*-isoprene has distinctly different mechanical properties from natural rubber as a result of this difference in configuration.

2.4.1.4 Polymer Structure In addition to their conformation and configuration, polymers can possess various overall structures (Fig. 2.27). As described above, they may be **linear**, with the repeat units joined in an end-to-end fashion. In contrast, some synthesis conditions produce side reactions that result in chains that branch off of the main polymer chain; these are termed **branched** polymers.

Both linear and branched polymers may be crosslinked. In **crosslinked polymers**, adjacent chains are joined at certain points via covalent bonds, forming a three-dimensional polymer network. Crosslinking can be induced during synthesis, or afterwards using a nonreversible chemical reaction. In one sense, crosslinking increases the molecular weight of the polymer chains as they are bonded together. An alternative method of producing polymer structures in three dimensions is through the use of **network polymers**, which, as explained earlier, have tri- or multifunctional mer units that can bind monomers or other polymers in more complicated formations than bifunctional monomers, which produce primarily linear polymers.

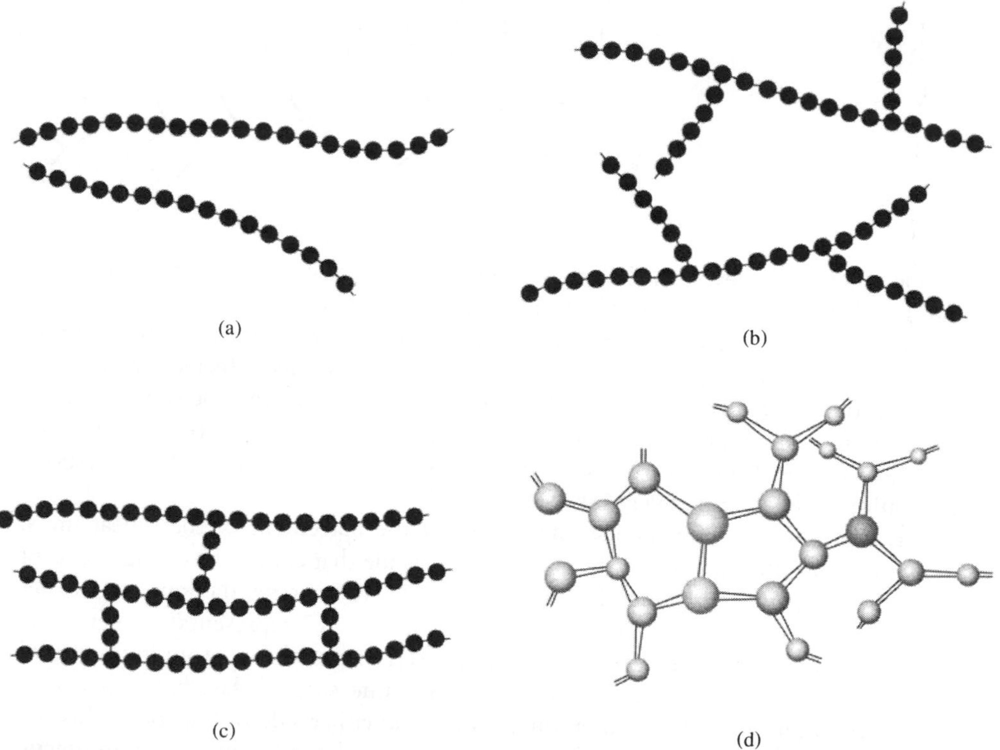

Figure 2.27
Overall structures of polymers. (a) Linear polymers have their repeat units joined in an end-to-end fashion. (b) Branched polymers are formed by synthesis conditions that encourage the formation of chains that branch off from the main polymer chain. (c) Crosslinked polymers possess adjacent chains that are joined at certain points via covalent bonds, forming a three-dimensional polymer network. Both linear and branched polymers may be crosslinked. (d) Network polymers have tri- or multifunctional mer units that can bind monomers or other polymers to produce three-dimensional network structures. (Adapted with permission from [4].)

EXAMPLE PROBLEM 2.7

Poly(ethylene) is a polymer used in a number of biomedical applications. One common application is the fabrication of wearing surfaces of orthopedic implants, such as the acetabular cup of a hip implant or the articulating surface of a knee implant. Consider a poly(ethylene) polymer chain with 25,000 mers.

(a) One method for estimating the length of a polymer chain is to model it as a chain stretched out end-to-end. Given that the angle between C–C covalent bonds is 109.5° and that the interatomic distance for a C–C bond is 1.54Å, calculate the length of the poly(ethylene) chain.

(b) More realistically, polymer chains can be modeled as random coils. The average end-to-end distance (L) of a randomly coiled polymer chain can be calculated from the relation $L = l\sqrt{m}$, where l is the interatomic distance and m is the number of bonds with that interatomic distance. Calculate the average end-to-end distance (L) for the poly(ethylene) chain, using the random coil model.

Solution:

(a) The bond angle ϕ is given as 109.5°. The bond length is given as 1.54Å, so ½ the bond length can be defined as r to be 0.77Å. The quantity y can be defined as the distance between two covalently bonded carbons, as projected on the chain axis.

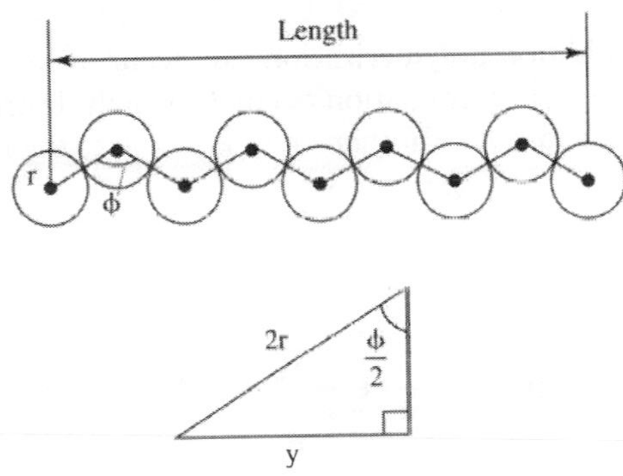

$$y = (2r)\sin(\phi/2)$$

$$y = (1.54\text{Å})\sin(54.75°)$$

$$y = 1.26\text{Å} = \text{projected bond length}$$

Since there are 25,000 mers in the polymer chain, the length of the polymer chain projected on the chain axis is as follows:

$$\text{Length} = (\text{Number of C–C bonds}) \times (\text{Projected C–C bond length})$$

$$\text{Length} = (2{*}25{,}000\text{-}1 \text{ Bonds}) \times (1.26\text{Å}) \text{ [There are 2 carbons/ mer.]}$$

$$\underline{\text{Length} = 62{,}999\text{Å} = 6.3\ \mu\text{m}}$$

(b) Using the random-coil end-to-end distance formula:

$$L = l\sqrt{m}$$

$$L = 1.54\text{Å}(2 \times 25{,}000\text{-}1)^{1/2}$$

$$\underline{L = 344\text{Å}}$$

■

2.4.2 Polymer Synthesis

Synthesis of polymers, also called **polymerization**, occurs through repeated chemical reactions that join individual mer units into a longer chain. There are three major types of polymerization: **addition polymerization, condensation polymerization,** and **polymer synthesis through genetic engineering**. The details of these reactions are described below.

2.4.2.1 Addition Polymerization The reaction of ethylene monomers to form poly(ethylene) via addition, or chain reaction, polymerization is shown in Fig. 2.28. Bifunctional monomers are required, and, unlike condensation polymerization, the product contains the same chemical structure as the mer unit. An initiator species is needed to commence the reaction, so an initiator molecule that easily forms free radicals or ions is often used. This is depicted as **I** in Fig. 2.28.

Addition polymerization reactions involve three distinct steps: initiation, propagation and termination. **Initiation** requires the activation of a monomer through reaction with either a radical species for free radical polymerization or an anionic or cationic species for anionic and cationic polymerization, respectively. Monomers continue to successively join the polymer chain and increase its molecular weight during the **propagation** step. It is important to note that during the propagation step the active site of the growing polymer chain is simultaneously transferred to the newly added monomer upon addition. This transfer allows for the continued growth of the polymer chain.

Termination of addition polymerization can occur in several ways. In the case of free radical polymerization, termination occurs through destruction of the active site by the reaction of free radicals. Another method involves the reaction of the activated

Initiation
$$I \xrightarrow{k_d} 2R\cdot$$
$$R\cdot + M \xrightarrow{k_i} M_1\cdot$$

Propagation
$$M_n\cdot + M \xrightarrow{k_p} M_{n+1}\cdot$$

Termination
$$M_n\cdot + M_m\cdot \xrightarrow{k_{tc}} M_{n+m} \quad \textit{Coupling}$$
$$M_n\cdot + M_m\cdot \xrightarrow{k_{td}} M_n + M_m \quad \textit{Disproportionation}$$

Figure 2.28
General reaction mechanism for addition, or chain reaction, polymerization. A radical species ($R\cdot$) needed to initiate the reaction is usually produced through dissociation of an initiator species (I). The radical is then added to a monomer molecule to produce a polymer chain initiating species ($M_1\cdot$) in the second part of initiation. Monomer molecules (M) are successively added to the activated chain end ($M_n\cdot$) to generate a polymer in the propagation step. Termination of chain growth may occur by a number of methods - two are depicted here: (1) reaction of the activated monomer ($M_n\cdot$ and $M_m\cdot$) on two propagating chains that react to form one longer chain (coupling) or (2) through disproportionation. Poly(ethylene), poly(propylene), poly(vinyl chloride) and poly(styrene) are examples of polymers synthesized via addition polymerization. The parameters k_d, k_i, k_p, k_{tc}, and k_{td} are the kinetic constants for the initiator dissociation, initiation, propagation, termination by coupling, and termination by disproportionation steps, respectively. (Adapted with permission from [10].)

end on two propagating chains ($M_n\cdot$ or $M_m\cdot$) to form a longer chain, thus ending the growth of both chains (see last section of Fig. 2.28). Another method of termination is through the reaction of the activated carbon on a propagating chain with a free radical of an initiator molecule. Chain growth can also terminate through transfer of a hydrogen atom from one growing chain to another in a process called disproportionation. In the case of anionic and cationic polymerization, however, termination generally occurs through reaction of the charged active site of the growing polymer with either trace amounts of water in the solvent in which the reaction is conducted or, depending on the nature of the solvent, with the solvent itself. Cationic polymerization can also terminate through various other side reactions, including anion-cation recombination and anion splitting.

Because termination is random with free radical polymerization, a variety of chain lengths are achieved using this method of polymerization, which leads to PI values >1.00. Poly(ethylene), poly(propylene), poly(vinyl chloride) and poly(styrene) are examples of polymers synthesized with free radical polymerization. The polymers generated through ionic polymerization are, in general, less polydisperse than those generated through free radical polymerization. Examples of polymers that are synthesized through anionic polymerization include poly(styrene), poly(methyl methacrylate) and poly(ethylene glycol). Additionally, poly(styrene) can be synthesized through cationic polymerization.

2.4.2.2 Condensation Polymerization Unlike addition polymerization, **condensation**, or step reaction, polymerization often involves more than one monomer species, and no radical initiator is required. Because of this, there is less distinction among initiation, propagation and termination stages, although the reaction does proceed in a stepwise manner. As shown in Fig. 2.29, the polymerization occurs through elimination of one molecule (usually water). Therefore, unlike addition polymerization, the product does not have the same chemical formula as either mer.

Long reaction times and nearly complete depletion of the monomer are needed to obtain high molecular weight substances from this polymerization method. During the reaction, chains with various lengths are produced, leading to *PI* values similar to those seen for addition polymerization. Nylons and poly(carbonates) are among the polymers formed in this way. Natural polymers, such as polysaccharides and proteins, are also a product of this synthetic reaction.

2.4.2.3 Polymer Production Via Genetic Engineering Addition and condensation polymerization generally result in the synthesis of polymers with a wide range of chain lengths and sequences, due to the probabilistic nature of the reactions involved.

(a)

$$n\text{A—A} + n\text{B—B} \longrightarrow \text{—}(\text{A—AB—B})_n\text{—}$$

$$n\text{H}_2\text{N—R—NH}_2 + n\text{HO}_2\text{C—R'—CO}_2\text{H} \longrightarrow \text{H}(\text{NH—R—NHCO—R'—CO})_n\text{OH} + (2n-1)\text{H}_2\text{O}$$

(b)

$$n\text{A—B} \longrightarrow \text{—}(\text{A—B})_n\text{—}$$

$$n\text{H}_2\text{N—R—CO}_2\text{H} \longrightarrow \text{H}(\text{NH—R—CO})_n\text{OH} + (n-1)\text{H}_2\text{O}$$

Figure 2.29
Condensation, or step reaction, polymerization mechanisms can be classified into two general groups, depending upon the types of monomers involved in the reaction. (a) The first group involves bifunctional or polyfunctional monomers, with each monomer possessing only one type of functional group. (b) The second group involves a single monomer species having both types of functional groups. In this figure, the general equation for each reaction mechanism (A and B are two different types of functional groups) is followed by an example reaction. (Adapted with permission from [10].)

Polymer production via genetic engineering, however, provides the potential for greater control over polymer architecture and weight distributions when synthesizing fibrous proteins and analogous natural polymers. However, it is not possible to create synthetic polymers, such as poly(ethylene) or poly(styrene), via this method.

Although a detailed account of this method is beyond the scope of this text, genetic engineering of protein polymers involves the expression within a host organism (usually bacteria) of a genetic vector that encodes the protein polymer of interest. This can be achieved by one of two general methods. First, DNA encoding the protein polymer can be isolated from an organism that naturally produces it, and the DNA coding units can be introduced into the DNA of the host bacteria for expression and polymer production. Alternatively, the DNA encoding the protein polymer can be chemically synthesized and subsequently introduced into the host organism. The second method is more widely used and allows for a high level of control over the sequence of the protein polymer. Additionally, the second method allows for optimization of the DNA sequence for maximal expression by the host organism used. Examples of polymers produced through genetic engineering include silks, collagens, viral proteins, and a variety of artificial structural proteins.

2.4.3 Copolymers

In the previous discussion, we have focused on the synthesis and structure of **homopolymers**, or polymers with one type of repeat unit. However, **copolymers** (those involving two or more repeat unit types) are often produced to create materials with improved properties. Copolymers can be formed by either traditional condensation or addition polymerization, using a blend of monomer types as the reactant species.

As shown in Fig. 2.30 with the different repeat units depicted in different colors, there are several types of copolymers. In **random copolymers**, the two mer units are distributed along the chain with no pattern. As the name indicates, mer types alternate

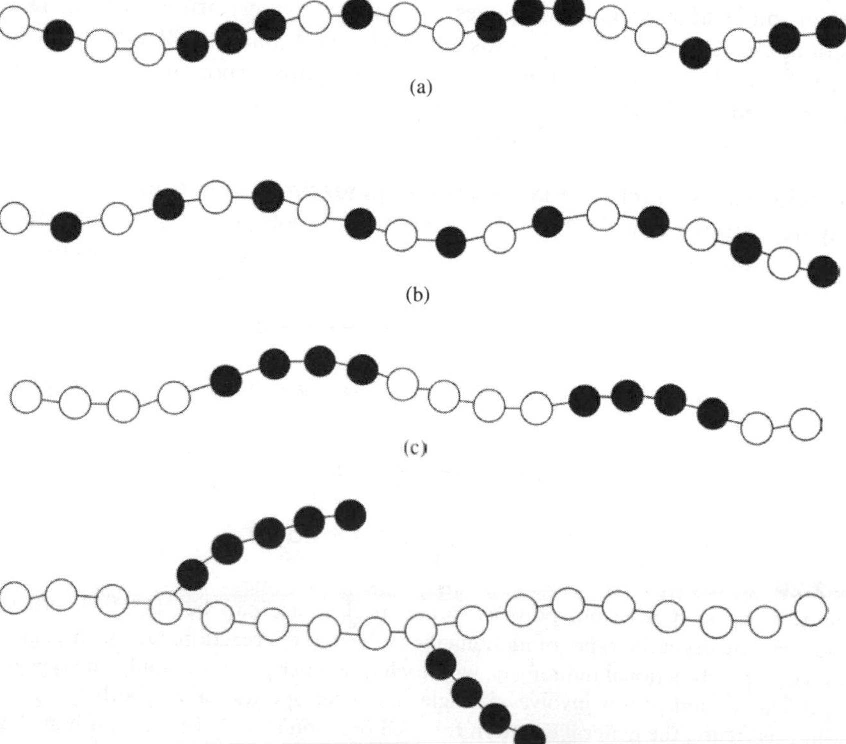

Figure 2.30
Types of copolymers. (a) Random copolymer—the two mer units are distributed along the chain with no pattern. (b) Alternating copolymer—mer types alternate. (c) Block copolymer—each type of repeat unit is clustered in regions (blocks) along the chain. (d) Graft copolymer—homopolymer chains are attached to a main homopolymer chain containing a different repeat unit. (Adapted with permission from [4].)

in an **alternating copolymer.** **Block copolymers** occur when each type of repeat unit is clustered in regions (blocks) along the chain. If homopolymer chains are attached as side chains to a main homopolymer chain containing a different repeat unit, this is called a **graft copolymer.** One of the most common examples of copolymers for biomedical applications is the random copolymerization of lactic acid and glycolic acid to form the biodegradable, synthetic polymer poly(lactic-*co*-glycolic acid), which is used in sutures, drug delivery devices, and tissue engineering scaffolds.

EXAMPLE PROBLEM 2.8

Given the molecular structure of the following copolymer poly(lactic-*co*-glycolic acid) (PLGA) commonly used in biodegradable sutures, determine the molecular weights for:

(a) Each repeat unit for the copolymer shown

$$HO{-}\left[C(=O){-}CH(CH_3){-}O\right]_n{-}\left[C(=O){-}CH_2{-}O\right]_m{-}H$$

(b) The copolymer when $n = 5$ and $m = 7$.
(c) The copolymer when $n = 7$ and $m = 3$.

Solution:

(a) The molecular weight for the repeat unit on the left (n) is as follows:

$$3 \text{ carbons } (12 \text{ g/mole C}) + 2 \text{ oxygens } (16 \text{ g/mole O}) + 4 \text{ hydrogens } (1 \text{ g/mole H}) = \underline{72 \text{ g/mole}}\ (n)$$

The molecular weight for the repeat unit on the right (m) is as follows:

$$2 \text{ carbons } (12 \text{ g/mole C}) + 2 \text{ oxygens } (16 \text{ g/mole O}) + 2 \text{ hydrogens } (1 \text{ g/mole H}) = \underline{58 \text{ g/mole}}\ (m)$$

(b) The molecular weight of the given copolymer is as follows:

$$5(72 \text{ g/mole } n) + 7(58 \text{ g/mole } m) + (16 \text{ g/mole oxygen}) + 2(1 \text{ g/mole hydrogen}) = \underline{784 \text{ g/mole}}$$

(c) The molecular weight of the given copolymer is as follows:

$$7(72 \text{ g/mole } n) + 3(58 \text{ g/mole } m) + (16 \text{ g/mole oxygen}) + 2(1 \text{ g/mole hydrogen}) = \underline{696 \text{ g/mole}}$$

■

2.4.4 Methods of Polymerization

A variety of polymerization methods exist for polymer production. The simplest method is **bulk polymerization,** in which only monomer and a monomer-soluble initiator are present in the reaction. This technique provides a high yield of high purity polymer, but tends to present difficulties with heat dissipation, especially in large-scale reactions, since most polymerization reactions are highly exothermic.

Problems in heat dissipation can be addressed by conducting the polymerization reaction in water or an appropriate organic solvent with high thermal conductivity in another method known as **solution polymerization.** In solution polymerization it is important that the monomer and initiator be soluble in the chosen solvent and that the solvent can be easily recovered following the reaction. Although solution polymerization addresses issues with heat dissipation, it generally has a small polymer yield per reaction volume and requires an additional step to remove the solvent.

Suspension polymerization is another method that presents high heat transfer capabilities. In this process, monomer and initiators that are not soluble in water are added under stirring to a reactor full of water. The insolubility of the monomer coupled with the mechanical agitation leads to the formation of monomer droplets containing initiator. These droplets can be stabilized with additives (colloids) and act as small reactors for polymerization. After the reaction, the resulting polymer beads can be recovered through filtration and washed.

A similar process, **emulsion polymerization,** involves the addition under stirring of a hydrophobic monomer, a water soluble initiator and a surfactant (emulsifier) to a reactor containing water. (See Chapter 7 for more on surfactants.) Emulsion polymerization results in the formation of polymer beads or rods, depending upon the reaction conditions and the surfactant used. The mechanism for emulsion polymerization is illustrated in Figure 2.31.

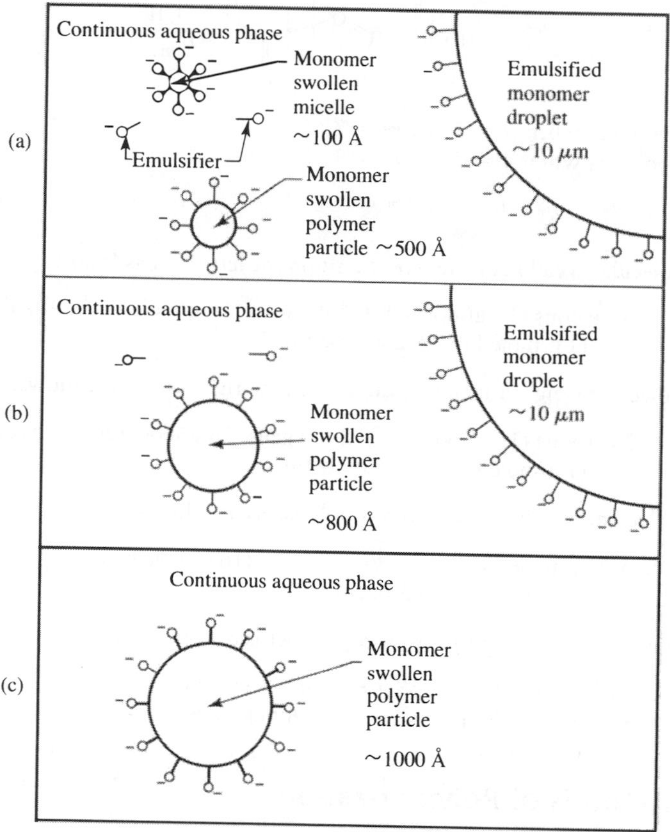

Figure 2.31
The mechanism for emulsion polymerization. This type of polymerization takes place in water with a water-soluble initiator, but involves a hydrophobic monomer. In order to disperse the hydrophobic monomer, a surfactant (emulsifier) is added. Because the surfactant possesses both hydrophilic and hydrophobic areas, it can be used as a coating for beads of the monomer and resulting polymer to promote their interaction with the aqueous environment. (a) At early stages of the reaction, three types of particles are present: emulsified monomer droplets, surfactant micelles containing solubilized monomer, and growing polymer particles stabilized by surfactant and swollen with monomer. (b) As the polymer particles grow, increasing amounts of surfactant are required to stabilize them until the surfactant micelles are depleted. (c) The polymer particles (swollen with monomer) continue to grow until the monomer in the emulsified monomer droplets is depleted and only surfactant stabilized polymer particles remain. (Reprinted with permission from [11].)

Additionally, polymerization can occur in the gas phase in **gaseous polymerization** and in the solid-state in **solid-state polymerization.** For solid-state polymerization, monomers in their crystalline state are polymerized through exposure to heat or irradiation. This process results in polymer chains that are oriented along the crystal structure. Lastly, polymerization can take place in a plasma environment in a process called **plasma polymerization.** This method is effective in depositing highly uniform thin films of polymer and can be used to alter surface properties, such as wettability (see Chapter 7).

2.4.5 Crystal Structures and Defects

2.4.5.1 Crystal Structures Like metals and ceramics, polymers can form crystalline structures, although their unit cells are more complex and contain more atoms than those for other types of materials. A number of aspects of a polymer's chemical structure affect its ability to crystallize. These include the polymer's tacticity (if it is isotactic, syndiotactic, or atactic) and its degree of branching. A large amount of branching reduces the crystallinity of a polymeric material, as does the presence of bulky side groups in its repeat unit. It is rare for polymers to be 100% crystalline; many are considered to be *semicrystalline.* A more in-depth discussion of polymer crystallinity is found in Chapter 3.

2.4.5.2 Point Defects and Impurities Point defects in the form of vacancies may occur in polymer crystals. In this case, a vacancy can be seen as the space between where one chain ends and the next begins. Polymer crystals usually have a large number of defects, but their presence has less of an effect on the overall properties of the material than defects in metals or ceramics. As with other types of biomaterials, impurities also exist in polymer crystals. In some situations, such as the synthesis of copolymers, these impurities have been added intentionally. (The effects of copolymerization on crystal structure are discussed in Chapter 3.)

2.5 Techniques: Introduction to Material Characterization

Characterization of properties relating to the chemical composition of a biomaterial can be accomplished through two major techniques, *spectroscopy* and *chromatography*. In ***spectroscopy***, one measures how compounds absorb different types of energy. As discussed in the previous chapter, due to the allowable energy states for electrons in the various orbitals, molecules absorb energy in discrete packets called **quanta.** The absorbed energy results in **excitation** of the sample by creating changes in electron or mechanical motion within the molecule.

Figure 2.32 and Table 2.7 depict the spectrum of energies that are employed in spectroscopy. (It is important to note in this figure that higher energy results in higher frequency and shorter wavelength radiation.) Each of the energy categories produces distinct changes in the atoms of a sample and thus provides different types of information about its chemical structure. In order of descending energy, X-rays promote electrons from inner subshells to outer ones, while ultraviolet/visible light excites only valence electrons (often from bonding to antibonding orbitals). Infrared energy causes vibration of bonds, and the lowest energy discussed here, radio waves (as used in nuclear magnetic resonance spectroscopy), produce transitions in nuclear spin.

In contrast to spectroscopy, ***chromatography*** uses various means to physically separate molecules on the basis of chemical characteristics such as charge or molecular weight. Both spectroscopic and chromatographic techniques are important in

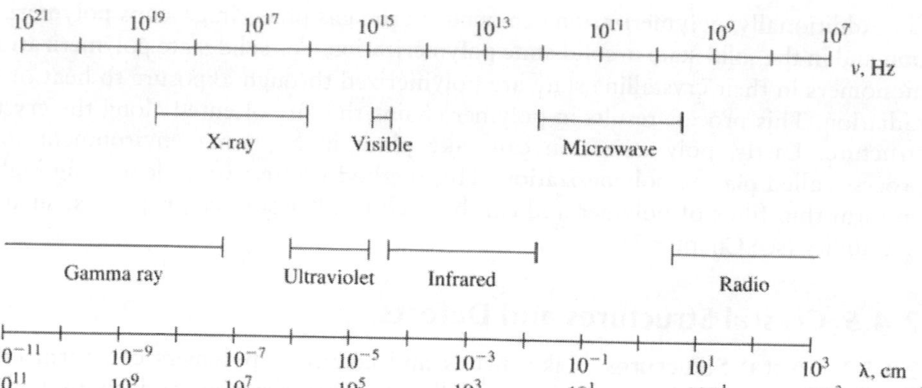

Figure 2.32
The spectrum of energies employed in spectroscopy. Note that higher energy results in higher frequency (ν) and shorter wavelength (λ) radiation. The parameter $\bar{\nu}$ refers to the wavenumber. (Reprinted with permission from [12])

defining chemical compositions of biomaterials, and often provide complementary data. As explained below, each technique reveals slightly different information, and some are preferred for certain materials over others. For example, since it is possible to learn about the composition of crystalline materials by knowing the type of crystal formed, X-ray diffraction is often used for metals and ceramics, while a number of other techniques such as ultraviolet, infrared, and nuclear magnetic resonance spectroscopy, as well as mass spectrometry and high performance liquid chromatography, provide information to address questions about the composition of polymers.

TABLE 2.7

Energies and Corresponding Atomic Transitions Found in Common Spectroscopic Techniques

Type Spectroscopy	Usual Wavelength Range*	Usual Wavenumber Range, cm^{-1}	Type of Quantum Transition
Gamma-ray emission	0.005–1.4Å	–	Nuclear
X-Ray absorption, emission, fluorescence, and diffraction	0.1–100Å	–	Inner electron
Vacuum ultraviolet absorption	10–180 nm	1×10^6 to 5×10^4	Bonding electrons
Ultraviolet visible absorption, emission, and fluorescence	180–780 nm	5×10^4 to 1.3×10^4	Bonding electrons
Infrared absorption and Raman scattering	0.78–300 μm	1.3×10^4 to 3.3×10^1	Rotation/vibration of molecules
Microwave absorption	0.75–3.75 mm	13–27	Rotation of molecules
Electron spin resonance	3 cm	0.33	Spin of electrons in a magnetic field
Nuclear magnetic resonance	0.6–10 m	1.7×10^{-2} to 1×10^3	Spin of nuclei in a magnetic field

*1 Å = 10^{-10} m = 10^{-8} cm
1 nm = 10^{-9} m = 10^{-7} cm
1 μm = 10^{-6} m = 10^{-4} cm
(Reprinted with permission from [12].)

2.5.1 X-Ray Diffraction

X-rays are a very high energy form of electromagnetic radiation used for a variety of characterization techniques. As mentioned above, X-rays are employed as a source for spectroscopic techniques to alter the energy state of core electrons. This is called **X-ray fluorescence**, of which there are two main types: *energy dispersive X-ray spectroscopy* (EDS) and *wavelength dispersive X-ray spectroscopy* (WDS). EDS is a more rapid spectroscopy method, but WDS has superior resolution. A more detailed description of these two methods is left to more advanced texts. X-rays are also important for biomaterial surface analysis in such techniques as electron spectroscopy for chemical analysis (ESCA), which will be discussed further in Chapter 7. A technique that uses X-rays for imaging is microcomputed tomography (μCT), and is discussed further in Chapter 14. In this section, we will focus on another characterization technique involving X-rays: **X-ray diffraction**. Rather than measuring how the absorbance of X-rays affects the sample, as in spectroscopic techniques, this method examines how X-rays, which can be viewed as waves like visible light, are diffracted from atoms in a material. X-ray diffraction is commonly used to determine structures of crystals, including calculation of Miller indices and unit cell size.

2.5.1.1 Basic Principles Because the wavelength of X-rays (0.5–50Å) is similar to the distance between atoms in a solid, they are ideal for exploring atomic arrangement in crystal structures. **Diffraction** of X-rays occurs when incident rays are scattered by atoms in a way that reinforces the waves. As seen in Fig. 2.33(a), if two waves (waves 1 and 2) of the same wavelength (λ) and amplitude (A) are in phase at point O/O' and are scattered so that they remain in phase (waves 1′ and 2′), they will combine in a reinforcing (or **constructive**) manner and the diffracted wave will have the same wavelength, but twice the amplitude ($2A$). This occurs only if the total distance traveled by waves 1 and 2 differ by an integer number of wavelengths.

On the other hand, as shown in Fig. 2.33(b), when the path lengths of two incident waves (waves 3 and 4) differ by a number of *half* wavelengths, after scattering, the waves (waves 3′ and 4′) are out of phase and there is **destructive interference**. The scattered waves cancel each other and no diffraction occurs. There are also a number of interactions that cause phase differences between these two extremes, leading to only partial reinforcement of incident waves.

When X-rays enter a sample, they are scattered in all directions by the electrons associated with each atom/ion. In most cases, this leads to destructive interference and no resulting X-rays can be measured. For certain atomic arrangements, however, diffraction occurs and X-ray patterns can be recorded. In Fig. 2.34, the planes of atoms marked A/A' and B/B' have the same Miller indices ($h\ k\ l$) and are separated by the distance d_{hkl} (interplanar spacing). Consider the path of parallel X-rays (waves 1 and 2) of wavelength λ that are in phase upon striking the sample at angle ϕ. Wave 1 is scattered by atom P, and wave 2 is scattered by atom Q. Since we know that for diffraction to occur, the total path length of the two waves must differ by an integral number of wavelengths, we can write

$$n\lambda = SQ + QT \tag{2.19}$$

where n is an integer. We can also rewrite this expression in terms of the crystal's interplanar spacing (d_{hkl}) using geometric relations:

$$n\lambda = d_{hkl}\sin\phi + d_{hkl}\sin\phi = 2d_{hkl}\sin\phi \tag{2.20}$$

a)

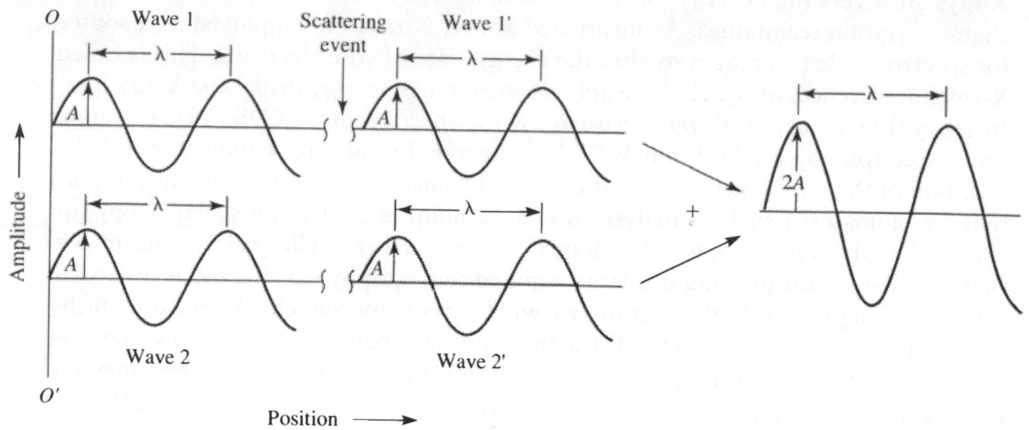

b)

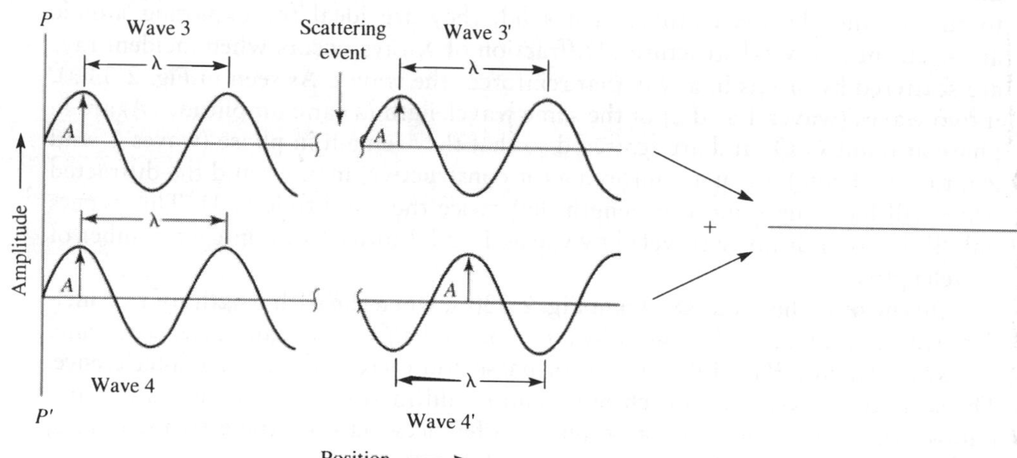

Figure 2.33
Constructive and destructive interference of X-rays. (a) If two waves (waves 1 and 2) of the same wavelength (λ) and amplitude (A) are in phase at point O/O' and are scattered so that they remain in phase (waves 1′ and 2′), they will combine in a constructive manner and diffraction will occur. The diffracted wave will have the same wavelength, but twice the amplitude ($2A$). This occurs only if the total distances traveled by waves 1 and 2 differ by an integer number of wavelengths. (b) When the path lengths of two incident waves (waves 3 and 4) differ by an odd number of *half* wavelengths, after scattering, the waves (waves 3′ and 4′) are out of phase and there is destructive interference. The scattered waves cancel each other and no diffraction occurs. (Adapted with permission from [4].)

This expression is known as **Bragg's law**, and if this condition is not met, there will be no diffraction resulting from this set of planes.

Interplanar spacing, as observed through X-ray diffraction experiments, is a function of a crystal's Miller indices and its lattice parameters. For cubic crystal systems, the relation is

$$d_{hkl} = \frac{a}{\sqrt{h^2 + k^2 + l^2}} \tag{2.21}$$

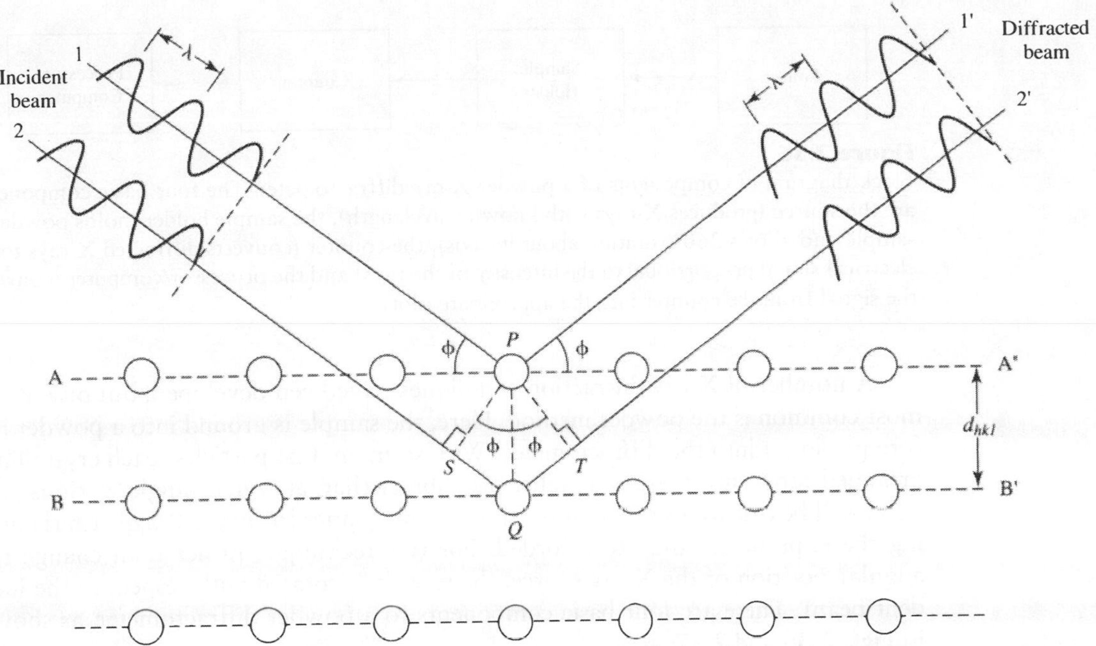

Figure 2.34
Scattering of X-rays by electrons in a crystalline material. The planes of atoms marked *A*/*A*′ and *B*/*B*′ have the same Miller indices (*h k l*) and are separated by the distance d_{hkl} (interplanar spacing). Waves 1 and 2 are parallel X-rays of wavelength λ that are in phase upon striking the sample at angle ϕ. Wave 1 is scattered by atom *P*, and wave 2 is scattered by atom *Q*. For diffraction to occur, the total path length of the two waves must differ by an integral number of wavelengths. This can be expressed in terms of the crystal's interplanar spacing (d_{hkl}): $n\lambda = d_{hkl} \sin \phi + d_{hkl} \sin \phi = 2d_{hkl} \sin \phi$ and is called Bragg's law. (Adapted with permission from [4].)

where *a* is the unit cell edge length. This relationship is more complex for other crystal systems. However, such equations can provide a means to determine the size of the unit cell and other important structural parameters based on X-ray diffraction data.

2.5.1.2 Instrumentation A typical X-ray diffraction pattern for aluminum powder is found in Fig. 2.35. Results are plotted as intensity (*y*-axis) as a function of 2θ (*x*-axis), where θ is the incident angle of the X-rays. Peaks are generated at angles that satisfy the Bragg criteria for a certain set of atomic planes. The figure includes the indices of such planes for aluminum.

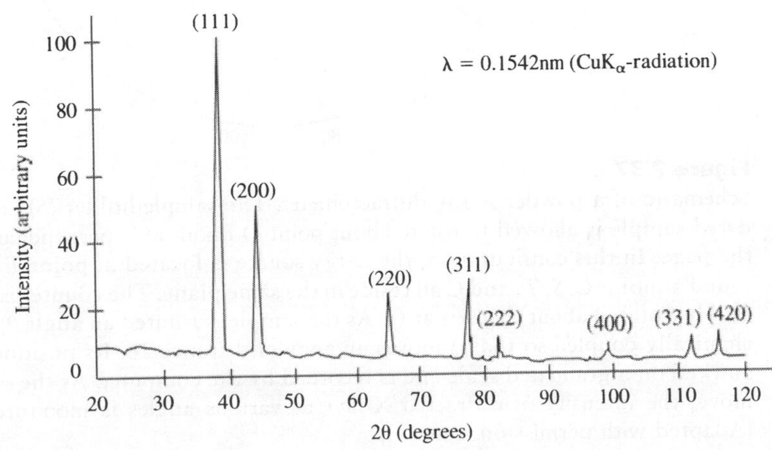

Figure 2.35
A typical X-ray diffraction pattern for aluminum powder. Peaks are generated at angles that satisfy the Bragg criteria for a certain set of atomic planes. The indices of these planes are noted in the figure. (Adapted with permission from [1].)

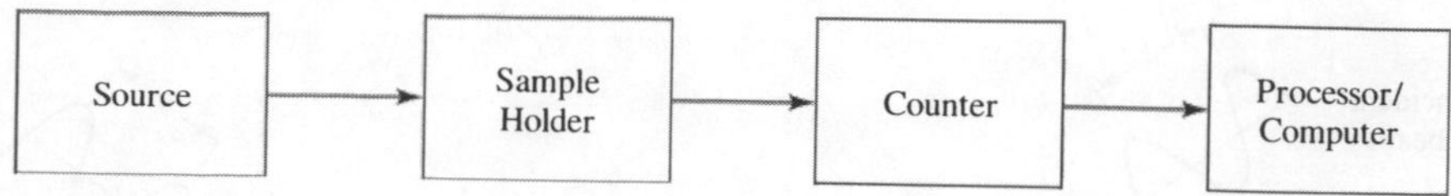

Figure 2.36
Block diagram of components of a powder X-ray diffractometer. The four basic components are the source (produces X-rays with known wavelength), the sample holder (holds powdered sample and allows 360° rotation about its axis), the counter (converts diffracted X-rays to an electrical signal proportional to the intensity of the rays) and the processor/computer (converts the signal from the counter into the appropriate plot).

A number of X-ray diffraction techniques have been developed, but one of the most common is the powder method. Here, the sample is ground into a powder before placing it into the **diffractometer**. With so many fine particles (each crystalline) arranged randomly, there is a higher probability that, at a given angle, various particles will be oriented so that all possible atomic planes fulfill the Bragg criteria during the experiment and are recorded. For this technique, rather than change the angular position of the X-ray source, the sample is rotated with respect to the incident beam. There are four basic components to a powder diffractometer, as shown in Figs. 2.36 and 2.37:

1. Source—produces X-rays with known wavelength.
2. Sample holder—holds powdered sample and allows 360° rotation about its axis.

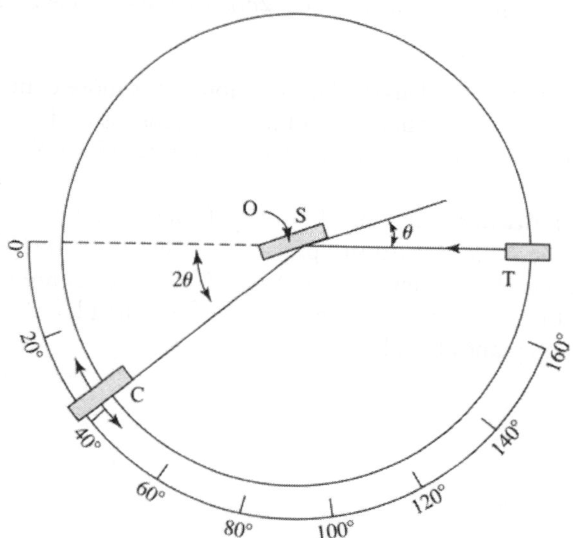

Figure 2.37
Schematic of a powder X-ray diffractometer. The sample holder (S) containing the powdered sample is allowed to rotate about point O on an axis perpendicular to the plane of the page. In this configuration, the X-ray source is located at point T and the counter is found at point C. S, T, and C all reside in the same plane. The counter is moveable and can also be rotated about the axis at O. As the sample is rotated an angle θ, the counter is mechanically coupled so that it moves an angular distance 2θ. Its position in terms of 2θ is marked on a graduated scale and is recorded by the computer. As the sample and counter move, the intensity of diffracted X-rays at various angles is monitored by the counter. (Adapted with permission from [4])

3. Counter—converts diffracted X-rays to an electrical signal proportional to the intensity of the rays. Rotates in conjunction with sample holder.
4. Processor (computer)—converts the signal from the counter into the appropriate plot.

As seen in the diagram (Fig. 2.37), the sample holder (*S*) containing the powdered sample is allowed to rotate about point O on an axis perpendicular to the plane of the page. In this configuration, the X-ray source is located at point *T* and the counter is found at point *C*. *S*, *T*, and *C* all reside in the same plane. The counter is moveable and can also be rotated about the axis at O. As the sample is rotated through an angle θ, the counter is mechanically coupled so that it moves a distance 2θ. Its position in terms of 2θ is marked on a graduated scale and is recorded by the computer. As the sample and counter move, the intensity of diffracted X-rays at various angles is monitored by the counter. At the end of the experiment, a summary of the diffraction pattern is plotted as a function of 2θ.

2.5.1.3 Information Provided X-ray diffraction is a powerful technique for exploring atomic and molecular arrangements in solids and can be used for all crystalline materials, including metals, ceramics and polymers. The size of a unit cell as well as its geometry can be determined from the angles at which peaks occur, and arrangement of atoms within the unit cell is indicated by the height of the peaks. In addition, compound identification may be carried out by comparing experimental results to diffraction patterns of known substances.

2.5.2 Ultraviolet and Visible Light Spectroscopy (UV-VIS)

2.5.2.1 Basic Principles The absorption of UV-VIS radiation [wavelength (λ): approximately 185–1100 nm] by a molecule (*M*) may promote one or more of its valence electrons to a higher energy state, resulting in molecular excitation to a new state (M^*)

$$M + h\nu = M^* \tag{2.22}$$

where ν is the frequency of radiation and h is the Planck's constant (6.6×10^{-34} J-s).

Usually, this involves the transition of electrons from σ or π bonding to antibonding molecular orbitals (see Chapter 1 for discussion of molecular orbitals). Since different amounts of energy are required for different transitions, absorption occurs at various wavelengths, depending on the chemical structure of the molecule. Figure 2.38 provides a general idea of the energies involved in common transitions.

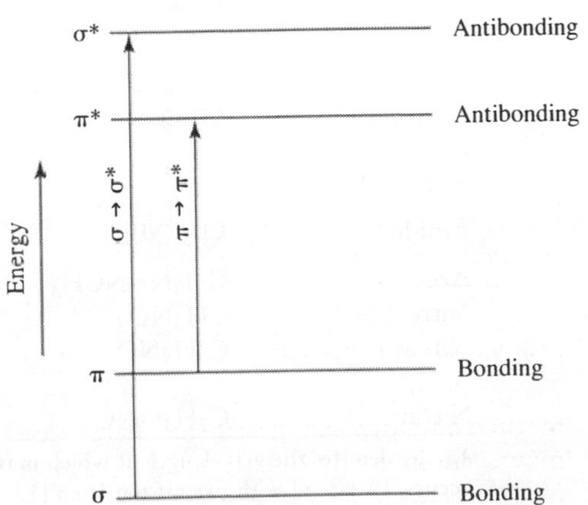

Figure 2.38
Excitation of molecules by UV-VIS radiation. Absorption of energy may promote one or more valence electrons from σ or π bonding to antibonding molecular orbitals. Since different amounts of energy are required for different transitions, absorption occurs at various wavelengths, depending on the chemical structure of the molecule. (Adapted with permission from [12].)

Examples of organic molecules that demonstrate characteristic absorption at a given wavelength are given in Table 2.8.

After excitation, the molecule returns to its ground state through the conversion of the excitation energy to another form, such as thermal energy (heat). This process is known as **relaxation**

$$M^* = M + heat \tag{2.23}$$

Return to the ground state can occur via a variety of means. An example of non-radiative relaxation is fluorescence, which will be discussed in Chapter 8 as a means to observe proteins.

2.5.2.2 Instrumentation A typical UV-VIS spectrum of poly(lactic-co-glycolic acid) (PLGA), a common suture material, is found in Fig. 2.39. UV-VIS spectra are generally plotted as absorbance (y-axis) as a function of wavelength (or wavenumber) on the x-axis. In order to obtain such a plot, many types of UV-VIS spectrophotometers have been developed. There are four basic components to a spectrophotometer, as shown in Fig. 2.40:

1. Source—provides energy over the wavelength range of interest.
2. Wavelength selector or filter—allows user to choose a specific wavelength if desired.
3. Detector—converts energy transmitted through the sample to an electrical signal.
4. Processor (computer)—converts the electrical signal into the appropriate spectrum.

TABLE 2.8

Common Chromophores and Corresponding Characteristic UV-VIS Absorption Wavelengths

Chromophore	Example	Solvent	$\lambda_{max\ abs}$(nm)
Alkene	$C_6H_{13}CH{=}CH_2$	*n*-Heptane	177
Alkyne	$C_5H_{11}C{\equiv}C{-}CH_3$	*n*-Heptane	178 196 225
Carbonyl	$CH_3C(=O)CH_3$	*n*-Hexane	186 280
	$CH_3C(=O)H$	*n*-Hexane	180 293
Carboxyl	$CH_3C(=O)OH$	Ethanol	204
Amido	$CH_3C(=O)NH_2$	Water	214
Azo	$CH_3N{=}NCH_3$	Ethanol	339
Nitro	CH_3NO_2	Isooctane	280
Nitroso	C_4H_9NO	Ethyl ether	300 665
Nitrate	$C_2H_5ONO_2$	Dioxane	270

λ_{maxabs} denotes the wavelength at which maximum absorption in the spectrum occurs. (Adapted with permission from [12].)

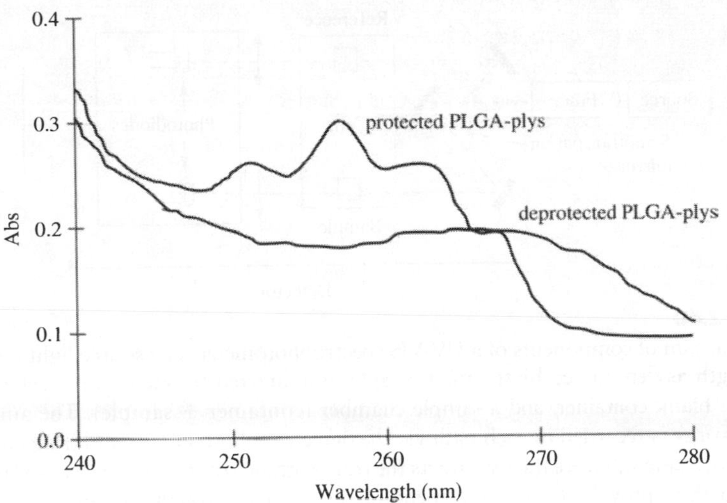

Protected PLGA-plys:

Deprotected PLGA-plys:

polylysine

Figure 2.39
UV-VIS spectra of poly(lactic-co-glycolic acid)-polylysine (PLGA-plys) before and after deprotection. The peak with the maximum at 257 nm corresponds to the presence of the CBZ (carbobenzoxy) protecting group on the protected polymer (the large ringed structure in the diagram). In the deprotection step, this chemical group is removed, as is evidenced by the decrease in this peak in the spectrum. PLGA-plys block copolymer was synthesized by coupling PLGA with a carboxyl end group to poly(ε-carbobenzoxy-L-lysine) and is an example of a polymer that possesses both biological molecules (an amino acid) and a synthetic polymer (PLGA). (Adapted with permission from [13].)

In UV-VIS spectroscopy, the sample is placed after the wavelength selector and before the detector. We will now focus our attention on one of the most common instruments: the double beam spectrophotometer (Fig. 2.40).

As shown in the diagram, the source light beam (at a given wavelength as determined by the settings of the filter) is split and directed through both a reference chamber, usually a blank container, and a sample chamber (container + sample). The amount of transmitted energy (transmittance) is recorded in each path via the photodiodes and transmitted to a computer. Processing software then subtracts the *transmittance* of the reference path from that of the sample path to provide the amount of energy transmitted through the sample, without interference that may arise from its holder or other environmental factors. Finally, fraction transmittance (F_t) is converted to fraction absorbance (F_a)($F_a = 1 - F_t$). The process is then

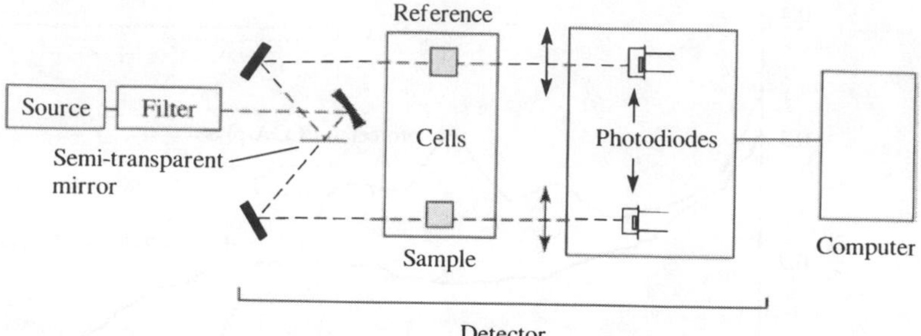

Figure 2.40
Block diagram of components of a UV-VIS spectrophotometer. The source light beam (at a given wavelength as determined by the filter) is split and directed through both a reference chamber, usually a blank container, and a sample chamber (container + sample). The amount of transmitted energy is recorded in each path via the detector (photodiodes) and transmitted to a computer. Processing software then subtracts the transmittance of the reference path from that of the sample path to provide the amount of energy transmitted through the sample, without interference that may arise from its holder or other environmental factors. The process is then repeated at the next wavelength, if desired. At the end of the wavelength scans, the entire spectrum is plotted for that sample. (Adapted with permission from [14].)

repeated at the next wavelength, if desired. At the end of the wavelength scans, the entire spectrum is plotted for that sample.

2.5.2.3 Information Provided The above description indicates that there are two main uses for UV-VIS spectroscopy. One is to produce spectra to help identify samples or chemical groups within samples. This is done by recording the absorbance over a wide range of wavelengths with successive scans by the spectrophotometer.

In addition, UV-VIS is often used to quantify the amount of a certain compound in a mixture or solution. Of course, this is only possible if the compound absorbs a significant amount of UV radiation at a certain wavelength, and if this wavelength is known. In this case repeated scans are not needed - the user simply chooses the appropriate wavelength and the computer records the absorbance value at that setting. Concentrations of both inorganic and organic substances can be quantified using this method, but it is more commonly used in the biomaterials field for organic materials (Table 2.8).

Quantification of a sample is made possible through the use of **Beer-Lambert's law**,

$$A = \varepsilon l C \tag{2.24}$$

where A is the absorbance measured by the spectrophotometer, l is the thickness of the sample through which the light is passed, C is the molar concentration of the compound, and ε is the molar absorption coefficient for that compound at a given wavelength. The parameter ε has been measured for many substances, and can be affected by temperature and the nature of the solvent, as well as the wavelength chosen.

A direct result of Beer-Lambert's law is that a standard curve of a given compound can be generated by measuring the absorbance at a fixed wavelength of the pure material at varying concentrations. An equation describing the linear relation over a certain range of absorbance and concentration can then be generated (Fig. 2.41). Using this relation, the concentration of that compound in an unknown sample can be determined

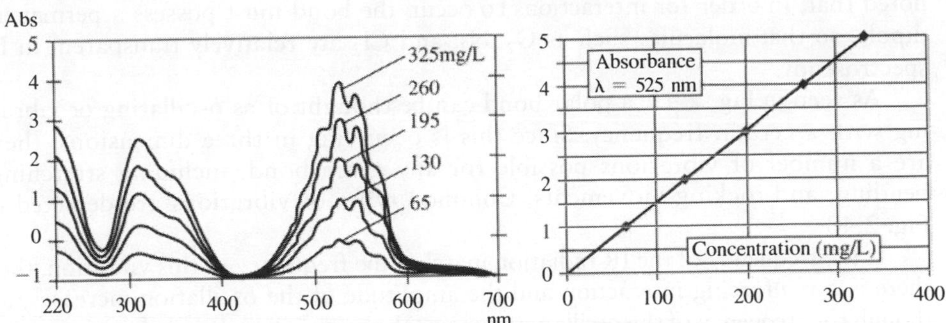

Figure 2.41
Standard curve for potassium permanganate. A standard curve is generated by measuring UV-VIS absorbance at a set wavelength of known concentrations (five concentrations in this example). Using Beer-Lambert's law, an equation describing the linear relation of absorbance and concentration can then be created. (Reprinted with permission from [14].)

by comparing the absorbance value of the unknown at the selected wavelength with values found in the standard curve.

The ease with which such quantification can take place using an UV-VIS system has made it a common technique in a variety of assays, including those for products of cellular function, as described in the second half of this book. In addition, UV-VIS detectors are often found as part of chromatographic techniques, such as HPLC (see section 2.5.6), to measure the amount of various compounds separated from a mixture injected into the instrument.

2.5.3 Infrared Spectroscopy (IR)

2.5.3.1 Basic Principles IR spectroscopy includes sources that produce radiation of wavelengths 0.78–1000 μm, but the majority of analysis takes place with energy of wavelengths 2.5–25 μm. Although interaction between IR radiation and analyte molecules is complex, the basic concepts can be understood by using a simple ball and spring model representing a bond between two atoms (Fig. 2.42). It should be

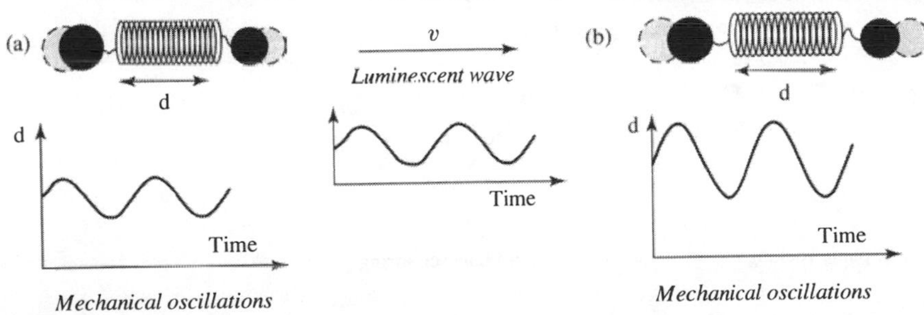

Figure 2.42
(a&b) Basic ball and spring model of IR energy interaction with chemical bonds. (It should be noted that, in order for interactions to occur, the bond must possess a permanent dipole.) As depicted above, a polar bond can be thought of as oscillating or vibrating with a certain frequency. If the frequency of the IR radiation matches the frequency of this vibration, then there is a reinforcing interaction and the amplitude of the oscillation increases, although the frequency of the oscillation remains the same. The result is that absorption at this IR frequency (wavelength) occurs for this material. (Adapted with permission from [14])

noted that, in order for interactions to occur, the bond must possess a permanent dipole, so that molecules such as O_2, N_2, and Cl_2 are relatively transparent in IR spectroscopy.

As seen in Fig. 2.43, a polar bond can be thought of as oscillating or vibrating with a certain frequency. Since this is occurring in three dimensions, there are a number of vibrations possible for any given bond, including stretching, bending, and rocking movements. Common types of vibrations are depicted in Fig. 2.43.

If the frequency of the IR radiation matches the frequency of this vibration, then there is a reinforcing interaction and the amplitude of the oscillation increases, although the frequency of the oscillation remains the same. The result is that absorption at this IR frequency (wavelength) is observed for this molecule. Since different types of bonds exist in a given sample, and there are multiple types of vibrations for each bond, absorption occurs at various wavelengths, depending on the chemical structure of the molecule. Table 2.9 provides a general idea of the frequencies absorbed for different chemical groups.

2.5.3.2 Instrumentation A typical IR spectrum of poly(styrene) is found in Fig. 2.44. In contrast to UV-VIS, IR spectra are generally plotted as percent transmittance (rather than absorbance) (y-axis), as a function of wavelength (or wavenumber) (x-axis). The basic instrumentation for IR spectroscopy is very similar to that for UV-VIS and includes an IR source, a wavelength selector, a detector and a processor [Fig. 2.45(a)]. Although double beam spectrophotometers are also often used for IR analysis, unlike UV-VIS, the sample is usually placed directly after the source, since the energies used in this type of analysis are not strong enough to damage the material.

Improvement in IR spectroscopy has come through the use of Fourier-transform techniques (FT-IR), which involve the inclusion of mirrors in the form of an

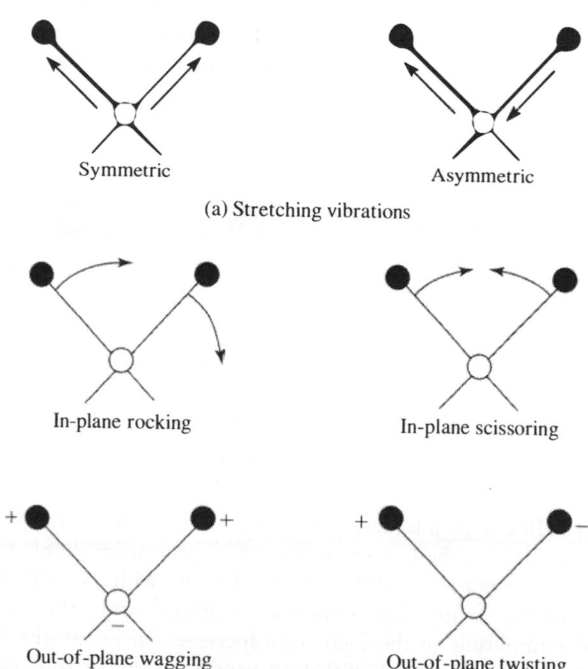

Figure 2.43
(a&b) Common types of three-dimensional vibrations in bonds between atoms. "+ indicates movement out of the plane of the page." (Adapted with permission from [12].)

TABLE 2.9

IR Frequencies Absorbed by Common Chemical Groups

Bond	Type of Compound	Frequency Range, cm^{-1}	Intensity
C—H	Alkanes	2850–2970	Strong
		1340–1470	Strong
C—H	Alkenes (>C=C<, H)	3010–3095	Medium
		675–995	Strong
C—H	Alkynes(–C≡C–H)	3300	Strong
C—H	Aromatic rings	3010–3100	Medium
		690–900	Strong
O—H	Monomeric alcohols, phenols	3590–3650	Variable
	Hydrogen bonded alcohols, phenols	3200–3600	Variable, sometimes broad
	Monomeric carboxylic acids	3500–3650	Medium
	Hydrogen-bonded carboxylic acids	2500–2700	Broad
N—H	Amines, amides	3300–3500	Medium
C=C	Alkenes	1610–1680	Variable
C=C	Aromatic rings	1500–1600	Variable
C≡C	Alkynes	2100–2260	Variable
C—N	Amines, amides	1180–1360	Strong
C≡N	Nitriles	2210–2280	Strong
C—O	Alcohols, ethers, carboxylic acids, esters	1050–1300	Strong
C=O	Aldehydes, ketones, carboxylic acids, esters	1690–1760	Strong
NO_2	Nitro compounds	1500–1570	Strong
		1300–1370	Strong

(Adapted with permission from [12].)

interferometer [Fig. 2.45(b) and 2.46]. Although the exact mechanism of interferometer function is beyond the scope of this book, the advantage of Fourier transform is that, since information for all wavelengths reaches the detector simultaneously, the scan time is significantly shortened. Thus, it is possible to perform more scans in a given time, which significantly increases the signal strength (signal to noise ratio). This advantage is particularly important in analyzing samples containing a small amount of material, such as is found when examining the surface of a biomaterial. The application of FT-IR to surface analysis will be discussed further in Chapter 7.

2.5.3.3 Information Provided Because samples analyzed by IR spectroscopy also follow Beer-Lambert's law, like UV-VIS, IR can be used to quantify amounts of substances. However, this technique has been most often employed in biomaterial characterization to record sample spectra, particularly of polymeric molecules. These spectra are unique for each material and form a sort of "molecular fingerprint," allowing identification of various materials via spectrum comparison. This type of analysis is very powerful, since IR provides more information about polymer structure and composition than most other characterization techniques.

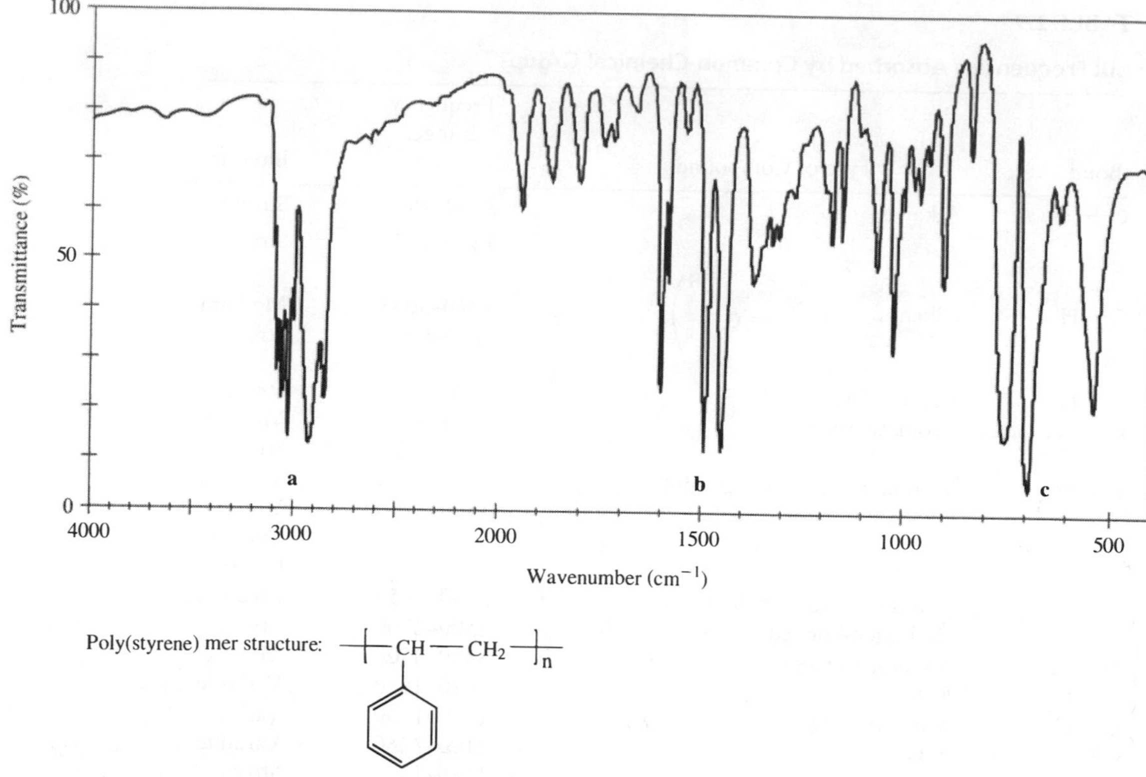

Figure 2.44
A typical IR spectrum of poly(styrene). In contrast to UV-VIS, IR spectra are generally plotted by percent transmittance (rather than absorbance) (y-axis), as a function of wavelength (or wavenumber) (x-axis) and, therefore, the peaks appear inverted. The IR spectrum, along with reference data such as shown in Table 2.9, is used to determine the structure of the material. For example, peaks are shown at 2800–3100 (a), 1400–1600 (b), and 600–900 (c) wavenumber. When used in conjunction with Table 2.9, it is evident that aromatic rings result in peaks between 3010–3100, 1500–1600, and 690–900. This would indicate that the material analyzed via IR spectroscopy contains an aromatic ring structure. This process is continued until the whole structure has been determined. (Adapted with permission from [15].)

Another common use for IR spectroscopy is to follow the relative change over time of certain peaks that correspond to specific types of bonds, as shown in Table 2.9. Examining the appearance of product peaks or disappearance of monomer peaks are two means to monitor a polymerization reaction, for example (Fig. 2.47).

2.5.4 Nuclear Magnetic Resonance Spectroscopy (NMR)

2.5.4.1 Basic Principles NMR utilizes radiation in the radio-frequency region (0.5–75 m) to excite molecules. However, in contrast to the types of spectroscopy previously discussed, NMR induces changes in the nucleus, rather than the electrons, of an atom. Additionally, the presence of a strong magnetic field is needed to observe the nuclear transitions.

As introduced in Chapter 1, quantum mechanical principles can be employed to describe the configurations of electrons around the nucleus, including the concept that each electron can be characterized in part by its angular momentum, or spin. In

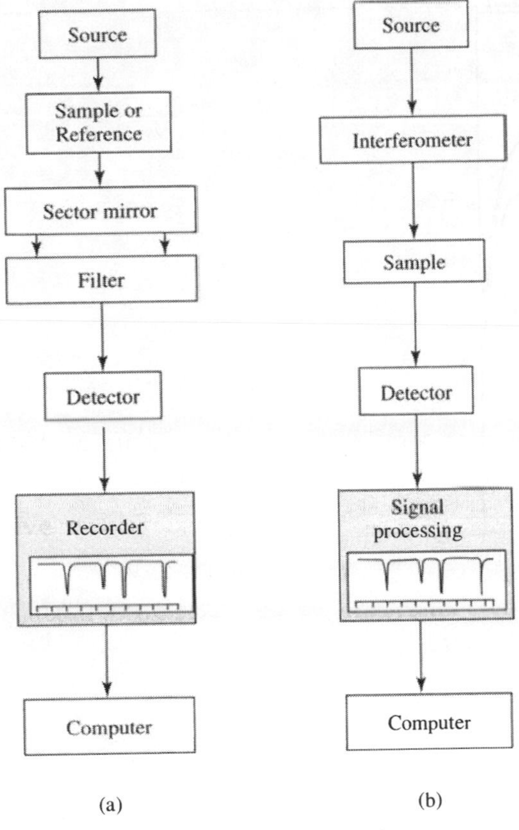

Figure 2.45
Block diagram of components of an IR spectrophotometer. (a) The basic instrumentation for IR spectroscopy is very similar to that for UV-VIS and includes an IR source, a wavelength selector, a detector and a processor. Unlike UV-VIS, the sample is usually placed directly after the source, since the energies used in this type of analysis are not strong enough to damage the material. (b) Improvement in IR spectroscopy has come through the use of Fourier-transform techniques (FT-IR), which involve the inclusion of mirrors in the form of an interferometer. The basic components of a FT-IR instrument are shown here. (Adapted with permission from [14].)

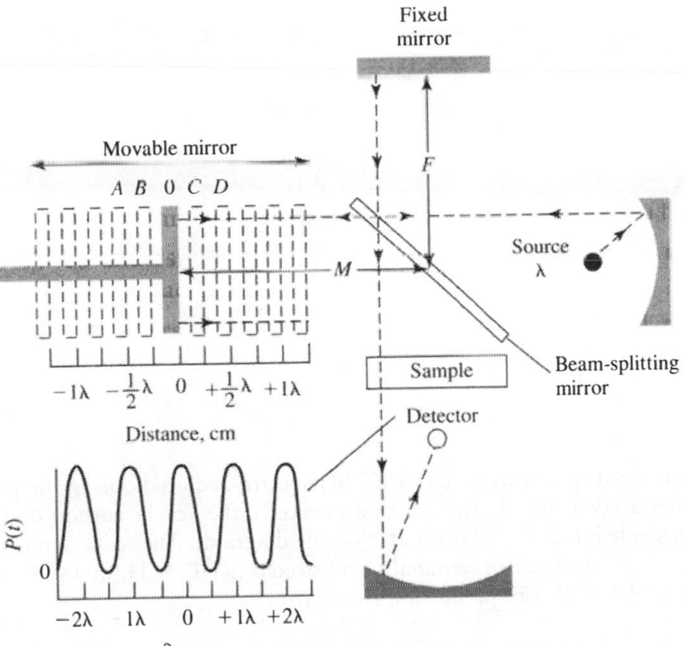

Figure 2.46
Detail of a Michelson interferometer. A source produces a beam of the proper wavelength that is then directed to a beam-splitting mirror, which transmits half the radiation and reflects the other half. The split beams are then reflected off mirrors (one fixed, one moveable) and are joined again at the beam splitter. When the two mirrors are equidistant from the beam splitter, the recombined beam is in phase and can be observed at the detector. However, if the distance of the two mirrors is off by 1/4 of a wavelength (total difference $1/2\lambda$), destructive interference occurs and nothing is registered at the detector. Because the recombined beam is passed through the sample, Fourier-transform techniques can then be used to convert information about absorbance of this beam into a traditional IR spectrum. The advantage of Fourier transform is that, since information for all wavelengths reaches the detector simultaneously, the scan time is significantly shortened and, thus, the signal to noise ratio is increased. (Adapted with permission from [12].)

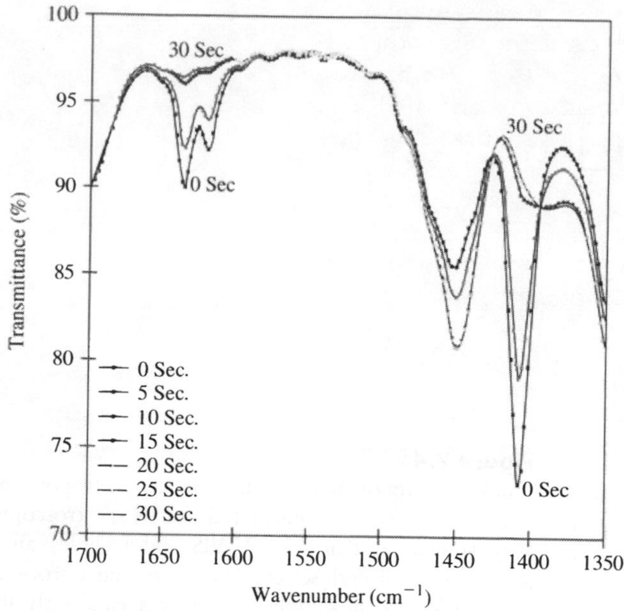

Poly(ethylene glycol) diacrylate:

Reaction of six molecules of poly(ethylene glycol) diacrylate:

Polymerization

Figure 2.47
Attenuated total internal reflectance Fourier-transform infrared spectroscopy (ATR/FT-IR) spectra acquired during the photopolymerization of poly(ethylene glycol) diacrylate using a UV lamp. As the reaction proceeds, the acrylic carbon double bound (C=C) (seen at 1 on the diagram) is converted to single bonds (C–C) (seen at 2 on the diagram). The reduction in the amount of this double bond was determined by measuring the decrease in terminal C=C stretch (RHC=CH) at 1635 cm^{-1} and C=C–H bending at 1410 cm^{-1} at several time points. (Adapted with permission from [16].)

an extension of these principles, many nuclei also behave as if they were spinning. Since nuclei are positively charged, their movement (spin) creates a small magnetic field, and each nucleus in an NMR experiment can be viewed as a small magnet. Like electrons, the nuclei of most interest to the biomaterialist (^1H and ^{13}C) have two theoretical orientations to their spin. Nuclei must have unequal numbers of protons and neutrons to produce a signal in NMR analysis.

Like little magnets, when the nuclei are placed in a larger, external magnetic field, their orientation can be in the same direction as the field, which is more energetically favorable and thus represents a lower energy state, or opposite to the field, which represents a higher energy state (Fig. 2.48). The difference in these two energy states increases with increasing strength of the magnetic field.

In a constant magnetic field, the addition of radio waves with just enough energy to bridge the gap in energy states will force some of the nuclei into the higher energy orientation. At this point, the nuclei are in **resonance.** This is indicated by absorbance of radio waves at a certain frequency, called the **resonance frequency.** After resonance has been achieved, as with other types of spectroscopy, molecular relaxation can occur through a variety of means.

When exposed to the same magnetic field, various molecules will require different amounts of energy to resonate (because they demonstrate different resonance frequencies). This is partially due to the local environment of the nucleus of interest (usually ^1H). To explain, we will discuss in more detail the cases of hydrogen bonded to fluorine, as in HF, and hydrogen bonded to carbon, as in CH_3.

In addition to the external magnetic field, the ^1H nucleus is also affected by smaller magnetic fields created by the circulation of electrons around it. The movement of these electrons creates a magnetic field whose strength is proportional to the electron density. This smaller field opposes the effects of the external field (Fig. 2.49). In the case of the H–C bond, there are more electrons nearby than would normally be found in a hydrogen atom, so the nucleus is said to be **shielded** from the strength of the external field. Therefore, less energy (lower frequency of radio waves) is needed to induce resonance in this molecule.

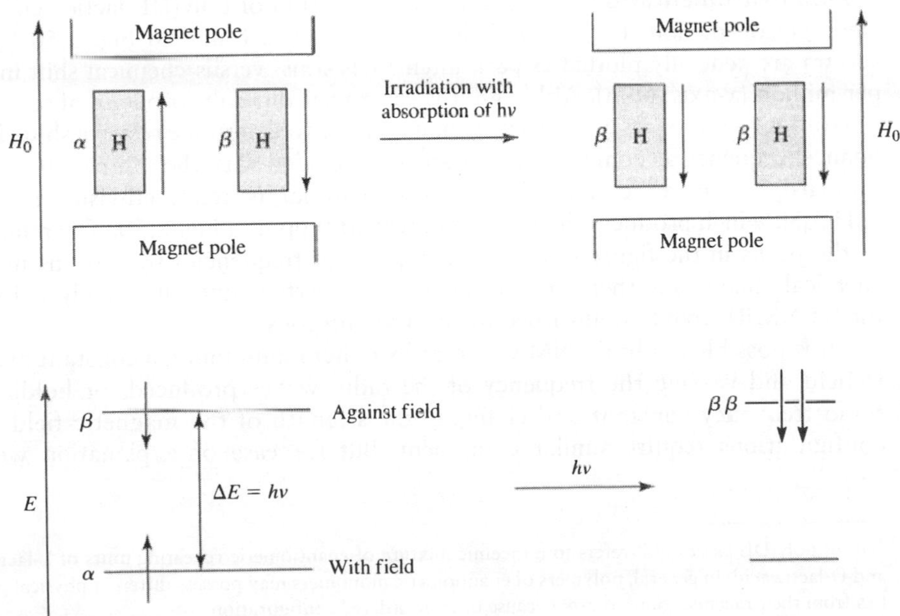

Figure 2.48
Theory behind nuclear magnetic resonance. When protons (H) are placed in a larger, external magnetic field, H_0 their spins can be oriented in the same direction as the field, which is more energetically favorable and thus represents a lower energy state (α), or with spin opposing the field (a higher energy state, β). The difference in energy ΔE between these two states is equal to $h\nu$. If exposed to radio energy of frequency ν (resonance frequency), then the nuclei will absorb this energy and the nuclear spin will be "flipped" from the α to the β state. At this point, the nuclei are in resonance. The resonance frequency depends strongly on the local environment of each nucleus. (Adapted with permission from [17].)

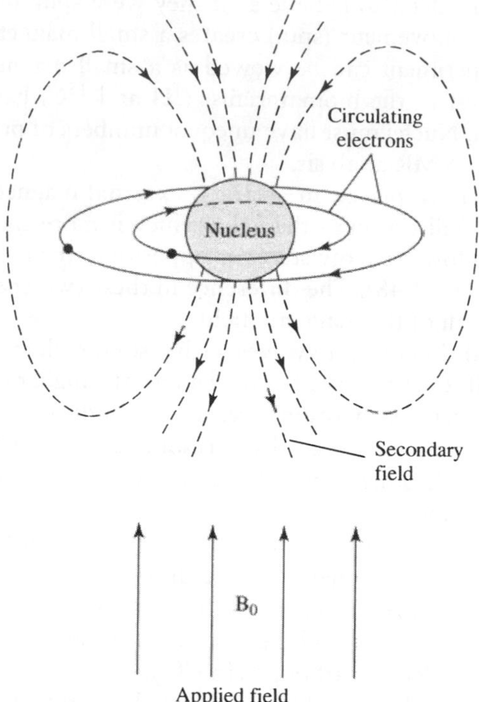

Figure 2.49
Effect of applied and secondary magnetic fields on the hydrogen nucleus. The nucleus is affected by small magnetic fields created by the circulation of electrons around it. This smaller field opposes the effects of the external field (B_0) and reduces the energy needed to induce resonance in the molecule. (Adapted with permission from [12].)

On other hand, if the hydrogen is bonded to a more electron-withdrawing (electronegative) atom such as fluorine (HF), the electron density around the hydrogen nucleus is less than normal, and the nucleus is **deshielded.** In this case, more energy is required and a higher resonance frequency than normal is recorded. These principles, along with more complicated aspects of a ^{1}H NMR spectrum, are used to determine molecular structure by identification of the localized environment of each proton in the sample.

2.5.4.2 Instrumentation A typical NMR spectrum of poly(DL-lactic acid-b-ethylene glycol)-monomethyl ether diblock copolymer is found in Fig. 2.50.[3] NMR spectra are generally plotted as peak intensity (y-axis) versus chemical shift in parts per million (x-axis, ppm). Although it is somewhat difficult to obtain absolute values for the x-axis of an NMR spectrum, it is easier to determine relative shifts in resonance frequency as compared to a standard included with the sample (an **internal standard**). In many cases, this reference material is tetramethylsilane (TMS), $(CH_3)_4Si$, which produces the large peak seen at 0 ppm in Fig. 2.50. The remainder of the peaks in the figure represent absorption of frequencies by protons in other chemical milieus, and therefore they are shifted a certain amount (usually 1–13 ppm for ^{1}H NMR) from that absorbed by the TMS protons.

It is possible to obtain NMR spectra by either maintaining a constant magnetic field and varying the frequency of the radio waves produced, or holding the radio frequency constant and changing the strength of the magnetic field. Both configurations require similar equipment, but for ease of explanation we will

[3]DL in poly(DL-lactic acid) refers to a racemic mixture of enantiomeric repeating units of L-lactic acid and D-lactic acid. In general, polymers of enantiomeric monomers may possess different physical properties from their racemic counterparts because of their ordered configuration.

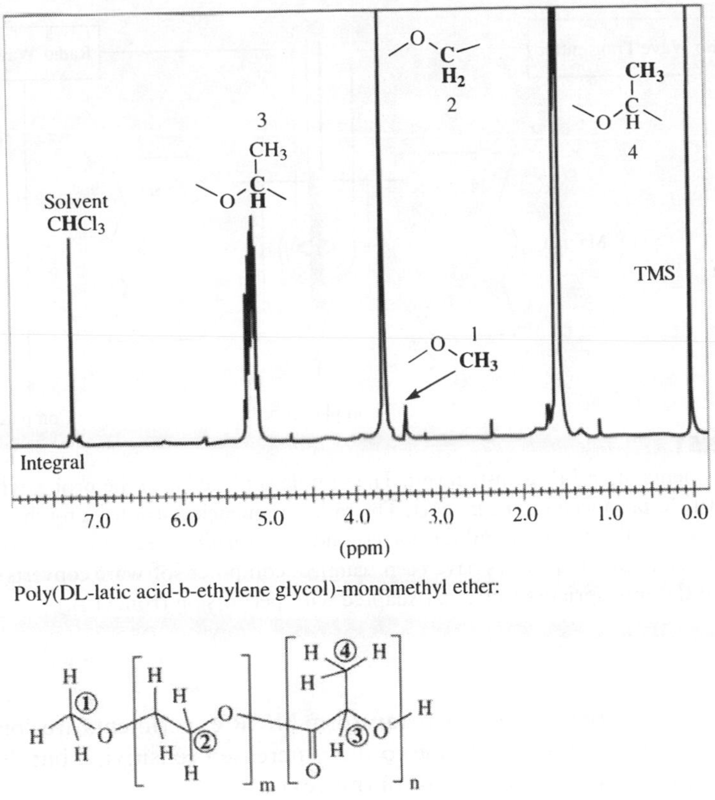

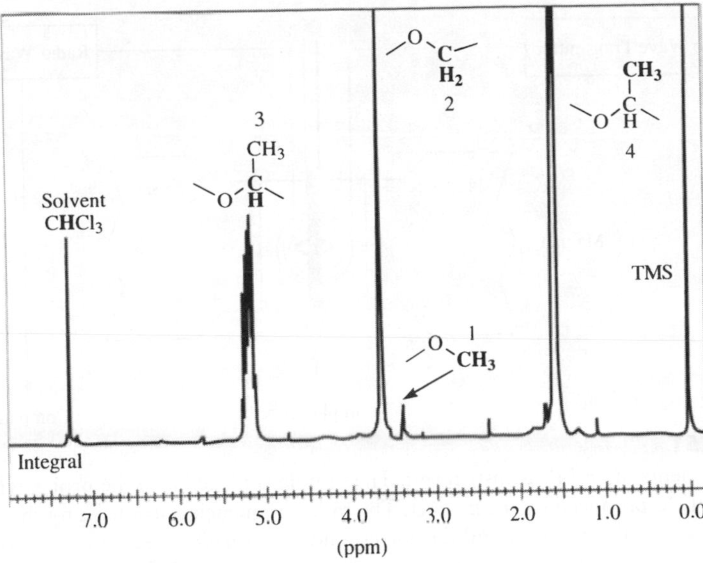

Poly(DL-latic acid-b-ethylene glycol)-monomethyl ether:

Figure 2.50
^{1}H-NMR spectrum of a poly(DL-lactic acid-b-ethylene glycol)-monomethyl ether diblock copolymer. Although it is somewhat difficult to obtain absolute values for the x-axis of a NMR spectrum, it is easier to determine relative shifts in resonance frequency as compared to a standard included with the sample (an internal standard). In many cases, this reference material is tetramethylsilane (TMS), $(CH_3)_4Si$, which produces the large peak seen at 0 ppm. As evidenced by the various peaks (1–4), the environment of the individual H atoms produces alterations in localized magnetic fields, resulting in different shifts that allow chemical structures to be distinguished. (Adapted with permission from [18].)

focus our attention on the former. There are five basic components to a NMR instrument, as shown in Fig. 2.51:

1. Magnet—produces a strong, uniform magnetic field.
2. Sample probe—allows for insertion of the sample into the magnetic field.
3. Radio wave transmitter—produces radio waves at a variety of frequencies.
4. Radio wave receiver/detector—converts the radio frequencies not absorbed by the sample into an electrical signal.
5. Processor (computer)—translates the output from the detector into the appropriate spectrum.

As shown in the diagram (Fig. 2.51), the sample is placed into the probe, which holds it in a constant field produced by the magnet. The radio frequencies produced by the transmitter are varied in a controlled manner, and the corresponding returning frequencies are recorded by the detector. After all the frequencies have been scanned, a computer converts the sample response into the appropriate spectrum.

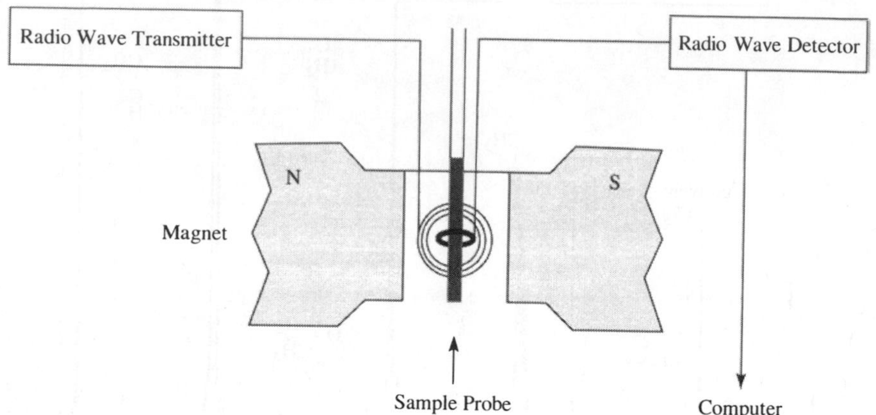

Figure 2.51
The components of an NMR instrument. The sample is placed into the probe, which holds it in a constant field produced by the magnet. The radio frequencies produced by the transmitter are varied in a controlled manner, and the corresponding returning frequencies are recorded by the detector. After all the frequencies have been scanned, computer software converts the sample response into the appropriate spectrum. (Adapted with permission from [14].)

Similar to IR spectroscopy, Fourier-transform NMR experiments are commonly performed in modern laboratories due to their increased sensitivity, but description of such techniques is beyond the scope of this text.

2.5.4.3 Information Provided NMR is a powerful tool for elucidating the structure of inorganic and organic molecules. Samples can be examined for the presence of certain types of bonds using characteristic chemical shifts for different groups, as listed in Table 2.10. Also, the relative amounts of atoms in various chemical states can be easily obtained. One of the most common uses of NMR in the biomaterials field is to characterize a polymer after a synthesis reaction to assure product quality and purity.

2.5.5 Mass Spectrometry

2.5.5.1 Basic Principles Despite the similarity of name and plot produced (also called a spectrum), mass spectrometry is not a type of spectroscopy, like X-ray, UV-VIS, IR or NMR, because it does not involve measuring the absorption of electromagnetic radiation. Instead, it determines the atomic or molecular masses of various species in a material. In order to accomplish this, the sample is first ionized though bombardment with high-energy particles (usually electrons). The resulting charged species are forced through a magnetic field, which interacts with them to deflect them from a linear path. Because lighter species are deflected more than heavier ones, the particles can be separated based on mass.[4] This technique is extremely sensitive to differences in mass, and can even distinguish between isotopes of the same element.

2.5.5.2 Instrumentation A typical mass spectrum of poly(methyl methacrylate) is found in Fig. 2.52. Mass spectra are generally plotted as relative intensity (y-axis) as

[4]Technically, in mass spectrometers, species are sorted on their mass to charge ratio (m/z ratio). However, since the ions often have a charge of $+1$ or -1, this is generally equivalent to separation by mass.

TABLE 2.10

Characteristic NMR Shifts for Common Chemical Groups

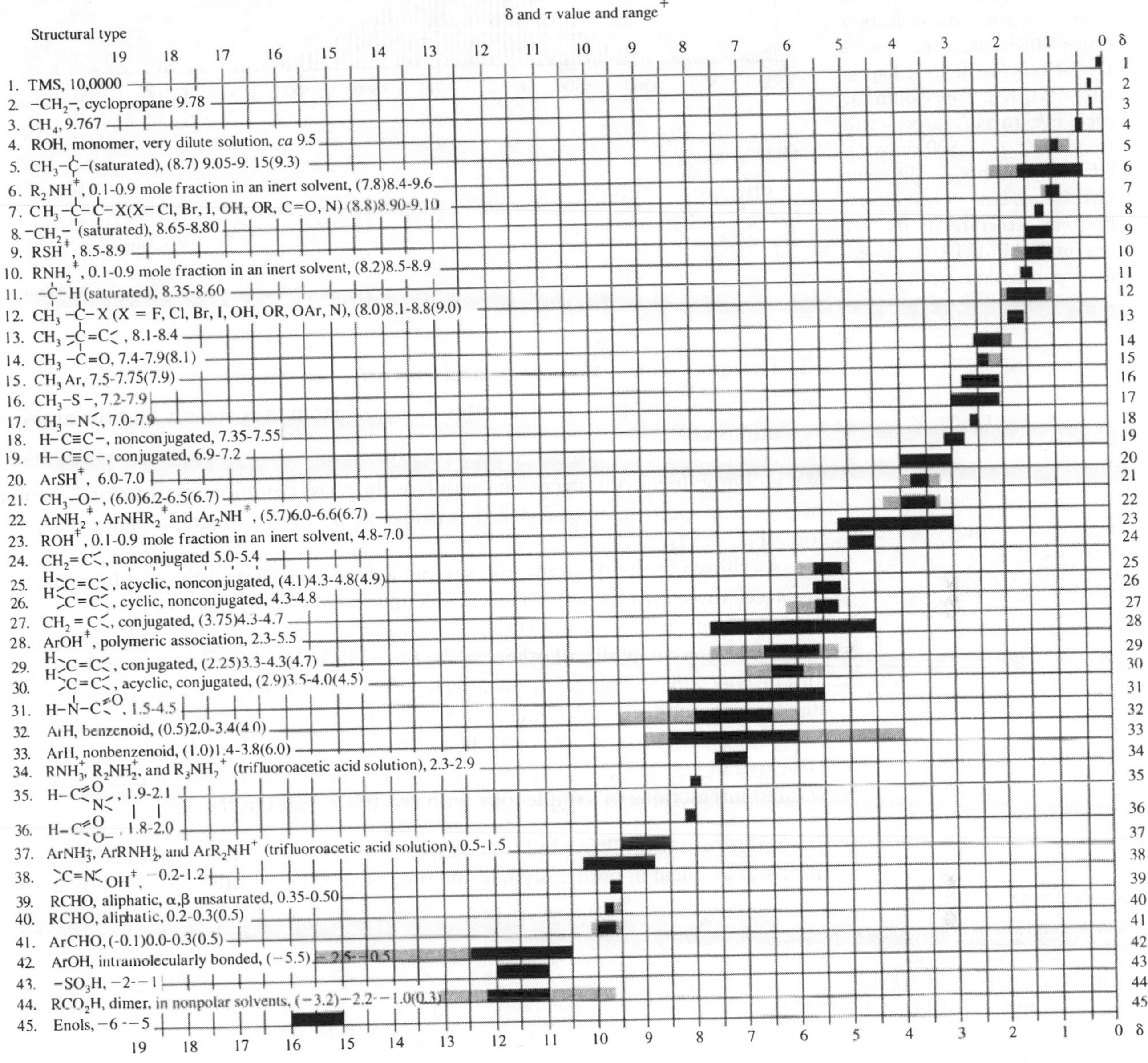

†Normally, absorptions for the functional groups indicated will be found within the range shown. Occasionally, a functional group will absorb outside this range. Approximate limits for this are indicated by absorption values in parentheses and by shading in the figure.

‡The absorption positions of these groups are concentration-dependent and are shifted to higher τ values in more dilute solutions.

(Adapted with permission from [19].)

a function of mass (x-axis). As with traditional spectroscopy techniques, a number of mass spectrometers have been developed. There are four basic components to a mass spectrometer, as shown in Figs. 2.53 and 2.54:

1. Inlet/ionization chamber—allows for insertion of the sample and its ionization via bombardment by high-energy particles.
2. Mass analyzer—uses a magnetic or electric field to separate the resulting ions based on mass.

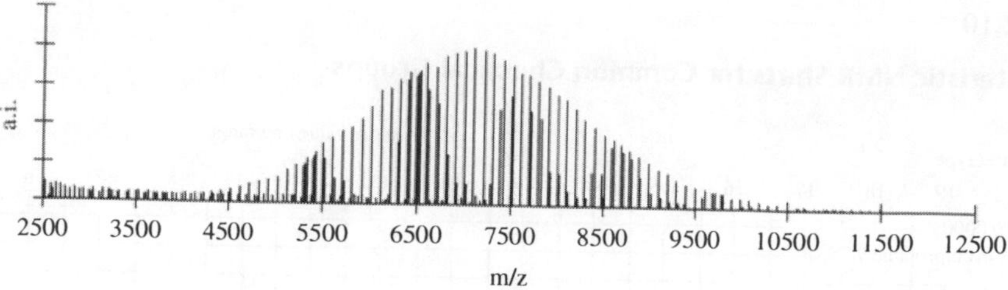

Figure 2.52
Spectrum from a type of mass spectrometry (matrix-assisted laser desorption/ionization time-of-flight mass spectrometry) of poly(methyl methacrylate) (PMMA). Top: Counts at each m/z (mass/charge) ratio from 2500 to 12,500 showing relative amounts of different PMMA ion fragments. Bottom: Structure of the repeat unit of PMMA. (Adapted with permission from [20].)

3. Detector—converts the impact of ions after separation into an electrical signal.
4. Processor (computer)—translates the signal from the detector into the appropriate spectrum.

We will now focus our attention on one of the most common instruments: the magnetic sector spectrometer, so called because it uses only a magnetic field to separate ions (Fig. 2.54).

As shown in the diagram, the sample is first ionized and the resulting particles are accelerated into the mass analyzer chamber. Because of the geometry of the mass analyzer and the strength of the magnet, only ions with a certain mass are allowed to hit the detector, while all others strike the walls of the chamber (see path of lighter and heavier ions in Fig. 2.54). By altering the magnetic field in a controlled manner, the detector can record the amount of ions having various masses. At the end of the sweep of magnetic field strength, the entire spectrum is plotted for that sample. As indicated in Fig. 2.53, mass spectrometry is performed under vacuum to prevent unwanted interactions of sample ions with reactive species in the air.

2.5.5.3 Information Provided Mass spectrometry can provide qualitative and quantitative assessment of both inorganic and organic molecules, although, for biomaterials,

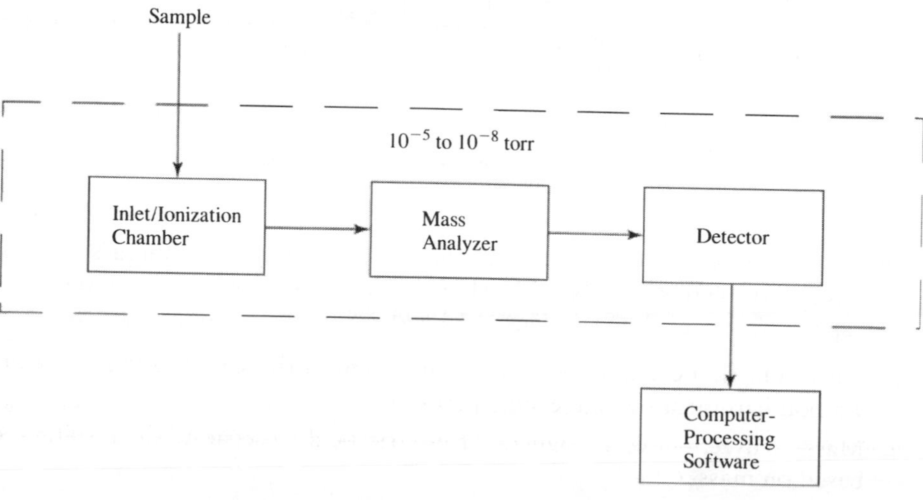

Figure 2.53
Block diagram of components of a mass spectrometer. The four basic components are the inlet/ionization chamber (allows for insertion of the sample and its ionization via bombardment by high-energy particles), the mass analyzer (uses a magnetic or electric field to separate the resulting ions based on mass), the detector (converts the impact of ions after separation into an electrical signal) and the processor/computer (translates the signal from the detector into the appropriate spectrum). (Adapted with permission from [12].)

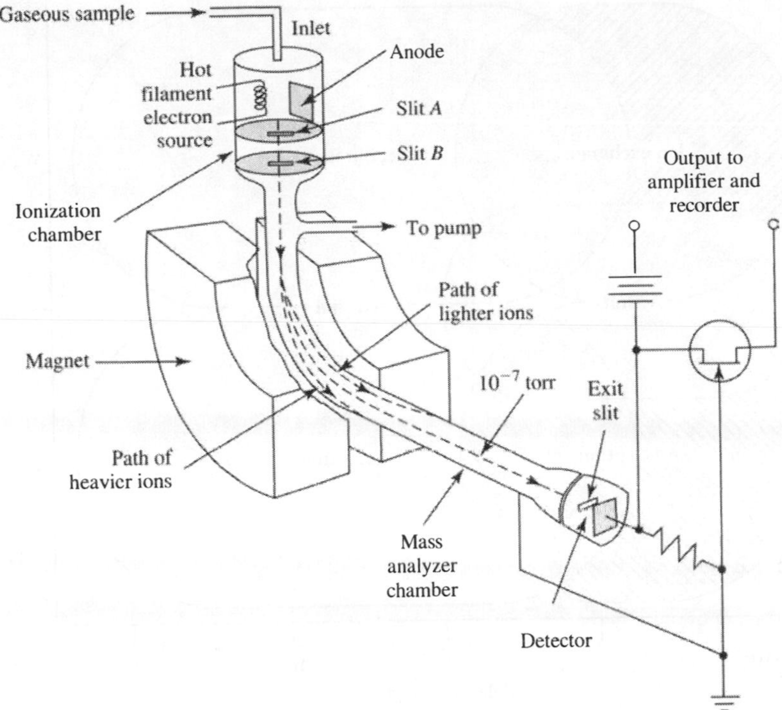

Figure 2.54
Schematic of a mass spectrometer. The sample is first ionized and the resulting particles are accelerated into the mass analyzer chamber. Because of the geometry of the mass analyzer and the strength of the magnet, only ions with a certain mass are allowed to hit the detector, while all others strike the walls of the chamber. By altering the magnetic field in a controlled manner, the detector can record the amount of ions having various masses. At the end of the sweep of magnetic field strength, the entire spectrum is plotted for that sample. (Adapted with permission from [12].)

it is primarily used for analysis of natural and synthetic polymers. In particular, this is one of the few methods that allows identification of isotope ratios within a substance. By examining the type of ions produced after bombardment, it is also possible to gain insight into the strength of various bonds in the molecule. Mass spectrometry can be combined with other methods, particularly chromatographic techniques, to provide more information about the separated compounds. A variant of this method, secondary ion mass spectrometry (SIMS), is often used for surface analysis of biomaterials, as discussed further in Chapter 7.

2.5.6 High-Performance Liquid Chromatography (HPLC): Size-Exclusion Chromatography

Like mass spectrometry, chromatography provides information based on separation of substances by chemical properties such as size or charge. Our discussion will focus on liquid chromatography, since this is the technique most commonly used for analysis of biomaterials, particularly natural and synthetic polymers. As shown in Fig. 2.55, there are many different types of liquid chromatography, but we will focus in this section on **size-exclusion chromatography** (SEC), which encompasses gel permeation and gel filtration chromatography. Affinity chromatography will be described in Chapter 8.

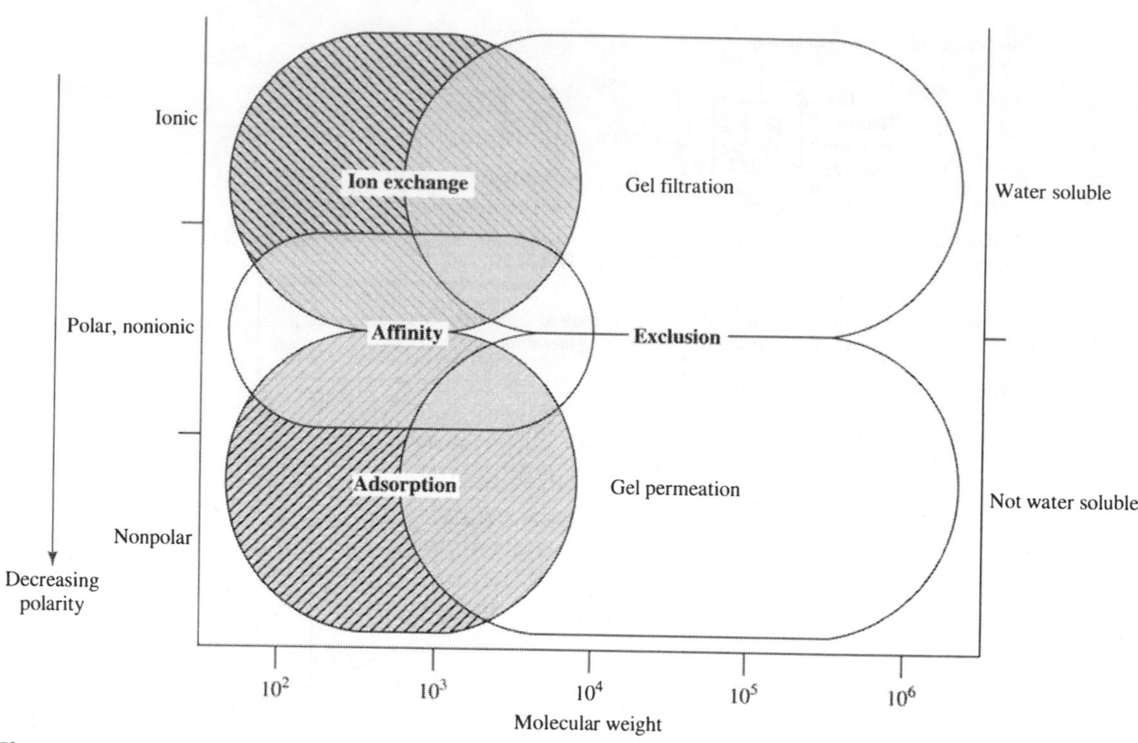

Figure 2.55
Classes of liquid chromatography. Chromatography provides information based on separation of substances by chemical properties such as size or charge.

2.5.6.1 Basic Principles SEC is based on the simple concept of filtration by size. A SEC system contains both a mobile and a stationary phase. The mobile phase is a liquid solvent into which the dissolved sample is injected. The stationary phase is composed of small (diameter ~10 μm) porous silica or polymer beads. The network of uniformly sized pores in the beads is open so that the sample and solvent can enter as the mobile phase is circulated through the system. While the analyte is in the porous structure, it is removed from the flow of the mobile phase and is thus considered to be **retained** in the stationary phase.

Retention time is highly affected by the size of the analyte. Molecules that are larger than the average pore size cannot enter and thus are not retained by the beads, while those that are very small can penetrate into the network and remain there for some time. Therefore, the first species to exit the stationary phase is the molecule with the largest size (highest molecular weight), and the smallest molecular weight compound exits (is **eluted**) last (Fig. 2.56). In between, molecules are retained for varying amounts of time depending on the extent of penetration of the porous network, which leads to separation of compounds by molecular weight.

2.5.6.2 Instrumentation Figure 2.57 is an example of a typical graph obtained from SEC analysis of poly(ethylene glycol) (PEG). Results are generally plotted as peak intensity (y-axis, units depend on type of detector) as a function of time (x-axis).

SEC can be divided into two subsets, both of which use the same instrumentation. **Gel filtration chromatography** (GFC) requires the use of aqueous solvents in the mobile phase and hydrophilic beads in the stationary phase. In contrast, **gel permeation chromatography** (GPC) employs organic solvents and a hydrophobic stationary phase.

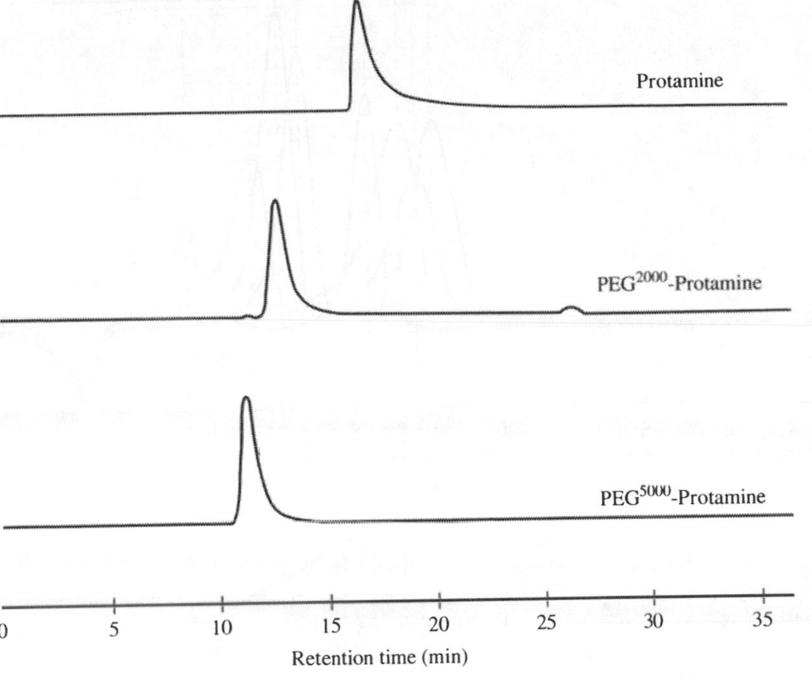

Figure 2.56
Size-exclusion chromatograms of a protein (protamine), the protein bonded to a synthetic polymer [poly(ethylene glycol) (PEG)] with a molecular weight of 2 kDa, and the protein bonded to PEG of 5 kDa. In size-exclusion chromatography, higher molecular weight substances are eluted earlier than smaller molecules. (Adapted with permission from [21].)

There are five basic components to an HPLC (SEC) instrument, as shown in Fig. 2.58:

1. Pump—causes circulation of the mobile phase.
2. Injector—injects a given amount of sample into the mobile phase.
3. Column—separates different sized molecules based on retention time.
4. Detector—translates the amount of analyte in the mobile phase to an electrical signal.
5. Processor (computer)— converts the signal from the detector into plots of peak intensity over time.

There are a wide variety of detectors for HPLC (SEC), many of which are based on techniques previously discussed, such as UV or IR (see above). Mass spectrometers as detectors are less common, but have found uses in certain systems. It should be noted that, in this list, "detector" is not used in the same manner as in lists of components for spectroscopy (see above). Here, the detector refers to the entire spectrophotometer, not just the device that converts transmitted light to an electrical signal.

The sample is injected into the mobile phase of the system, a degassed solvent. Degassing is required to prevent any bubbles from becoming trapped in the instrument. The solvent and analyte are then pumped through a separation column at a constant flow rate. The sample is retained through interactions with the beads packing the column until it finally reaches the end, where it passes through the detector. After all of the sample has exited the column, processing software produces a plot of peak intensity vs. time.

2.5.6.3 Information Provided A main use of SEC is to determine the molecular weight of synthetic and natural polymers. This can be done in a quantitative manner using standards of the polymer of interest with known molecular weights. As explained

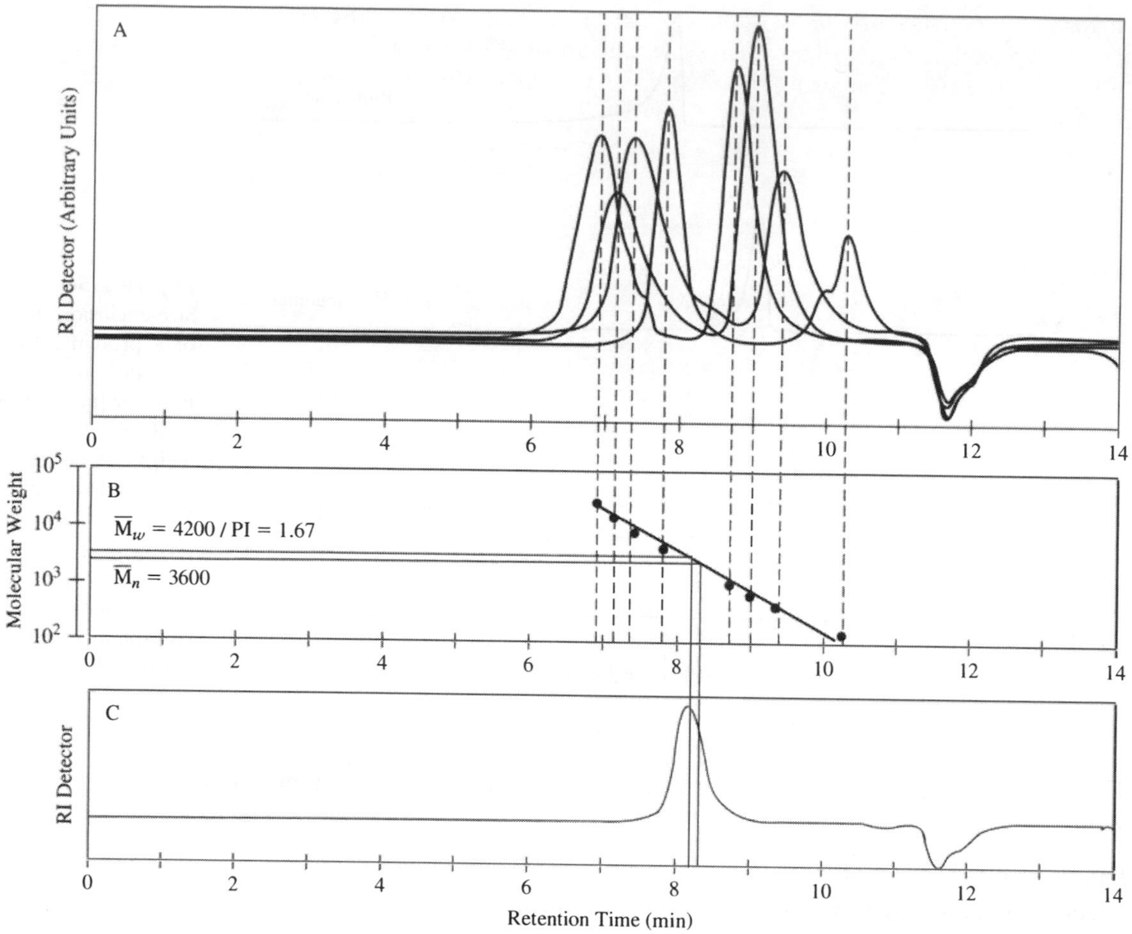

Figure 2.57

Results from SEC analysis of poly(ethylene glycol) (PEG). (A) Size-exclusion chromatographs of eight PEG standards of known molecular weight. This data can then be used to create a calibration curve (B), which is used to determine the weight ($\overline{M}_w$) and number ($\overline{M}_n$) average molecular weight of an unknown sample. To generate the calibration curve, the retention time for each peak of the known samples is plotted against their known molecular weight [as seen in (B)]. An unknown sample can then be run through the SEC (C), and using the retention time and the calibration curve created in (B), the $\overline{M}_w$ and $\overline{M}_n$ of the sample can be determined. The sample's polydispersity index (*PI*) can then be calculated from $\overline{M}_w/\overline{M}_n$.

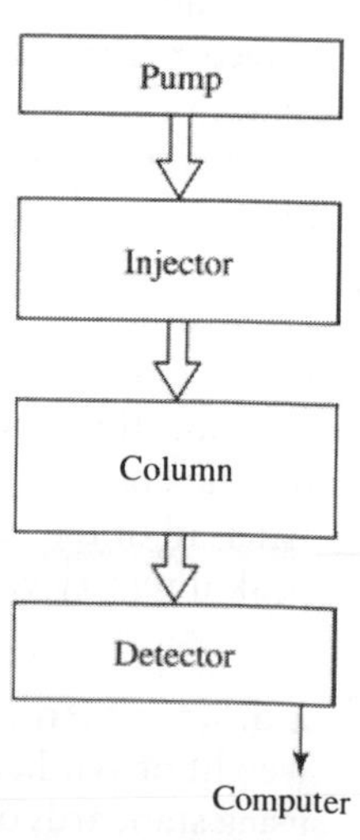

Figure 2.58

Block diagram of components of an HPLC instrument (SEC). The basic components are the pump (causes circulation of the mobile phase), the injector (injects a given amount of sample into the mobile phase), the column (separates different sized molecules based on retention time), the detector (translates the amount of analyte in the mobile phase to an electrical signal), and the processor/computer (converts the signal from the detector into plots of peak intensity over time). It should be noted that, here, the "detector" refers to the entire spectrophotometer, not just the device that converts transmitted light to an electrical signal. (Adapted with permission from [14].)

above for UV-VIS spectroscopy, a standard curve of molecular weight vs. time can be created (Fig. 2.57). By comparing the elution time for the unknown sample to that on the standard curve, the molecular weight of the unknown can be determined.

A curve generated via SEC for a polymer sample is really a version of the graphs of weight or number fraction vs. molecular weight seen in section 2.4.1.2 (Fig. 2.22). Because of this, software programs use similar methods to those described earlier to calculate values for $\overline{M}_n$, $\overline{M}_w$, and PI. This includes determination of the fraction of the total polymer that is eluted between two elution times as well as the average molecular weight for that fraction (using the values from the standard curve). Once this information is determined, equations are used to calculate the desired values. SEC is often employed as a means to monitor polymerization and/or assure the consistency of a product from a synthesis reaction.

Summary

- The molecular structure of a material can be classified as crystalline if the constituent atoms are arranged in such a manner that long-range order is present on the molecular level. Alternatively, materials that lack such long-range order can be classified as amorphous. Various materials, including some polymers, contain both crystalline and amorphous regions and are called semicrystalline.
- Both metals and ceramic materials are crystalline; however, due to the ionic nature of ceramics, the crystal structures are thought of as being composed of ions rather than atoms. A wider range of crystal structures are possible in ceramics than in metals, due to the vast variety of chemical compositions possible in ceramic materials. Ceramic materials can have AX crystal structures, in which the anion and cation have the same charge, or A_mX_p crystal structures, in which the charges are not equal. Carbon-based materials such as graphite and single walled carbon nanotubes can be considered to be ceramics.
- Various crystal structures can be characterized by their unit cells and represented by their lattice structures. Seven primary combinations of the lattice parameters (a, b and c) and angles (α, β and γ) describe the most common crystal systems; namely, cubic, tetragonal, orthorhombic, rhombohedral, hexagonal, monoclinic and triclinic. Miller indices can be used to notate points and planes in a lattice structure.
- Crystal structures in metals and ceramics typically contain various defects and impurities that can affect the chemical and mechanical properties of the material. Point defects in metals include vacancies (absent atoms) and self-interstitials (extra atoms) in the crystal structure. An impurity (solute) can fill spaces between the host metal (solvent) in interstitial solutions or replace solvent atoms in substitutional solutions. The atomic radii, electronegativities, and valence charges of the atoms involved strongly influence the type of impurities that may occur. Alloys are an example of materials in which impurities have been introduced in a controlled manner to impart beneficial properties.

- One type of defect in ceramic materials is the Schottky defect, in which the vacancies in both anions and cations are in the correct ratio to maintain neutrality. Frenkel defects are found in the creation of a vacancy/interstitial pair to maintain electroneutrality in a ceramic material. As with metals, impurities can be found in ceramics, but the charge of the host material and of the impurity strongly influence the stability of the impurities.
- The transport of material by atomic motion is known as diffusion. Diffusion that occurs in solid materials is known as solid state diffusion and can include vacancy and interstitial diffusion. In the case of steady-state diffusion, diffusion flux (J) does not change with time.
- Polymeric materials are generally long chains based upon covalently bonded hydrocarbons. The smallest building block of a polymer is a mer, a fixed number of atoms in a given structure that is repeated over and over to form the polymer. A large variety of mechanical and chemical properties are possible with polymeric materials.
- A number of reaction mechanisms can result in polymer production from the constituent monomers, including addition polymerization and condensation polymerization mechanisms. Addition polymerization reactions, which can involve either an activated radical (free radical polymerization) or ionic moiety (ionic polymerization), involve a number of distinct steps. Condensation polymerization occurs through the elimination of a molecule (usually water). Additionally, proteins such as silk and elastin can be polymerized through genetic engineering approaches using a host organism.
- Polymers can be crystalline, amorphous, or semicrystalline and can contain point defects in the form of vacancies between polymer chain ends. Parameters such as the chemical composition, tacticity and degree of branching of a polymer strongly influence the ability of the polymer to form crystals. Bulky side groups along the polymer chain as well as high degrees of polymer branching impede the ability of the chains to reside close enough to one another to form crystal structures.
- Various techniques may be employed to characterize the chemical composition of a biomaterial. One broad class of techniques is spectroscopy, in which the absorption of different types of energy by the compound of interest is measured. Examples of spectroscopic techniques include X-ray diffraction, ultraviolet and visible light spectroscopy, infrared spectroscopy, nuclear magnetic resonance spectroscopy and mass spectrometry. Another broad class of techniques of characterization is chromatography, in which molecules are physically separated based upon chemical characteristics, such as charge or molecular weight. Examples of chromatographic techniques include gel permeation chromatography and gel filtration chromatography.

Problems

2.1 You are evaluating a variety of new materials for use in the femoral stem of a hip joint replacement.

(a) A diagram of the crystal structure of materials (a) and (b) are shown below. Identify each crystal structure. For each structure calculate the coordination number, derive the relation between r (radius of sphere) and a (length of cube side), and determine the APF of each.

(a) (b)

(b) You are given a third material (c), which has not been characterized. What analytical technique would you use to determine the crystal structure and unit cell size?

(c) You determine that material (c) has a hexagonal close-packed structure, which is shown below. Calculate the APF of this material. The c-to-a ratio is 1.633. (Note: The center layer consists of the equivalent of three total atoms within the unit cell, and the radius of the atom is r.)

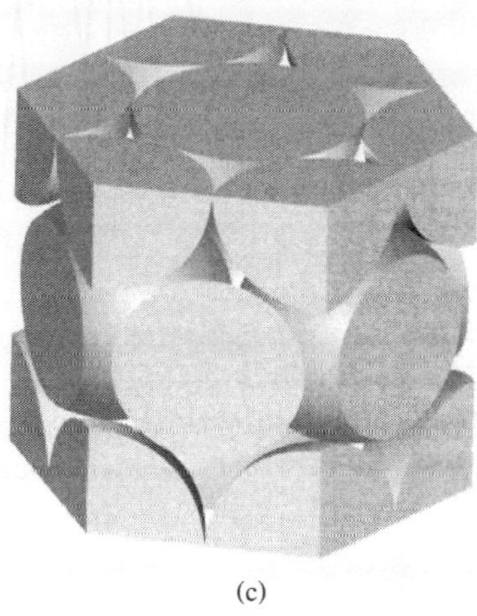

(c)

(d) Would you be likely to find interstitial defects in any of these three materials? Why?

2.2 You are examining a copolymer for its potential as a material for a vascular graft. You are trying to determine whether you want a high or low degree of crystallinity in the material. What type of structures for copolymers have a higher probability for crystallization?

2.3 Poly(ε-capralactone) is being considered as a potential material for a vascular graft. After a particular batch has been made, someone gives you the following fractional distribution data and asks you to calculate $\overline{M}_n$, $\overline{M}_w$ and PI for this polymer:

W_i	0.10	0.10	0.30	0.40	0.10
M_i (kg/mol)	25	30	40	70	100

2.4 You are given four additional polymeric materials (A, B, C, D) to examine for potential as a vascular graft material, and you are told to use size-exclusion chromatography to determine the approximate molecular weights of the unknown polymers. You obtain the following information for the first three samples (A, B, C):

(a) Assuming monodisperse samples, what is the molecular weight of each?
Standard 1: Molecular weight 50,000 g/mol
Standard 2: Molecular weight 40,000 g/mol
Standard 3: Molecular weight 35,000 g/mol
Standard 4: Molecular weight 20,000 g/mol
Standard 5: Molecular weight 10,000 g/mol
Unknown A: Peak amount polymer eluted at 7.4 min
Unknown B: Peak amount polymer eluted at 8.4 min
Unknown C: Peak amount polymer eluted at 9.6 min

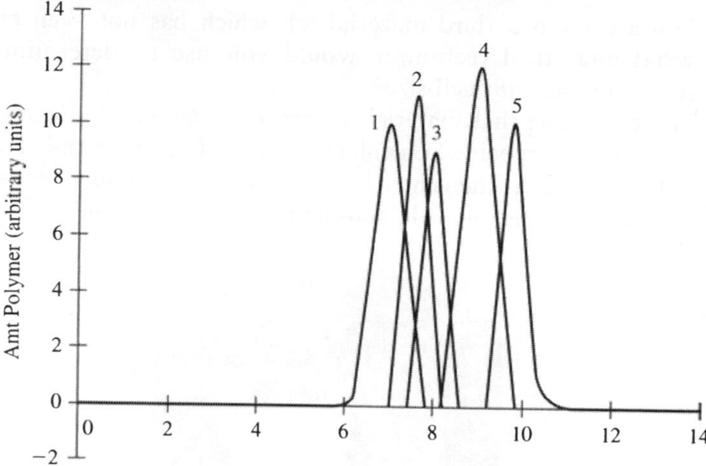

(b) A problem commonly encountered in SEC is overloading of the chromatography column by injection of a highly concentrated sample, which results in broadening of the peak on the chromatogram. You injected a highly concentrated sample of unknown D into the chromatography column. Which

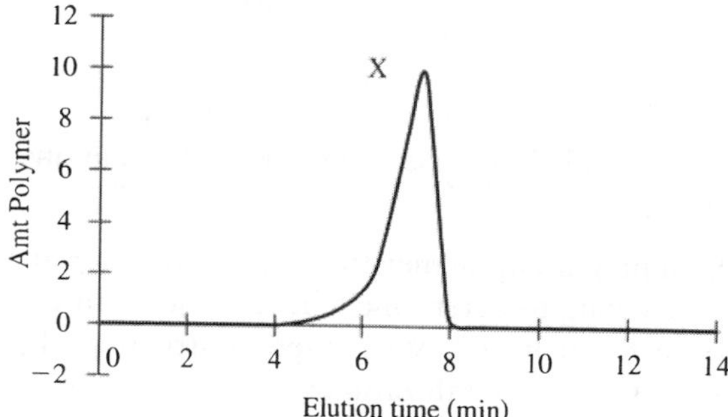

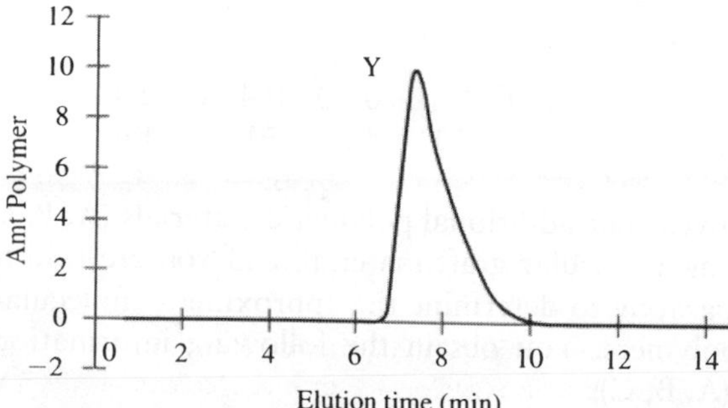

of the following curves would result? Pick X or Y and describe why, based on molecular interactions of the sample with the column.

2.5 Calculate the Miller indices for the following planes and include the steps necessary to arrive at your conclusion. (Note: $x = a$ axis, $y = b$ axis, $z = c$ axis)

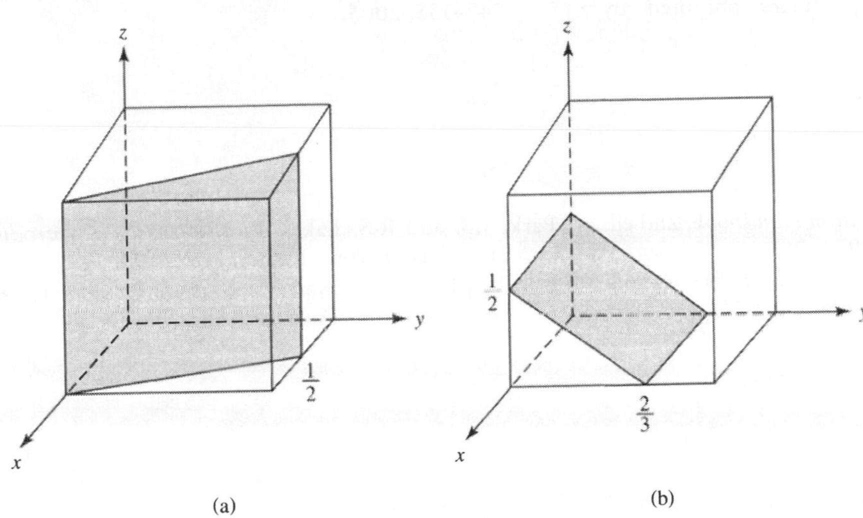

References

1. Shackelford, J.F. *Introduction to Materials Science for Engineers*, 5th ed. Upper Saddle River: Prentice Hall, 2000.
2. Shackelford, J.F., *Introduction to Materials Science for Engineers*, 4th ed. Upper Saddle River: Prentice Hall, 1996.
3. Atkins, P. and L. Jones, *Chemistry: Molecules, Matter, and Change*, 3rd ed, New York: Freeman, 1997.
4. Callister, Jr., W.D. *Materials Science and Engineering: An Introduction*, 3rd ed. New York: John Wiley and Sons, 1994.
5. Schaffer, J.P., A. Saxena, S.D. Antolovich, T.H. Sanders Jr., and S.B. Warner. *The Science and Design of Engineering Materials*, 2nd ed. Boston: McGraw-Hill, 1999.
6. Kingery, W.D., et al., *Introduction to Ceramics*, 2nd ed. New York: John Wiley & Sons, 1976.
7. Engelberg, I. and J. Kohn. "Physico-Mechanical Properties of Degradable Polymers Used in Medical Applications: A Comparative Study," in *Biomaterials*, vol. 12, pp. 292–304, 1991.
8. Askeland, Donald R. *The Science and Engineering of Materials*, 2nd edition, Boston: PWS-KENT Publishing Company, 1989.
9. Treloar, L.R.G., *The Physics of Rubber Elasticity*, 2nd ed, Oxford: Oxford University Press, 1958.
10. Odian, G. *Principles of Polymerization*, 3rd ed. New York: John Wiley and Sons, 1991.
11. Ray, W.H. and R.L. Laurence. "Polymerization Reaction Engineering," in *Chemical Reactor Theory: A Review*, L. Lapidus and N.R. Amundson, Eds. Englewood Cliffs: Prentice Hall, pp. 532–582, 1977.
12. Skoog, D.A. and J.J. Leary. *Principles of Instrumental Analysis*, 4th ed. Orlando: Saunders College Publishing, 1992.
13. Lavik, E.B., J.S. Hrkach, N. Lotan, R. Nazarov, and R. Langer. "A Simple Synthetic Route to the Formation of a Block Copolymer of Poly(Lactic-Co-Glycolic Acid) and Polylysine for the Fabrication of Functionalized, Degradable Structures for Biomedical Applications," in *Journal of Biomedical Materials Research*, vol. 58, pp. 291–294, 2001.
14. Rouessac, F. and A. Rouessac. *Chemical Analysis: Modern Instrumental Methods and Techniques*. New York: John Wiley and Sons, 2000.
15. SDBS, National Institute of Advanced Industrial Science and Technology(Japan).
16. Mellott, M.B., K. Searcy, and M.V. Pishko. "Release of Protein from Highly Cross-Linked Hydrogels of Poly(Ethylene Glycol) Diacrylate Fabricated by UV Polymerization," in *Biomaterials*, vol. 22, pp. 929–941, 2001.
17. Vollhardt, K.P.C. and N.E. Schore. *Organic Chemistry*, 2nd ed. New York: W. H. Freeman, 1994.
18. Lucke, A., J. Tessmar, E. Schnell, G. Schmeer, and A. Gopferich. "Biodegradable Poly(D,L-Lactic Acid)-Poly(Ethylene Glycol)-Monomethyl Ether Diblock Copolymers: Structures and Surface Properties Relevant

to Their Use as Biomaterials," in *Biomaterials*, vol. 21, pp. 2361–2370, 2000.

19. Taylor, *Applications of Absorption Spectroscopy by Organic Compounds*. Englewood Clifffs, NJ: Prentice Hall, 1965.
20. Wetzel, SJ, CM, Guttman, JE Girad, "The influnce of matrix and laser energy on the molecular mass distribution of synthetic polymers obtained by MALDI-TOFMS," *Int J.Mass Spect*, vol 238, pp.215–225, 2004.
21. Chang, L.C., H.F. Lee, M.J. Chung, and V.C. Yang. "PEG-Modified Protamine with Improved Pharmacological/Pharmaceutical Properties as a Potential Protamine Substitute: Synthesis and in Vitro Evaluation," in *Bioconjugate Chemistry*, vol. 16, pp. 147–155, 2005.

Additional Reading

Ewing, G.W *Analytical Instrumentation Handbook*, 2nd ed. New York: Marcel Dekker, 1997.

Park, J.B. and J.D. Bronzino. *Biomaterials: Principles and Applications*. Boca Raton: CRC Press, 2003.

Park, J.B. and R.S. Lakes. *Biomaterials: An Introduction*, 2nd ed. New York: Plenum Press, 1992.

Rabek, J.F. *Experimental Methods in Polymer Chemistry*. New York: John Wiley and Sons, 1980.

Physical Properties of Biomaterials

CHAPTER 3

Main Objective

To understand how material subunits from Chapter 2 interact to make bulk materials and to comprehend how the thermal treatment of various materials affects their three-dimensional structure.

Specific Objectives

1. To compare and contrast linear, planar and volume defects in crystals.
2. To draw and use Burger's vector notation to determine type of linear dislocations.
3. To understand how dislocations lead to the possibility of material deformation for crystalline materials and to contrast this with deformation in amorphous materials (viscous flow).
4. To compare and contrast the types of planar defects in crystals and understand how their presence affects chemical reactivity of the material.
5. To give examples and uses for three-dimensional (volume) defects.
6. To understand models for crystalline structure in polymers.
7. To understand the difference between the types of thermal transitions for crystalline and noncrystalline materials.
8. To understand the basic theory behind differential scanning calorimetry (a thermal analysis technique).

3.1 Introduction: From Atomic Groupings to Bulk Materials

In this chapter, we move from how atoms interact to make biomaterial subunits to how the subunits interact to form bulk materials. For metals and ceramics, which are usually polycrystalline materials, the interactions of multiple crystals define the material's physical properties. Although the term "physical properties" can encompass a variety of characteristics, two of the most important for these materials are the amount and type of dislocations that occur within or between crystals. These characteristics, discussed in the first sections of this chapter, can affect mechanical properties and material processability (see Chapters 4 and 6).

For polymers, the subunits are sections of mers, and how they interact to create crystalline and amorphous regions also defines the physical properties of this material type. In this case, one of the most important physical characteristics is the percent crystallinity of the polymer. Polymer crystallinity, discussed in more detail later in the chapter, impacts mechanical and degradative properties of the final material (see Chapters 4 and 5).

Another key aspect of all materials is how their physical properties change in response to temperature. Thermal transitions of both crystalline and amorphous materials will be explained at the molecular level in the later sections of this chapter. These properties are particularly important to the processing of biomaterials (see Chapter 6).

3.2 Crystallinity and Linear Defects

As discussed in the previous chapter, crystalline materials contain point defects that can affect their mechanical properties. In addition, several other defect types that involve larger areas of the crystal are possible. These include linear defects and planar defects. It is estimated that, in a metallic material, only five atoms in 100,000,000 lie on a linear defect. However, despite their low occurrence, linear defects have a large impact on the final strength of the material. It is also important to note that the presence of these defects, particularly in metals, is what allows for their fabrication into complex shapes (see Chapter 6).

3.2.1 Dislocations

3.2.1.1 Edge Dislocations Crystals can possess several types of linear, or one-dimensional, defects. One of these is an **edge dislocation**, shown in Fig. 3.1. This occurs when an extra portion of a plane of atoms (half-plane) terminates in a crystal. In this case, the defect is actually the line that defines the end of the extra half-plane, called the **dislocation line**. In the figure, this line would be perpendicular to the

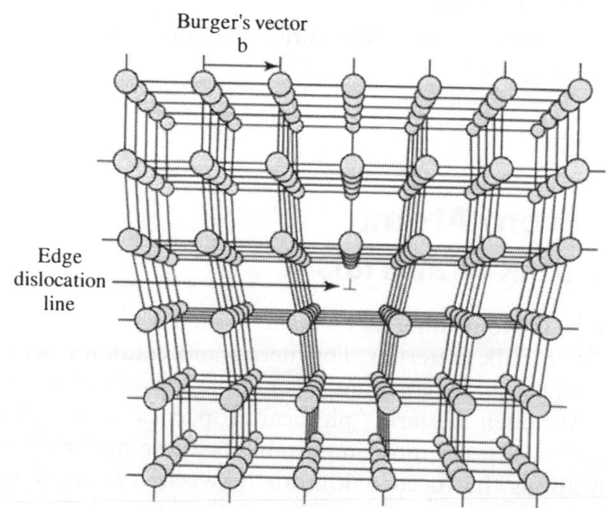

Figure 3.1
Schematic of an edge dislocation, a type of linear defect in crystals, which occurs when an extra portion of a plane of atoms (half-plane) terminates in a crystal. In this case, the defect is actually the line that defines the end of the extra half-plane, called the dislocation line; it would be perpendicular to the plane of the page. The symbol ⊥ is used to designate an edge dislocation, with the cross of the "⊥" representing the position of the dislocation line. (Adapted with permission from [1].)

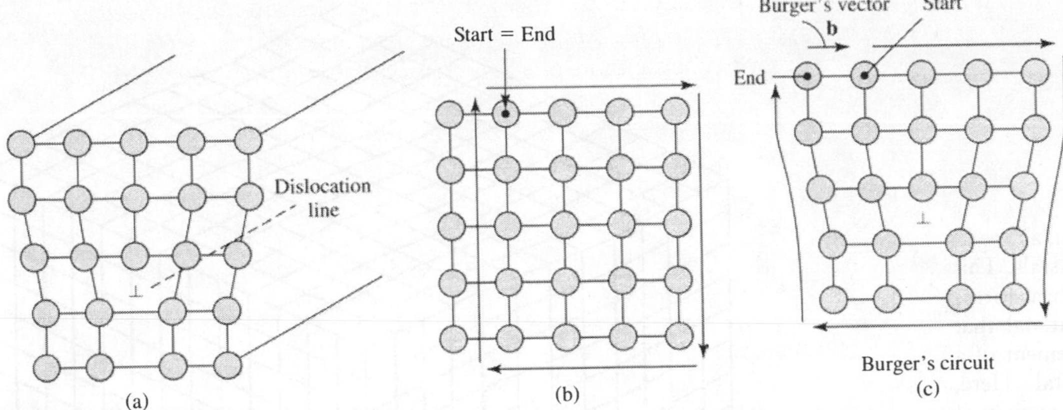

Figure 3.2
Depiction of Burger's vector. An edge dislocation is shown in (a), compared to the defect-free section seen in (b). The magnitude and direction of atomic displacement in a linear defect can be ascertained by drawing a circuit around the area of the crystal containing the dislocation. This circuit has the same number of atomic steps as for a similar circuit in a defect-free region. Therefore, the circuit should close on itself, except for the presence of the defect. However, due to the defect, an additional vector (Burger's vector) must be drawn to complete the atomic circuit (c). (Adapted with permission from [1].)

plane of the page. The symbol ⊥ is used to designate an edge dislocation, with the cross of the "⊥" representing the position of the dislocation line. The addition of the half-plane of atoms in a crystal can occur for a variety of reasons, including accidents in the crystal growth process, internal stresses from other defects in the crystal, or the interaction of resident dislocations during plastic deformation (discussed in greater depth later in the chapter).

Two important characteristics of dislocations are the magnitude and direction of atomic displacement. These can be ascertained by drawing a circuit around the area of the crystal containing the dislocation. As depicted in Fig. 3.2, this circuit has the same number of atomic steps as a similar circuit in a defect-free region. Therefore, the circuit should close on itself, except for the presence of the defect. However, due to the defect, an additional vector must be drawn to complete the atomic circuit. This is called the **Burger's vector** (**b**) for that dislocation. For an edge dislocation, the Burger's vector is perpendicular to the dislocation line (Fig. 3.1).

3.2.1.2 Screw and Mixed Dislocations Another type of linear defect is the **screw dislocation.** This can be conceptualized as the result of shear forces on part of the material that caused the displacement of a portion of the crystal. In Fig. 3.3 a part of the top section of the crystal has been moved one atomic distance to the right relative to the bottom half of the crystal. This type of dislocation is so named because of the helical pattern that the planes of atoms follow around the dislocation line. A screw dislocation is indicated with a ↻ (Fig. 3.3), and, in this case, the Burger's vector is parallel to the dislocation line.

Most linear defects exhibit both edge and screw qualities and are called **mixed dislocations.** Such a dislocation is shown in Fig. 3.4. In between the two faces where the dislocation is neither pure screw nor pure edge, the defect has a mixed character. This is best demonstrated by examining the orientation of the Burger's vector, which remains constant for a given defect. For more complex defects, such as that in Fig. 3.4,

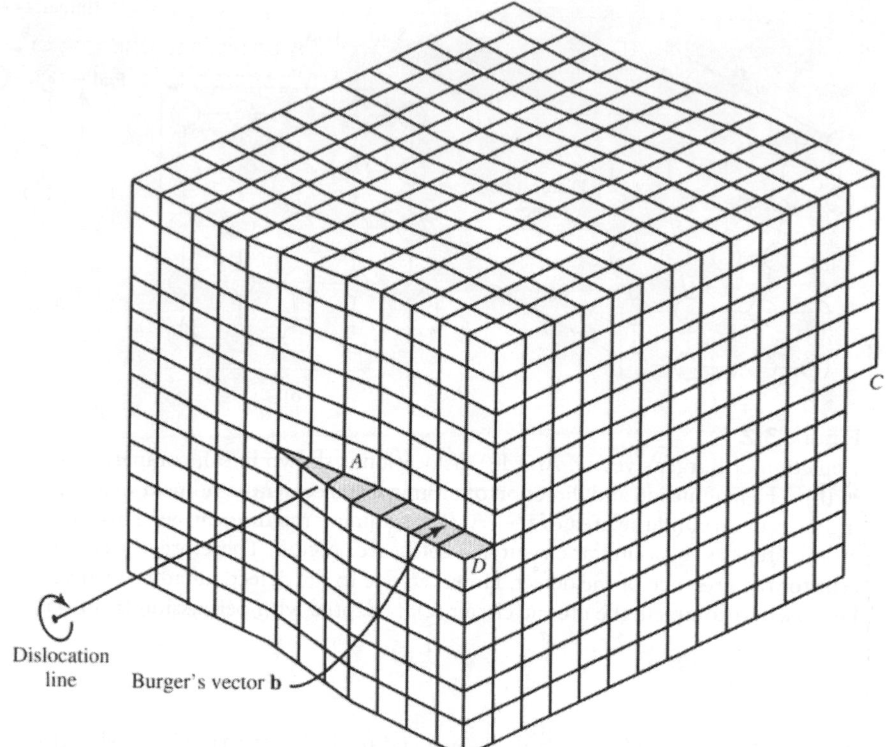

Figure 3.3
A screw dislocation, a type of linear defect in crystals. This can be caused by shear forces on part of the material that caused the displacement of a portion of the crystal. Here, a part of the top section of the crystal has been moved one atomic distance to the right relative to the bottom half of the crystal. This type of dislocation is so named because of the helical pattern that the planes of atoms follow around the dislocation line. A screw dislocation is indicated with a ↻. (Adapted with permission from [2].)

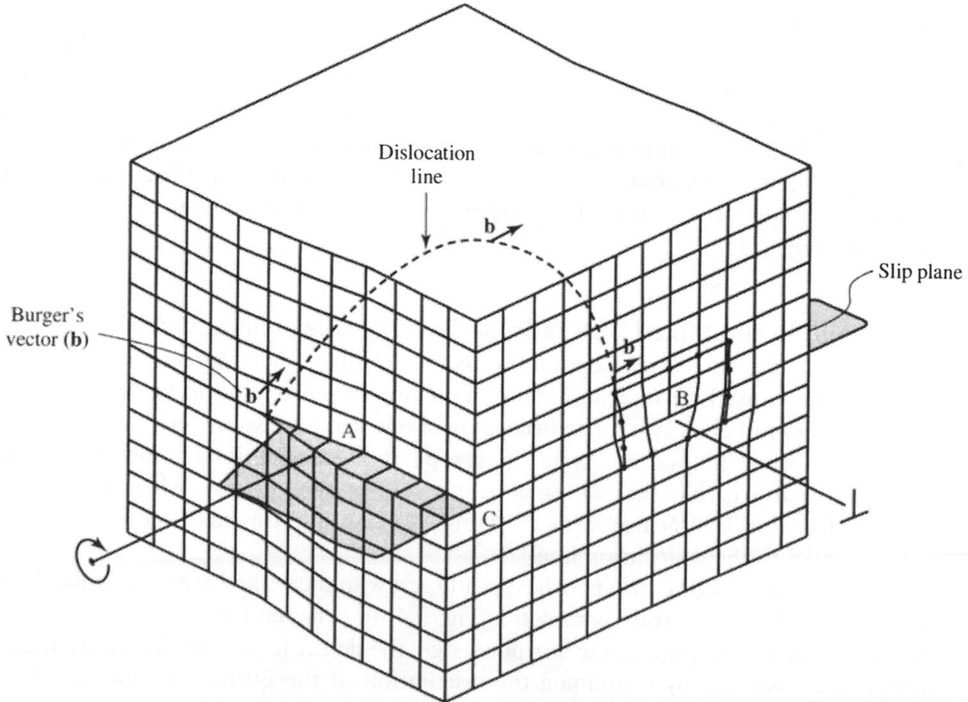

Figure 3.4
A mixed dislocation, a type of linear defect in crystals. The orientation of the dislocation line with respect to the Burger's vector changes in different areas of the crystal. For an edge dislocation, the dislocation line is perpendicular to the Burger's vector (section near point *B* in above figure) and for a screw dislocation the dislocation line is parallel to the Burger's vector (section near point *A* in above figure). When it is neither completely perpendicular nor completely parallel, this is the region of the mixed dislocation. (Adapted with permission from [2].)

the dislocation line changes so that it is oriented differently with respect to the Burger's vector in different areas of the crystal. When it is neither completely perpendicular nor completely parallel to the Burger's vector, this is the region of the mixed dislocation.

3.2.1.3 Characteristics of Dislocations There are a number of key characteristics associated with dislocations, no matter what their classification. These are summarized below:

1. Localized lattice strains develop as a result of the dislocation. For example, in an edge dislocation, the atoms above the dislocation line are compressed together, and those below are pulled apart.
2. The classification of a dislocation is dependent on the relationship between the Burger's vector and the dislocation line.
3. The Burger's vector is invariant (does not change for a given defect).
4. A dislocation cannot end in a defect-free region of a crystal. Instead, it ends on the crystal surface, on itself, or connects with another dislocation.
5. The plane on which a dislocation may move (slip) contains both the Burger's vector and the dislocation line and is a plane of high atomic density (see below for a discussion of slip planes).

EXAMPLE PROBLEM 3.1

Given the crystal structure illustrated below, locate the dislocation and draw the Burger's circuit around it. Draw the Burger's vector for the dislocation. Indicate the type of dislocation and rationalize your answer using the Burger's vector that you identified. Mark the dislocation with the proper dislocation symbol.

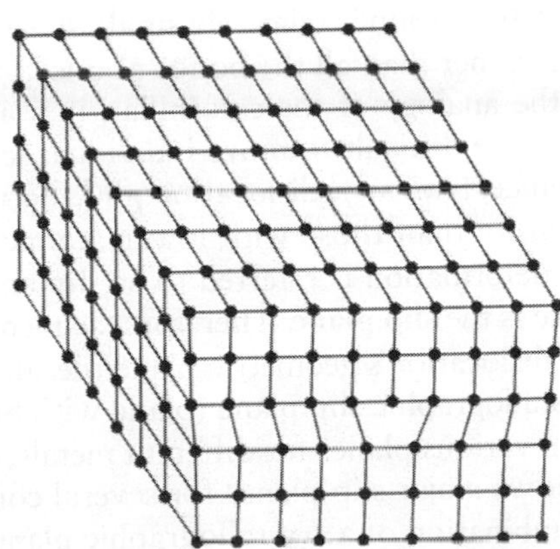

Solution: The dislocation present is an edge dislocation, as the Burger's vector is perpendicular to the dislocation line.

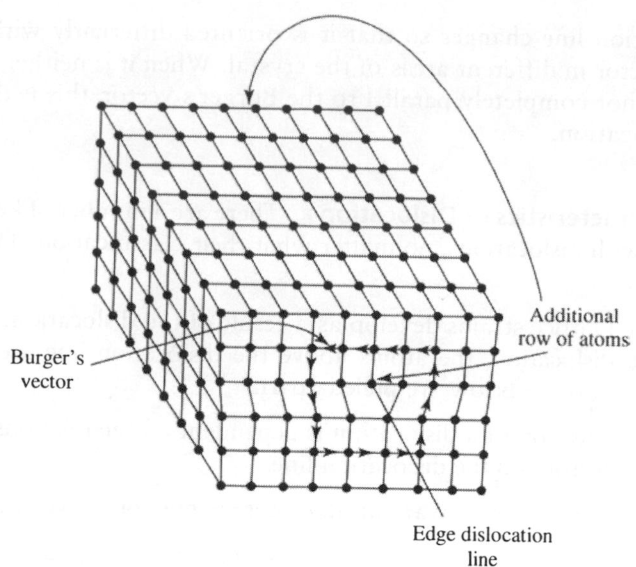

■

3.2.2 Deformation

As mentioned earlier, the presence of even a small number of linear defects has a large effect on the mechanical properties of the overall material. This is mainly due to the fact that these dislocations allow plastic (permanent) deformation of a crystalline material. Plastic deformation occurs by movement of dislocations, or **dislocation glide.**

As shown in Fig. 3.5, if a shear stress (τ) is applied to a crystal having an edge dislocation, there is energy added to the system that can cause the breaking of bonds between atoms in row C and row A and the formation of bonds between atoms in row B and row A. This leaves the atoms in row C without the correct coordination number and marks the new position of the edge defect (it was previously located by atoms in row B). In this manner, a dislocation can glide by one atomic spacing at a time until it exits a crystal, much as a caterpillar moves one section of its body at a time to effect total displacement (Fig. 3.5). Using this model, the amount of shear stress needed to cause deformation is relatively small, since only one row of bonds at a time must be broken, rather than all the bonds at once.

Continuing with the analogy of the caterpillar, it is apparent that if there are larger steps, it will be more difficult to move individual sections of the caterpillar's body the required distance. Similarly, dislocation glide occurs more easily on planes with higher atomic density than those with lower atomic density. When speaking about crystals, plastic deformation is referred to as **slip** and the plane in which the deformation takes place is the **slip plane.** Therefore, as mentioned above, slip occurs in a crystal only if the dislocation's geometric plane (defined by the Burger's vector) coincides with the crystallographic slip plane (plane with highest atomic density).

Slip planes occur in various planes for different metals, depending on the crystal structure. Table 3.1 shows major slip planes for several common crystal structures. A **slip system** is the combination of a crystallographic plane through which slip can occur and the number of directions slip can take place along this plane. It is interesting to note that those metals with a higher number of slip systems, such as aluminum, are more deformable (ductile), while those having only a few, such as magnesium, break with little deformation (are brittle).

As discussed in the previous chapter with point defects, similar types of linear defects are found in ceramics, but their movement is limited by the requirement

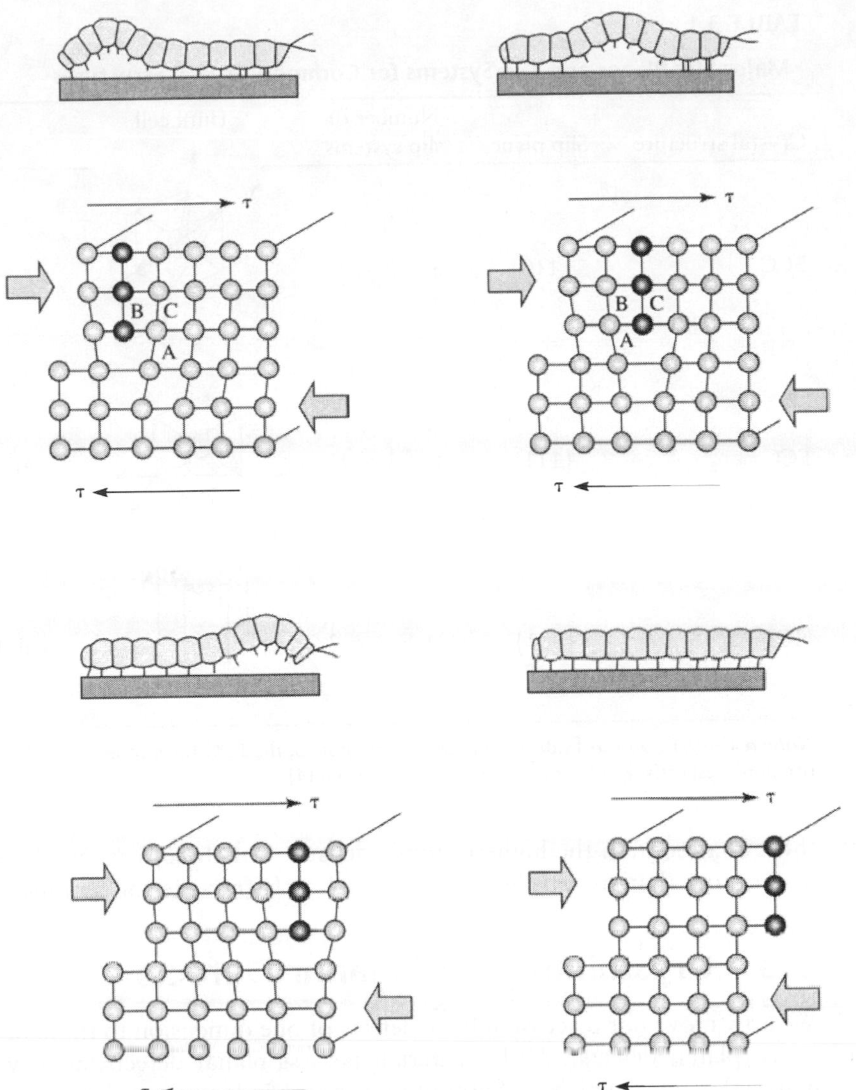

Figure 3.5
Diagram of dislocation glide in crystalline materials (end-on view). If enough energy is added to the system, the bonds between atoms in row C (rows extend out of the plane of the page) and row A will break and bonds between atoms in row B and row A will form. This leaves the atoms in row C without the correct coordination number and marks the new position of the edge defect (previously located by atoms in row B). In this manner, dislocations can glide by one atomic spacing at a time until they exit a crystal, much as a caterpillar moves one section of its body at a time to effect total displacement. (Adapted with permission from [1], p. 152, and [3].)

of electroneutrality. This generally means that the Burger's vectors are longer for ceramics than metals (Fig. 3.6) and that the planes on which slip can occur (that for example, do not place two atoms of like charge next to each other) are not

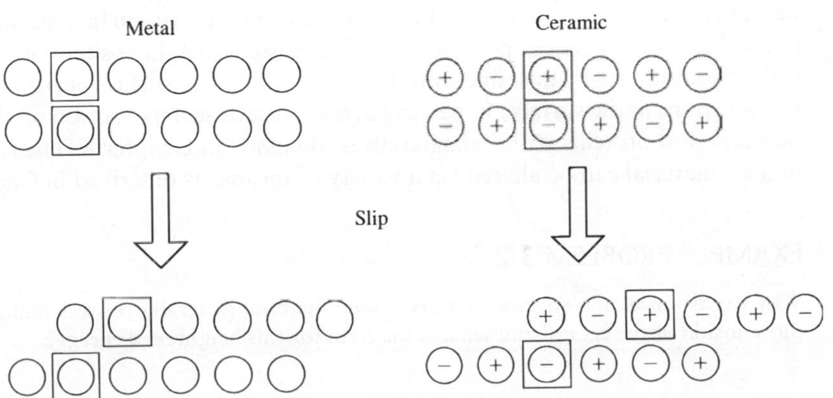

Figure 3.6
Diagram showing the variation in slip between metals and ceramics. In a metal, the dislocation can move by one atomic position, whereas with a ceramic the dislocation must occur over two atomic positions, due to the electroneutrality requirement. This leads to a larger Burger's vector in ceramics when compared to metals. The amount of movement can be seen by the variation in the location of the squares, with each pair indicating a relating pair of atoms.

TABLE 3.1

Major Slip Planes and Slip Systems for Common Crystal Structures

Crystal structure	Slip plane	Number of slip systems	Until cell	Examples
BCC	{110}	$6 \times 2 = 12$		α-Fe, Mo, W
FCC	{111}	$4 \times 3 = 12$		Al, Cu, γ-Fe, Ni
HCP	{001}	$1 \times 3 = 3$		Cd, Mg, α-Ti, Zn

Note: α-Fe, γ-Fe and α-Ti denote the BCC form of iron, the FCC form of iron and the HCP form of titanium, respectively. (Adapted with permission from [4].)

those that contain the highest atomic density. For these reasons, there is less slip in ceramics than metals, leading to more brittle fracture for ceramic materials.

3.3 Crystallinity and Planar Defects

We now move our discussion from defects of one dimension to those of two dimensions (planar defects). All biomaterials possess planar defects, as they include the material surface, which is of utmost importance in biocompatibility (see Chapter 7). Other examples of planar defects include grain boundaries in metals and ceramics.

3.3.1 External Surface

Atoms at the surface of a material are not bonded to the maximum possible number of nearest neighbors, so they possess higher energy than those atoms located inside a crystal. This extra energy is called the surface free energy or **surface tension** and is expressed in units of energy per unit area. The existence of these sites with higher energy is thermodynamically unstable, and the need to minimize surface energy leads to chemical reactions at the surface. In particular, the effect of surface tension on the interaction of water and proteins with biomaterials is discussed in Chapter 8. The surface tension of a biomaterial can be altered via a variety of means, as described in Chapter 7.

EXAMPLE PROBLEM 3.2

Why do atoms at the surface of a crystalline material generally possess higher energy than those inside of the crystal and what is the term for this heightened energy?

Solution: Unlike most atoms in the interior of a crystalline material, atoms at the surface of a crystalline material are not bonded to the maximum number of nearest neighbor atoms. Consequently, the atoms at the surface generally have a higher energy than comparable atoms within the material. The term for the heightened energy of atoms at the surface of a crystalline material is "surface tension." ■

3.3.2 Grain Boundaries

Most metals and ceramics are polycrystalline, composed of a large number of small, randomly oriented crystals, or grains. The interface between these grains is called the **grain boundary**. Because of the disorder of these regions, grain boundary atoms do not usually attain the optimal coordination number. Thus, as with the external surface, these atoms are in a higher energy state than comparable atoms in the center of the grain. This leads to higher chemical reactivity in these regions. For example, corrosive attack often occurs first at grain boundaries in metals (see Chapter 5). The total interfacial energy is lower in materials with larger grains, since there are fewer boundary areas than for materials with smaller grains.

There are two types of grain boundaries that can be distinguished via microscopic observation (see Fig. 3.7). If the grains on either side of the boundary have similar orientations (only a few degrees different), this is a **small-angle grain boundary**. Grains with more severe misalignment form **high-angle grain boundaries.** Since the increase in energy at the grain boundary is a result of atomic mismatch, the greater the degree of misorientation, the higher the energy of the boundary. Two common small-angle grain boundaries are the **tilt boundary**, which is composed of aligned edge dislocations, and the **twist boundary**, which is composed of aligned screw dislocations. A diagram showing how a series of edge dislocations can lead to a tilt boundary with tilt angle θ is found in Fig. 3.8.

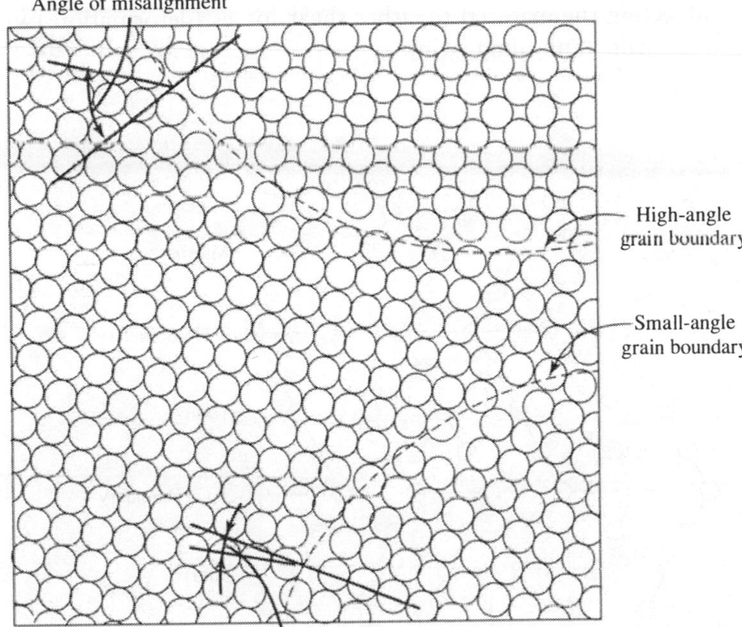

Figure 3.7
Classes of grain boundaries. If the grains on either side of the boundary have similar orientations (only a few degrees' difference), this is termed a small-angle grain boundary. Grains with more severe misalignment form high-angle grain boundaries. Since the increase in energy at the grain boundary is a result of atomic mismatch, the greater the degree of misorientation, the higher the energy of the boundary. (Adapted with permission from [3].)

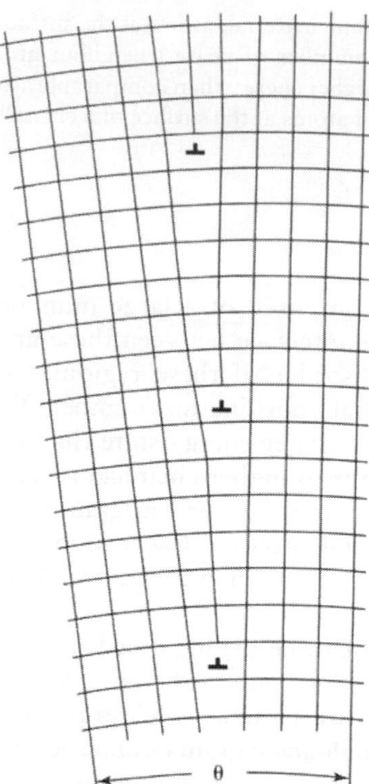

Figure 3.8
Formation of a tilt grain boundary. A series of edge dislocation can lead to a tilt boundary with tilt angle θ. (Adapted with permission from [3].)

A special type of grain boundary defect is termed a **twin boundary**. This occurs when there is a mirror image of atomic placement across the boundary. The area of material between two of these boundaries is called a **twin** (Fig. 3.9). The basic crystal structure is the same both inside and outside the twin. Twinning can be caused by subjecting the material to either shear forces (deformation twin) or annealing heat treatments (annealing twin).

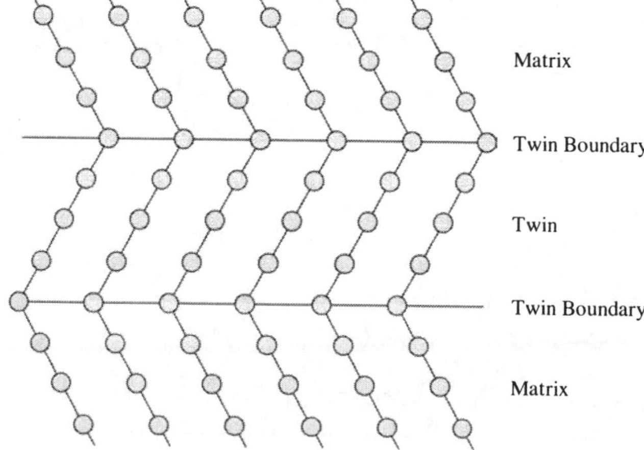

Figure 3.9
A twin boundary, a special type of grain boundary defect that contains a mirror image of atomic placement across the boundary. The area of material between two of these boundaries is called a twin. The basic crystal structure is the same both inside and outside the twin. (Adapted with permission from [1].)

EXAMPLE PROBLEM 3.3

Consider the two metal samples indicated below, each composed of the same metal. The only difference between the two samples is the size of the grains in the material. Which sample has the higher total interfacial energy? Why?

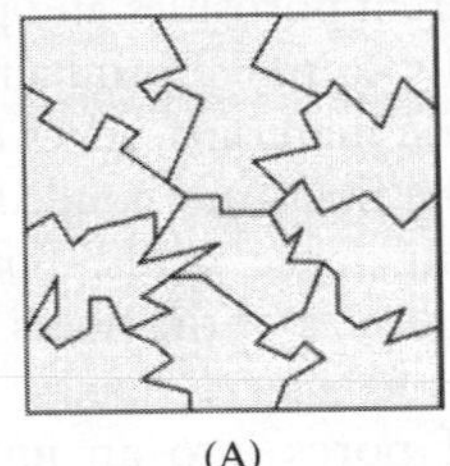
(A)

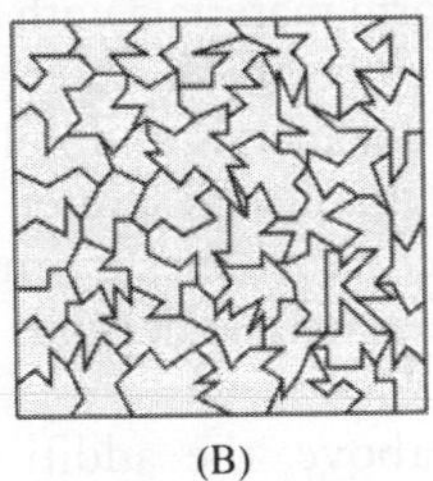
(B)

Solution: The sample with the smaller grains (B) would have the higher total interfacial energy due to the larger amount of boundary area present between grains. As the size of the grains decreases, the total amount of interface between grains increases. Since the energy of atoms at grain boundaries is generally higher than that of atoms at the center of a grain, the total interfacial energy would be higher. ■

EXAMPLE PROBLEM 3.4

Consider a polycrystalline rod of iron submerged in a beaker of brine (saltwater solution). Would one expect corrosive attack to begin first at the grain boundaries or at the center of grains? Why?

Solution: As the atoms at the grain boundaries are generally at a higher energy state than those at the center of a grain, they are generally more reactive. Thus, one could reasonably expect that corrosive attack would begin first with the atoms at the grain boundaries. ■

3.4 Crystallinity and Volume Defects

As the name implies, volume defects are three-dimensional regions in which the long-range order of the crystal is lost. Examples of volume defects include **precipitates** and **voids**. Precipitates are clusters of substitutional or interstitial impurities, while voids are three-dimensional aggregates of vacancies.

Voids are of particular importance in biomaterials, because in addition to their accidental formation due to the clustering of point defects, it is possible to create void space (pores) in a controlled manner to alter the biological response to the material. This is usually accomplished through the addition of porogens at some point during the fabrication of the implant, or via the creation of fibers that are then made into highly porous three-dimensional meshes.

Porogens can either be solid or gaseous. Common solid porogens include salt (NaCl), collagen-based materials (gelatin) or waxy materials such as lipids or paraffin. The concept behind the use of these porogens is that they are solid when mixed with the material, but can be easily extracted after fabrication of the implant to leave behind large void spaces (pores). Extraction can occur through dissolution in water (NaCl) or via a temperature change that transforms solid porogens into liquid (gelatin or waxes). Porogens such as these have been explored mainly for use with polymeric biomaterials. Another option for ceramic materials is the addition of a second ceramic phase that decomposes during the processing procedure to leave pores in the remaining material. In either case, the amount of solid porogen included affects the porosity of the final material, while the pore geometry is determined by the shape of the porogen chosen.

Gaseous porogens such as N_2 or CO_2 are most often employed to form void spaces in polymeric biomaterials. These gases can be liberated during polymerization, or can be bubbled through the polymer while it is in a molten state to form three-dimensional foams upon cooling. The amount, rate, and timing of gas introduction can be altered to form materials with different porosities and pore geometries.

Fibers have also been used successfully to make products with large void volumes, particularly for metals and polymeric materials. After drawing the appropriate material into a fiber (see Chapter 6), the fibers are bonded or woven together to form a three-dimensional mesh containing large voids. Both porosity and pore geometry for these materials depends on the size of the fibers and how densely they can be packed.

As indicated above, the addition of pores into an implant can be accomplished in some manner for all types of biomaterials. Advantages of porous structures are that they allow for the exchange of fluids and gases deep within the material and that they encourage tissue ingrowth and implant anchoring. Allowing nearly unhampered diffusion of nutrients and waste products enables the foams to be seeded with cells for a myriad of tissue engineering applications. However, the presence of pores decreases the mechanical properties of the material and alters both the biodegradation and corrosion properties of the implant. Therefore, for a given material, the percent porosity must be optimized, keeping in mind the intended final application.

3.5 Crystallinity and Polymeric Materials

A key physical property of polymers is their percent crystallinity. The amount of crystallinity in polymeric materials varies much more than for metals and many ceramics, which are virtually all crystalline. As discussed briefly in Chapter 2, polymers form crystals that are significantly different in structure than those in other materials. Due to the large molecules involved, polymeric unit cells are relatively complex. A typical unit cell for poly(ethylene) (orthorhombic geometry) and its relationship to the polymer chains is shown in Fig. 3.10. As with other crystalline materials, information about the structure of polymeric crystals can be obtained through X-ray diffraction experiments (see Chapter 2 for a description of this technique).

3.5.1 Percent Crystallinity

The fraction of crystalline areas in a polymeric material is highly dependent on the chemical structure of its mer as well as the polymer's configuration. Anything that prevents chain alignment (such as kinks) or discourages secondary bonding between chains will reduce polymer crystallinity. The following factors can influence percent crystallinity:

1. mer side groups
2. chain branching
3. tacticity
4. regularity of mer placement in copolymers

Side groups (groups of atoms that project from the backbone) are important in crystallization because if they are large and bulky, this prevents neighboring chains from coming close enough to form a crystalline structure. For example, poly(styrene), with its pendant benzene ring, is an amorphous polymer. For similar reasons, branched polymers exhibit lower percent crystallinity than linear polymers.

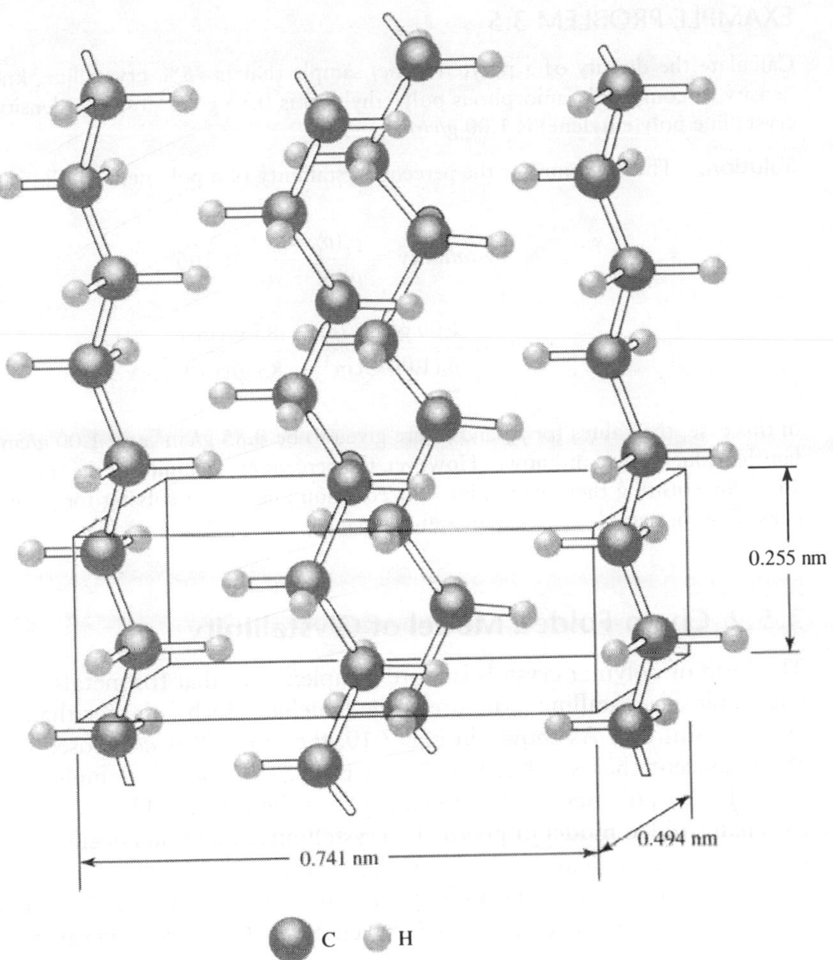

Figure 3.10
A typical unit cell for poly(ethylene) (orthorhombic geometry) and its relationship to constituent polymer chains. The unit cell is composed of atoms from adjacent chains. (Adapted with permission from [5].)

The location of the side groups is also important. Atactic polymers are much more difficult to crystallize than isotactic or syndiotactic polymers, since the random placement of the side groups prevents sections of neighboring polymer chains from coming together in an ordered fashion. Extending this idea to copolymers, if the two different mers are more regularly arranged, such as for alternating and block copolymers, there is a higher probability of the formation of crystalline regions.

It is rare for a polymeric material to be 100% crystalline. This is due to the large size and flexibility of the molecules involved, which significantly increases the possibility that they will fold back on themselves or intermingle with other chains to form complex, nonordered entanglements. Calculation of percent polymer crystallinity therefore provides useful information about the physical structure of these materials. This calculation is based on the fact that crystalline regions of a polymer are denser than amorphous regions (up to 20% difference in density) because the chains are more closely packed in the crystalline regions. Therefore, with careful density measurements of the polymer sample (ρ_s), the same polymer in its (nearly) completely crystalline form (ρ_c), and the polymer in its completely amorphous form (ρ_a), percent *crystallinity* may be determined via the following equation:

$$\%\ crystallinity = \frac{\rho_c(\rho_s - \rho_a)}{\rho_s(\rho_c - \rho_a)} \times 100 \qquad (3.1)$$

EXAMPLE PROBLEM 3.5

Calculate the density of a poly(ethylene) sample that is 75% crystalline, knowing that the density of completely amorphous poly(ethylene) is 0.85 g/cm^3 and the density of completely crystalline poly(ethylene) is 1.00 g/cm^3.

Solution: The equation for the percent crystallinity of a polymer samples is as follows:

$$\%\ crystallinity = \frac{\rho_c(\rho_s - \rho_a)}{\rho_s(\rho_c - \rho_a)} \times 100$$

$$75\% = \frac{1.00\ \text{g/cm}^3\ (\rho_s - .85\ \text{g/cm}^3)}{\rho_s(1.00\ \text{g/cm}^3 - .85\ \text{g/cm}^3)} \times 100$$

In this case, the values for ρ_a and ρ_c are given to be 0.85 g/cm^3 and 1.00 g/cm^3, respectively, but the value of ρ_s is unknown. However, the percent crystallinity of the sample is given to be 75%. Substituting these values into the equation above and solving for ρ_s, we find that the density of the sample is approximately 0.96 g/cm^3. ■

3.5.2 Chain-Folded Model of Crystallinity

The form of polymer crystals is more complex than that for metals or ceramics. The basic unit of crystalline structure is the lamella, which is larger than the polymeric crystal's unit cell. As shown in Fig. 3.10, the unit cell is composed of a few atoms from adjacent chains, while Fig. 3.11 depicts a portion of a lamella, which contains a number of polymer chains folded back on themselves. This model is thus named the **chain-folded model** of polymeric crystallinity. The folds occur at the faces, with regularly aligned chain sections within the lamella.

Although Fig. 3.11 shows an idealized concept of a lamella, in reality, folding may be much more complicated, given that there are several polymer chains found within each lamella. A more realistic visualization may be found in Fig. 3.12. This figure includes several intermingled chains, each of which has crystalline regions located inside the lamellar structure and non-crystalline regions found outside.

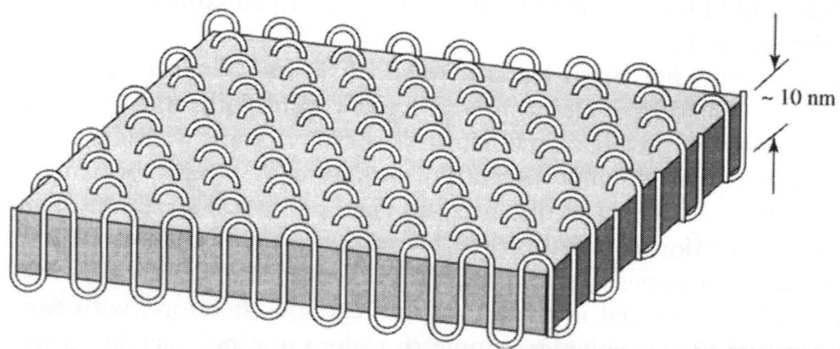

Figure 3.11
A portion of a lamella, the basic unit of crystal structure in polymers. The lamella is larger than the polymeric crystal's unit cell and contains a number of polymer chains folded back on themselves. The folds occur at the faces, with regularly aligned chain sections found inside the lamella. (Adapted with permission from [3].)

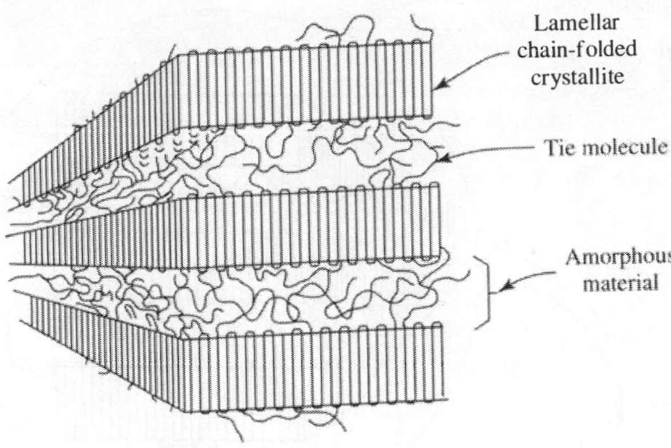

Figure 3.12
Folding in polymer lamella including multiple chains. Although the previous figure shows an idealized concept of a lamella, in reality folding may be much more complicated, given that there are several polymer chains found within each lamella. This figure includes several intermingled chains where each has crystalline regions located inside the lamellar structure and noncrystalline regions found outside. (Adapted with permission from [3])

When a polymer is crystallized from a molten state, the formation of **spherulites** is observed. As shown in Fig. 3.13, these are three-dimensional aggregates of lamellae. The lamellae form radial lines, with the folds oriented perpendicular to the radial direction. Lamellae are separated by amorphous regions that include chain folds and the tie molecules that bind lamellae into aggregates.

As shown in Fig. 3.14, as the spherulites grow, they impinge on one another and deviate from their spherical shape. In this type of crystal formation, the spherulites are analogous to grains in polycrystalline metals and ceramics, although they actually contain many crystalline lamellae as well as amorphous areas.

EXAMPLE PROBLEM 3.6

Consider the following copolymer chains:

(a) -A-B-A-B-A-B-A-B-A-B-A-B-A-B-A-B-
(b) -A-B-B-B-A-A-B-A-B-A-A-A-B-A-B-B-

Which chain is an alternating copolymer, and which is a random copolymer? Which chain would have a higher probability of forming crystalline regions? Why?

Solution: The mers alternate regularly in chain (a), whereas the mers appear randomly arranged in (b). It follows that chain (a) is an alternating copolymer, while chain (b) is a random copolymer. Chain (a) would thus present a higher probability of forming crystalline regions due to the regular arrangement of its mers, relative to chain (b). ■

3.5.3 Defects in Polymer Crystals

3.5.3.1 Linear Defects As in metals and ceramics, dislocations can also occur in crystalline regions of polymers. However, because of the size of the unit cell, the Burger's vectors produced are longer than those for either metals or ceramics. Since the covalent bonds within the polymer chains are stronger than the secondary forces between chains, slip usually takes place along the axis of polymer chains. Unlike

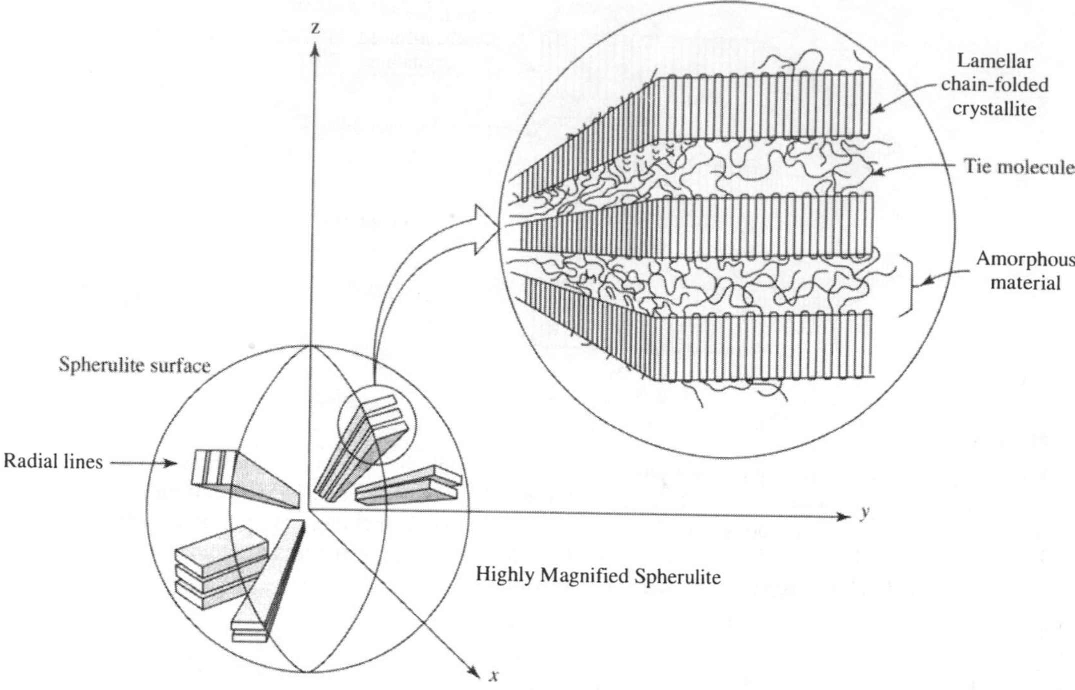

Figure 3.13
Composition of spherulites. When a polymer is crystallized from a molten state, the formation of spherulites is observed. As shown above, these are three-dimensional aggregates of lamellae. The lamellae form radial lines, with the folds oriented perpendicular to the radial direction. Lamellae are separated by amorphous regions that include chain folds and the tie molecules that bind lamellae into aggregates. (Adapted with permission from [3].)

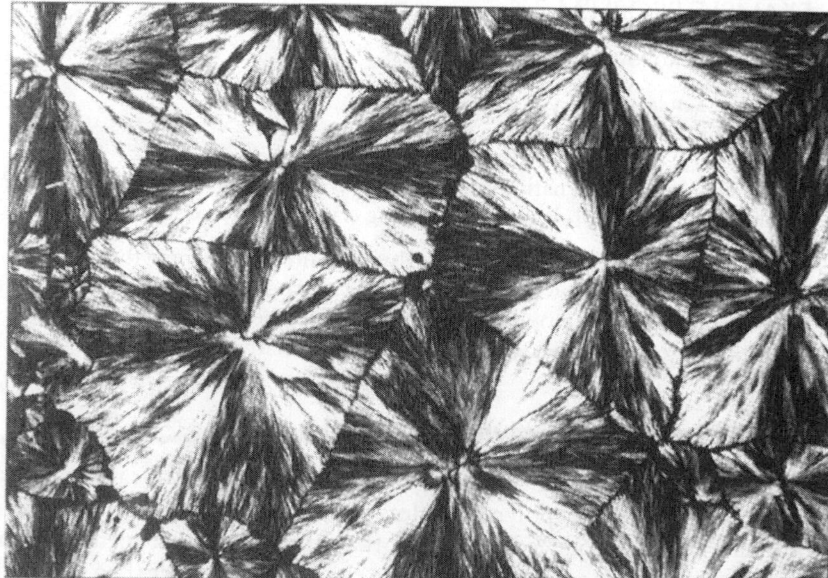

Figure 3.14
Polymer spherulites under polarized light. Using this type of microscopy, each spherulite appears to contain a Maltese cross. As shown here, when the spherulites grow, they impinge on one another and deviate from their spherical shape. (Reprinted with permission from [1].)

metals and ceramics, dislocations do not play a large role in the deformation of polymeric materials. The unique causes of deformation in crystalline and semi-crystalline polymers will be discussed further in the next chapter.

3.5.3.2 Planar and Volume Defects Like linear defects, planar crystal defects also exist in polymeric materials. Polymeric implants possess surfaces with additional energy, similar to metals and ceramics. In addition, boundaries between spherulites can be considered akin to grain boundaries in metals and ceramics. As mentioned earlier, both solid and gaseous porogens can be added to polymers to form voids, a type of volume defect.

3.6 Thermal Transitions of Crystalline and Non-Crystalline Materials

A final physical property that is of interest for all types of biomaterials is how the material subunits described in this chapter are affected by changes in temperature. This is particularly important to processing and fabrication of biomedical implants, since, for example, there is a significant difference in how crystalline and amorphous materials behave in response to temperature changes. The definitions of several thermal transition points are based on changes in how the material deforms. Therefore, we will begin this section with a discussion of viscosity and material deformation.

3.6.1 Viscous Flow

As mentioned earlier in the chapter, plastic deformation takes place due to dislocation movement in crystalline materials. However, since there is no regular structure in noncrystalline materials, a different mechanism of deformation, called **viscous flow** occurs. In viscous flow, the same type of deformation that liquids undergo, the *rate* of deformation is proportional to the applied stress (this will be discussed more fully in the following chapter). This can be written as

$$\tau = \eta\dot{\gamma} \tag{3.2}$$

where τ is the (shear) stress applied to the material; η is the proportionality constant, also referred to as the **viscosity** of the material; and $\dot{\gamma}$ is the rate of applied (shear) strain, or rate of deformation. Viscosity, which is measured in poise (P) or pascal-seconds (Pa-s), represents a material's ability to resist deformation. The wide range of viscosities possible and the effect of viscosity on handleability (ease of handling) is easily demonstrated by comparing the properties of water (η = 0.01 P) and caramel (η = 50 P). At the upper extreme, glasses have a very high viscosity (10^{25} P) due to the presence of strong interatomic bonds.

3.6.2 Thermal Transitions

3.6.2.1 Metals and Crystalline Ceramics The characteristic thermal transition for crystalline materials is the **melting point** (T_m). This is the temperature above which atomic movement is large enough to break the material's highly ordered structure. At temperatures higher than T_m, the material behaves as liquid and deforms via viscous flow. Below this temperature, the substance is a highly ordered solid, with its crystal structure and grain boundaries intact.

3.6.2.2 Amorphous Ceramics (Glasses) In contrast to crystalline materials, glasses do not solidify below a certain temperature (there is no distinct T_m). Instead, the material becomes more and more viscous with decreasing temperature until it can be treated as solid. In the "solid" state, there is very little atomic movement. However, although there is no exact T_m for glasses, this and other thermal transitions can be defined in terms of the viscosity of the material.

The transitions shown in Fig. 3.15 are arbitrarily chosen, but are quite important to glass-shaping operations (see Chapter 6 for a more detailed discussion of glass processing). From highest temperature to lowest, T_m is the temperature when the viscosity of the material is 100 P. Above this temperature, the material can be handled as a liquid. The **working point** is defined as the temperature at which the viscosity of the glass is 10^4 P. At this temperature, the material is easily deformed, but maintains some solid-like properties. At lower temperatures, the material becomes more and more like a solid. The **glass transition temperature** (**T_g**) is the temperature below which the material is considered to be a glass (solid).

3.6.2.3 Polymers Polymers may behave like a liquid, a rubbery solid, or a glass depending on their temperature and molecular structure. Figure 3.16 depicts the effect of molecular weight and temperature on polymer properties (and T_m and T_g).

Like other crystalline materials, crystalline polymers can undergo melting at a defined T_m. Below this temperature, the crystals are highly ordered, while above it, there is a random ordering of chains with no repeating structure. This occurs when

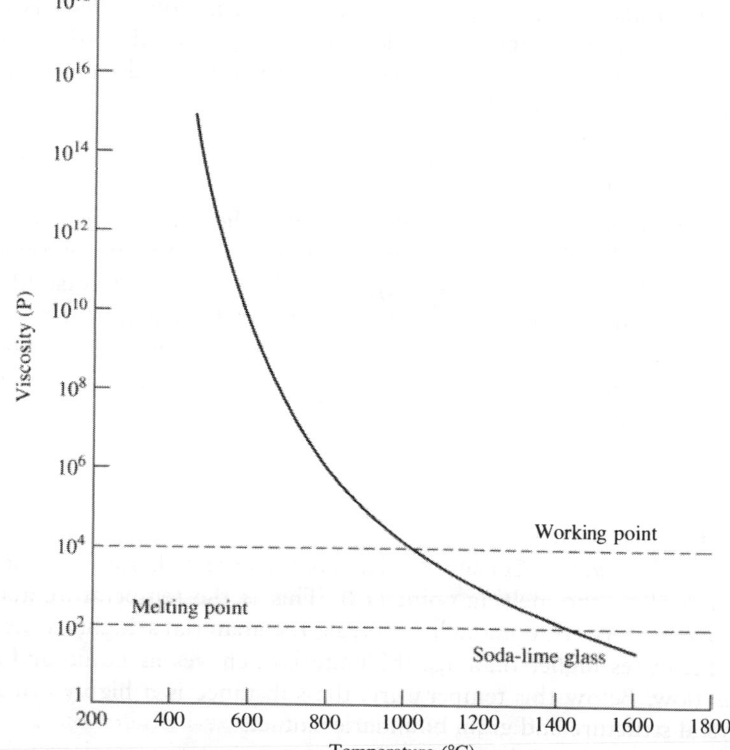

Figure 3.15
Thermal transitions for glasses. The transitions shown here are arbitrarily chosen, but are quite important to glass-shaping operations. The melting point (T_m) is the temperature when the viscosity of the material is 100 P. Above this temperature, the material can be handled as a liquid. The working point is defined as the temperature at which the viscosity of the glass is 10^4 P. At this temperature, the material is easily deformed, but maintains some solid-like properties. At lower temperatures, the material becomes more and more like a solid. (Adapted with permission from [6].)

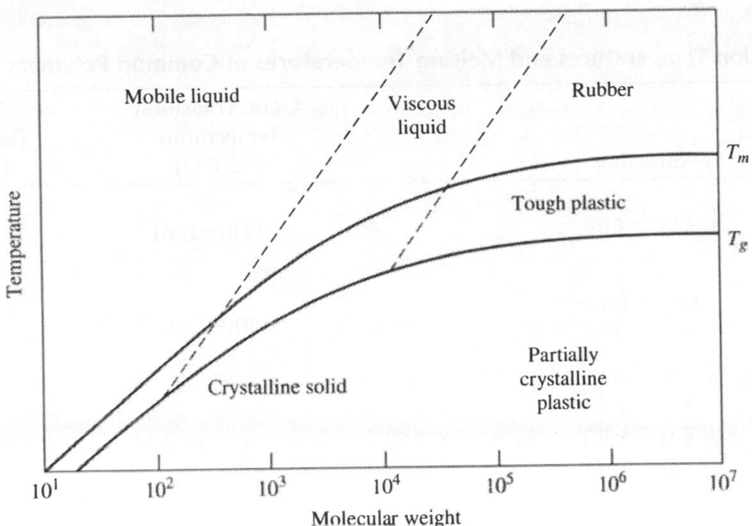

Figure 3.16
Effect of molecular weight and temperature on polymer properties (T_g and T_m). Polymers may behave like a liquid, a rubbery solid, or a glass depending on their temperature and molecular structure. Crystalline polymers can undergo melting at a defined T_m. Below this temperature, the crystals are highly ordered, while above it, there is a random ordering of chains with no repeating structure. T_m increases with increasing molecular weight. Alternatively, those polymers that are amorphous possess a glass transition point (T_g). T_g generally occurs at lower temperatures than T_m. Below the glass transition, the polymeric material is glassy and brittle, while above it, the chains are mobile enough to produce a rubbery, elastic material. Like T_m, a polymer's T_g increases with increasing molecular weight. (Adapted with permission from [7].)

there are enough atoms or chain segments vibrating with sufficient energy to become coordinated and result in overall chain motion (translational motion). This motion then can overcome the secondary bonds that are formed between chains and disrupt the long-range order of the crystal.

Because of this, factors that influence a polymer's ability to form secondary bonds will impact the T_m. These include many of the factors affecting the percent crystallinity of a polymer (discussed previously), such as the degree of branching, and other concerns, such as the molecular weight. For example, with more chain branching, the molecules are less densely packed and therefore cannot form van der Waals interactions or hydrogen bonds as easily. This results in a decrease in T_m with increasing amounts of branching.

In contrast, T_m increases with increasing molecular weight (Fig. 3.16). This is due to the fact that with higher molecular weight, there are fewer polymer chain ends. Because chain ends are more free to move than other parts of the macromolecule, more energy is needed to produce the motion required to release the chains from their ordered structure if the chains have a higher molecular weight.

Alternatively, those polymers that are amorphous possess a glass transition point (T_g) similar to that of ceramic glasses. T_g generally occurs at lower temperatures than T_m (see Table 3.2). Below the glass transition, the polymeric material is glassy and brittle, while above it, the chains are mobile enough to produce a rubbery, elastic material. This occurs when there is a high enough temperature to impart sufficient energy to cause molecular motion around the polymer backbone. The ratio of T_m to T_g of a polymer, in the absence of any solvent and where temperature is in degrees Kelvin, usually falls between 1.4 and 2.0, with a few exceptions [8].

TABLE 3.2

Comparison of Typical Glass Transition Temperatures and Melting Temperatures of Common Polymers

Material	Structure	Glass Transition Temperature [°C (°F)]	Melting Temperature [°C (°F)]
Poly(ethylene) (low density)	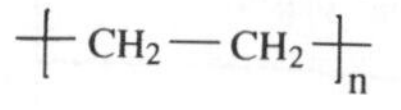 $-[CH_2-CH_2]_n-$	−110(−166)	115 (239)
Poly(ethylene) (high density)	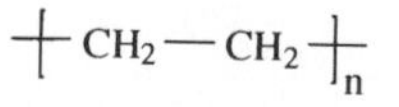 $-[CH_2-CH_2]_n-$	−90(−130)	137 (279)
Poly(tetrafluoro-ethylene)	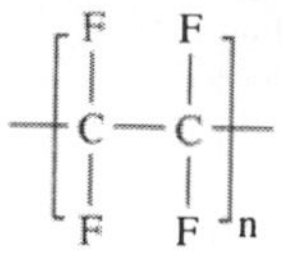 $-[CF_2-CF_2]_n-$	−90(−130)	327 (621)
Poly(propylene)	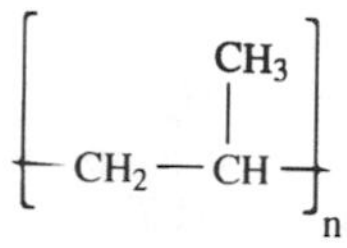 $-[CH_2-CH(CH_3)]_n-$	−20(−4)	175 (347)
Nylon 6,6	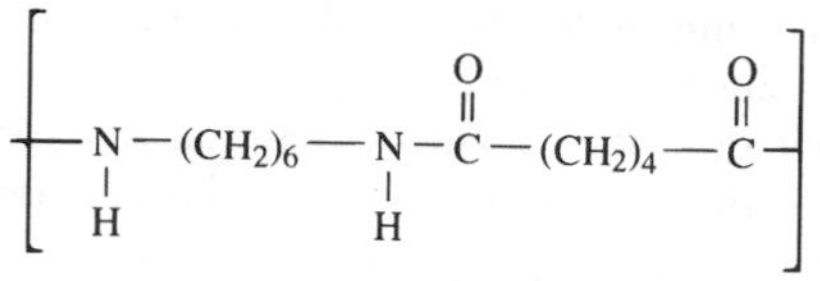 $-[NH-(CH_2)_6-NH-C(=O)-(CH_2)_4-C(=O)]-$	57 (135)	265 (509)
Poly(ethylene terephthalate)	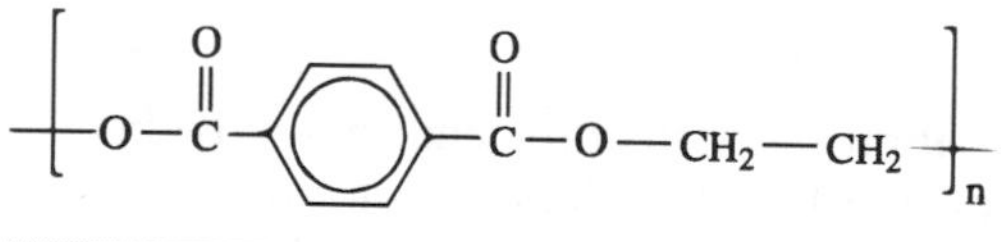 $-[O-C(=O)-C_6H_4-C(=O)-O-CH_2-CH_2]_n-$	73 (163)	265 (509)

(Adapted with permission from [3].)

Factors that influence chain vibration and rotation have a large effect on the T_g of a polymer. Chain flexibility is one of the major determinants of the glass transition point, since more flexibility results in a greater possibility for molecular motion. Therefore, a polymer with more flexible chains will require less energy to achieve the required movement around the backbone and its T_g will be lower.

Chemical constituents have the largest effect on chain flexibility. C–O bonds rotate more easily than C–C bonds, so the presence of these bonds reduces T_g, while the addition of bulky side groups reduces movement around the backbone and increases T_g. Polar side groups that promote chain interactions also increase T_g. For the same reasons as described for T_m, a polymer's T_g is higher at higher molecular weight (Table 3.3). In the same vein, crosslinking reduces overall molecular motion and thus increases T_g.

As may be assumed, semicrystalline polymers that contain both crystalline and amorphous regions can have both glass transition and melting points. However, T_m may be undetectable for polymers with low percent crystallinity.

For those polymers possessing the ability to crystallize, at a characteristic temperature above T_g known as the **crystallization temperature** (**T_c**), the polymer chains will have sufficient energy to move into a highly ordered crystalline state. This arrangement of the polymer chains into a crystalline state is an exothermic process. A polymer can be annealed by raising the temperature of the sample to its

TABLE 3.3

Comparison of Glass Transition Temperatures and Melting Temperatures of Poly(Lactic Acid) with Two Different Molecular Weights

Weight average molecular weight (Da)	Glass Transition Temperature (°C)	Melting Temperature (°C)
50,000	54	170
300,000	59	178

(Adapted with permission from [9])

T_c, maintaining this temperature for some time t and then lowering the temperature very slowly. The degree of crystallinity of the polymer developed at time t, $X(t)$, is described by the Avrami equation as

$$X(t) = 1 - e^{-kt^n} \tag{3.3}$$

where k is the kinetic rate constant of crystal growth and n is a number characteristic of the mechanism of crystal nucleation and growth. Upon further heating of the polymer at temperatures above T_c, the melting temperature T_m of the polymer will be reached and the crystal structure will become disrupted. More details about measurement of these transitions are provided in the following section.

EXAMPLE PROBLEM 3.7

Given that the kinetic rate constant of a particular polymer sample is 2.5×10^{-6} 1/s^3 and that the value of n is 3 for the crystallization of this particular polymer sample in the given conditions, plot the degree of crystallinity of the sample from time $t = 0$ through 125 s. What is the degree of crystallinity of the sample at time $t = 3$ hours?

Solution: At three hours, the time in seconds equals (3 hr) * (60 min/hr) * (60 s/min) = 10800 s. Substituting this value along with the other given values into the Avrami equation and solving for X_c, we find that the degree of crystallinity is approximately 1. This value makes sense, as the degree of crystallinity of a sample cannot exceed a value of 1, which reflects 100% crystallinity. ■

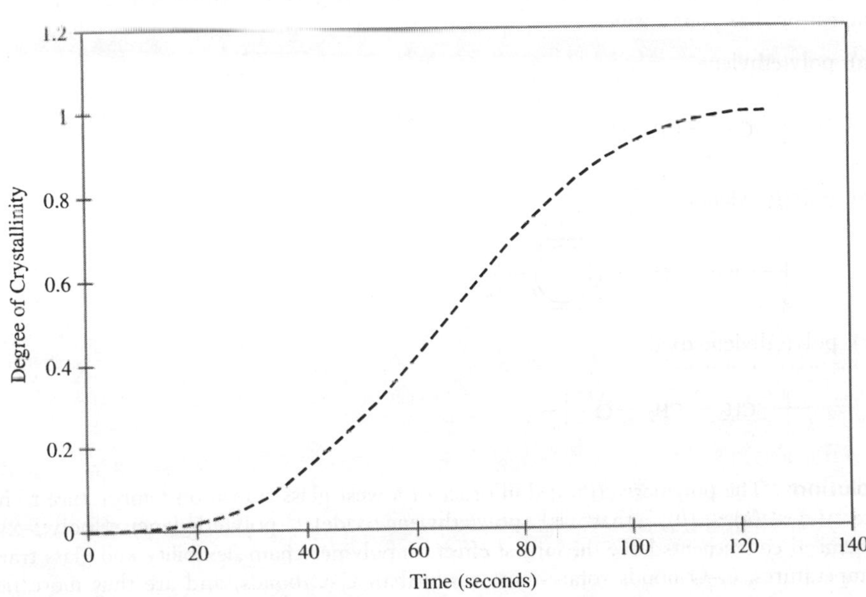

EXAMPLE PROBLEM 3.8

Some researchers utilize the following form of the Avrami equation in their experimental studies:

$$\ln\left(\ln\left(\frac{1}{1 - X_c}\right)\right) = \ln(k) + n \cdot \ln(t)$$

Derive this form of the Avrami equation from the form of the equation given in the text.

Solution: $X_c = 1 - e^{-kt^n}$

Subtracting 1 from each side of the equation and then multiplying each side of the equation by -1 yields

$$1 - X_c = e^{-kt^n}$$

Taking the natural log of both sides of the equation gives

$$\ln(1 - X_c) = -kt^n$$

Multiplying each side of the equation by -1 produces

$$-\ln(1 - X_c) = kt^n$$

Recalling that $-\ln(x) = \ln(1/x)$, we obtain

$$\ln\left(\frac{1}{1 - X_c}\right) = kt^n$$

Taking the natural log of both sides of the equation and recalling that $\ln(x \cdot y) = \ln(x) + \ln(y)$ and that $\ln(x^y) = y \cdot \ln(x)$ results in

$$\ln\left(\ln\left(\frac{1}{1 - X_c}\right)\right) = \ln(k) + n \cdot \ln(t)$$ ■

EXAMPLE PROBLEM 3.9

Assuming that there are amorphous regions in materials made from each of the following polymers, place the three polymers in order of lowest glass transition temperature to highest and rationalize your answer:

(a) poly(ethylene)

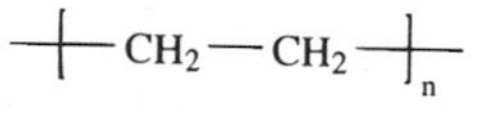

$$\left[CH_2 - CH_2 \right]_n$$

(b) poly(p-xylene)

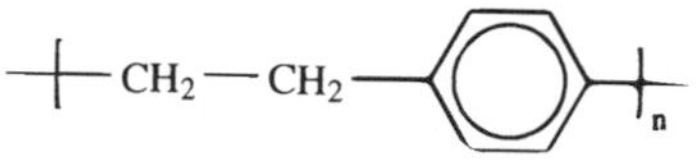

$$\left[CH_2 - CH_2 - C_6H_4 \right]_n$$

(c) poly(ethylene oxide)

$$\left[CH_2 - CH_2 - O \right]_n$$

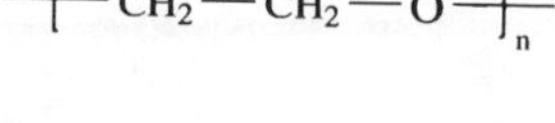

Solution: The polymers arranged in order of lowest glass transition temperature to highest are $(c) < (a) < (b)$, that is poly(ethylene oxide) < poly(ethylene) < poly(p-xylene). Chemical constituents have the largest effect on polymer chain flexibility and glass transition temperatures. C–O bonds rotate more easily than C–C bonds, and are thus more flexible.

However, bulky groups in the chain, such as the benzene ring in the poly(*p*-xylene), prevent rotation around the polymer backbone, and result in a higher T_g. In this case the C–O bond in the poly(ethylene oxide) chain makes it the most flexible polymer of the three (lowest T_g), and the benzene ring in the poly(*p*-xylene) chain makes it the least flexible (highest T_g) polymer of the three, all other factors being equal. ■

3.7 Techniques: Introduction to Thermal Analysis

As mentioned earlier in this chapter, how materials respond to temperature changes is important for their processing and final application. In a controlled environment, a material's response to change in temperature can also provide useful information about the chemical or physical makeup of the material. **Thermal analysis** consists of a group of characterization techniques that involve the measurement of the physical properties of a material (and/or reaction products) as a function of temperature as the sample is subjected to controlled changes in temperature.

Thermal analysis encompasses many well-known techniques, such as **thermogravimetric analysis (TGA)**, **dynamic mechanical analysis (DMA)**, and others, but the one that we shall focus on in this section is **differential scanning calorimetry (DSC)**. DSC has become one of the most popular thermal techniques since it can provide a variety of information about a material, including melting and glass transitions and percent crystallinity of polymeric materials.

3.7.1 Differential Scanning Calorimetry

3.7.1.1 Basic Principles In DSC, the difference in heat flow into a sample and reference material is recorded as a function of temperature while the two are exposed to a controlled temperature ramp. There are two types of DSC experiments: **power-compensated DSC** and **heat-flux DSC**. For power-compensated DSC, the sample and reference cells are heated by individual heaters and the temperature difference between the cells is kept near zero. The power needed to maintain this equal temperature is then compared. In heat-flux DSC, the sample and reference are heated from the same heater and the temperature difference between the two cells is measured. The temperature difference is then converted to heat flow. This difference is depicted in Fig. 3.17. In the following section, we will focus on the operation of the power-compensated DSC.

3.7.1.2 Instrumentation A typical plot produced from a DSC experiment is found in Fig. 3.18. Results are generally plotted as heat flow in units of power/mass (*y*-axis) as a function of temperature (*x*-axis). Thermal transitions are characterized as endothermic (requiring energy to proceed) or exothermic (releasing energy during the process).

There are three basic components to a differential scanning calorimeter, as shown in Fig. 3.19:

1. Furnace(s)—heats sample and reference material with parameters specified by processor (computer).
2. DSC sensors—hold sample and reference and record changes in power to maintain temperatures of each cell.
3. Processor (computer)—controls ramp time and final temperature of the furnaces. Uses the electrical signal from the sensors to control the temperature of the samples in real time via the furnaces. Produces final plotted results.

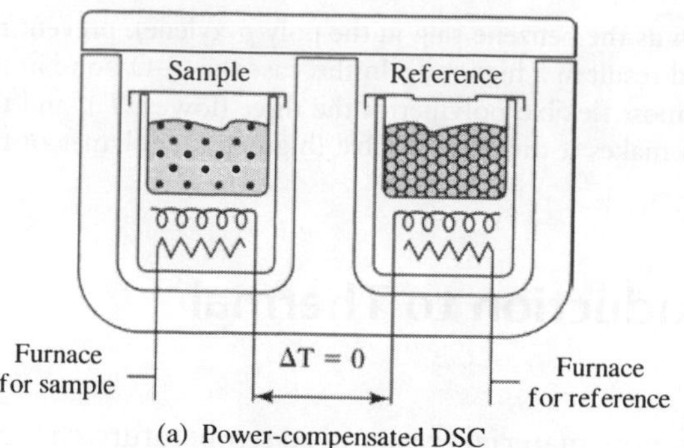

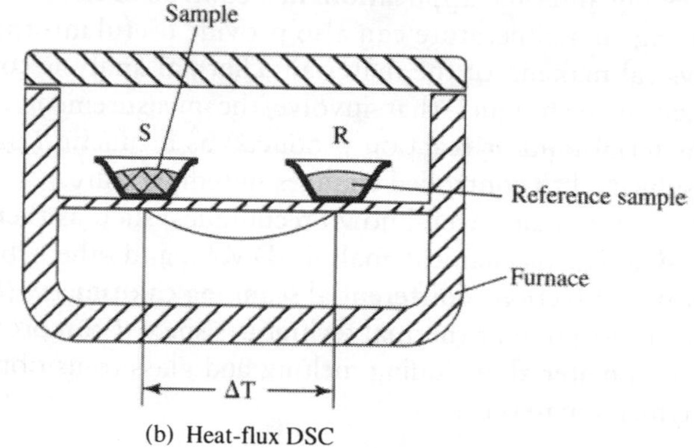

Figure 3.17
Different types of DSC. (a) For power-compensated DSC, the sample and reference cells are heated by individual heaters and the temperature difference between the cells is kept near zero. The power needed to maintain this equal temperature is then compared. (b) In heat-flux DSC, the sample and reference are heated from the same heater and the temperature difference between the two cells is measured. The temperature difference is then converted to heat flow. (Adapted with permission from [10].)

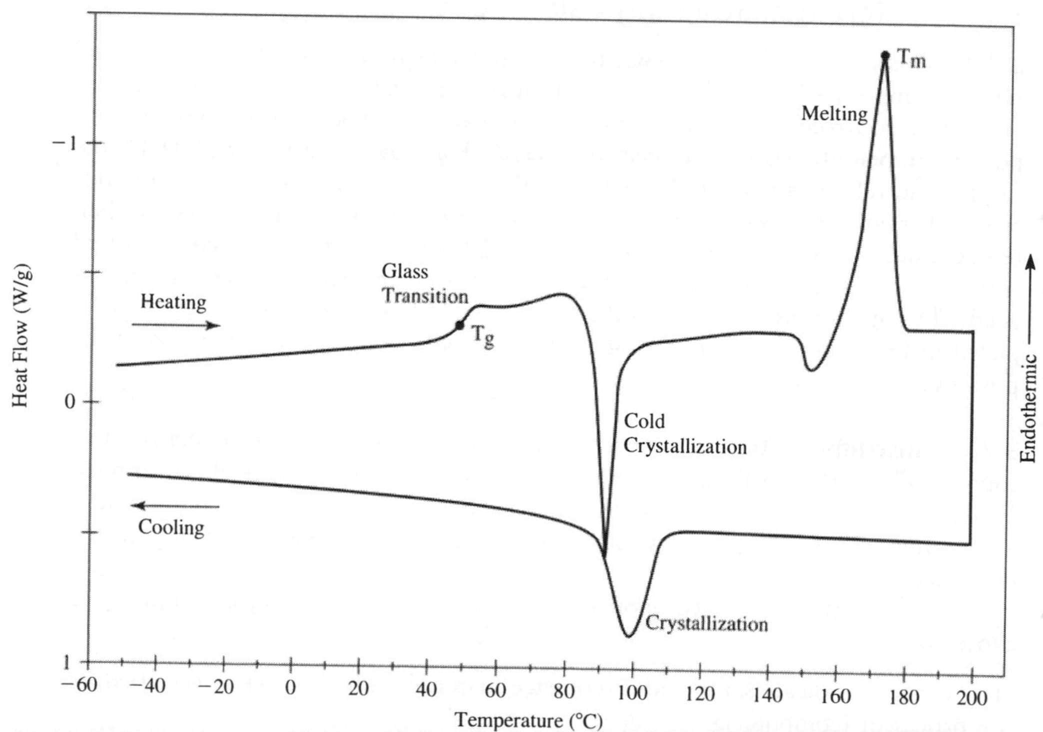

Figure 3.18
DSC thermogram of poly(L-lactic acid) (PLLA). During the heating ramp (10°C/min) the glass transition, cold crystallization and melting of the material occur and during the cooling (10°C/min) the crystallization of the material is observed. The glass transition temperature (T_g) and melting temperature (T_m) are indicated in the figure. (Adapted with permission from [11].)

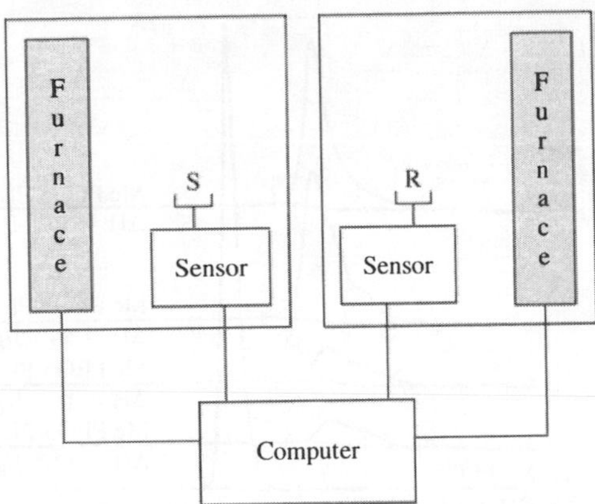

Figure 3.19
Block diagram of components of a differential scanning calorimeter. For a DSC measurement, the sample (S) is first placed in a holding pan made of a metal with high thermal conductivity and hermetically sealed to produce a controlled environment. The reference material (R) is often an empty pan, but can contain a material with known thermal properties. As shown in the diagram, for power-compensated DSC, the two pans are heated with separate furnaces, while processing software controls the furnaces and thus the temperature of the samples. As part of its control mechanism, the computer (via the sensors holding the samples) records how much power is required to maintain a similar temperature in the two pans and plots this as a function of temperature after the temperature ramp has been completed. (Adapted with permission from [12].)

For a DSC measurement, the sample is first placed in a holding pan made of a metal with high thermal conductivity and hermetically sealed to produce a controlled environment. The reference material is often an empty pan, but can contain a material with known thermal properties. As shown in the diagram, for power-compensated DSC, the two pans are heated with separate furnaces, while processing software controls the furnaces and thus the temperature of the samples. As part of its control mechanism, the computer records how much power is required to maintain a similar temperature in the two pans and plots this as a function of temperature after the temperature ramp has been completed. Certain differential scanning calorimeters are also equipped with a cooling device, so temperature ramps can be increasing, decreasing, or even cyclical.

3.7.1.3 Information Provided As seen in Fig. 3.18, both T_g and T_m can be determined via DSC. At T_g, the heat capacity of the sample increases since energy is absorbed by chain rearrangement. T_m refers to the peak temperature. Melting of polymers in general occurs over a range of temperatures due to the presence of crystals of different sizes. Although it may be possible to observe these changes for all types of materials, the working temperature limit on many DSC furnaces makes this technique useful primarily for the characterization of polymeric materials.

DSC is especially useful in determining percent crystallinity of polymers. Since the T_m endotherm is affected by the amount of crystalline material present, comparing the area under the curve representing T_m for a semicrystalline polymer with that for the same polymer in its crystalline form can provide an accurate measure of the percent crystallinity of the semicrystalline polymer (Fig. 3.20).

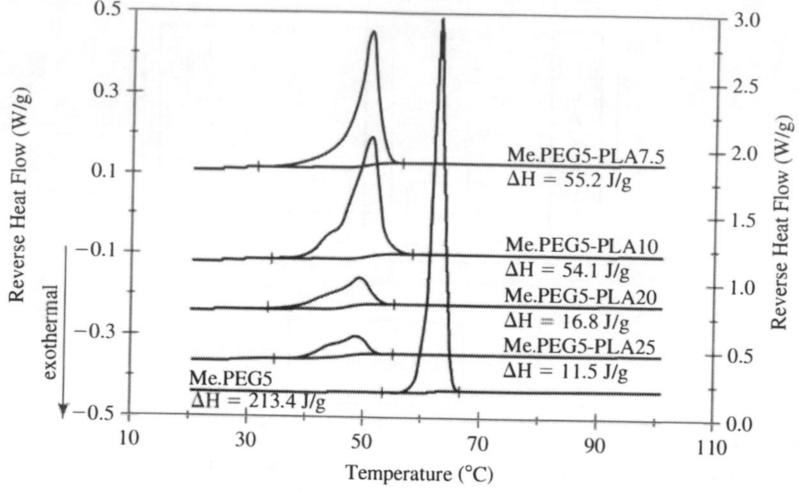

Figure 3.20
DSC thermograms of poly(D,L-lactic acid)-poly(ethylene glycol)-monomethyl ether diblock copolymers obtained by DSC measurements (left y-axis). The structure of these polymers (Me.PEG-PLAs—numbers indicate the molecular weight of the corresponding polymer blocks in kDa) is found in the bottom panel. Since the T_m endotherm is affected by amount of crystalline material present, by comparing the area under the curve representing T_m for a semicrystalline polymer (Me.PEG-PLA) with that for a similar polymer in its crystalline form (Me.PEG5), an accurate measure of the percent crystallinity of the semicrystalline polymer may be obtained. In the graph, crystalline Me.PEG5 is used as a control (right y-axis). In comparison, it can be seen that the crystallinity of the Me.PEG-PLA increases with decreasing molecular weight of the PLA block (from 25 kDa to 7.5kDa). As the PLA molecular weight is reduced, this increases the relative amount of the crystalline Me.PEG5 within the copolymer. (Adapted with permission from [13].)

EXAMPLE PROBLEM 3.10

Consider the following DSC thermogram of a polycrystalline polymer. Match the transition temperatures (A, B, and C) with the proper landmarks: (T_g, T_m, and T_c). Based on information

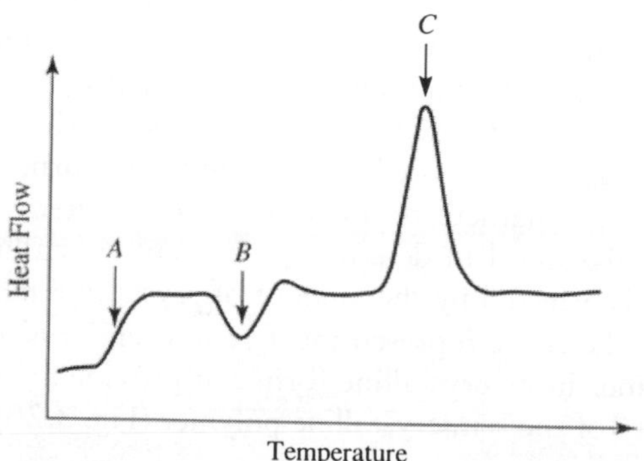

provided in the thermogram, is the T_c peak endothermic or exothermic? Support your answer. Similarly, is the T_m peak endothermic or exothermic? Why?

Solution: *A* corresponds with the T_g (glass transition temperature), while *B* denotes the T_c (crystallization temperature) and *C* marks the T_m (melting temperature). The T_c transition is marked by an exothermic peak (flow of heat out of the sample) as the polymer chains arrange into a crystalline state. The T_m transition is marked by an endothermic peak (flow of heat into the sample) as additional energy is required to disrupt the crystal structure of the polymer. ■

Summary

- Defects in crystal structures include those occurring in one dimension (linear defects), two dimensions (planar defects), and three dimensions (volume defects).
- Several types of linear defects can be present in crystal structures, including edge dislocations, screw dislocations and mixed dislocations (exhibiting both edge and screw characteristics). The Burger's vector can be used to classify a dislocation and to map the motion of linear defects in a crystal.
- The presence of linear defects causes localized strains in the crystal lattice and can lead to plastic deformation of the material through movement of the dislocations. Amorphous materials, however, do not present highly ordered structure and deform by viscous flow, in which the rate of deformation is proportional to the applied stress.
- Planar defects include the material surface and grain boundaries. Atoms at the external surface of a material do not attain the optimal coordination number and consequently possess excess energy, which leads to chemical reactions at the material surface. Most metals and ceramics are composed of randomly oriented crystals, known as grains, of various sizes. The atoms at the disordered interface between grains (grain boundary) are not at the optimal coordination number and thus possess higher energy than comparable atoms within the grain. The higher energy at grain boundaries results in higher chemical reactivity at these sites, relative to the bulk material.
- Volume defects are three-dimensional regions in which the long-range order of the crystal is lost. Volume defects include precipitates (aggregates of impurities) and voids (aggregates of vacancies). Processing to increase void defects is particularly important for tissue engineering applications, as void volume provides a space into which new tissue may grow.
- The form of polymer crystals is generally much more complex than with metals or ceramics. The chain-folded model of polymeric crystallinity holds that the polymer chains fold back on themselves at the faces of lamellae and are regularly aligned within lamellae. Spherulites are three-dimensional aggregates of lamellae and are analogous to grains in ceramic and metallic crystals.
- The melting point (T_m) of a crystalline metal or ceramic is the temperature above which sufficient atomic movement is present to break the highly ordered structure of the material and allow viscous flow and below which the material is solid. Amorphous ceramics (glasses) do not solidify below a certain temperature and do not present a distinct melting temperature, so T_m is defined in terms of the viscosity of the material. Likewise, the glass transition temperature (T_g) for amorphous ceramics is defined as the temperature below which the material is sufficiently viscous to be considered a glass (solid).

- For crystalline polymers, the melting point is the temperature above which the vibrational energy of the polymer chains is sufficient to overcome secondary bonds between the chains and to allow for translational chain motion. Similarly, amorphous polymers possess a glass transition point above which the polymer chains have sufficient energy to cause molecular motion around the polymer backbone, resulting in a rubbery material. T_g generally occurs at a lower temperature than T_m. For semicrystalline polymers, between T_g and T_m the chains increase in energy and mobility, which can lead to a highly ordered crystalline state.
- Techniques of thermal analysis allow for measurement of the physical properties of a material as a function of temperature and enable the characterization of the thermal transitions of a material. Differential scanning calorimetry is one such technique that allows for characterization of T_m, T_g, and other transitions as well as the percent crystallinity of a polymer under the proper conditions.

Problems

3.1 Would a perfect metallic crystal be brittle or ductile? Why?

3.2 During the normal function of a femoral stem component of a hip joint implant, would you expect slip to occur?

3.3 Below are three polymers to be examined for use as vascular graft materials:

(i) Poly(styrene)

```
   H    H    H    H    H    H    H    H
   |    |    |    |    |    |    |    |
 — C —  C —  C —  C —  C —  C —  C —  C —
   |    |    |    |    |    |    |    |
  Ph    H   Ph    H   Ph    H   Ph    H
```

(ii) Poly(acrylonitrile)

```
  CN    H   CN    H    H    H   CN    H
   |    |    |    |    |    |    |    |
 — C —  C —  C —  C —  C —  C —  C —  C —
   |    |    |    |    |    |    |    |
   H    H    H    H   CN    H    H    H
```

(iii) Poly(tetrafluoroethylene)

```
   F    F    F    F    F    F    F    F
   |    |    |    |    |    |    |    |
 — C —  C —  C —  C —  C —  C —  C —  C —
   |    |    |    |    |    |    |    |
   F    F    F    F    F    F    F    F
```

(a) Which two do you believe would exhibit the highest and the lowest degree crystallinity, respectively, and why?
(b) What analytical technique would you use to determine the crystallinity of each material?
(c) Assume that the values below represent the T_g and T_m for each of the three materials:

Material	(i)	(ii)	(iii)
T_m (°C)	38	52	102
T_g (°C)	30	28	45

Based on this information, which of these materials would you select for this application?
(d) What structural characteristics of these polymers have an effect on the melting and glass transition temperatures?
(e) You are given another polymer to examine for this application. For a preliminary test, you run DSC on a sample, the results of which are shown below (Note: endothermic reactions are shown as positive on this graph). What are the T_m and T_g of the sample? Would this material be suitable?

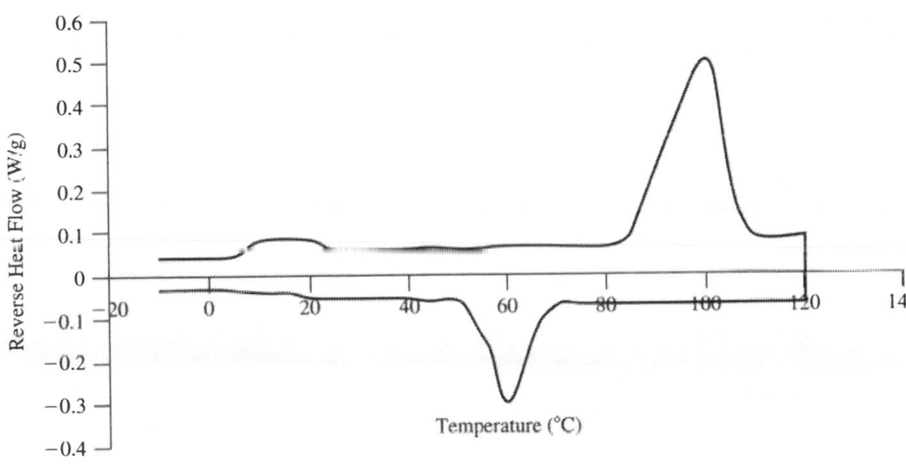

References

1. Schaffer, J.P., A. Saxena, S.D. Antolovich, J. Sanders, T.H., and S.B. Warner, *The Science and Design of Engineering Materials*, 2nd ed. Boston: McGraw-Hill, 1999.
2. Shackelford, J.F. *Introduction to Materials Science for Engineers*, 4th ed. Upper Saddle River: Prentice Hall, 1996.
3. Callister, Jr., W.D. *Materials Science and Engineering: An Introduction*, 3rd ed. New York: John Wiley and Sons, 1994.
4. Shackelford, J.F. *Introduction to Materials Science for Engineers*, 5th ed. Upper Saddle River: Prentice Hall, 2000.
5. Bunn, C.W., *Chemical Crystallography*, Oxford: Oxford University Press, 1945.
6. Kingery, W.D., et al., *Introduction to Ceramics*, 2nd ed. New York: John Wiley & Sons, 1976.
7. Park, J.B. and R.S. Lakes, *Biomaterials: An Introduction*, 2nd ed. New York: Plenum Press, 1992.

8. Peppas, N.A. *Structure and Properties of Polymeric Materials: A Study Guide for Students of Che 544.* West Lafayette: Purdue University, 1984.
9. Engelberg, I. and J. Kohn. "Physico-Mechanical Properties of Degradable Polymers Used in Medical Applications: A Comparative Study" *Biomaterials*, vol. 12, pp. 292–304, 1991.
10. Hemminger, W., and S.M. Serge, "Definitions, Nomencature, Terms, and Literature" in *Handbook of Thermal Analysis and Chemistry*, vol.1, pp. 1–74, Amsterdam: Elsevier, 1998.
11. Ljungberg N. and Wesslen, B. "Tributyl Citrate Oligomers as Plasticizers for Poly (Lactic Acid): Thermo-Mechanical Film Properties and Aging." *Polymer*, vol. 44, pp. 7679–7688, 2003.
12. Haines, P.J. *Thermal Methods of Analysis: Principles, Applications, and Problems*, 1st ed. New York: Blackie Academic and Professional, 1995.
13. Lucke, A., J. Tessmar, E. Schnell, G. Schmeer, and A. Gopferich. "Biodegradable Poly(D,L-Lactic Acid)-Poly(Ethylene Glycol)-Monomethyl Ether Diblock Copolymers: Structures and Surface Properties Relevant to Their Use as Biomaterials." *Biomaterials*, vol. 21, pp. 2361–2370, 2000.

Additional Reading

Park, J.B. and J.D. Bronzino. *Biomaterials: Principles and Applications.* Boca Raton: CRC Press, 2003.

Rabek, J.F. *Experimental Methods in Polymer Chemistry.* New York: John Wiley and Sons, 1980.

Skoog, D.A., F.J. Holler, and S.R. Crouch. *Principles of Instrumental Analysis*, 6th ed. Boston: Brooks Cole, 2006.

Young, R.J. and P.A. Lovell. *Introduction to Polymers*, 2nd ed. London: Chapman and Hall, 1991.

Mechanical Properties of Biomaterials

CHAPTER 4

Main Objective

To understand the molecular mechanisms behind the mechanical properties for each class of material as well as the principles behind events that strengthen and weaken biomaterials.

Specific Objectives

1. To understand and apply equations for calculation of engineering stress and strain, shear stress and strain, and true stress and strain.
2. To complete calculations based on stress-strain curves.
3. To understand the molecular mechanisms of elastic and plastic deformation in metals, ceramics and polymers.
4. To understand the need and the experimental setup for bending tests.
5. To understand the molecular mechanisms of viscoelastic behavior in metals, ceramics and polymers.
6. To create simple models of viscoelastic behavior in biomaterials.
7. To understand the molecular reasons for biomaterial weakening through degradation or due to the inclusion of pores.
8. To compare and contrast types of fracture and explain the role of stress raisers.
9. To understand how fatigue failure is different from other modes of failure and the factors that affect fatigue life.
10. To understand the molecular mechanisms behind material strengthening techniques.
11. To understand the basic theory behind and possible limitations to the mechanical testing of materials.

4.1 Introduction: Modes of Mechanical Testing

Previous chapters have discussed the chemical makeup of various biomaterials and how this affects physical properties such as crystallinity and thermal transitions. This chapter will address how the nature of their bonds and sub-unit structures translates into distinct mechanical properties for each class of biomaterials. Mechanical properties of materials include

1. Tensile/compressive properties
2. Shear/torsion properties
3. Bending properties
4. Viscoelastic properties
5. Hardness

This chapter will focus on the first four of those listed, as they are of particular interest for general biomedical applications. Specifically, testing methods and the molecular causes of each set of properties will be discussed.

4.2 Mechanical Testing Methods, Results and Calculations

Mechanical assessment of materials is performed with a **mechanical testing frame** like that seen in Fig. 4.1. While the specific mechanisms of its operation are discussed in more detail at the end of this chapter, in general, different fixtures can be attached to accommodate various testing modes. The design of the device allows for controlled loading in a well-defined environment for all testing modes. A number of

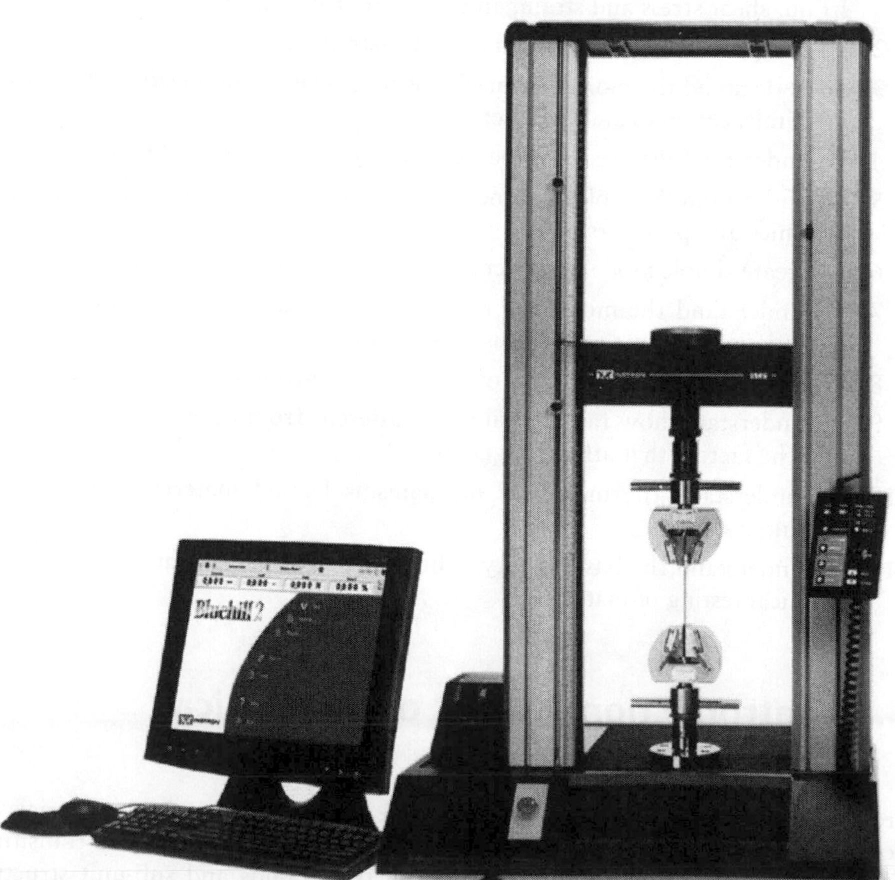

Figure 4.1
A mechanical testing frame used for determining the mechanical properties of various materials. (Reprinted with permission from Instron Corporation [1].)

ASTM standards (created by ASTM International) provide guidelines for most testing modes and material types. Of particular interest for biomaterials applications, the machine design allows samples to be tested in the wet state, thus approximating *in vivo* conditions much more accurately.

4.2.1 Tensile and Shear Properties

4.2.1.1 Calculations for Tensile and Shear Tests As shown in Fig. 4.2(a-c), in mechanical testing, force can be applied as tensile, compressive, or shear. **Tensile testing** is one of the most common testing methods. A diagram of a specimen undergoing tensile testing is found in Fig. 4.3. From ASTM standards, typically, the tensile sample is shaped into a "dog-bone" geometry, with either a round or rectangular cross-section (Fig. 4.4). During testing, the sample is placed in the mechanical testing frame so that one end is attached to a moveable platform, which loads the specimen along the longitudinal axis. Further details about the operation of the loading frame can be found at the end of this chapter.

The two important parameters measured during tensile testing are load and specimen elongation. From these, engineering stress (σ) and engineering strain (ε)

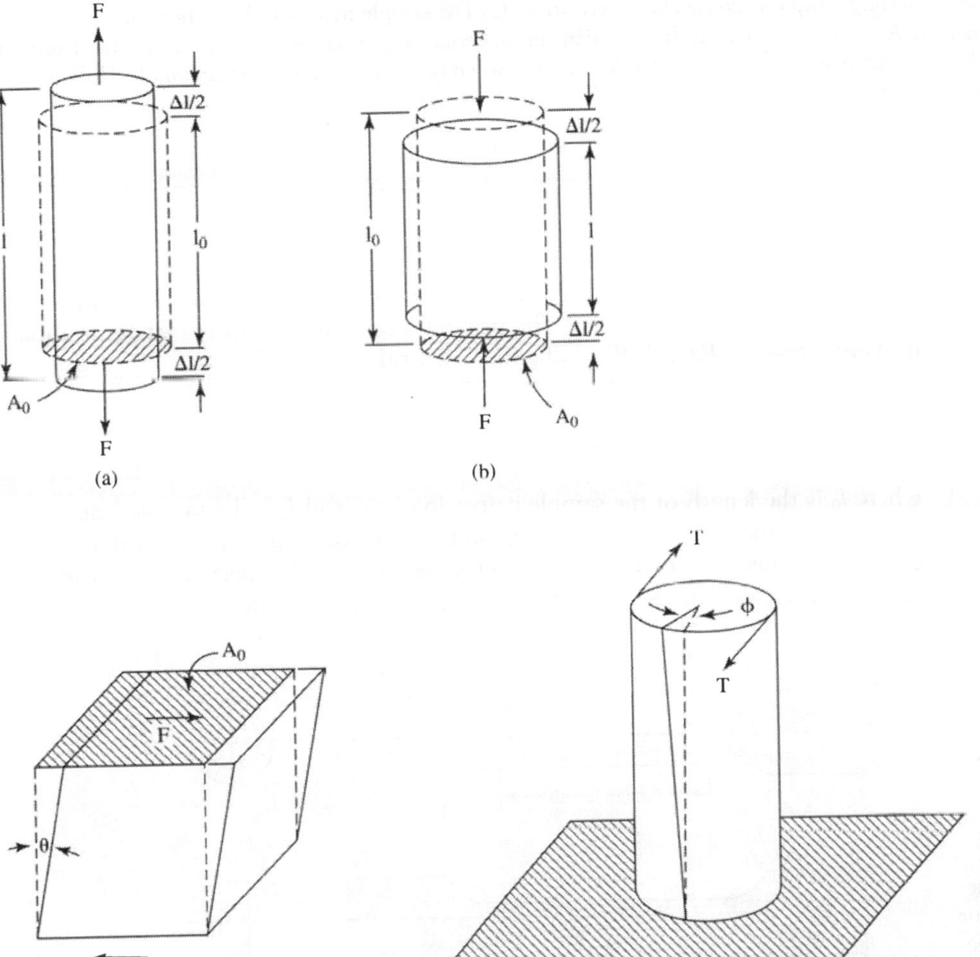

Figure 4.2
Types of forces that can be applied to a material: (a) tensile, (b) compressive, (c) shear, and (d) torsion. (Adapted with permission from [2].)

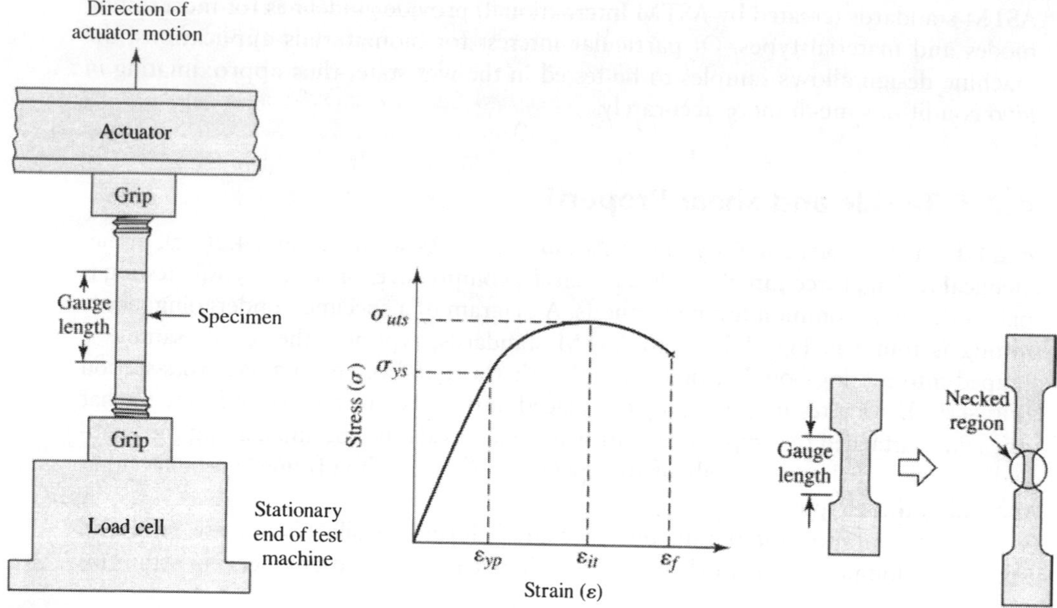

Figure 4.3
A sample testing setup for tensile characterization. (a) The sample material placed in a mechanical testing frame. (b) A stress-strain curve, from which the material properties of the sample can be determined. (c) A gross example of what occurs to the material when tension is applied to the sample. (Adapted with permission from [3].)

can be calculated. Engineering stress is

$$\sigma = \frac{F}{A_0} \tag{4.1}$$

where F is the force applied perpendicular to the cross-section of the sample at any point during the test and A_0 is the original cross-sectional area of the sample. SI units of stress are Pascals (Pa). Engineering strain is

$$\varepsilon = \frac{l_i - l_o}{l_o} \tag{4.2}$$

where l_0 is the length of the sample before loading, and l_i is the sample length at any point during the testing procedure. As seen in the equation, strain is a dimensionless quantity. Because they take into account the geometry of the specimen, stress and strain values can (ideally) be used to compare materials that were tested in different shapes.

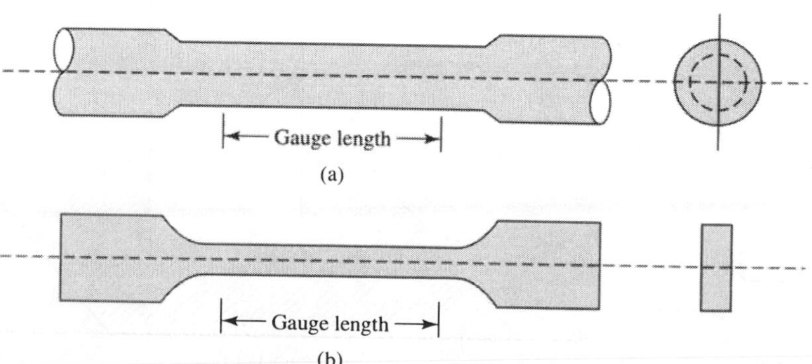

Figure 4.4
The dog-bone shaped geometry used for tensile testing for (a) round materials and (b) rectangular materials. (Adapted with permission from [2].)

Compression testing is also often performed on biomaterials [Fig. 4.2(b)], particularly if they are to be subjected to compressive forces while in use, such as for orthopedic implants. Typical compressive specimens are cylindrical, with a length at least twice that of their diameter. The same equations are used to calculate stress and strain as for tensile tests, but since the compressive force acts in the opposite direction to the tensile force, F is taken to be negative, resulting in a negative stress. Additionally, since the sample becomes smaller along the axis of the stress, l_0 is larger than l_i, and the calculated strain is negative.

Unlike tensile or compressive modes, **shear testing** produces forces that are parallel to the top and bottom faces of the sample [Fig. 4.2(c)]. Shear stress (τ) can be calculated by

$$\tau = \frac{F}{A_0} \tag{4.3}$$

In this case, F is the force imparted parallel to the upper and lower faces, while A_0 is the area of these faces.

As seen in Fig. 4.2(c), the shear force causes sample deformation of angle θ. Therefore, shear strain (γ) is defined as

$$\gamma = \tan \theta \tag{4.4}$$

In many cases, instead of pure shear, **torsion forces** may be applied to the sample. As depicted in Fig. 4.2(d), a torque force (T) twists a cylindrical specimen to cause deformation of angle ϕ on one end relative to the other end. Calculation of shear stress and strain is completed via modification of equations 4.3 and 4.4.

4.2.1.2 Stress-Strain Curves and Elastic Deformation A composite diagram showing a range of stress-strain responses for various materials is found in Fig. 4.5. Looking at Material I of Fig. 4.5 and at Fig. 4.6, it can be seen that the stress and strain are proportional to each other at all values. This relationship is known as **Hooke's law** and can be written

$$\sigma = E\varepsilon \tag{4.5}$$

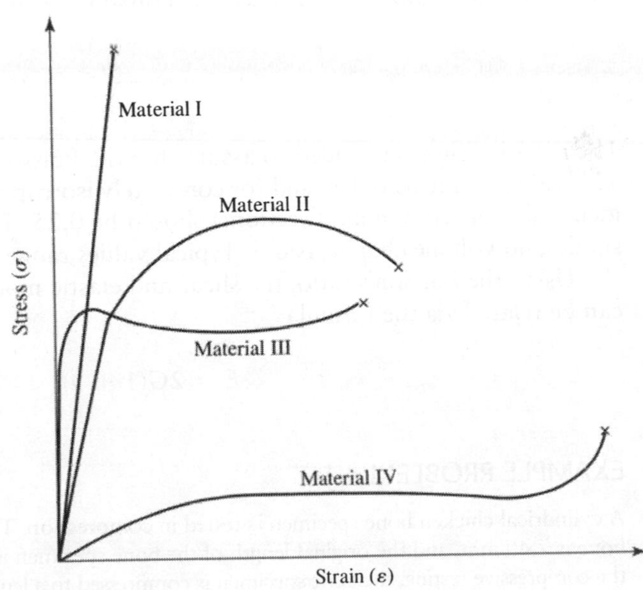

Figure 4.5
The wide variations possible on the stress-strain curve depending on the tested material. Ceramics are often brittle and demonstrate behavior similar to Material I, while metals produce curves similar to Material II. Polymers fall into a wide range of categories, from very brittle materials (Material I), to materials exhibiting plastic deformation (Material III), to highly elastic materials (Material IV). (Adapted with permission from [2] and [3].)

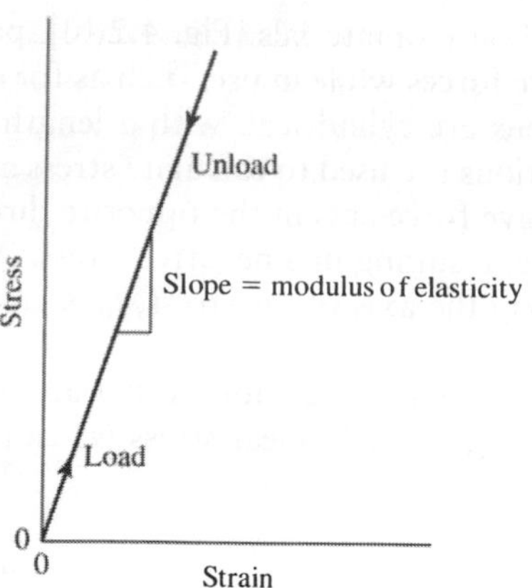

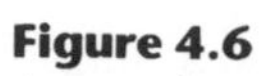
Figure 4.6
A sample stress-strain curve showing a linear relationship, from which the modulus of elasticity can be calculated (slope of the curve). (Adapted with permission from [2].)

where E is the **modulus of elasticity** or **Young's modulus** (MPa). In the area of the curve where the stress and strain follow this linear relationship, the sample undergoes **elastic deformation.** The slope of the curve in this region is the modulus of elasticity, or stiffness of the material. For materials with high E, a large stress is required before deformation will occur. Elastic deformation is not permanent; upon release of the load, the sample returns to its original shape.

The relationship described above is valid for both tensile and compressive testing. Similarly, shear stress and strain can be related by

$$\tau = G\gamma \tag{4.6}$$

where G is the **shear modulus,** which, as for tensile/compressive testing, also represents the slope of the stress-strain curve in the elastic region.

As shown in Fig. 4.7, when elastic elongation occurs along the axis of loading, there is contraction in the directions perpendicular to this loading. For cylindrical specimens, this perpendicular (transverse) strain is represented as $\varepsilon_t = \Delta d/d_0$, where Δd is the change in diameter and d_0 is the original diameter of the specimen. The ratio of the strain that occurs in the transverse direction to the strain that occurs along the loading axis (ε_a) is called the **Poisson's ratio** (ν):

$$\nu = -\frac{\varepsilon_t}{\varepsilon_a} \tag{4.7}$$

Figure 4.7
Schematic showing the radial contraction that occurs when a material undergoes tensile deformation. The ratio of the strain in the transverse direction to the strain in the longitudinal direction (direction of the applied force F) is the Poisson's ratio. (Adapted with permission from [3].)

The negative sign is included to assure that the Poisson's ratio is a positive number. This value is dimensionless and for completely isotropic materials (those which have identical properties in all directions) should be 0.25. The theoretical maximum, assuming no volume change, is 0.5. Typical values range from 0.25 to 0.35.

Using the Poisson's ratio, the shear and elastic moduli for an isotropic material can be related via the formula

$$E = 2G(1 + \nu) \tag{4.8}$$

EXAMPLE PROBLEM 4.1

A cylindrical chicken bone specimen is tested in compression. The original outer diameter of the bone is 7.40 mm, and the original length of the bone specimen is 45.00 mm. At one point during the compressive testing, the bone specimen is compressed to a length of 42.75 mm. One researcher hypothesizes that the Poisson's ratio of the sample at this point is 0.3. What would the outer diameter of the bone specimen need to be at this point for the Poisson's ratio of 0.3 to be correct?

Solution: The Poisson's ratio is defined as the ratio of the strain of a sample in the transverse direction to the strain in the axial direction: $\nu = -\varepsilon_t/\varepsilon_a$. In this case, the strain in the axial direction can be calculated from the information given and is

$$\varepsilon_a = (42.75\text{ mm} - 45.00\text{ mm})/(45.00\text{ mm}) = -0.05$$

Since the hypothesized Poisson's ratio is given to be 0.3, and the axial strain has been calculated to be −0.05, the transverse strain can be calculated as follows:

$$\varepsilon_t = -(\nu\varepsilon_a) = -(0.3(-0.05)) = 0.015$$

Recalling that $\varepsilon_t = (\Delta d/d_o)$, where d_o equals 7.40 mm in this case, the equation can be solved to find the outer diameter of the sample required to give the hypothesized Poisson's ratio as follows:

$$\varepsilon_t = (d_t - 7.40\text{ mm})/(7.40\text{ mm}) = 0.015$$

$$0.111\text{ mm} + 7.40\text{ mm} = d_t$$

$$d_t = \underline{7.511\text{ mm}}$$

■

4.2.1.3 Molecular Causes of Elastic Deformation On a molecular level, elastic deformation is a result of small changes in atomic spacing and stretching of bonds. The resistance to this deformation is provided by the interatomic bonding forces. Those materials with stronger bonds will be less easily deformed (have a higher modulus of elasticity). Revisiting the force-separation curves described in Chapter 1 (Fig. 1.10), it is found that E is proportional to the slope of these curves at the equilibrium bond length r_0:

$$E \propto \left(\frac{dF}{dr}\right)_{r_0} \tag{4.9}$$

As can be seen in Fig. 4.8, those materials that possess a high E (very stiff materials) demonstrate a force-separation curve with very steep sides, so more energy is required to move the atoms away from their equilibrium positions. As a result of the nature of their chemical bonds, values for E are generally greater for ceramics than metals, and both ceramics and metals are stiffer than most polymers. It should be noted, however, that due to the structure of their chains, mechanical properties in polymeric materials are highly direction dependent. Therefore, along the axis of the chain, where primary (covalent) bonds exist between atoms, polymers can possess similar strength and stiffness to metals or ceramics. However, in other directions, where the material is held together mainly by secondary forces, mechanical properties are usually significantly lower.

4.2.1.4 Stress-Strain Curves and Plastic Deformation As mentioned in Chapter 3, **plastic deformation** can also occur and plays a large role in forming operations, particularly for metals and polymers. In contrast to elastic deformation, plastic deformation is permanent, so that the sample never returns completely to its original shape. Evidence of plastic deformation is apparent for Materials II, III, and IV in Fig. 4.5 in the nonlinear portion after the elastic region.

In the following discussion, plastic deformation of materials in tension is considered. The beginning of plastic deformation is the point where the stress-strain

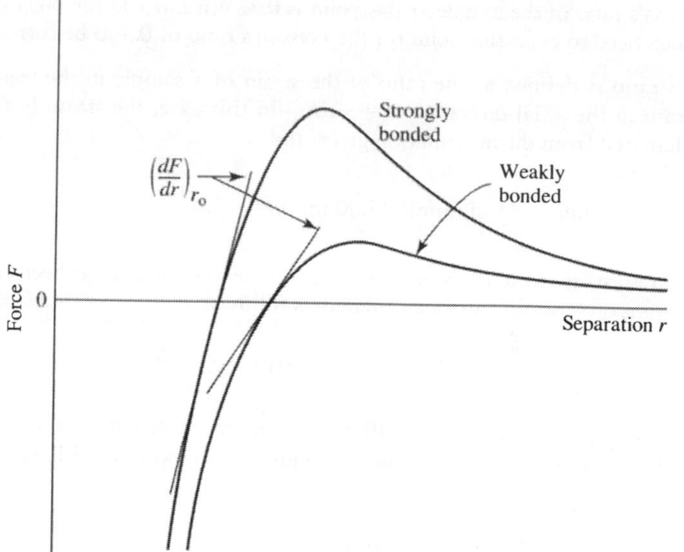

Figure 4.8
Diagram showing the relationship between elastic modulus (E) and bond strength. E is proportional to $\frac{dF}{dr}$ at r_o so materials that possess a high E (are stiffer) demonstrate a force-separation curve with very steep sides, and more energy is required to move the atoms away from their equilibrium positions. (Adapted with permission from [2].)

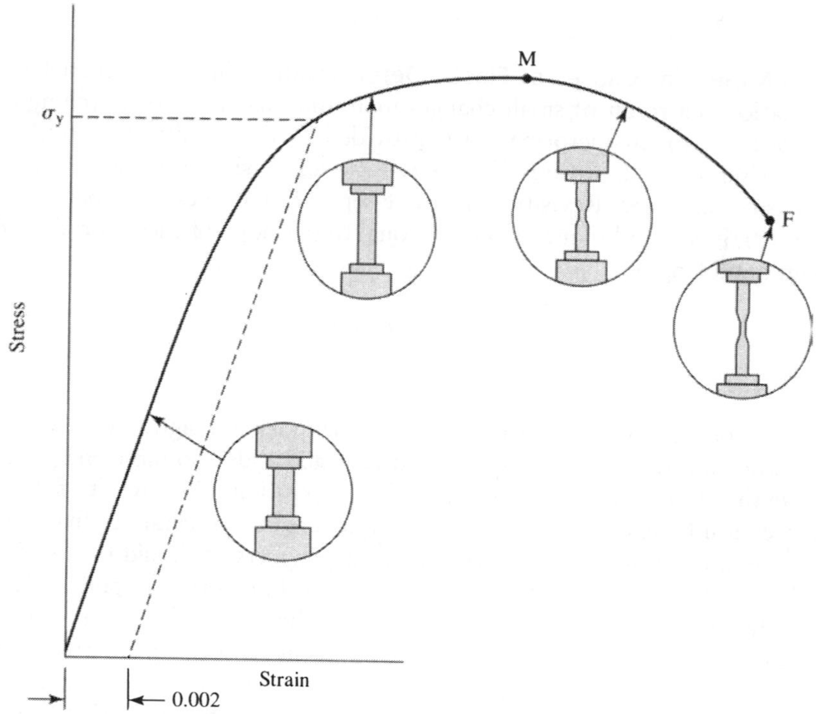

Figure 4.9
Stress vs. strain curve showing elastic and plastic deformation of a material. During the elastic region no necking of the sample occurs, and if the stress is removed, the sample will return to its original state. In this scenario, it is difficult to find the point between the linear and non-linear regions, so a 0.2% strain offset is used. To do this, a line parallel to the elastic portion is created, with the origin of the line having an offset of 0.002 (0.2%) strain. Where this line connects with the curve is considered the yield point, and is used to determine the yield strength (σ_y). From this point until the ultimate tensile strength (point M), plastic deformation occurs, meaning that if the stress is removed, the sample will not return to its native state. After this point, necking will occur in the sample until fracture (point F). (Adapted with permission from [2].)

relationship no longer follows Hooke's law, hence the curve changes from a linear region to a nonlinear region. The stress corresponding to the end of the elastic region of the curve is known as the **yield strength** (σ_y) and the strain at this value is the **yield point strain** (ε_{yp}). However, this transition is not always readily apparent for certain materials and the change can be difficult to pinpoint (Fig. 4.9). In this case, it is common to use a 0.2% strain offset to determine the yield point.

After yielding, there is an increase in stress required to continue plastic deformation until a maximum is reached (the **ultimate tensile strength** or just **tensile strength,** σ_{uts}). After this value, necking of the specimen occurs (Fig. 4.9) and there is no longer uniform strain across the entire specimen (deformation occurs at the necked area only). With the onset of necking, the stress required to cause further plastic deformation decreases until the point of material fracture (**fracture strength,** σ_f). It should be noted that of these values, the yield strength is often used as a key design parameter, since by the time the material reaches its ultimate tensile strength, it has undergone significant plastic deformation and may no longer meet the shape requirements for the application.

An important property associated with plastic deformation is the ductility of a material. **Ductility** reflects the ability of a material to deform plastically before breaking. Those materials that have low ductility will fracture with very little plastic deformation (Fig. 4.10) and are considered **brittle.** Many ceramics behave in this manner.

Ductility values can be calculated as % elongation ($\%EL$) or % area reduction ($\%AR$). The former gives

$$\%EL = \frac{l_f - l_0}{l_0} \cdot 100 \tag{4.10}$$

where l_f is the length at fracture and l_0 is the gauge length (the original length of the thin portion of the dog-bone specimen; see Fig. 4.4). The latter yields

$$\%AR = \frac{A_0 - A_f}{A_0} \cdot 100 \tag{4.11}$$

where A_0 is the original sample's cross-sectional area and A_f is the cross-sectional area at fracture. $\%EL$ depends on the gauge length of the specimen and this information should be included when reporting these results. In contrast, $\%AR$ is independent of sample parameters. $\%EL$ and $\%AR$ are not expected to be equal for a given sample.

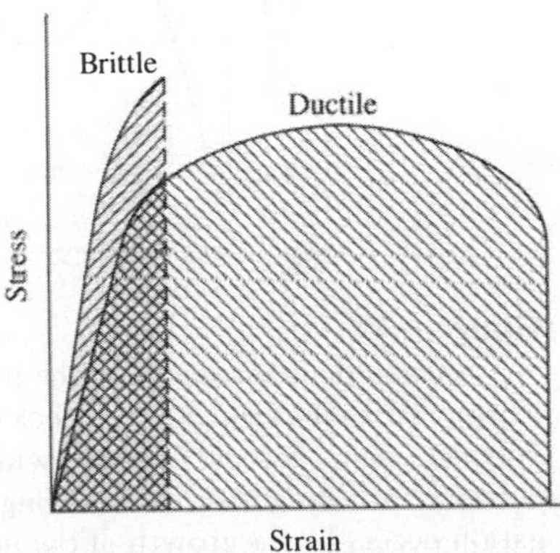

Figure 4.10
Stress-strain diagram of a brittle and ductile material. Note that the area under the curve is small in the brittle material compared to the ductile material. (Adapted with permission from [2].)

It should be noted that plastic deformation for polymers, particularly semicrystalline polymers, is slightly different from what was described above for crystalline materials such as metals (Fig. 4.9). Figure 4.11 depicts macroscopic deformation of a semicrystalline polymer in tension. After the yield point, a neck develops, like that seen for metals. However, within this neck, the polymer chains become oriented with the direction of the load. As mentioned above, the chains have more of an ability to resist deformation along their axes due to strong primary bond interactions. Therefore, specimen elongation occurs by the growth of the necked region along the gauge length, with an accompanying increase in chain order in this region. This contrasts with sample deformation in metals, in which the extension is confined only to the original necked area (Fig. 4.9). Just before fracture, there is a dramatic increase in stress needed to deform the polymer sample, which corresponds to the energy needed to overcome the strength of the primary bonds within the aligned chains.

Although this discussion of plastic deformation has focused on changes associated with tensile loading, similar stress-strain curves are found for materials undergoing compressive, shear or torsional loading. In each of these cases, the stages of deformation and fracture may differ from those seen in tension. For example, there is no maximum strength after yield for compressive testing, since there is no necking of the specimen.

To this point, calculations of stress and strain have been based on the original sample dimensions, assuming that there is negligible change in size during testing. These values are referred to as **engineering stress and strain**. However, these are not entirely accurate, especially once specimen necking begins. Therefore, it is sometimes more useful to speak of **true stress and strain**. True stress (σ_t) is the force (F) divided by the area at any point (instantaneous area, A_{in}):

$$\sigma_t = \frac{F}{A_{in}} \tag{4.12}$$

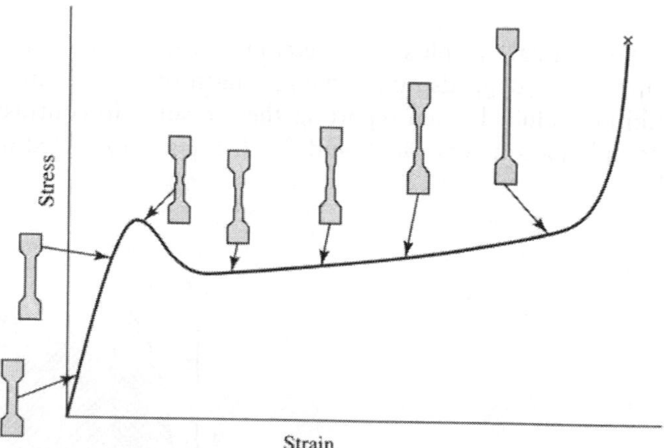

Figure 4.11
Stress-strain diagram depicting the macroscopic deformation of a semicrystalline polymer in tension. After the yield point, a neck develops, like that seen for metals. Within this neck, the polymer chains become oriented with the direction of the load, due to their ability to resist deformation along their axes (strong primary bond interactions). Therefore, specimen elongation occurs by the growth of the necked region along the gauge length, with an accompanying increase in chain order in this region. (Adapted with permission from [3] and [4].)

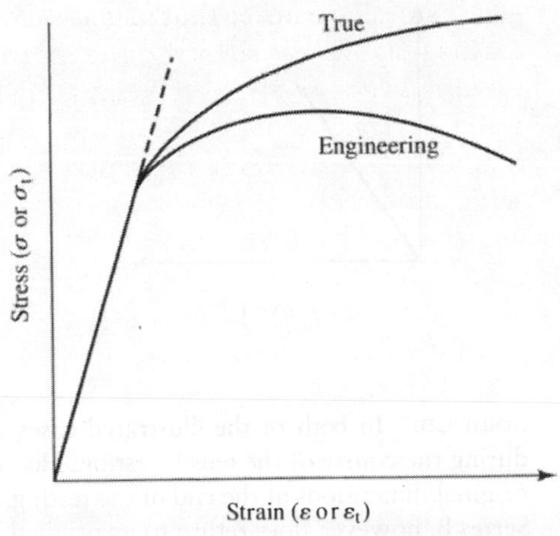

Figure 4.12
Diagram demonstrating the difference between an engineering stress-strain curve and a true stress-strain curve. Note that there is no decrease in stress throughout the test on the actual sample; this decrease is simply an artifact of the engineering stress-strain calculations. (Adapted with permission from [3].)

Similarly, the expression for the true strain (ε_t) can be derived from that for engineering strain (eq. 4.2, restated here as 4.13):

$$\varepsilon = \frac{l_i - l_0}{l_0} \tag{4.13}$$

Modifying this equation from the reference of a single point in the testing procedure, the numerator becomes the differential change in length (dl_i) and the denominator, rather than the original length, is the instantaneous length at that point in time (l_i). To find the total strain up to that moment in the test, an integral is needed:

$$\varepsilon_t = \int_{l_0}^{l_i} \frac{dl}{l} \tag{4.14}$$

This can be reduced to

$$\varepsilon_t = \ln\left(\frac{l_i}{l_0}\right) \tag{4.15}$$

where l_0 is the original length of the sample. Figure 4.12 demonstrates the difference between a typical engineering stress-strain curve and its corresponding true stress-strain values.

EXAMPLE PROBLEM 4.2

Consider the following test specimens that were subjected to tensile testing. Label each series with the type of deformation that occurs and justify your answer. Match each series to the corresponding stress-strain curve. For which series is the mechanical deformation subject to Hooke's Law throughout the testing illustrated?

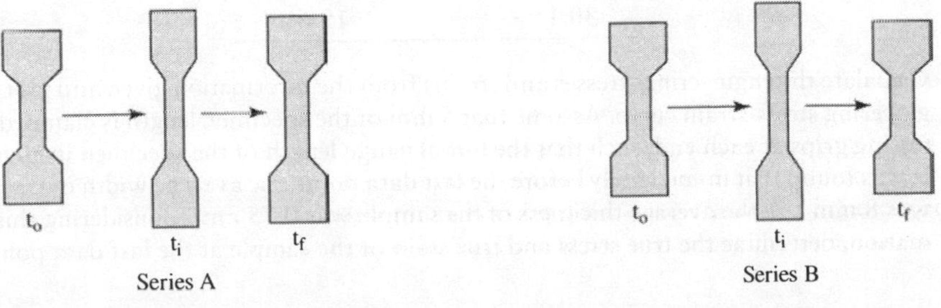

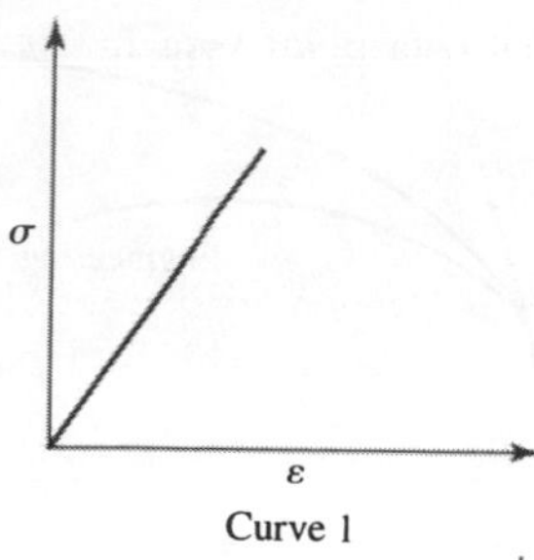

Curve 1

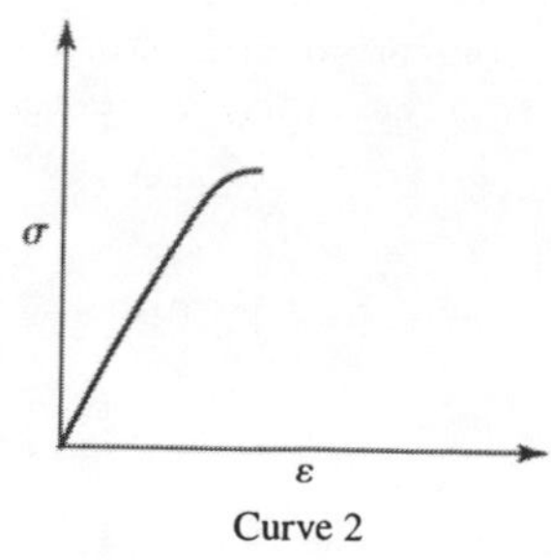

Curve 2

Solution: In both of the illustrated cases, the sample changes from its original dimensions during the course of the tensile testing. However, in Series A, the sample does not return to its original dimensions at the end of the testing. Thus, Series A demonstrates plastic deformation. Series B, however, does return to its original dimensions at the end of the tensile testing. Thus, Series B demonstrates elastic deformation. Consequently, Series B was subject to Hooke's Law throughout the testing, as this applies to samples that remain within the region of linear elasticity. Curve 1 illustrates elastic deformation, as the curve remains linear throughout. Curve 2, on the other hand, demonstrates plastic deformation, as the curve deviates from the region of linearity at higher strains as the sample begins to yield. Thus, Curve 1 corresponds with Series B, and Curve 2 corresponds with Series A. ■

EXAMPLE PROBLEM 4.3

A strip of chicken skin was excised for mechanical testing in tension. The initial dimensions of the rectangular specimen were 30 mm long and 15 mm wide, with an average thickness of 3 mm. The mechanical testing was conducted at a rate of 5 mm/sec. The following data were obtained:

Gauge length (mm)	Force (N)
20.0	0.0
20.5	0.1
21.0	0.3
21.5	0.5
22.0	0.8
22.5	1.1
23.1	1.6
23.6	2.0
24.2	2.7
24.6	3.6
25.2	4.7
25.7	6.2
26.3	7.9
26.8	9.7
27.4	11.4
27.9	12.9
28.5	14.5
29.0	16.4
29.6	18.3
30.1	19.6

(a) Calculate the engineering stresses and strains from the information given and plot the engineering stress-strain curve. Assume that 5 mm of the specimen length is clamped by the testing grips at each end, such that the initial gauge length of the specimen is 20 mm.

(b) It was found that immediately before the last data point, the average width of the sample was 8 mm and the average thickness of the sample was 0.75 mm. Considering this information, determine the true stress and true stain of the sample at the last data point.

(c) Compare the true stress and strain values for the final data point with the engineering stress and strain values for the final data point.

Solution:

(a) Since the initial gauge length of the specimen is given to be 20 mm and the gauge length for each data point is given, the engineering strain can be calculated at each point as follows:

$$\varepsilon = (l_i - l_o)/l_o$$
$$\varepsilon = (l_i - 20 \text{ mm})/20 \text{ mm}$$

The engineering stress can be calculated by dividing the force at each point by the cross-sectional area of the sample. In this case, the cross-sectional area of the sample is the width of the sample (15 mm) times the average thickness of the sample (3 mm). Thus,

$$A = 15 \text{ mm} \cdot 3 \text{ mm} = 45 \text{ mm}^2$$
$$\sigma = F/A_o = F/45 \text{ mm}^2$$

The calculated stresses and strains are as follows:

Strain	Stress (N/mm^2)
0.00	0.00
0.02	0.00
0.05	0.01
0.07	0.01
0.10	0.02
0.12	0.02
0.15	0.03
0.18	0.05
0.21	0.06
0.23	0.08
0.26	0.10
0.29	0.14
0.31	0.18
0.34	0.22
0.37	0.25
0.39	0.29
0.42	0.32
0.45	0.36
0.48	0.41
0.51	0.44

The engineering stress-strain plot is as follows:

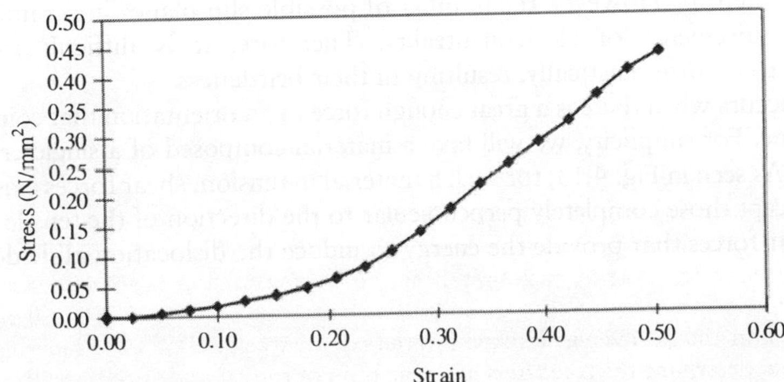

(b) The true stress of a sample takes into account the changes in the sample dimensions that may occur with time. As a result, the true stress is determined by the formula

$$\sigma_t = F/A_t,$$

where A_t is the cross-sectional area at the time of interest. In this case, the dimensions of the sample at time t are given to be 8 mm in width and 0.75 mm in thickness. Thus, the cross-sectional area of the sample at the time point of interest is (8 mm)(0.75 mm) = 6 mm^2.

So, the true stress at this point can be calculated as follows:

$$\sigma_t = (19.6 \text{ N})/(6 \text{ mm}^2) = \underline{3.27 \text{ N/mm}^2}$$

The true strain of the sample at the final point can be calculated from the equation $\varepsilon_t = ln(l_i/l_o)$ as follows:

$$\varepsilon_t = \ln(30.1 \text{ mm}/20 \text{ mm}) = \underline{0.41}$$

(c) The calculated true stress of 3.27 N/mm^2 is much greater than the engineering stress of 0.51 N/mm^2 for the last data point. The difference is due mainly to the large changes in the cross-sectional area of the sample from the initial value (changed from the initial value of 45 mm^2 to 6 mm^2). If a given force is distributed across a smaller cross-sectional area, as was the case in this exercise, then the stress increases. There was little difference observed between the engineering strain and the true strain for the sample at the final point. ■

4.2.1.5 Molecular Causes of Plastic Deformation Figure 4.5 depicts the stress-strain response for a number of material types. As mentioned previously, ceramics are often brittle and demonstrate behavior similar to Material I, while metals produce curves similar to Material II. Polymers fall into a wide range of categories, from very brittle materials (like Material I) to materials exhibiting plastic deformation (like Material III) to highly elastic materials (like Material IV).

Although the first two types of polymer mechanical behavior are similar to those discussed for ceramics and metals, the third type, **elasticity**, is characteristic only of a subset of polymers called **elastomers**. The most common elastomer is rubber. Elastic materials are defined as those that allow large recoverable strains at low stress levels. The molecular causes for this particular mechanical behavior are discussed below.

4.2.1.6 Causes of Plastic Deformation—Metals and Crystalline Ceramics At this point, a detailed look at what happens on an atomic scale to produce plastic deformation of the various classes of materials is warranted. As discussed in Chapter 3, metals and crystalline ceramics undergo deformation due to dislocation glide along a plane called the **slip plane**. The slip plane is usually the plane with the highest atomic density. However, the number of possible slip planes in ceramics is limited by requirements of electroneutrality. Therefore, it is difficult for ceramic materials to deform plastically, resulting in their brittleness.

Slip occurs when there is a great enough force in an orientation that coincides with a slip plane. For simplicity, we will take a material composed of a single crystal as an example. As seen in Fig. 4.13, for such a material in tension, shear forces exist along all planes except those completely perpendicular to the direction of the tensile force. It is these shear forces that provide the energy to induce the dislocation glide described in

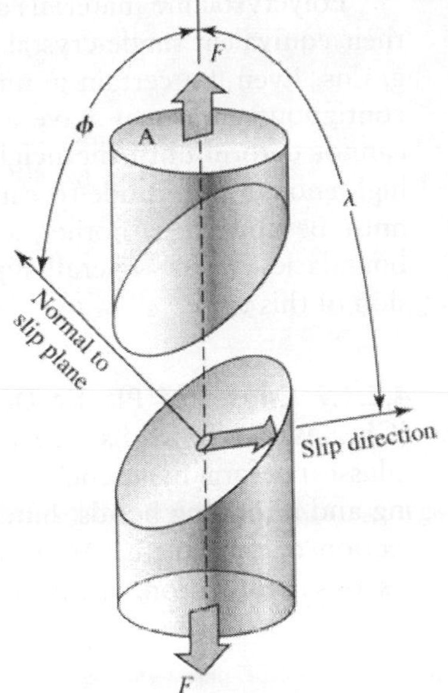

Figure 4.13
Schematic showing slip in a tensile specimen. Slip is caused by shear stress in a tensile specimen, which can occur in any direction with the exception of perpendicular to the tensile force. This stress in the slip plane can be calculated using the tensile stress on the sample, and the two angles shown in the figure (ϕ and λ). (Adapted with permission from [2].)

the previous chapter. Therefore, the magnitude of the shear stress felt by the slip plane (**resolved shear stress,** τ_r) is of particular interest and can be determined by the equation

$$\tau_r = \sigma \cos \phi \cos \lambda \qquad (4.16)$$

where σ is the tensile stress, ϕ is the angle between the normal to the slip plane and the direction of applied force, and λ is the angle between the slip direction and the direction of applied force. When the resolved shear stress along a slip plane exceeds a certain value, called the critical resolved shear stress (τ_{crss}), slip is initiated. τ_{crss} varies according to the material and is a factor in determining the yield strength of the material.

Deformation of polycrystalline materials is more complex, since each grain is oriented randomly. Therefore, some grains may be arranged favorably with the applied force to allow slip, while others may not. For each grain, slip occurs along the plane with the most appropriate orientation. As shown in Fig. 4.14, macroscopic deformation of polycrystalline materials occurs due to deformation of individual grains, rather than alterations or opening of grain boundaries.

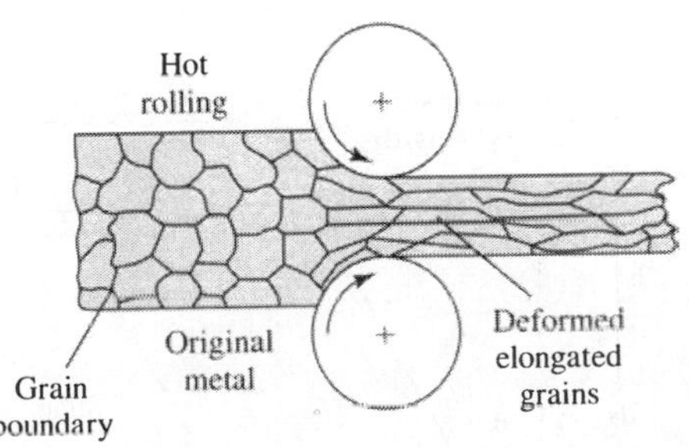

Figure 4.14
During hot rolling of metals, which is used to produce a final product with smaller cross-sectional area (see Chapter 6), macroscopic elongation occurs. As shown in this diagram, this is due to deformation of individual grains, rather than opening of the grain boundaries. (Adapted with permission from [5].)

Polycrystalline materials are usually stronger (have higher yield strengths) than their equivalent single-crystal materials due to constraints imposed by neighboring grains. Even if a certain grain is orientated to allow slip at a low level of stress, a contiguous grain may have a much less favorable orientation, and the first grain cannot deform until the neighboring grain also deforms. Therefore, a stress with high enough magnitude to cause deformation of the less-favorably arranged grains must be applied. (Another way of thinking of this is that the presence of grain boundaries hinders overall slip in the material—see Section 4.5 for further discussion of this topic.)

4.2.1.7 Causes of Plastic Deformation—Amorphous Polymers and Ceramics (Glasses) Also as discussed in Chapter 3, noncrystalline polymers and ceramics (glasses) deform by viscous flow. Here, atoms or ions slide past each other by breaking and reforming bonds, but, in contrast to dislocations, there is no prescribed direction of movement. As with slip, shear stress also plays an important role in viscous deformation. From Chapter 3, we have seen that

$$\tau = \eta\dot{\gamma} \tag{4.17}$$

or, in viscous flow, the *rate* of deformation is proportional to the applied stress. The proportionality constant η is the viscosity of the sample, and $\dot{\gamma}$ is the rate of shear deformation $\left(\frac{d\gamma}{dt}\right)$. This is called **Newton's law.**

Now that we understand more about the different types of mechanical properties of materials, we can derive this relationship. Newton's law can be seen as an extension of the shear stress/shear strain relationship for solids discussed above (Fig. 4.15):

$$\tau = G\gamma \tag{4.18}$$

As depicted in Fig. 4.15, here, another form of γ is used:

$$\gamma = \tan\theta = \frac{dy}{dx} \tag{4.19}$$

However, as discussed in the previous chapter, amorphous materials can be thought of as cooled liquids, so when we replace the solid sample in the figure with an equal volume of liquid, we obtain a relationship like that shown in Fig. 4.16. In this case, the shear force does not cause a single strain value, but the deformation

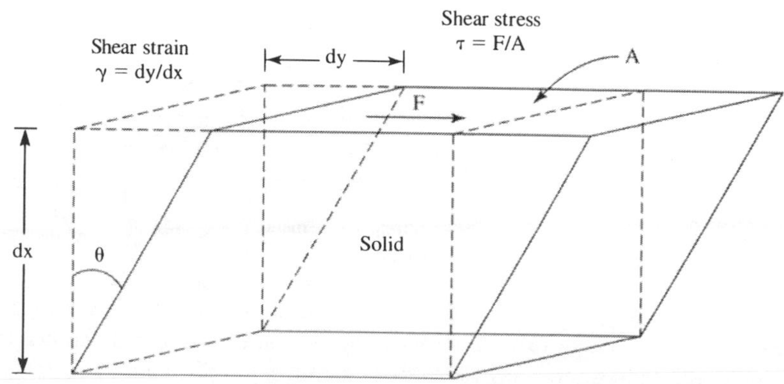

Figure 4.15
Schematic of the deformation that occurs when a crystalline material undergoes shear stress. (Adapted with permission from [3].)

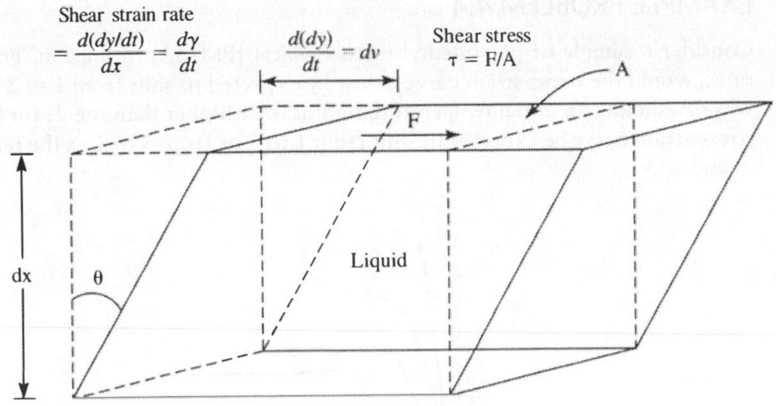

Figure 4.16 Schematic of the deformation that occurs when an amorphous material undergoes shear stress. (Adapted with permission from [3].)

continues with time. The rate of deformation [$(d(dy/dt))$] is proportional to the shear force F:

$$F \propto d(dy/dt) \tag{4.20}$$

If the force is normalized by the area to obtain shear stress (τ) and the displacement rate is normalized by the height (dx) the expression becomes

$$\tau \propto \frac{d(dy/dt)}{dx} \tag{4.21}$$

Because dx is a constant, the equation can be rearranged:

$$\tau \propto \frac{d(dy/dx)}{dt} \tag{4.22}$$

Replacing dy/dx with γ, and including η as a constant of proportionality yields

$$\tau = \eta\left(\frac{d\gamma}{dt}\right) = \eta\dot{\gamma} \tag{4.23}$$

4.2.1.8 Causes of Plastic Deformation—Polymers (General) The results of mechanical testing of polymers are more dependent on testing conditions than are the results for metals and ceramics. Temperature has striking effects on the behavior of the material. Similarly, the properties observed can be influenced by the rate of testing. Either increasing the testing temperature or decreasing the strain rate causes a reduction in E, a decrease in tensile strength and an increase in ductility. The molecular reasons for these phenomena are described below.

For all polymers containing amorphous regions, whether the material is tested at temperatures above or below its T_g has a very large impact on its mechanical properties. Below T_g, the polymer chains are "frozen" and the resulting material is brittle. Above T_g, the polymer chains begin to rotate around their backbones and move relative to one another, so the material becomes more ductile.

The effect of strain rate on mechanical properties can be related, in part, to the necking phenomenon described earlier. If a polymeric sample is pulled too quickly, the chains do not have enough time to rearrange and orient themselves along the axis of loading in the neck region. Therefore, at higher strain rates, less deformation occurs, and the specimen behaves in a more brittle manner and has a higher overall strength.

EXAMPLE PROBLEM 4.4

Consider a sample of poly(methyl methacrylate) (PMMA) in tension. For increasing strain rates, would the stress-strain curve below be expected to shift from 1 to 3 or from 3 to 1 and why? Assuming an initial temperature significantly higher than the T_g for PMMA, would the stress-strain curve be expected to shift from 1 to 3 or from 3 to 1 as the temperature decreases and why?

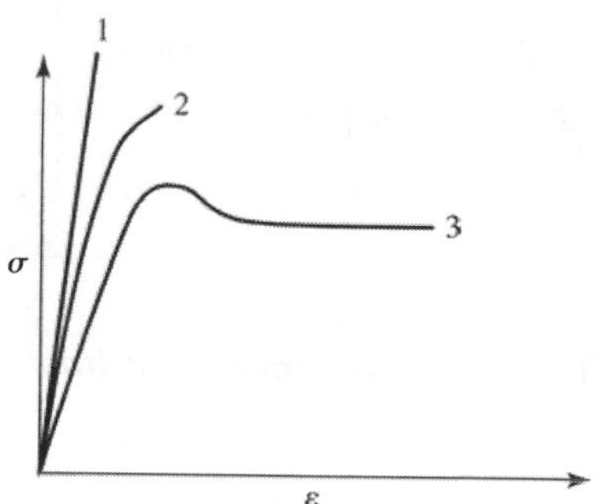

Solution: For increasing strain rates, the stress-strain curve would be expected to shift from 3 to 1. As the strain rate increases, the polymer chains are given less time to orient themselves along the axis of loading. Thus, at higher strain rates, the sample behaves in an increasingly brittle manner and with a higher strength. Starting at a temperature much higher than T_g for PMMA, the sample would behave in a manner similar to curve 3, as the polymer chains have a large amount of energy to rearrange with the applied force. As the temperature decreases toward T_g, one would expect the stress-strain curve to shift toward curve 1, as the energy available for polymer chain movement decreases and the material acts in a more brittle manner. ■

4.2.1.9 Causes of Plastic Deformation—Semi-Crystalline Polymers and Elastomers Because two particular subclasses of polymers, semicrystalline polymers and elastomers, possess unique stress-strain properties, their deformation is discussed here in more detail. This description follows that of Callister [2] for both polymer types. Semicrystalline polymers are composed of spherulites, as depicted in Fig. 3.12. These spherulites contain crystalline lamellar regions that radiate from the center. In between the lamellae are amorphous regions that contain tie molecules to connect neighboring lamellae.

Plastic deformation for these polymers can be conceptualized as interactions between the lamellar and amorphous regions in response to a tensile force. As shown in Fig. 4.17, there are several stages of elongation. In the first stage, the tie chains extend and the lamellae slide past each other. In the second stage, the lamellae themselves become reoriented so that the chain folds are aligned along the axis of loading. After this, blocks of the crystalline phases separate from each other. However, adjacent lamellae within the blocks are still attached via the tie molecules. Finally, the blocks and tie molecules become oriented along the axis of the applied tensile force. In this way, tensile forces can induce significant chain orientation in semicrystalline polymers (as seen in the necking phenomena described above). As in grains in polycrystalline metals and ceramics, this also induces a change in shape of the spherulites.

An interesting aspect to semicrystalline polymers is that synthesis and processing parameters can easily affect their deformation behavior, as seen in Fig. 4.18. Any changes that inhibit chain motion within these polymers increase the observed strength and decrease the ductility. Such changes include increasing the polymer

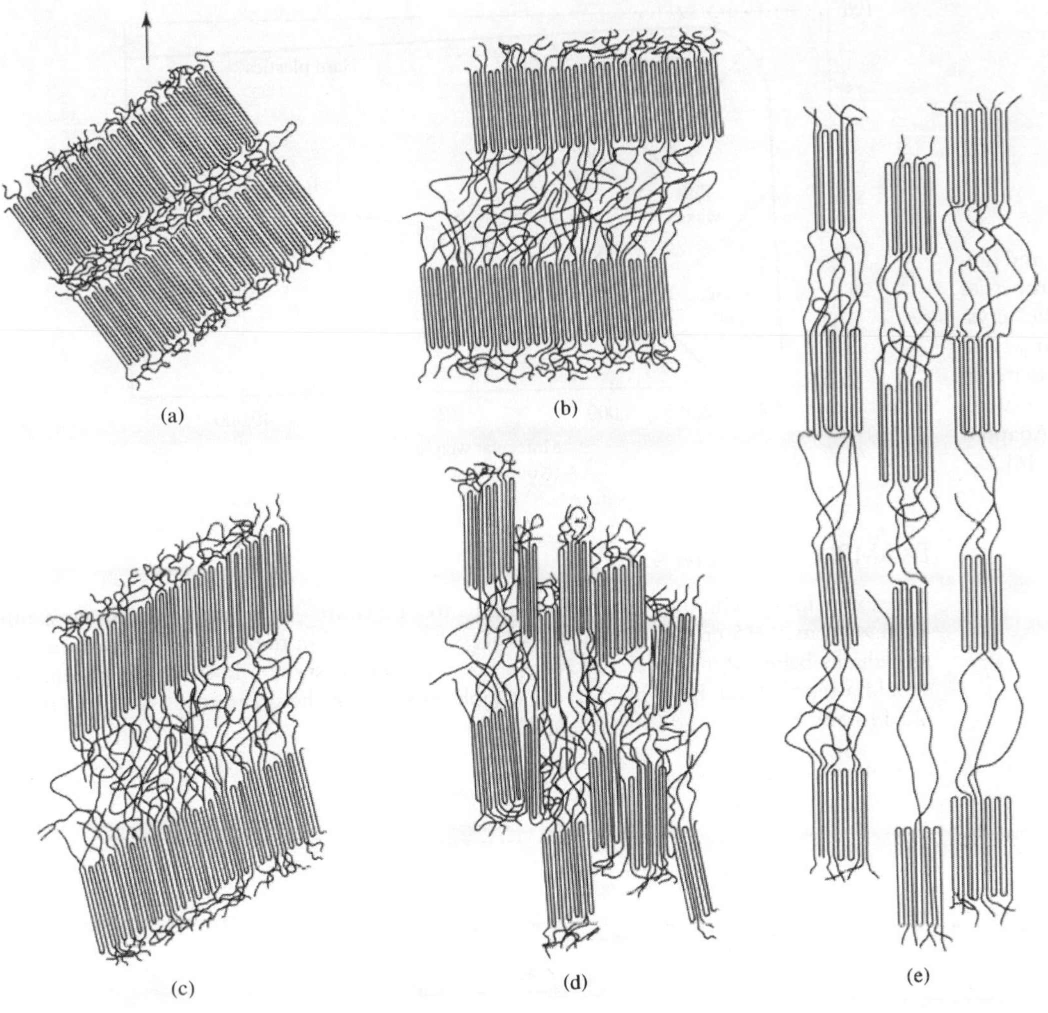

Figure 4.17
Plastic deformation for semicrystalline polymers (a) can be conceptualized as interactions between the lamellar and amorphous regions in response to a tensile force. There are several stages of elongation. (b) In the first stage, the tie chains extend and the lamellae slide past each other. (c) In the second stage, the lamellae themselves become re-oriented so that the chain folds are aligned along the axis of loading. (d) After this, blocks of the crystalline phases separate from each other. However, adjacent lamellae within the blocks are still attached via the tie molecules. (e) Finally, the blocks and tie molecules become oriented along the axis of the applied tensile force. In this way, tensile forces can induce significant chain orientation in semicrystalline polymers. (Adapted with permission from [4].)

crystallinity, increasing the molecular weight, or crosslinking the polymer. Secondary bonds that exist in crystalline areas where the chains are more tightly packed are effective in restricting chain motion. Thus, percent crystallinity can have a significant effect on the mechanical properties of a polymer. An increase in molecular weight will also strengthen a polymer, since physical entanglements between larger chains will inhibit chain movement (Fig. 4.18). Finally, covalent linkages, such as those formed during crosslinking, will also prevent chain movement and increase the strength and brittleness of the polymer.

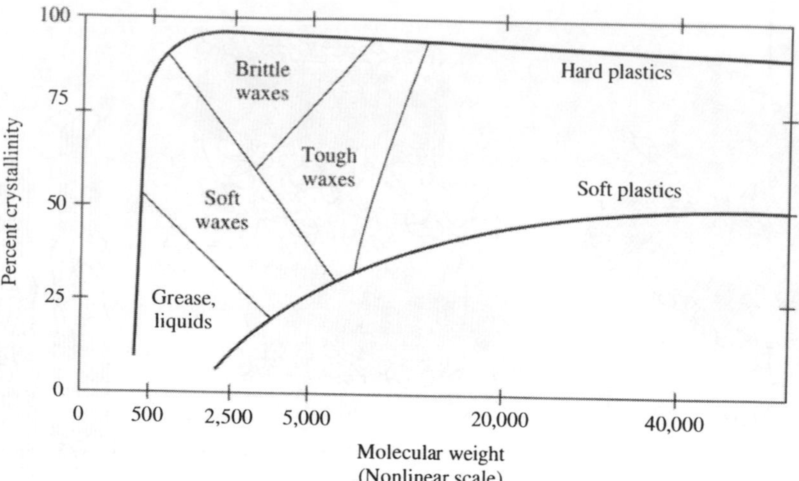

Figure 4.18
Effect of crystallinity and molecular weight on properties of polymers. As the crystallinity and molecular weight increase, the same material can be found in liquid, wax, or stiff solid form. (Adapted with permission from [6].)

EXAMPLE PROBLEM 4.5

An extrusion technique was employed to fabricate a square polymer sample 4 cm × 4 cm × 0.5 cm. The extrusion process has resulted in the vast majority of the polymer chains being aligned preferentially in one direction as shown. In which direction, then, should a tensile force be applied to the sample to result in the greatest resistance to the applied force? Why?

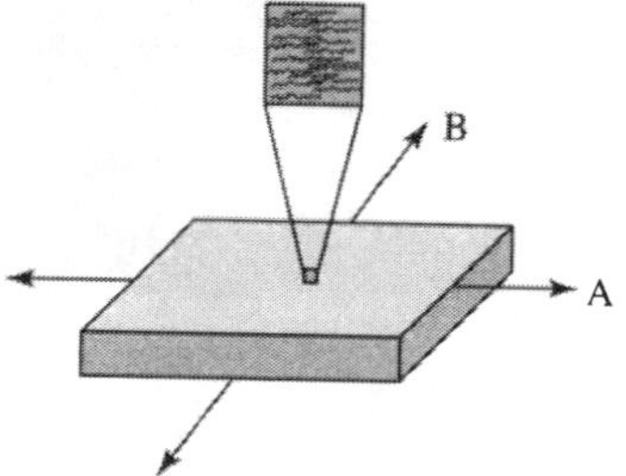

Solution: The tensile force should be applied along the direction indicated by arrow "A" as this direction is parallel to the axis of orientation of the majority of the polymer chains in the material, as illustrated. Although secondary forces may exist between the polymer chains, the strongest forces in the material are found in the molecular bonds along the backbones of the polymer chains. In this case, the majority of the polymer chains are oriented along one axis; thus the greatest resistance to force would occur along this axis. The resistance to force in the direction of arrow "B" would stem primarily from chain entanglements and any secondary forces that might be present between the polymer chains. These forces are much weaker than the covalent forces found in the polymer chains themselves.

■

As depicted in Material IV in Fig. 4.5, elastomers are unique in that they allow large elastic deformation at low stresses, due to their distinctive chain structure. Elastomers are amorphous materials in their unstressed state, composed of coiled chains with nearly free bond rotations around the backbone, as shown in Fig. 4.19. The chains are crosslinked at given points to prevent chains from slipping past each other, which would result in plastic deformation of the material.

An example of an elastomer found in the human body is **elastin**, which confers resiliency and extensibility to many tissues (see Chapter 9 for more information on elastin). Elastin is a particularly important constituent of tissues that must undergo

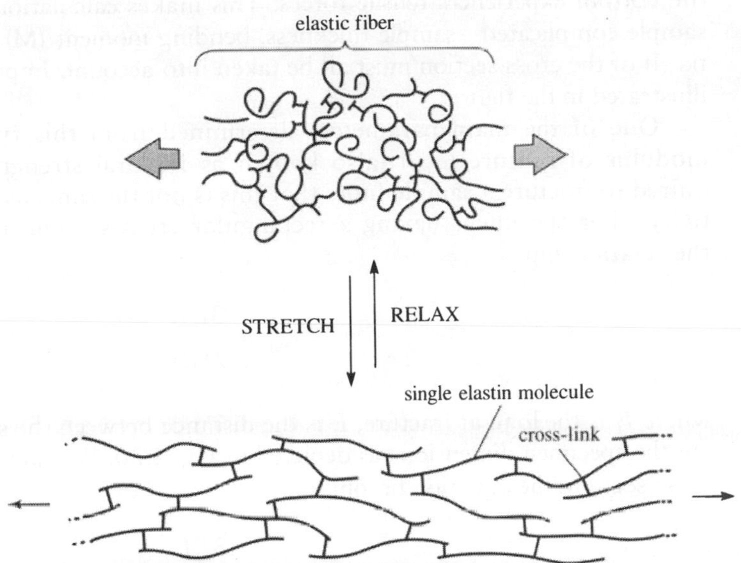

Figure 4.19
Diagram of elastin, a type of elastomer, showing its relaxed and stressed states. Elastomers are amorphous materials in their unstressed state, composed of coiled chains with nearly free bond rotations around the backbone. Tensile forces cause the individual elastin molecules to unfold and align in the direction of loading. The network is held together by the cross links between the elastin molecules. If the applied stress is removed, the elastin will return to its unstretched state due to thermodynamic considerations. (Adapted with permission from [7].)

many stretch-relaxation cycles, such as the air sacs in the lungs. Like other elastomers, elastin fibers exist as crosslinked coiled protein chains.

When elastomers are above their T_g, a tensile force applied to the sample will cause the uncoiling of the chains and their alignment along the axis of tension, as seen in Fig. 4.19. The driving force for the elastomer to return to its prestressed state after the removal of the tensile force is thermodynamic. The entropy of the system is greater in the amorphous than the ordered state that occurs after tension. Since greater disorder is favored, entropic concerns cause the material to return to its original state. Elastomers can be modeled as little springs that obey Hooke's law. This model and its uses will be explained further in the next section.

4.2.2 Bending Properties

The stress-strain behavior of materials can also be determined through bending tests. While these tests can be performed on a variety of materials, they are usually used on ceramics, due to the inherent brittleness of the material (simply clamping a ceramic specimen can lead to fracture, hence it is a difficult material to test under tension).

Bending tests can be performed on specimens having rectangular or circular cross-sections, as shown in Fig. 4.20. The sample can be subjected to three-point (seen in figure) or four-point bending. A disadvantage of bending tests is that the magnitude and type of stress is not constant across the sample. For the experiment shown in the figure, the top of the specimen experiences compressive forces, while

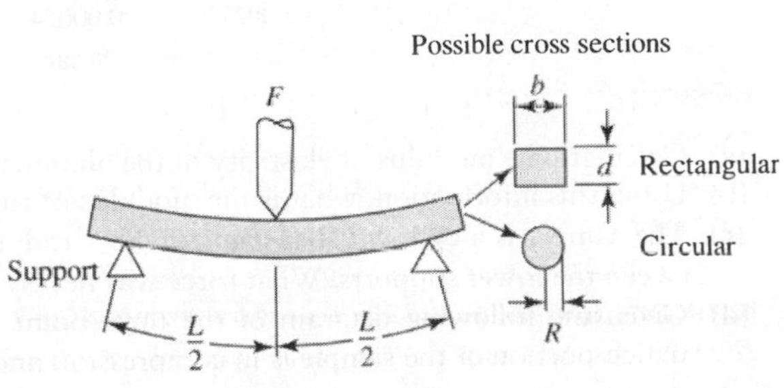

Figure 4.20
Schematic of a three-point bending test. If the applied load F causes fracture of the specimen, then the modulus of rupture can be calculated. This test can be carried out with either rectangular or cylindrical specimens (see inset of cross-sections). (Adapted with permission from [2].)

the bottom experiences tensile forces. This makes calculation of the stress on the sample complicated—sample thickness, bending moment (M) and moment of inertia (I) of the cross-section must all be taken into account. Important parameters are illustrated in the figure.

One of the main parameters determined from this type of testing is the **modulus of rupture** (σ_{mr}) (also known as flexural strength), or the stress required to fracture a sample (note that this is not the same as the modulus of elasticity). For specimens having a rectangular cross-section, this is calculated via the relationship

$$\sigma_{mr} = \frac{3F_f L}{2bd^2} \tag{4.24}$$

where F_f is the load at fracture, L is the distance between the supports and b and d are the specimen dimensions as depicted in Fig. 4.20. For samples having a circular cross-section, the equation becomes

$$\sigma_{mr} = \frac{3F_f L}{\pi R^3} \tag{4.25}$$

where R is the radius of the sample.

Stress-strain curves similar to those resulting from tensile tests can be produced from bending data. Since there is little plastic deformation of these materials, there exists a linear relationship between stress and strain until sample fracture. As with tensile testing, the slope of this curve is the modulus of elasticity.

EXAMPLE PROBLEM 4.6

The following is a stress-strain curve resulting from a three-point bending test on an alumina (ceramic) test sample:

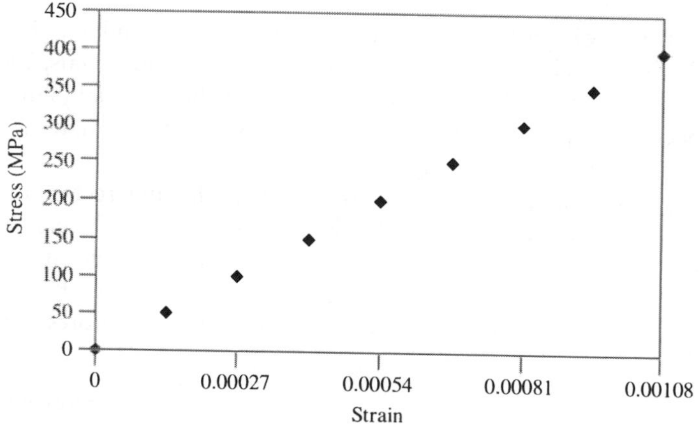

(a) Calculate the modulus of elasticity of the alumina sample.

(b) Using this information, what is the modulus of rupture?

(c) The sample is a cylindrical specimen with a radius of 1 cm and a distance of 10 cm between the lower supports. What force was necessary to cause this fracture?

(d) Given the following diagram of the three-point bending test of a rectangular sample, which portion of the sample is in compression and which portion is in tension?

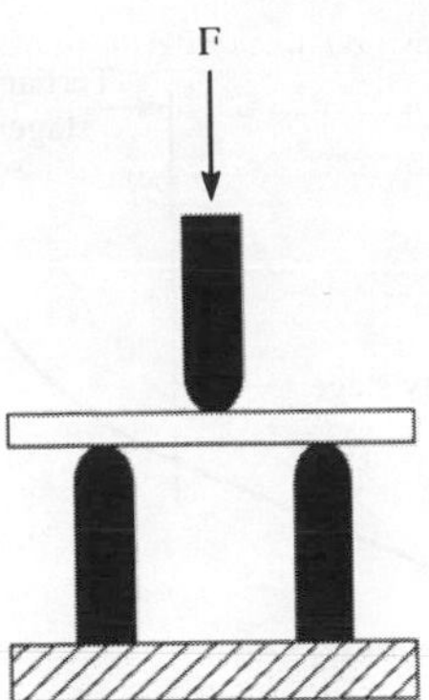

Solution:

(a) The modulus of elasticity can be determined from the slope of the linear portion of the stress-strain curve:

$$E = \frac{\Delta\sigma}{\Delta\varepsilon} = \frac{400 \quad 0\ \text{MPa}}{0.00108 - 0} = 370\ \text{GPa}$$

(b) The modulus of rupture is the stress at the point of fracture, around 400MPa.

(c) Solve equation 4.25 for F_f and determine the force at fracture:

$$F_f = \frac{\sigma_{mr}\pi R^3}{3L} = \frac{400000\pi 0.01^3}{3 \times 0.1} \approx 4.2\text{N}$$

(d) The portion of the sample at the top facing the indenting attachment is in compression, while the portion of the sample at the bottom facing the two supporting points is in tension under the load. ■

4.2.3 Time-Dependent Properties

Traditional mechanical tests like those described above do not provide a full picture of the stress-strain behavior of materials, since they measure response to loading over a relatively short time. However, some materials experience changes at the molecular level that result in alterations in mechanical properties when loaded for longer times. Two of these time-dependent properties, creep and stress relaxation, are described in the following sections.

4.2.3.1 Creep Creep can be defined as plastic deformation of a sample under constant load over time. Creep can be observed in all materials, but it is usually only a concern at temperatures greater than $0.4T_m$ (T_m = absolute melting temperature) for metals and even higher temperatures for ceramics. In contrast, creep can occur at or around room temperature for some polymer systems.

Creep tests are performed by exerting a constant (usually tensile) load on the specimen while maintaining the system at a fixed temperature. The resulting strain is recorded as a function of time. A typical creep curve for metal and ceramic materials is found in Fig. 4.21.

This curve can be divided into three distinct regions. After the initial deformation, the first stage, **primary creep**, is characterized by an increase in strain with time, while the creep rate (the slope of the curve) decreases. This is due to repositioning of aspects of the material, such as dislocations, in response to loading. As the load continues, an equilibrium is established within the material substructure and a minimum creep rate is attained. This is **secondary creep**, and in this area, there is a linear relationship between creep strain and time. Secondary creep usually lasts for

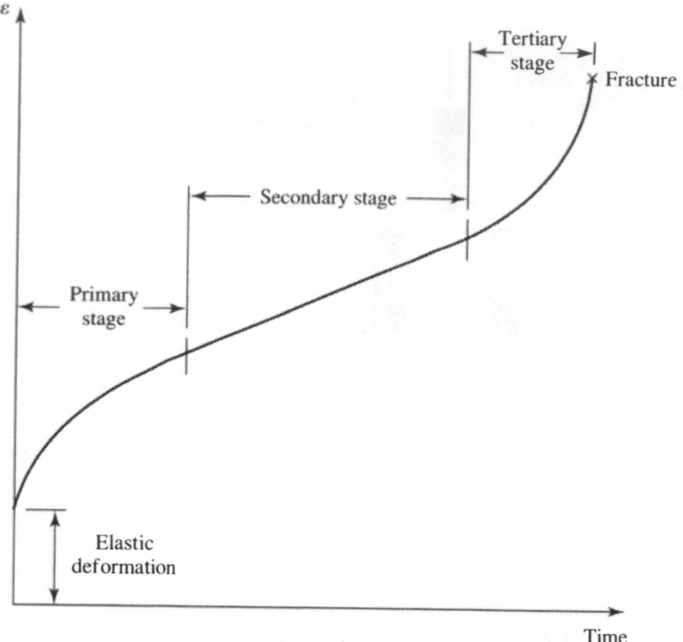

Figure 4.21
A typical creep curve for a metal or ceramic material. The strain observed by the sample varies as a function of time. This curve can be divided into three distinct regions. After the initial deformation, the first stage, primary creep, is characterized by an increase in strain with time, while the creep rate (slope of curve) decreases. As the load continues, an equilibrium is established within the material substructure and secondary creep is achieved. In this area, there is a linear relationship between creep strain and time. Finally, tertiary creep leads rapidly to failure. (Adapted with permission from [3].)

the longest period. Finally, **tertiary creep** leads to failure. In this stage, gross defects appear inside the material, such as grain boundary separation, cracks, or voids. Here, elongation proceeds rapidly until material failure.

Important parameters obtained from creep testing are the **steady state creep rate, $\dot{\varepsilon}$,** and the time to rupture (t_r). $\dot{\varepsilon}$ is calculated by taking the slope of the creep curve in the secondary stage. However, because both the applied stress and the testing temperature have a large effect on a material's creep response, these parameters must be specified for each value of $\dot{\varepsilon}$ and t_r. As seen in Fig. 4.22, $\dot{\varepsilon}$ increases with increasing stress and increasing temperature. In contrast, t_r decreases at higher temperatures or stresses.

Creep curves for polymers, like those shown in Fig. 4.23, are similar to those for metals and ceramics, but with less distinct stages of creep deformation. This figure also demonstrates that creep in polymeric materials can be a concern even at relatively low temperatures and stresses. The possibility of creep at body temperature is extremely important to recall when designing polymeric implants that must maintain specific dimensions in order to function. For example, one of the reasons for failure of polymer-based ligament replacements over years in the body is creep of the material, which leads to the inability of the device to maintain the joint in its proper position.

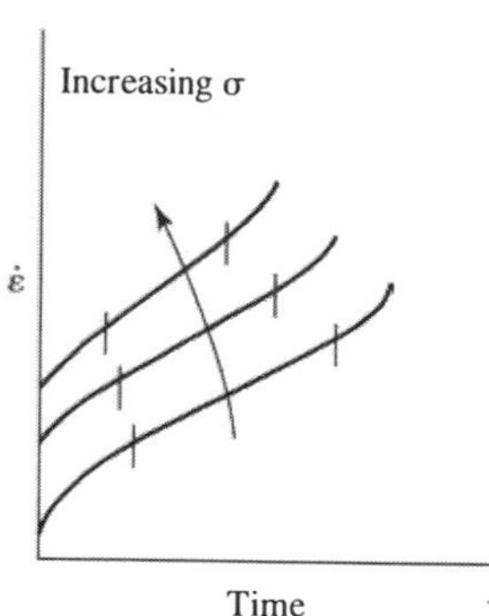

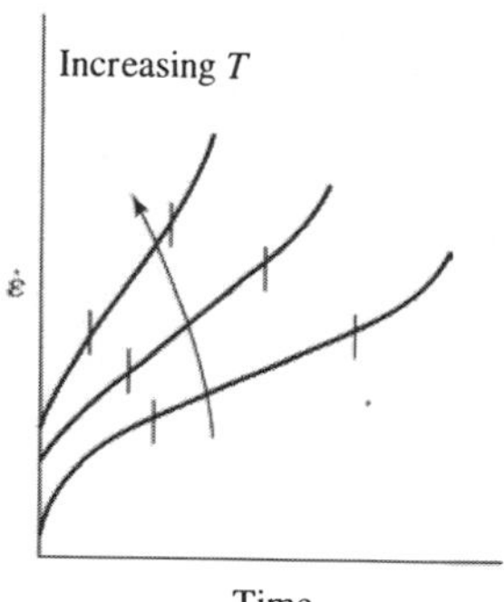

Figure 4.22
Effect of stress and temperature on creep response. Steady state creep rate ($\dot{\varepsilon}$) increases with increasing stress and increasing temperature. (Adapted with permission from [8].)

4.2.3.2 Molecular Causes of Creep—Metals On an atomic scale, creep is caused by a variety of mechanisms, depending on the material type. In metals, creep can be a result of grain boundaries sliding relative to one another, or migration of vacancies. Vacancy migration is promoted at high temperatures due to greater atomic diffusion with increasing temperature (see Chapter 2). In particular, there are two main creep mechanisms involving vacancy migration: stress-induced vacancy diffusion and dislocation climb.

Stress-induced vacancy diffusion is depicted in Fig. 4.24. As a result of loading, extra vacancies are produced on the faces of the grains perpendicular to the applied stress (AB and CD), and these have a tendency to migrate to the faces parallel to the stress axis (AC and BD). As with all vacancy diffusion, atomic diffusion is in the opposite direction, resulting in an elongation of the grain along the line of applied

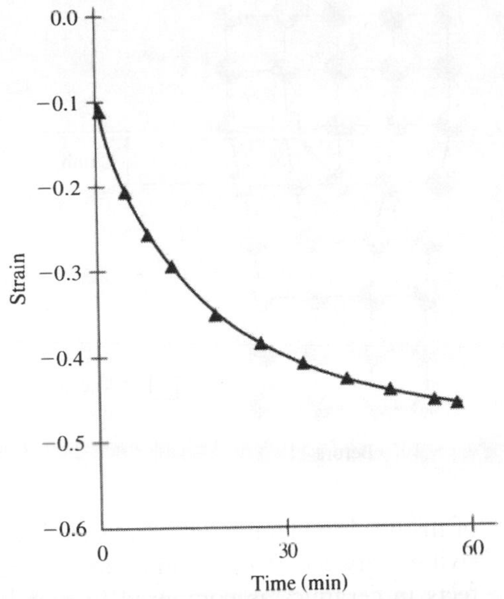

Figure 4.23
A typical creep curve for a porous polymeric material (poly(lactic-co-glycolic acid), PLGA 50:50) under applied stress of 9.5 kPa. (In this case, strain is negative because the load applied was compressive, rather than tensile, but the continual change in length with time still occurs.) Creep curves for polymers are similar to those for metals and ceramics, but with less distinct stages of creep deformation. Creep in polymeric materials can be a concern even at relatively low temperatures and stresses. (Adapted with permission from [9].)

stress. This type of stress-induced vacancy diffusion is called **Nabarro-Herring creep.** If the vacancies migrate along the grain boundaries rather than through the bulk of the grain, this is termed **Coble creep.**

As the name implies, in **dislocation climb** a dislocation moves (climbs) one atomic spacing by diffusion of an entire row of vacancies to the extra partial plane of atoms found in an edge dislocation. Atomic movement is opposite to this, as shown in Fig. 4.25.

4.2.3.3 Molecular Causes of Creep—Ceramics Creep mechanisms for ceramics are similar to those in metals, but ceramics are more resistant to creep deformation for a variety of reasons. Ion and vacancy diffusion are more difficult in ceramics because

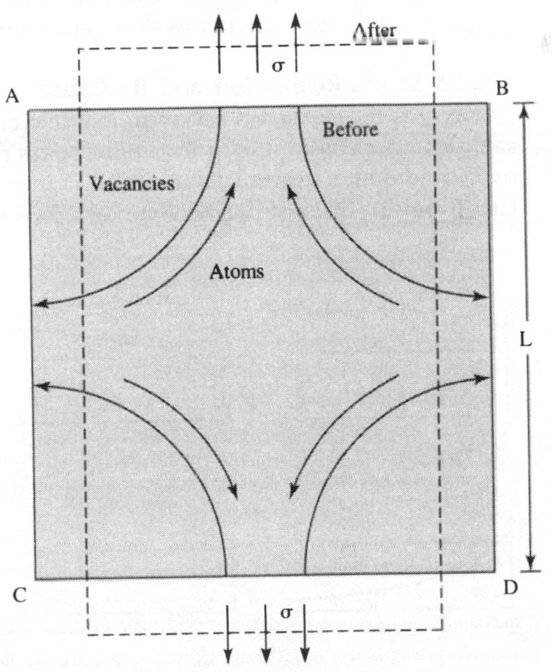

Figure 4.24
A schematic of stress-induced vacancy diffusion. As a result of loading, extra vacancies are produced on the faces of the grains perpendicular to the applied stress (AB and CD), and these have a tendency to migrate to the faces parallel to the stress axis (AC and BD). As with all vacancy diffusion, atomic diffusion is in the opposite direction, resulting in an elongation of the grain along the line of applied stress. The parameter L is the original length of the grain and σ is the applied stress. (Adapted with permission from [3].)

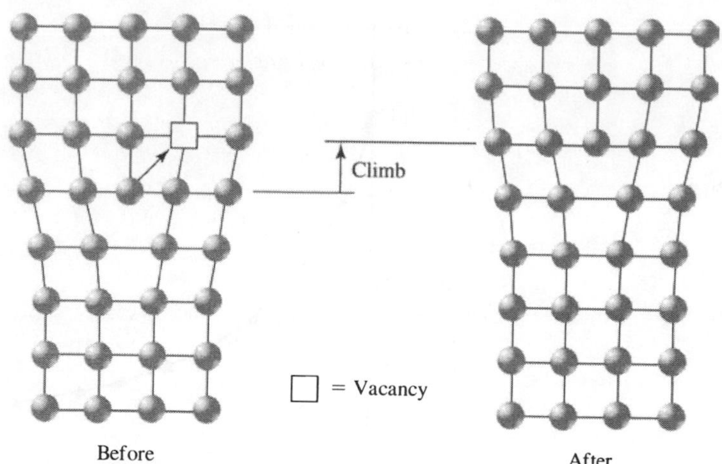

Figure 4.25
A diagram of dislocation climb (end-on view). In this scenario, a dislocation moves (climbs) one atomic spacing by diffusion of an entire row of vacancies to the extra partial plane of atoms found in an edge dislocation. (Adapted with permission from [3].)

of the need to maintain electroneutrality of the material, and the difference in diffusivities between cations and anions. In addition, there are generally fewer point defects in ceramics as compared to metals. With these constraints, grain boundary sliding is a main means for microstructural rearrangement and creep deformation in this class of biomaterials.

4.2.3.4 Molecular Causes of Creep—Polymers Creep deformation in semicrystalline and amorphous polymers depends on movement of chains in the amorphous regions via viscous flow. Therefore, the percent crystallinity and whether testing occurs above or below the polymer's T_g has a large influence on the creep properties observed. Susceptibility to creep decreases as the crystallinity of the polymer increases since there is a smaller fraction of amorphous areas in more highly crystalline samples. Below T_g, the chains in the amorphous regions are not able to rotate or slide and no time-dependent deformation is observed. At these temperatures, generally only elastic deformation is recorded up to the point of fracture. On the other hand, above T_g, the polymer chains can move past each other, so time-dependent properties indicative of viscous flow (creep and stress relaxation) can be seen.

4.2.3.5 Stress Relaxation and its Causes A related time-dependent mechanical property is termed **stress relaxation.** While creep involves plastic deformation of a sample under constant load over time, stress relaxation is the decrease in stress seen over time under constant strain, and is most often found in polymeric materials. Creep and stress relaxation behavior are depicted graphically in Fig. 4.26. A common

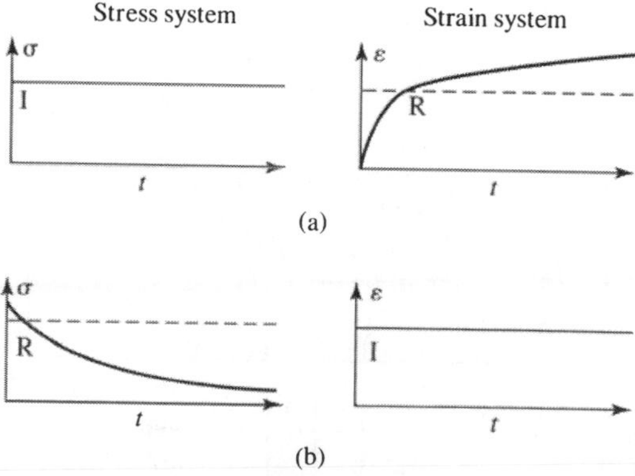

Figure 4.26
(a) The creep response of a polymeric material, which involves plastic deformation (increased strain) of a sample under constant load over time. (b) Stress relaxation response in a polymeric material, where a decrease in stress is seen over time under constant strain. *I* represents the input on the sample and *R* indicates the response of the material. (Adapted with permission from [10].)

example of stress relaxation is provided by a rubber band binding a stack of items for a period of time. As time progresses, the rubber band relaxes and no longer tightly binds the stack.

Stress relaxation experiments are conducted in a similar manner to creep experiments. However, in this case, the specimen is loaded with sufficient stress to produce a small strain. The changes in stress needed to maintain a constant strain are then monitored as a function of time as the system is maintained at a constant temperature.

The molecular causes for stress relaxation involve movement of chains in the amorphous regions of the polymer, as for creep. Therefore, the percent crystallinity and testing temperature relative to the T_g of the polymer also affect stress relaxation behavior. Like creep, stress relaxation behavior is observed only at temperatures above T_g, where viscous flow of the polymer chains is possible.

4.2.3.6 Mathematical Models of Viscoelastic Behavior At temperatures below T_g, polymers behave mainly as elastic solids, and at temperatures above T_m, they are viscous liquids. However, at temperatures between T_g and T_m, polymeric materials exhibit both viscous and elastic properties, and thus are considered to be **viscoelastic.** Fig. 4.27 depicts the difference in responses between the three types of materials. For the applied step load shown in Fig. 4.27(a), the strain in the entirely elastic material occurs instantaneously and remains constant [Fig. 4.27(b)], while the strain in the entirely viscous material increases linearly with time [Fig. 4.27(d)]. The viscoelastic material demonstrates intermediate properties—an instantaneous strain occurs, but it is followed by further deformation, the magnitude of which is time-dependent [Fig. 4.27(c)]. Thus, the nature of viscoelastic materials leads to the demonstration of time-dependent mechanical properties such as creep and stress relaxation, described in the preceding section.

A common example of a viscoelastic substance is a silicone-based polymer known by the brand name as Silly Putty.® If one forms this material into a ball and throws it, it will bounce (behave elastically). However, one can also pull it slowly and it will elongate/flow like a viscous liquid. As with other viscoelastic materials, the rate of strain in Silly Putty determines how it behaves. At high rates of deformation (strain), such as during bouncing, the elastic component of the response dominates. At slower deformation rates, the viscous portion dominates.

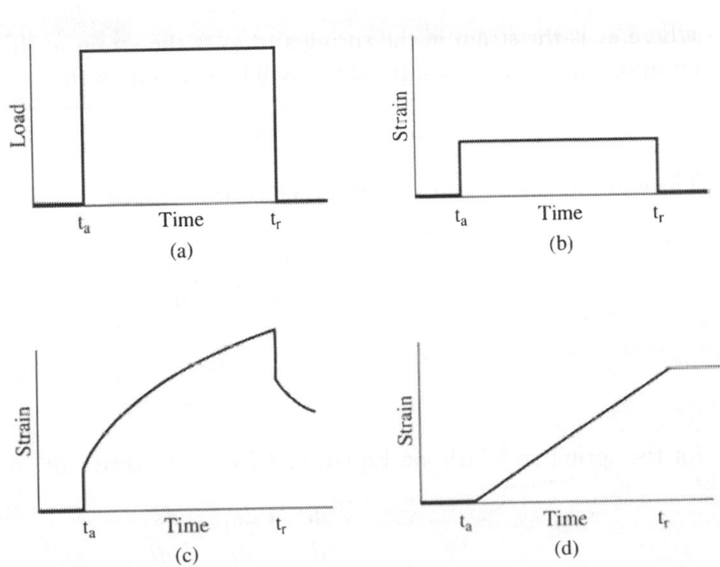

Figure 4.27
A schematic of the response of different materials to a step load. The parameter t_a indicates when the step load is applied and t_r indicates when the load is released. (a) The applied step load. (b) The strain seen in an entirely elastic material, which is instantaneous and remains constant. (c) The strain seen in a viscoelastic material, which demonstrates intermediate properties—an instantaneous strain occurs, but it is followed by further deformation, the magnitude of which is time-dependent. (d) The strain seen in an entirely viscous material, which increases linearly with time. (Adapted with permission from [2].)

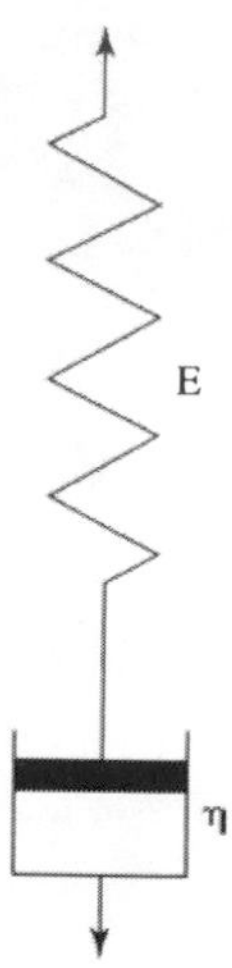

Figure 4.28
Schematic of the Maxwell model, which consists of a spring and dashpot in series (A dashpot can be likened to a shock absorber in a car, which contains a damping fluid and thus has a similar time-dependent response). E represents the elastic modulus of the elastic portion of the response, while η represents the viscosity of the viscous portion of the response. (Adapted with permission from [10].)

To more fully explore viscoelastic responses such as creep and stress relaxation, a number of models have been developed. The following discussion is based on that of [2]. For an idealized model, it is assumed that the elastic component of the response obeys Hooke's law. It is modeled with a mechanical analog, a **spring**, whose deformation follows the equation

$$\sigma = E\varepsilon \tag{4.26}$$

or, in differential form,

$$\frac{d\sigma}{dt} = E\frac{d\varepsilon}{dt} \tag{4.27}$$

Similarly, the viscous portion of the response is assumed to follow Newton's law and its mechanical model is a **dashpot** (Fig. 4.28). (A dashpot can be likened to a shock absorber in a car, which contains a damping fluid and thus has a similar time-dependent response.) For these simplified models, no distinction is made between shear stress and strain and tensile/compressive stress and strain. Instead, it is the nature of the relationship between the stress and strain that is of most importance. Therefore, for ease of notation, Newton's law can be rewritten as

$$\tau = \eta\frac{d\gamma}{dt} = \sigma = \eta\frac{d\varepsilon}{dt} \tag{4.28}$$

There are many different ways to combine these elements to model viscoelastic behavior. Complicated models involving multiple springs and dashpots have been derived, but we will focus in this section on two simple models: the Maxwell model and the Voigt model.

4.2.3.7 Viscoelastic Behavior—Maxwell Model The **Maxwell model** proposes a spring and dashpot in series, as shown in Fig. 4.28. When a stress σ is applied, there will be a resulting strain ε in the system that is the addition of the strain in each of the components; that is,

$$\varepsilon = \varepsilon_1 + \varepsilon_2 \tag{4.29}$$

where ε_1 is the strain in the spring and ε_2 is the strain in the dashpot. Because the components are in series, the stress will be equal in each:

$$\sigma_1 = \sigma_2 = \sigma \tag{4.30}$$

The equations 4.27 and 4.28 can then be rewritten as

$$\frac{d\sigma}{dt} = E\frac{d\varepsilon_1}{dt} \tag{4.31}$$

$$\sigma = \eta\frac{d\varepsilon_2}{dt} \tag{4.32}$$

for the spring and dashpot. Equation 4.29 can be differentiated to give

$$\frac{d\varepsilon}{dt} = \frac{d\varepsilon_1}{dt} + \frac{d\varepsilon_2}{dt} \tag{4.33}$$

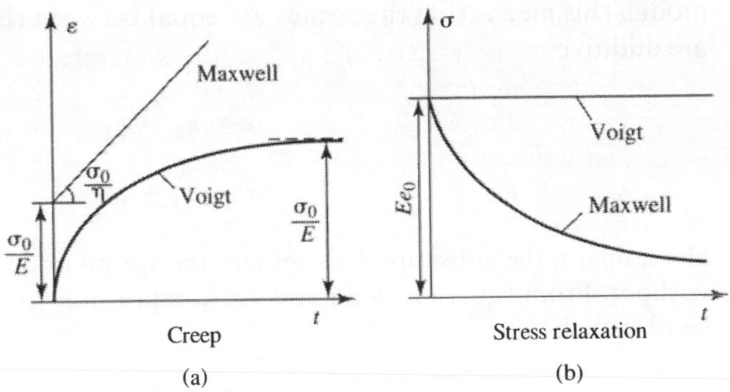

Figure 4.29
The responses predicted by the Maxwell model and the Voigt model for both (a) creep and (b) stress relaxation. (Adapted with permission from [10].)

Substitution of the expressions for $d\varepsilon_1/dt$ and $d\varepsilon_2/dt$ results in

$$\frac{d\varepsilon}{dt} = \frac{1}{E}\frac{d\sigma}{dt} + \frac{\sigma}{\eta} \tag{4.34}$$

The validity of this model in predicting behavior of polymers can be examined by applying it to creep and stress relaxation situations. During creep, the stress is held constant at σ_0 and, thus, $d\sigma/dt = 0$. The above equation can then be written

$$\frac{d\varepsilon}{dt} = \frac{\sigma_0}{\eta} \tag{4.35}$$

This equation shows that the Maxwell model predicts Newtonian flow during creep, and the strain would then be expected to increase linearly with time. This is obviously not what occurs [Fig. 4.26(a)], so this model has minimal predictive value for creep conditions.

However, during stress relaxation, a constant strain is maintained $\varepsilon = \varepsilon_0$ and, therefore, $d\varepsilon/dt = 0$. In this case, the equation becomes

$$0 = \frac{1}{E}\frac{d\sigma}{dt} + \frac{\sigma}{\eta} \tag{4.36}$$

or

$$\frac{d\sigma}{\sigma} = -\frac{E}{\eta}dt \tag{4.37}$$

Assuming that at $t = 0$, $\sigma = \sigma_0$, this expression can be integrated to give

$$\sigma = \sigma_0 e^{\frac{-Et}{\eta}} \tag{4.38}$$

so an exponential decrease in stress is expected over time, as is observed in polymers during stress relaxation [Fig. 4.26(b)]. The responses predicted by the Maxwell model for both creep and stress relaxation are depicted in Fig. 4.29.

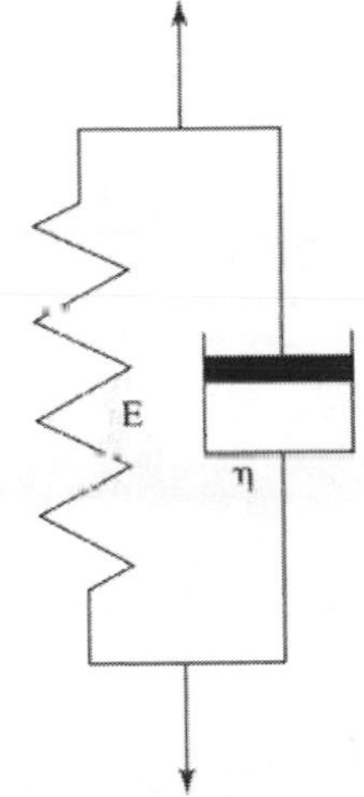

Figure 4.30
Schematic of the Voigt model, which consists of a spring and dashpot in parallel. E represents the elastic modulus of the elastic portion of the response, while η represents the viscosity of the viscous portion of the response. (Adapted with permission from [10].)

4.2.3.8 Viscoelastic Behavior—Voigt Model The Voigt (or Kelvin) **model** uses the same components as the Maxwell model, but in a different order. As seen in Fig. 4.30, in this system, the elements are in parallel. In contrast to the previous model, this means that the strains are equal between the elements, but the stresses are additive:

$$\varepsilon = \varepsilon_1 = \varepsilon_2 \tag{4.39}$$

$$\sigma = \sigma_1 + \sigma_2 \tag{4.40}$$

Here, again, the subscript 1 designates the spring and the subscript 2 refers to the dashpot. From equations 4.26 and 4.27, expressions for the stresses σ_1 and σ_2 can be obtained:

$$\sigma_1 = E\varepsilon \tag{4.41}$$

and

$$\sigma_2 = \eta \frac{d\varepsilon}{dt} \tag{4.42}$$

These can be placed into equation 4.40 to yield

$$\sigma = E\varepsilon + \eta \frac{d\varepsilon}{dt} \tag{4.43}$$

or

$$\frac{d\varepsilon}{dt} = \frac{\sigma}{\eta} - \frac{E\varepsilon}{\eta} \tag{4.44}$$

As with the Maxwell model, the validity of the Voigt model can be examined for both creep and stress relaxation phenomena. During creep, $\sigma = \sigma_0$ and the above equation 4.44 becomes

$$\frac{d\varepsilon}{dt} = \frac{\sigma_0}{\eta} - \frac{E\varepsilon}{\eta} \tag{4.45}$$

The solution to this equation is

$$\varepsilon = \frac{\sigma_0}{E}\left(1 - e^{\frac{-Et}{\eta}}\right) \tag{4.46}$$

which shows an exponential increase in strain over time, as is observed during creep experiments. The predicted response is shown in Fig. 4.29.

However, this model does not hold for stress relaxation conditions. When the strain is held constant at ε_0 and $d\varepsilon/dt = 0$, equation 4.45 becomes

$$\frac{\sigma}{\eta} = \frac{E\varepsilon_0}{\eta} \tag{4.47}$$

or

$$\sigma = E\varepsilon_0 \tag{4.48}$$

This is Hooke's law, so in this case, the Voigt model does not take into account the viscous portion of the response (Fig. 4.29) and thus is not useful for predicting polymer behavior under these conditions.

From the above discussion, it is clear that the Maxwell system can provide a simple model of polymeric stress relaxation behavior, while the Voigt model can be employed for creep conditions. In this vein, several combinations of these models have been developed to simultaneously predict creep and stress relaxation behavior. A simple combination called the **standard linear solid model** is shown in Fig. 4.31. It should be noted that, regardless of the complexity of the model, spring-dashpot systems can be used to describe the general behavior of a polymer, but do not provide information about the molecular causes for the time-dependent phenomena observed.

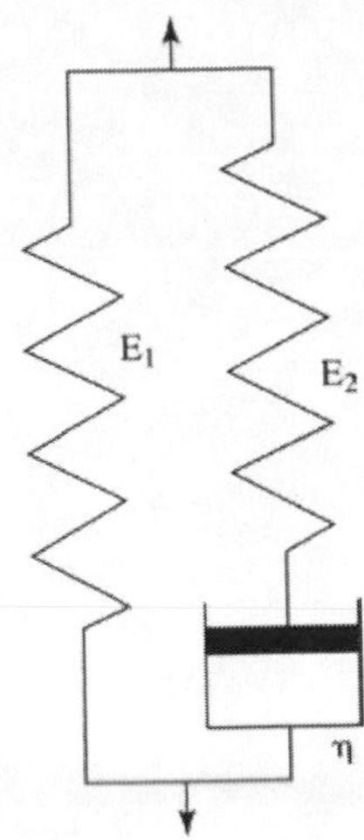

Figure 4.31
Schematic of the standard linear solid model, which is a combination of the Maxwell and Voigt models. E represents the elastic modulus of the elastic portion of the response, while η represents the viscosity of the viscous portion of the response. (Adapted with permission from [10].)

EXAMPLE PROBLEM 4.7

Consider the standard linear solid model illustrated in Fig. 4.31. Derive the differential equation for this model and use this equation to explore (a) the case of stress relaxation and (b) the case of creep for this system.

Solution:

$$E_1 = \sigma_1/\varepsilon_1$$

$$E_2 = \sigma_2/\varepsilon_2$$

$$\eta = \sigma_\eta/(d\varepsilon_\eta/dt)$$

$$\varepsilon_1 = \varepsilon_2 + \varepsilon_\eta = \varepsilon \rightarrow \varepsilon = \varepsilon_1 \text{ and } d\varepsilon/dt = d\varepsilon_1/dt$$

$$d\varepsilon_1/dt = d\varepsilon_2/dt + d\varepsilon_\eta/dt = d\varepsilon/dt$$

$$\sigma_2 = \sigma_\eta$$

$$\sigma = \sigma_2 + \sigma_1 = \sigma_\eta + \sigma_1$$

$$d\sigma/dt = d\sigma_2/dt + d\sigma_1/dt = d\sigma_\eta/dt + d\sigma_1/dt$$

$$d\varepsilon/dt = \sigma_\eta/\eta + [d\sigma_2/dt]/E_2$$

$$\sigma_\eta = [d\varepsilon/dt - [d\sigma_2/dt]/E_2]\eta$$

$$d\sigma_2/dt = d\sigma/dt - d\sigma_1/dt$$

$$\sigma_1 = E_1\varepsilon_1 = E_1\varepsilon$$

$$d\sigma_1/dt = E_1 d\varepsilon_1/dt = E_1 d\varepsilon/dt$$

$$\rightarrow \sigma_\eta = [d\varepsilon/dt - (d\sigma/dt - E_1 d\varepsilon/dt)/E_2]\eta$$

$$\sigma_{E1} = E_1\varepsilon_1$$

$$\rightarrow \sigma = [d\varepsilon/dt - (d\sigma/dt - E_1 d\varepsilon/dt)/E_2]\eta + E_1\varepsilon$$

$$\sigma/\eta = d\varepsilon/dt - (d\sigma/dt - E_1 d\varepsilon/dt)/E_2 + E_1\varepsilon/\eta$$

$$\sigma(E_2/\eta) = E_2 d\varepsilon/dt - d\sigma/dt + E_1 d\varepsilon/dt + (E_1E_2/\eta)\varepsilon$$

$$\rightarrow \underline{d\sigma/dt + \sigma(E_2/\eta) = d\varepsilon/dt(E_1 + E_2) + \varepsilon(E_1E_2/\eta)}$$

For the case of stress relaxation, $\varepsilon = \varepsilon_o$ and $d\varepsilon/dt = 0$.
Plugging these conditions into the differential equation above yields

$$d\sigma/dt + \sigma(E_2/\eta) = \varepsilon_o(E_1E_2/\eta)$$

$$d\sigma/dt = \varepsilon_o(E_1E_2/\eta) - (E_2/\eta)\sigma$$

$d\sigma/dt = (1/\eta)[E_1E_2\varepsilon_o - E_2\sigma]$

$[d\sigma/dt]/[E_2\sigma - E_1E_2\varepsilon_o] = -(1/\eta)$

$d/dt(\ln|\sigma E_2 - E_1E_2\varepsilon_o|) = -E_2/\eta$

$\ln|\sigma E_2 - E_1E_2\varepsilon_o| = (-E_2/\eta)t + C$, where C is a constant

$|\sigma E_2 - E_1E_2\varepsilon_o| = e^C \exp[(-E_2/\eta)t]$

$\sigma E_2 = E_1E_2\varepsilon_o + k \exp[(-E_2/\eta)t]$, where k is a constant

$\sigma(t) = E_1\varepsilon_o + K \exp[(-E_2/\eta)t]$, where K is a real constant greater than zero.

For the case of creep, $\sigma = \sigma_o$ and $d\sigma/dt = 0$.
Plugging these conditions into the differential equation above gives

$d\sigma/dt = -\sigma_o(E_2/\eta) + d\varepsilon/dt(E_1 + E_2) + \varepsilon(E_1E_2/\eta) = 0$

$d\varepsilon/dt(E_1 + E_2) + \varepsilon(E_1E_2/\eta) = \sigma_o(E_2/\eta)$

$d\varepsilon/dt + [E_1E_2\varepsilon]/[\eta(E_1 + E_2)] = \sigma_oE_2/[\eta(E_1 + E_2)]$

$d\varepsilon/dt = -[E_1E_2\varepsilon]/[\eta(E_1 + E_2)] + \sigma_oE_2/[\eta(E_1 + E_2)]$

$(d\varepsilon/dt)/[E_1E_2\varepsilon - \sigma_oE_2] = -1/[\eta(E_1 + E_2)]$

$d/dt(\ln|E_1E_2\varepsilon - \sigma_oE_2|) = -(E_1E_2)/[\eta(E_1 + E_2)]$

$\ln|E_1E_2\varepsilon - \sigma_oE_2| = -(E_1E_2)/[\eta(E_1 + E_2)]t + C$, where C is a constant

$|E_1E_2\varepsilon - \sigma_oE_2| = e^C \exp[-(E_1E_2)t/[\eta(E_1 + E_2)]]$

$\varepsilon E_1E_2 = \sigma_oE_2 + k \exp[-(E_1E_2)t/[\eta(E_1 + E_2)]]$, where k is a constant

$\varepsilon = \sigma_o/E_1 + k \exp[-(E_1E_2)t/[\eta(E_1 + E_2)]]$

$\varepsilon(t) = \sigma_o/E_1 + K \exp[-(E_1E_2)t/[\eta(E_1 + E_2)]]$, where K is a real constant greater than zero.

■

4.2.4 Influence of Porosity and Degradation on Mechanical Properties

As discussed in Chapter 3, pores can be created in a biomaterial in a controlled manner through the addition of porogens. Alternatively, they may be an unwanted by-product of material processing in which gas was trapped in the sample, or in which incomplete sintering occurred (metals and ceramics only, see Chapter 6). No matter what their origin, the presence of pores will decrease the elastic modulus and the strength of a biomaterial. Fracture strength is reduced with the addition of pores for two main reasons. Pores decrease the cross-sectional area across which the sample is loaded. In addition, they act as stress concentrators (see section 4.3.3) and can increase significantly the stress applied to localized areas of the sample.

The use of biodegradable materials for implants is particularly challenging, since their mechanical properties vary with time. For example, poly(glycolic acid) of 50% crystallinity, used as a biodegradable suture, loses most of its mechanical strength after two to four weeks of degradation (Fig. 4.32) [11]. Many parameters, including chemical structure and the presence of pores, can affect the degradation rate (this is discussed further in Chapter 5). These must be taken into account when designing a tissue engineering scaffold so that it maintains sufficient mechanical properties until enough tissue has been generated to take over the function of the

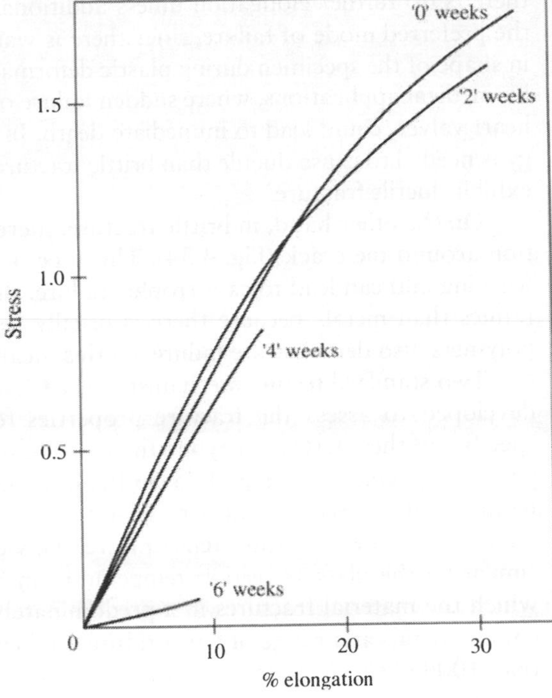

Figure 4.32
Change in mechanical properties of poly(glycolic acid) of 50% crystallinity with time. Degradation of the polymer over two to four weeks results in a loss of the majority of its mechanical strength. (Adapted with permission from [11].)

scaffold. Thus, the timing of degradation and the concomitant decrease in mechanical properties is a crucial design parameter for biodegradable implants.

4.3 Fracture and Failure

4.3.1 Ductile and Brittle Fracture

If either time-dependent or time-independent deformation is continued, eventually the material will fracture. If the material undergoes plastic deformation before breaking, it experiences **ductile fracture.** If there is little plastic deformation, the material demonstrates **brittle fracture.** For simplicity, in the following section we will focus on fracture that occurs during tensile testing only.

Ductile failure is characterized by plastic deformation in the area of the crack, as demonstrated by the cone-shaped appearance of the fractured specimen in Fig. 4.33. Crack propagation occurs fairly slowly, and the crack is considered to be **stable,** since

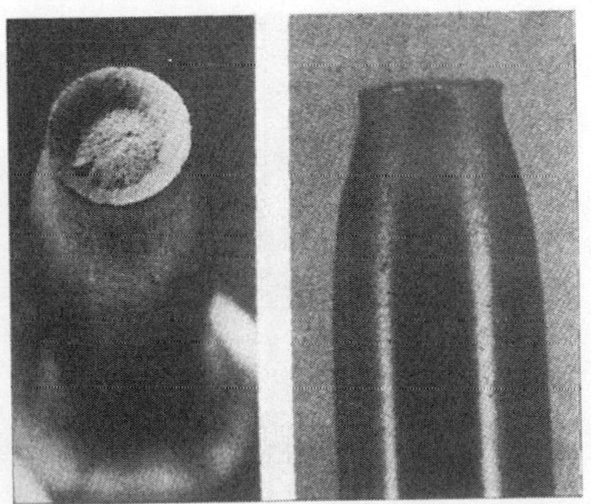

Figure 4.33
Ductile failure in a metallic material, which is characterized by plastic deformation in the area of the crack, as demonstrated by the cone-shaped appearance at the fracture of the specimen. (Reprinted with permission from [12].)

there is no further elongation unless additional stress is applied. Ductile fracture is the preferred mode of failure, since there is warning available in the form of change in shape of the specimen during plastic deformation. This is particularly important in biomedical applications, where sudden failure of certain devices, such as replacement heart valves, could lead to immediate death. In addition, generally more strain energy is needed to cause ductile than brittle fracture. Metals and some types of polymers exhibit ductile fracture.

On the other hand, in brittle fracture, there is little evidence of plastic deformation around the crack (Fig. 4.34). This type of fracture proceeds quickly with little warning and can lead to catastrophic failure. Brittle fracture is more common in ceramics than metals because there is usually less slip in ceramics. Certain types of polymers also demonstrate failure via this means.

Two standard testing mechanisms, the **Charpy and Izod impact tests**, have been developed to assess the fracture properties for various materials. Although the specifics of these tests are beyond the scope of this text, the general experimental apparatus is depicted in Fig. 4.35 and is designed to measure impact energy as the hammer hits the sample. In particular, these experiments are used to determine the **ductile-to-brittle transition temperature.** This characteristic temperature, which is similar to the glass transition temperature in polymers, is the temperature below which the material fractures in a predominately brittle manner. This transition occurs in metals at a range of temperatures and ceramics only at temperatures greater than 1000°C.

4.3.2 Polymer Crazing

As mentioned above, polymers can undergo ductile or brittle fracture, depending on their chemical composition and the temperature of the specimen. **Crazing** is another phenomenon that can be involved in the fracture of some amorphous thermoplastic polymers (polymers that can be cooled and heated repeatedly—see section 6.6.1). Like cracks, crazes are initiated in regions near scratches or other flaws that are exposed to high levels of stress. Crazes are generally found perpendicular to the axis of tensile stress.

As a part of crazing, there are areas of localized yielding, which cause the formation of fibrils containing oriented polymer chains. Interconnected small void areas are also created. Unlike cracks, crazes can support a load, but the maximum before fracture is less than that for the noncrazed material. If the stress applied is great enough, the fibrillar structure will degrade and the voids will expand, leading to crack formation in the crazed area.

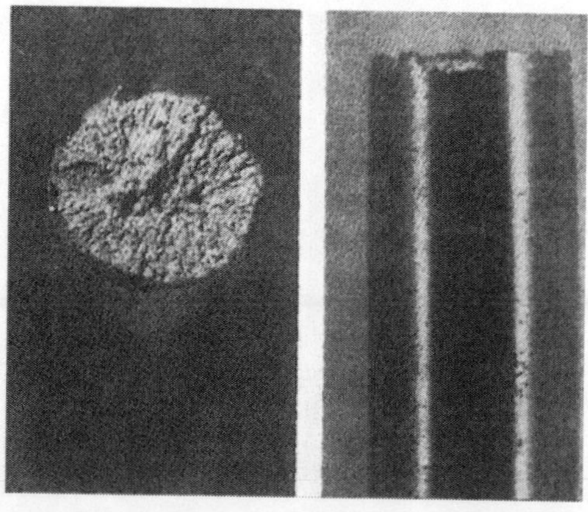

Figure 4.34
Brittle fracture in a metallic material, which is characterized by little evidence of plastic deformation around the crack. (Reprinted with permission from [12].)

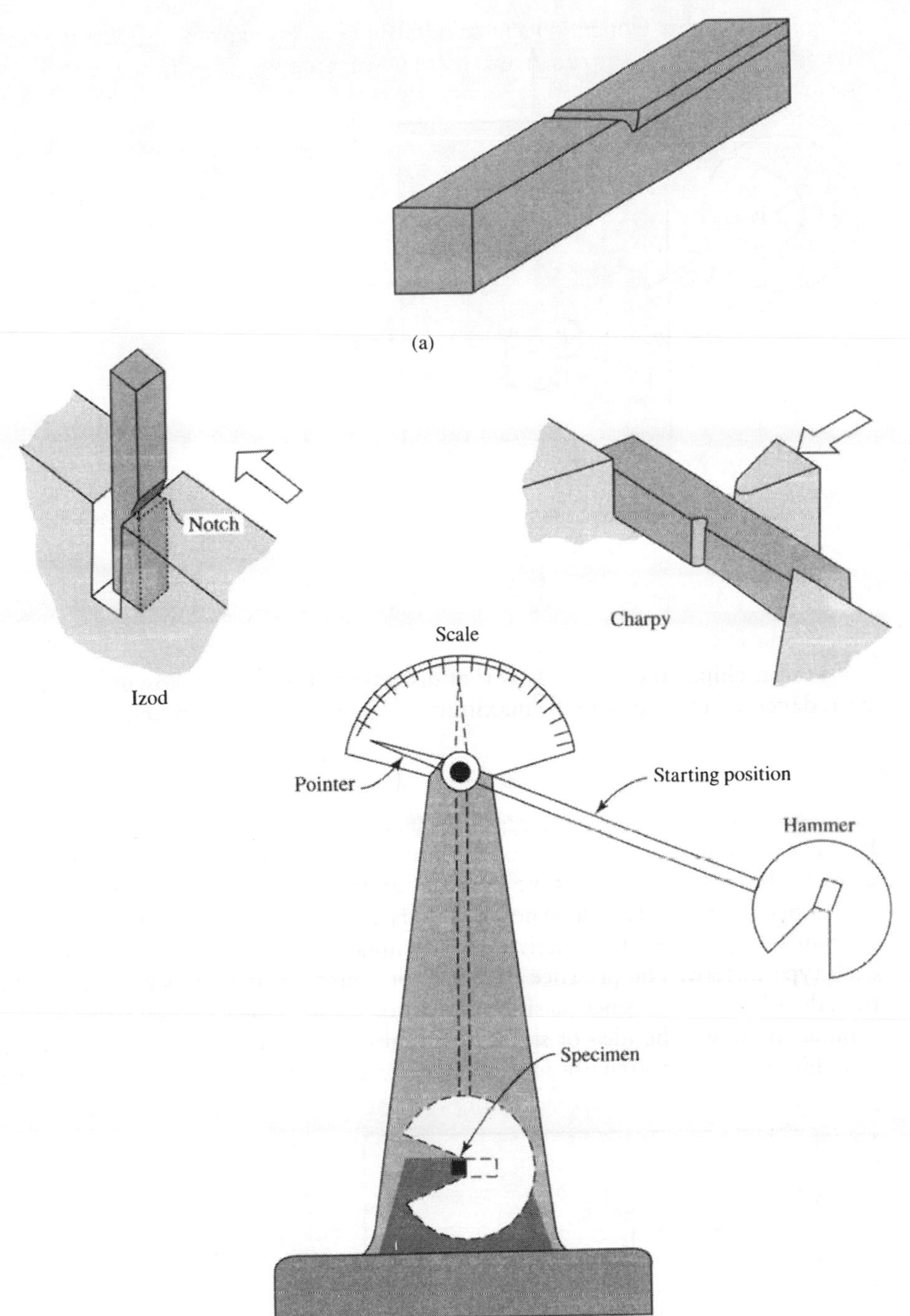

Figure 4.35
Charpy and Izod impact tests. (a) Test specimen. (b) Testing machine/setup. Although the specimen configuration varies between the Charpy and Izod tests, in both cases, the testing hammer is raised to various heights until the height necessary for specimen fracture is determined, and the corresponding impact energy can be then read from the scale. (Adapted with permission from [13].)

4.3.3 Stress Concentrators

As mentioned in the previous section, small flaws or cracks in a material can cause the formation of larger cracks or crazes in neighboring regions. This is because the applied stress can be amplified at the tip of the flaw. Fig. 4.36 depicts an elliptical crack in the center of a material and Fig. 4.37 shows the corresponding increase in stress at the edges of the crack. Farther away, the stress is reduced to a value equal to the overall applied stress (σ_0). Because these flaws cause a localized increase in stress, they are termed **stress concentrators** or **stress raisers**.

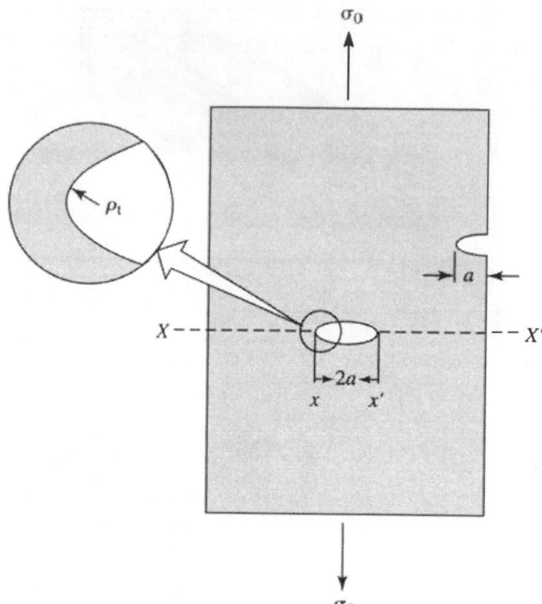

Figure 4.36
Schematic showing an elliptical crack in the center of a material. This crack is responsible for an effective local stress that is greater than σ_0. (Adapted with permission from [2].)

For an elliptical crack such as that discussed above, the following equation has been developed to estimate the maximum stress at the crack tip (σ_m):

$$\sigma_m = 2\sigma_0\left(\frac{a}{\rho_t}\right)^{1/2} \tag{4.49}$$

In this equation, ρ_t is the radius of curvature of the crack tip, and a is the length of a crack on the surface or half the length of an internal crack (Fig. 4.36).

Other stress raisers include notches, sharp corners, and pores (discussed previously). Similar equations can be derived to determine the maximum stress experienced for each type of flaw. The presence of stress concentrators is more significant in brittle than ductile materials, since plastic deformation reduces the localized stress in the area around the flaw. The idea of stress raisers also helps explain why ceramics usually have higher fracture strengths in compression than in tension. Although stress-raising

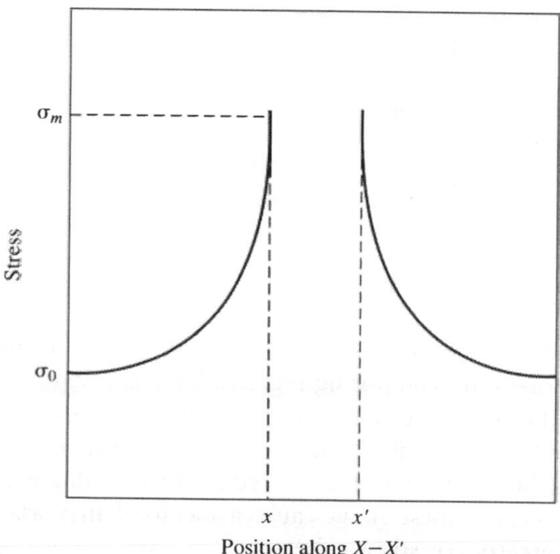

Figure 4.37
Diagram showing the increase in stress at the edge of the crack in Fig. 4.36. The parameter σ_0 is the overall applied stress on the material and σ_m is the maximum stress, seen at the crack tip. (Adapted with permission from [2].)

flaws occur in both cases, there is lower localized stress amplification in compression than tension, resulting in a higher applied stress (σ_0) before failure for compression.

4.4 Fatigue and Fatigue Testing

4.4.1 Fatigue

Another mechanical property of extreme importance is how biomaterials behave under repeated loading as would occur in the use of many medical devices. Repeated loading can lead to failure at stresses significantly less than the tensile or yield strengths as determined by the static testing methods described previously. This type of failure, known as **fatigue fracture**, occurs suddenly after the material has been subjected to many cycles of altering stress or strain. Fatigue is the cause of up to 90% of metallic fractures, and both ceramics and polymers can also undergo this type of failure.

Fatigue fracture is brittle, with little plastic deformation around the fracture, even in ductile materials. Although loading can actually strengthen a crystalline (or semicrystalline) material (see Chapter 6 for further discussion of this phenomenon, called strain hardening), repeated stress increases the number of dislocations and creates more and more imperfections in the crystal structure. These flaws then can act to nucleate cracks, which eventually lead to failure of the material. Fatigue failure occurs in three main stages:

1. Crack initiation—a small crack is created at an area of high stress.
2. Crack propagation—the crack increases in size with each successive loading cycle.
3. Final failure—occurs rapidly after the crack has reached a certain size.

Therefore, the fatigue life (N_f, see section 4.4.2) of a material can be estimated as the number of cycles required for crack initiation (N_i) plus the number of cycles needed for propagation to the critical size for failure (N_p):

$$N_f = N_i + N_p \tag{4.50}$$

4.4.2 Fatigue Testing

Material fatigue testing is completed using a rotating-bending apparatus like that shown in Fig. 4.38 or a uniaxial tension-compression machine, which employs a mechanical testing frame like that described at the end of this chapter. In this testing

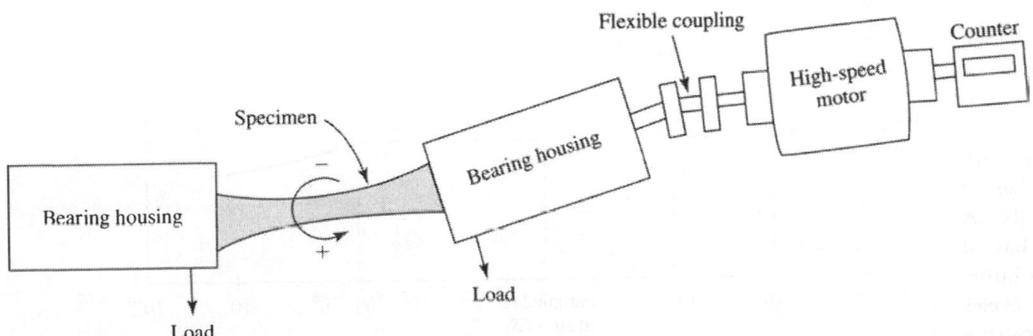

Figure 4.38
A rotating-bending apparatus used for material fatigue testing. In this example, both tensile and torsion forces are applied to the sample. (Adapted with permission from [14].)

procedure, specimens are exposed to cycles of stress at relatively high stress values (usually two-thirds of the static tensile strength) and the number of cycles to failure are observed. Other specimens are subjected to lower levels of stress and the corresponding number of cycles is recorded for each set of samples. This allows the generation of stress (S) vs. number of cycles to failure (N) plots. For such graphs, S usually represents the **stress amplitude**, or the difference in the maximum (σ_{max}) and minimum (σ_{min}) applied stress divided by two:

$$S = \frac{\sigma_{max} - \sigma_{min}}{2} \tag{4.51}$$

Two typical S–N curves are shown in Fig. 4.39. For some metals, including certain titanium alloys, below a certain stress level fatigue failure will not occur, regardless of the number of cycles the sample experiences. This stress value is called

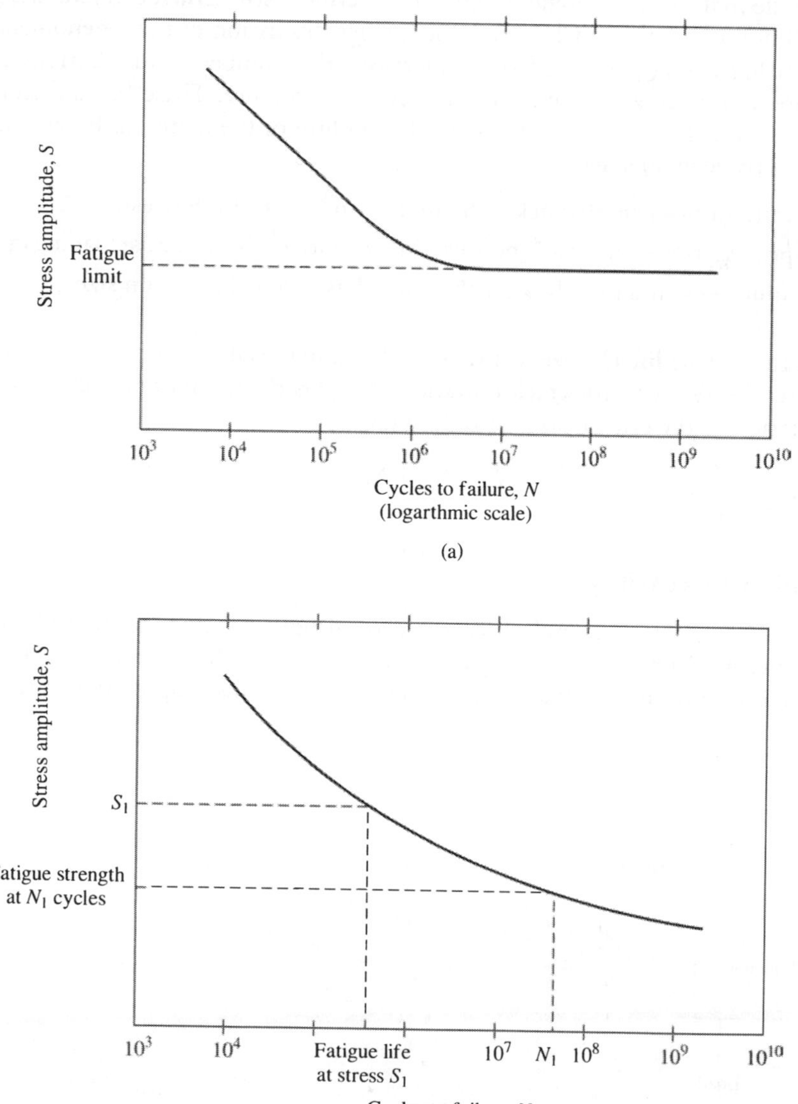

Figure 4.39
Two typical S–N curves seen in fatigue testing. (a) A material that demonstrates a fatigue limit (it will not fracture under a certain load, regardless of the number of cycles experienced). (b) A material that does not have a fatigue limit. From this information the number of cycles necessary for fatigue fracture at a certain stress can be determined. (Adapted with permission from [2].)

the **fatigue limit** or endurance limit, and the S–N graph becomes horizontal at this level [Fig. 4.39(a)].

In contrast, many alloys containing metals such as aluminum do not demonstrate a clear fatigue limit, but the curve continues downward with decreasing values of applied stress. These materials are instead characterized by their **fatigue strength,** which is defined as the stress level that will cause failure after a given number of cycles. Figure 4.39(b) depicts the fatigue strength for N_1 cycles.

As mentioned above, **fatigue life** (N_f) is an important parameter for all types of materials. This is the number of cycles required to cause fatigue fracture at a specified stress [Fig. 4.39(b)], and it depends on the kinetics of crack propagation, as explained earlier.

4.4.3 Factors that Affect Fatigue Life

As with other types of failure, increased stress resulting from flaws in a biomaterial can act to nucleate cracks, which eventually result in fatigue fracture. Therefore, anything that acts to increase regional stresses can impact the fatigue life of the device. As seen from the S–N curves in Fig. 4.39, one of these factors is the amplitude of the applied stress. With increasing stress, the number of cycles to failure decreases significantly.

Since in many cases the maximum stress occurs at the surface of a component, impurities in the surface region can also reduce fatigue life. Therefore, particular care should be taken to understand how surface treatments of biomaterials may affect the localized stress experienced in this region. In the same vein, the avoidance of other stress raisers, such as notches or sharp corners, in the design of the implant is encouraged in order to improve fatigue life. Biodegradable materials may be particularly susceptible to fatigue fracture at later time points due to a combined decrease in mechanical properties and potential production of flaws within the implant due to the degradation process.

In addition to internal parameters, the environment of the implant may affect its fatigue properties. As discussed in more detail in the next chapter, the body's tissues contain a number of active substances, including water, salts and proteins, that can react chemically with biomaterials. Failure that occurs because of the presence of cyclic stresses in combination with chemical attack is called **corrosion fatigue,** and this type of fracture is a serious concern for implants designed to remain in the body for long periods of time.

4.5 Methods to Improve Mechanical Properties

As discussed earlier in the chapter, metals, crystalline ceramics, and polymers undergo plastic deformation due to dislocation glide or slip. Therefore, to strengthen these materials, it is necessary to reduce the movement of dislocations. A detailed discussion of various methods to do this is reserved for Chapter 6. However, a brief overview is presented in this section, with particular emphasis on concepts described in this chapter.

Slip can be reduced in materials either by the inclusion of additives or through various processing techniques. Additives include metal alloys, since the impurity atoms can help to cancel the lattice strains that result from dislocations and thus "stabilize" the dislocation and prevent its movement. In polymers, **fillers** can be added. Fillers (usually particulates of ceramics or other polymers) increase strength by acting as additional entanglements or crosslinks and thus restricting chain motion. A popular class of fillers for mechanical reinforcement are the single-walled carbon nanotubes discussed in Chapter 2.

Processing can also affect the ease of dislocation motion in a sample. As mentioned previously, polycrystalline materials are generally stronger than those composed of only one crystal, in part because grain boundaries discourage dislocation movement. Materials with smaller grains have more grain boundaries per volume, and thus are usually stronger than materials with larger grains. In metals and ceramics, the cooling rate of the material (after it has been formed into a specific shape, for example) affects the grain size, with grain growth preferred at higher temperatures.

As in metals and ceramics, the cooling rate also influences the strength of polymeric materials. For polymers, crystalline regions have more interactions between adjacent chains and, thus, the higher percent crystallinity of a semicrystalline polymer, the stronger it is expected to be. A plot of strength as a function of percent crystallinity of poly(ethylene) is found in Fig. 4.40. In this case, the polymer chains must be allowed time to align to form crystalline structures, so very rapid cooling may result in a low percent crystallinity and reduce the overall strength of the material.

From these examples, it can be seen that the thermal history of a material can have a large impact on its mechanical properties. This is explored further in the discussion of processing of biomaterials found in Chapter 6.

EXAMPLE PROBLEM 4.8

Assume that a pure and perfectly crystalline (no crystal defects or impurities) aluminum bar can be formed.

(a) Would more or less energy be required to break the perfect aluminum bar when compared with a real aluminum bar (containing defects and impurities), all other things being equal (dimensions, temperature, strain rate, etc.)?
(b) If one were to start with an aluminum bar with a sufficient number of defects such that an average person could bend it easily with their hands, would one expect the bar to become more or less difficult to bend as the number of bending cycles increases? Why?
(c) Would the slope of the elastic portion of the stress-strain curve be higher for the perfect aluminum bar or the real aluminum? Why?

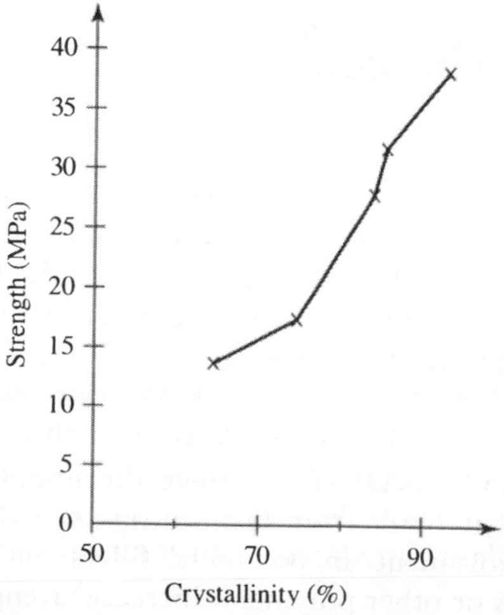

Figure 4.40
A plot of strength as related to percent crystallinity of poly(ethylene). Crystalline regions have more interactions between adjacent chains and, thus, the higher percent crystallinity of a semicrystalline polymer, the stronger it is expected to be. (Adapted with permission from [15].)

Solution:

(a) A perfect aluminum bar would have no impurities or defects, thus it would have a perfect crystal structure. Normally, impurities and defects are present in the metal, and the movement of these defects and impurities allows for material deformation without necessarily having to break bonds between the metal atoms. In this way, the macroscopic mechanical properties of metals are conferred by the defects present in the metal. However, in the case of a crystal with absolutely no defects, deformation of the material with applied force would break the atomic bonds in a plane of the crystal. Thus, a much higher energy would be required to break the perfect aluminum bar.

(b) Starting with an aluminum bar with a number of dislocations and defects just sufficient to allow for bending of the bar, the bar could initially bend quite easily as the defects and dislocations do not have many interactions. However, as the bar is bent, the dislocations move and additional edge and line defects are created. As the bending cycles continue, the movement of the bar becomes increasingly difficult, as the increasing defect interactions raise the energy barrier needed to continue to bend the bar. One can think of the work-hardening a blacksmith imparts upon a piece of metal while hot through repeated hammerings as an analogous example. With each stroke of the hammer, more defects and dislocations are created and the number of interaction between these defects increases, thereby increasing the hardness of the material.

(c) The slope of the elastic portion of the stress-strain curve would be the same for the perfect aluminum bar and the real aluminum bar because the slope reflects the strengths of interatomic bonds within the material. In this case, the atomic composition of both materials is the same; it is the absence or presence of defects that is different. ■

4.6 Techniques: Introduction to Mechanical Analysis

The major piece of equipment for mechanical testing as described in this chapter is the mechanical testing frame shown in Fig. 4.1. Although it was already described briefly, this method is treated in more depth here for comparison with characterization techniques discussed in other chapters. It should be noted that a common means of obtaining mechanical properties during oscillatory loading is **dynamic mechanical analysis (DMA)**, but a description of this method is beyond the scope of this text.

4.6.1 Mechanical Testing

4.6.1.1 Basic Principles The testing frame is designed to subject a sample to uniaxial loading at a controlled amplitude and rate. This can occur once per sample, or can be repeated, as in fatigue testing. The shape of the sample is dictated by ASTM standards, taking into account the amount of material available and the form it will take in the final application. For tensile testing, a rod or film is often shaped into a "dog-bone" geometry, as shown in Fig. 4.4. This effectively raises the stress in the portion with the smaller cross-section and causes a reproducible region of breakage in all samples. This geometry mitigates artifacts, such as specimen fracture near the gripping mechanisms due to stress raisers caused by the clamps. Mechanical tests are normally **destructive** - that is, the test continues until the specimen breaks.

4.6.1.2 Instrumentation A typical plot produced from a mechanical testing experiment is found in Fig. 4.5. Results are generally plotted as stress (y-axis) as a function of strain (x-axis). Equations to calculate stress and strain were presented earlier in this chapter (equations 4.1 and 4.2).

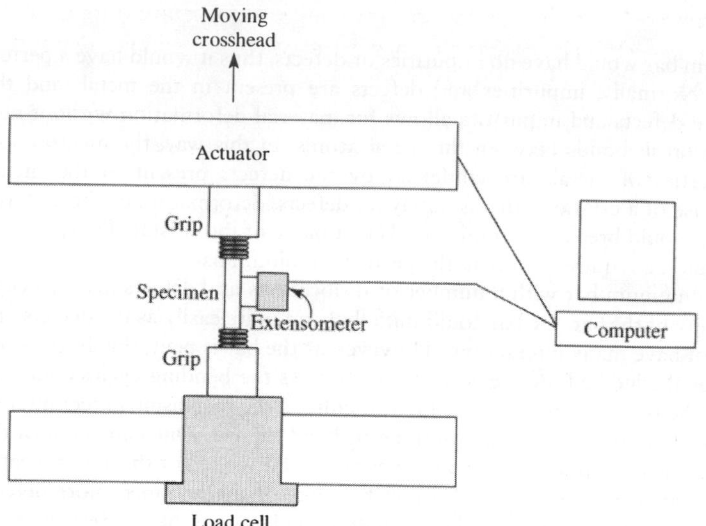

Figure 4.41
A block diagram of a mechanical testing apparatus. (Adapted with permission from [16].)

The basic components to the mechanical testing apparatus, as shown in Fig. 4.41 are as follows:

1. Grips/actuator—holds sample; through the movement of the grip attached to the actuator, load is applied along the axis of the sample.
2. Load cell—records instantaneous load on the sample and sends this information to the processor/computer.
3. Extensometer—records instantaneous length of the sample and sends this information to the processor/computer.
4. Processor (computer)— converts the electrical signals from the load cell and extensometer into a stress-strain plot.

During testing, the sample is placed in the mechanical testing frame and clamped tightly with the grips. As depicted in Fig. 4.41, one of the grips is attached to a moveable platform (actuator), which moves at a constant speed, thus loading the specimen along the longitudinal axis. As the actuator moves, the load cell records the load on the sample, while another transducer, the extensometer, measures the change in length of the specimen. The computer then converts load-elongation information into a stress-strain curve.

4.6.1.3 Information Provided Mechanical testing produces stress vs. strain or stress/strain vs. time curves for a variety of testing modes. The most common of these are tensile, compressive, bending, creep, and stress relaxation tests. From these curves, a number of characteristic values, such as modulus and yield and tensile strengths, can be calculated. As mentioned earlier, fatigue life and other parameters can be determined from uniaxial fatigue experiments performed on a mechanical testing frame. Mechanical testing is crucial to determine if a biomaterial will be suitable for a certain application, given the loading parameters of the tissue of interest.

Summary

- The mechanical properties of a material can be characterized through mechanical testing in tension, compression, bending, shear, or torsion. During tensile testing, the load and specimen elongation are measured and can be normalized with respect to specimen geometry to give stress (force/area) and strain (length/length), respectively. Stress-strain curves can vary widely, depending upon the nature of the material tested.

- Elastic deformation of a sample occurs when, upon release of the load, the sample returns to its original shape. The linear portion of a stress-strain curve in which the curve obeys Hooke's law ($\sigma = E\varepsilon$) represents elastic deformation of the sample. The slope of this linear region is known as the modulus of elasticity (force/area) or Young's modulus of the material.
- Elastic deformation results from slight changes in atomic spacing and stretching of bonds. The stiffness of a material directly reflects the amount of energy required to move atoms in a material from their equilibrium positions. Thus, ceramics are generally stiffer than metals. The stiffness of polymers is typically directionally dependent.
- Plastic deformation is permanent deformation from which the sample cannot return to its original shape following loading. The stress corresponding to the end of the elastic region is called the yield stress, and the strain at this value is the yield point strain. Beyond the yield point, an increase in stress is required to continue plastic deformation until the ultimate tensile strength is met. After this point, further stress results in necking of the specimen and finally fracture.
- Metals and crystalline ceramics deform plastically through dislocation glide along a slip plane. Requirements of electroneutrality in ceramics limit the number of possible slip planes, thus ceramics are typically brittle. Plastic deformation of polycrystalline materials occurs through deformation of individual grains rather than alternations or openings of grain boundaries.
- Plastic deformation of semicrystalline polymers occurs through interactions between amorphous regions and lamellae in response to the load. First, tie chains extend and lamellae slide past one another. Then, the lamellae reorient so that the chain folds are aligned along the axis of loading and blocks of the crystalline phases separate from each other. Finally, the blocks and tie chains orient along the axis of applied force.
- Amorphous polymers and ceramics deform plastically by viscous flow, in which atoms slide past one another through the breaking and reforming of bonds. However, unlike deformation in crystalline materials, there is no prescribed direction of movement.
- Three- or four-point bending tests are often used with ceramic materials as an alternative to tensile testing to determine the modulus of rupture (stress at fracture).
- Some materials present time-dependent mechanical properties. Creep is one such property, in which the sample deforms plastically with time under constant load. Stress relaxation is another such property, in which the stress of a sample decreases with time under constant strain.
- Creep in metals can result from grain boundaries sliding relative to one another or from migration of vacancies. Although mechanisms of creep in ceramics are similar to those in metals, ceramics are generally more resistant to creep, due in part to requirements of electroneutrality. Creep deformation in semicrystalline and amorphous polymers depends upon the movement of chains in the amorphous regions of the material via viscous flow.
- A number of models have been developed to more fully explore viscoelastic responses of materials. The Maxwell model consists of a spring and dashpot in series and is typically appropriate for predicting stress-relaxation behavior.

The Voigt model consists of a spring and dashpot in parallel and is typically appropriate for predicting creep behavior.

- Various modes of material fracture exist. If a material undergoes plastic deformation before it fractures, then it experiences ductile fracture. Fractures that involve little plastic deformation are called brittle fractures. Small flaws or cracks in a material that cause a localized increase in stress are called stress raisers. The presence of stress concentrators is more significant in brittle than ductile materials, since plastic deformation reduces the localized stress in the area around the flaw.
- Voids or pores in biomaterials, necessary for many tissue engineering applications, act as stress raisers and considerably weaken the overall material. In addition, degradation *in vivo* can decrease mechanical properties significantly and must be taken into account in the original implant design.
- Fatigue failure of a material occurs following repeated cycles of stress or strain. The repeated stresses of fatigue testing result in an increased number of imperfections and dislocations in the crystal structure of a material. These flaws can act to nucleate cracks, which can propagate and lead ultimately to the failure of the material. Any factor that acts to increase regional stresses can impact the fatigue life of the material.
- Various methods can be employed to improve the mechanical properties of materials, such as the inclusion of fillers in polymers to increase chain entanglements.
- Although a variety of mechanical testing modes are possible, a typical mechanical testing apparatus includes grips, an actuator, load cell, extensometer and a data processor.

Problems

4.1 You are instructed to choose a class of polymer for use in a vascular graft, with the most significant concern being that the material has the ability to expand and contract in circumference during the pulsatile flow of blood.

(a) Which class do you believe would be ideal for this application and why?

(b) Design an *in vitro* experimental setup to examine the susceptibility of the material in a vascular tube form to fatigue along the circumference. You will need to include a method to simulate the mechanical stresses and physiologic conditions the material will experience *in vivo*. What are the important parameters to consider in this setup?

(c) You are given another material that could be used for this application, Dacron®, and are instructed to determine the tensile strength of this material. Using a normal dog-bone geometry, you test the polymer at a rate of 1 mm/min and find it has an elastic modulus of 3 GPa. You repeat the test at 5 mm/min. Would you expect the tensile modulus to be on the order of 0.3 GPa or 30 GPa? Why? (Please explain from a molecular perspective.)

4.2 You want to examine the possibility of using a polymeric material as an artificial load bearing surface for articulating joints. But the deformation of this material under loading is a concern. You have been informed that if the material has a Poisson's ratio under 0.1, then it can undergo further testing for this application. You are given a cylindrical sample that is 10 mm in diameter and 3 mm in height. During compression testing, you apply a strain of 20% in the axial direction, and the diameter of the cylindrical sample increases by 0.4 mm at its widest point. What is the Poisson's ratio of the sample? Does it pass or fail the screening test?

4.3 As mentioned in problem 1.2 from Chapter 1, if you stand on one leg the load exerted on the hip joint is 2.4 times your body weight. Assuming a simple cylindrical model for the implant, calculate the corresponding stress (in MPa) on a hip implant in a 175lb. individual with a hip implant with a cross-sectional area of 5.6 cm^2. If the hip implant is made of Ti6Al4V (124 GPa elastic modulus), what is the strain for the given loading conditions?

4.4 Someone brings you the femoral stem of a hip joint prosthesis that has fractured in its midsection after 15 years in a patient.

(a) Using your knowledge to date, what is the most likely cause for this failure? Would you expect this fracture to be more brittle or ductile in character?

(b) After determining that the above material is no longer suitable for a femoral stem, you decide to examine a new material. Tensile testing results are shown below. A cylindrical dog-bone specimen with a diameter of 12.8 mm and a length of 60 mm in the testing region was used. What is the elastic modulus for this material? What is the maximum stress you would want to apply to this material before it would fail for this application? What is the ultimate tensile strength?

Force (N)	Length (mm)
0	60.00
15442	60.06
30883	60.12
46325	60.18
61766	60.24
77208	60.30
92649	60.36
105517	60.42
107834	60.48
109506	60.54
110150	60.60
110664	60.66
108992	60.72
106547	60.78

(c) You want to increase the stiffness of this material. Knowing that the material is poured into a cast, removed, and then allowed to cool at room temperature, how would you change the processing? Why would this change the modulus of the material?

(d) A colleague proposes the idea of using one of the following two shapes instead of the typical dog-bone shape for tensile testing of your modified material. Is either of these a viable option? Why or why not?

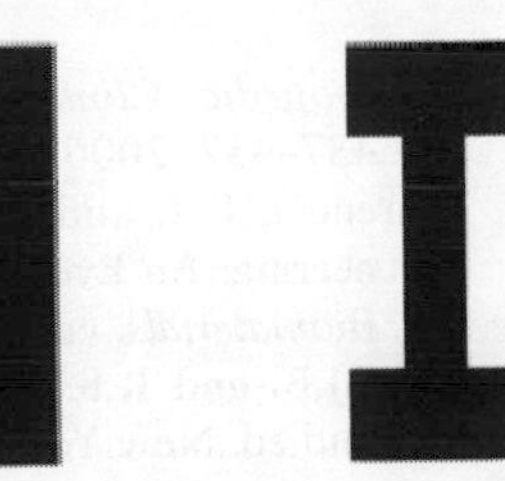

4.5 You are comparing two different processing methods used for forming Ti6Al4V into a femoral stem of a hip joint prothesis. The following diagram shows the structures that result from the two methods:

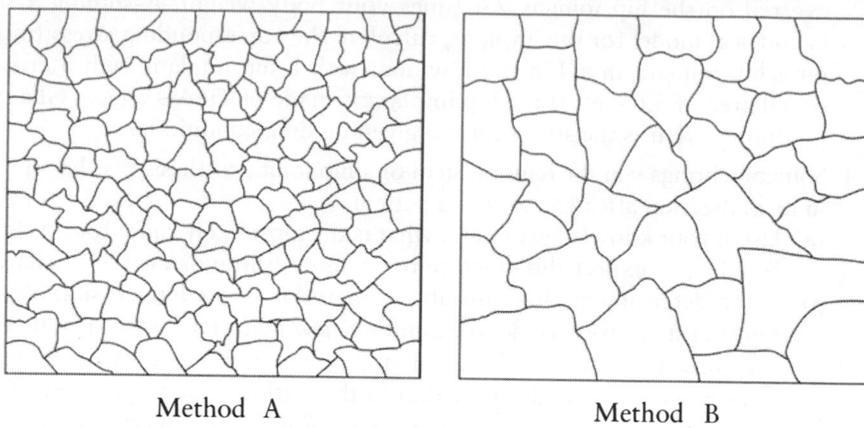

Which of the two processing methods results in a material with a higher ultimate tensile strength? Why?

References

1. Instron Corporation, www.*instron.com*.
2. Callister, Jr., W.D. *Materials Science and Engineering: An Introduction*, 3rd ed. New York: John Wiley and Sons, 1994.
3. Schaffer, J.P., A. Saxena, S.D. Antolovich, T.H. Sanders, Jr., and S.B. Warner. *The Science and Design of Engineering Materials*, 2nd ed. Boston: McGraw-Hill, 1999.
4. Schultz, J.M., *Polymer Materials Science*, 1st, ed. Englewood Cliffs, NJ: Prentice Hall, 1974.
5. Kalpakjian, S., *Manufacturing Engineering and Technology* 2nd ed. New York: Addison-Wesley, 1991.
6. Richards, R.B. "Polyethylene—Structure, Crystallinity and Properties," *J Appl Chem*, vol. 1, p. 370, 1951.
7. Alberts, B., D. Bray, J. Lewis, M. Raff, K. Roberts, and J. Watson. *Molecular Biology of the Cell*, 3rd ed. New York: Garland Publishing, 1994.
8. Shackelford, J.F. *Introduction to Materials Science for Engineers*, 5th ed. Upper Saddle River: Prentice Hall, 2000.
9. Mikos, A.G., G. Sarakinos, S.M. Leite, J.P. Vacanti, and R. Langer. "Laminated Three-Dimensional Biodegradable Foams for Use in Tissue Engineering." *Biomaterials*, vol. 14, pp. 323–330, 1993.
10. Young, R.J. and P.A. Lovell. *Introduction to Polymers*, 2nd ed. London: Chapman and Hall, 1991.
11. Mark, J.E. *Physical Properties of Polymers Handbook*. Woodbury: American Institute of Physics, 1996.
12. *Metals Handbook*, 9th ed., Vol. 11, "Failure Analysis and Prevention," Materials Park, OH: ASM International, 1986.
13. Pollack, H.W. *Materials Science and Metallurgy*, 4th ed. Englewood Cliffs, NJ: Prentice-Hall, 1998.
14. Keyser, C.A. *Materials Science in Engineering*, 4th ed., New York: Macmillan, 1986.
15. Boeing, H.V. *Polyolefins: Structure and Properties*, Lausanne: Elsevier Press, 1966.
16. Shackelford, J.F. *Introduction to Materials Science for Engineers*, 4th ed. Upper Saddle River NJ: Prentice Hall, 1996.

Additional Reading

Cooke, F.W. "Bulk Properties of Materials." In *Biomaterials Science: An Introduction to Materials in Medicine*, B.D. Ratner, A.S. Hoffman, F.J. Schoen, and J.E. Lemons, Eds., 2nd ed. San Diego: Elsevier Academic Press, pp. 23–32, 2004.

Koski, J.A., C. Ibarra, and S.A. Rodeo. "Tissue-Engineered Ligament: Cells, Matrix, and Growth Factors." *The Orthopedic Clinics of North America*, vol. 31, pp. 437–452, 2000.

Laurencin, C.T. and J.W. Freeman. "Ligament Tissue Engineering: An Evolutionary Materials Science Approach." *Biomaterials*, vol. 26, pp. 7530–7536, 2005.

Park, J.B. and R.S. Lakes. *Biomaterials: An Introduction*, 2nd ed. New York: Plenum Press, 1992.

Biomaterial Degradation

CHAPTER 5

Main Objective

To understand the molecular mechanisms behind environmental degradation of metals, ceramics, and polymers in the human body.

Specific Objectives

1. To distinguish between controlled and uncontrolled material degradation.
2. To understand how redox reactions cause corrosion.
3. To compare and contrast types of corrosion.
4. To understand the contribution of the location of the implant to its corrosion rate.
5. To compare and contrast the degradation of metals, ceramics, and polymers.
6. To distinguish between polymer chain scission by hydrolysis and by oxidation.
7. To understand the factors that influence controlled polymer and ceramic degradation.
8. To distinguish between bulk and surface erosion of biodegradable polymer systems.

5.1 Introduction: Degradation in the Biological Environment

In the previous chapters, we have explained how the physical and mechanical properties of different classes of biomaterials are dependent on the atomic/molecular structure of the materials. In this chapter, we will describe how the degradation of materials in the body is also affected by this structure, and how the degradation process affects the physical and mechanical properties of the overall material.

Biomaterial degradation can occur in an **uncontrolled** manner, which is usually undesirable because it often leads to structural breakdown of the material and premature failure of the device. In contrast, some materials have been designed to degrade in a **controlled** manner, and these are often employed in tissue engineering or drug delivery applications, where the overall goal is temporary tissue replacement and/or release of bioactive factors. This chapter begins with a discussion of undesired

TABLE 5.1

Concentration of Various Ionic Components of Blood Plasma and Extracellular Fluid

Anion, cation	Blood plasma (mM)	Extracellular fluid (mM)
Cl^-	96–111	112–120
HCO_3^-	16–31	25.3–29.7
HPO_4^{2-}	1–1.5	1.93–2
SO_4^{2-}	0.35–1	0.4
$H_2PO_4^-$	2	—
Na^+	131–155	141–145
Mg^{2+}	0.7–1.9	1.3
Ca^{2+}	1.9–3	1.4–1.55
K^+	3.5–5.6	3.5–4

(Adapted with permission from [1].)

biomaterial degradation and closes with a section on materials in which biodegradation is expected as a part of device function.

Although the body provides a relatively mild environment with a neutral pH and constant temperature, the presence of aqueous media containing ions (see Table 5.1 for the composition of blood and extracellular fluid) facilitates the corrosion of metallic implants. Also, specific reactions, such as the actions of inflammatory cells, can change the local chemistry around a device after implantation. As discussed further in Chapter 10, specific inflammatory cells may attach to the biomaterial surface and excrete strong oxidizing agents, such as peroxides, as well as lower the pH drastically in the area, which can further encourage corrosion or degradation of the material.

These unique properties of the biological environment make it difficult to predict the extent of decomposition *in vivo* for materials undergoing either controlled or uncontrolled degradation. Therefore, *in vivo* testing of new biomaterials is necessary to assess degradation at the site of proposed implantation before they can be used clinically (see the last section in this chapter for more information on this topic).

5.2 Corrosion/Degradation of Metals and Ceramics

Given the chemical composition of physiologic fluids, metals are, in general, more susceptible to degradation *in vivo* than ceramic-based materials. Degradation of metals is referred to as **corrosion**, and, due to its common occurrence in biomedical implants, will be the subject of a large portion of this section. Characterization and prediction of corrosion is very important in order to forecast how long the metal may stay in the body before it undergoes structural changes or failure. However, knowledge of corrosion is also crucial in predicting the biocompatibility of an implant. During corrosion, leaching of ions from the metallic surface into the surroundings may have deleterious short- or long-term biological consequences that must be taken into account when determining the suitability of a certain metal for use in the body.

5.2.1 Fundamentals of Corrosion

5.2.1.1 Oxidation-Reduction Reactions Corrosion is an **electrochemical** process that involves transfer of electrons from one substance to another. Corrosion occurs through coupling of two reactions: **oxidation**, which generates electrons, and **reduction**, which consumes electrons. Combined, these are termed **redox** reactions. For a metal M with n valence electrons, oxidation can be represented as

$$M \longrightarrow M^{n+} + ne^-$$

where e^- indicates a free electron. The place where oxidation occurs is called the **anode.**

The corresponding reduction reaction depends on the environment in which the corrosion is taking place. If the milieu is acidic (such as may occur under or around inflammatory cells attached to biomaterials), H^+ ions are reduced to form hydrogen gas:

$$2H^+ + 2e^- \longrightarrow H_2$$

Since dissolved oxygen is also present in body fluids, alternate reactions include the reduction of oxygen in acidic solutions, namely,

$$O_2 + 4H^+ + 4e^- \longrightarrow 2H_2O$$

or, in neutral or basic solutions,

$$O_2 + 2H_2O + 4e^- \longrightarrow 4(OH^-)$$

These reduction reactions take place at the **cathode.**

A simple example of coupled redox reactions is the formation of an electrochemical (or galvanic) cell, also called a battery, using a strip of solid zinc immersed in a solution containing zinc ions and a strip of copper in a separate container with a solution of copper ions (Fig. 5.1). The two solutions are connected with a **salt bridge** composed of a substance that readily dissociates into ions, such as KCl. The circuit is completed by connecting the two metal strips (**electrodes**) with a wire so that electrons can flow from one piece of metal to the other. A voltmeter is also placed in the circuit to record the potential difference between the electrodes.

In each compartment (called a **half-cell**), a reaction occurs. In this example, zinc is oxidized:

$$Zn \longrightarrow Zn^{2+} + 2e^-$$

while, in the other half-cell, copper ions are reduced:

$$Cu^{2+} + 2e^- \longrightarrow Cu$$

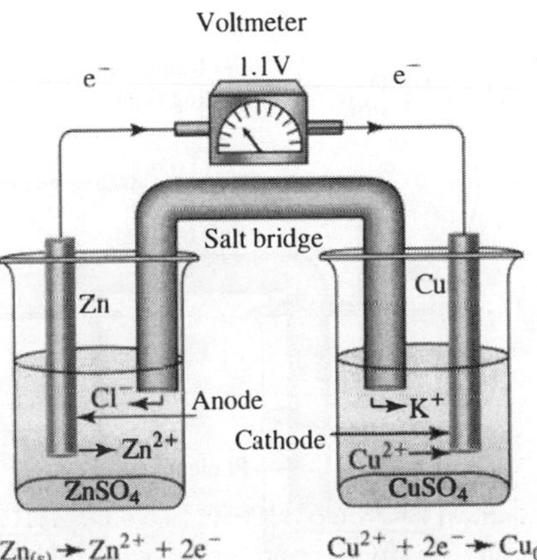

Figure 5.1
An electrochemical (or galvanic) cell. A strip of solid zinc and solid copper are immersed in corresponding solutions containing zinc ions and copper ions, respectively. The two solutions are connected with a salt bridge composed of a substance that readily dissociates into ions, such as KCl. A completed circuit is formed by connecting the two metal strips (electrodes) with a wire so that electrons can flow from one piece of metal to the other. A voltmeter is used to record the potential difference between the electrodes—in this case, 1.1V. (Adapted with permission from [2].)

This results in slow dissolution of the solid zinc anode, with concomitant deposition of copper at the cathode. The role of the salt bridge is to provide ions that maintain a neutral charge in each half-cell. If the concentrations of the solutions in each compartment are 1M and the cell is tested at room temperature (**standard conditions**), the voltmeter in the circuit should read 1.1V.

5.2.1.2 Half-Cell Potentials Why is it that for the system depicted in Fig. 5.1, zinc is always the anode and the copper the cathode? This depends on how easily each metal will release electrons (be oxidized). In order to rank the oxidation behavior of different metals, the concept of **standard reduction potentials** for half-cells was developed. In this case, the potential difference for each metal is measured with respect to a **standard hydrogen electrode.** As illustrated in Fig. 5.2, a hydrogen electrode is formed by bubbling hydrogen through a 1M solution of HCl containing a strip of platinum. The solid platinum does not participate in the reaction, but provides a surface on which the hydrogen ions can be oxidized or reduced.

The use of the standard electrode in an electrochemical cell (Fig. 5.2) is the same as that described for the zinc-copper system described previously. This set-up has been employed to determine the reduction potentials for a number of metals, some of which are listed in Table 5.2. As one moves down the table [called the **standard electromotive force (emf) series**], the metals' propensity for oxidation becomes higher and they are more active (anodic), as indicated in the table. As demonstrated by the zinc-copper example, the metal with the more negative standard reduction potential will always act as the anode.

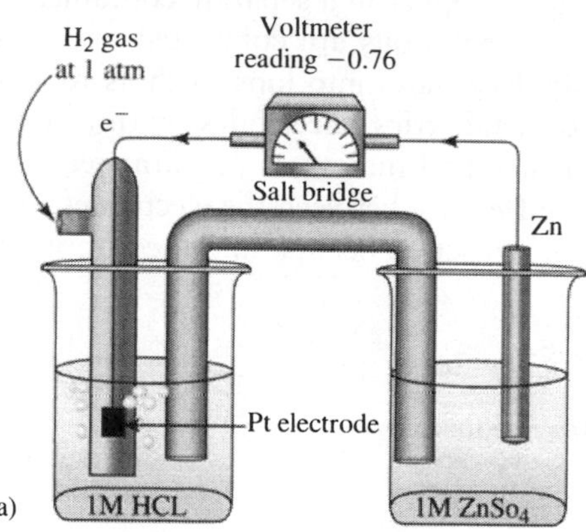

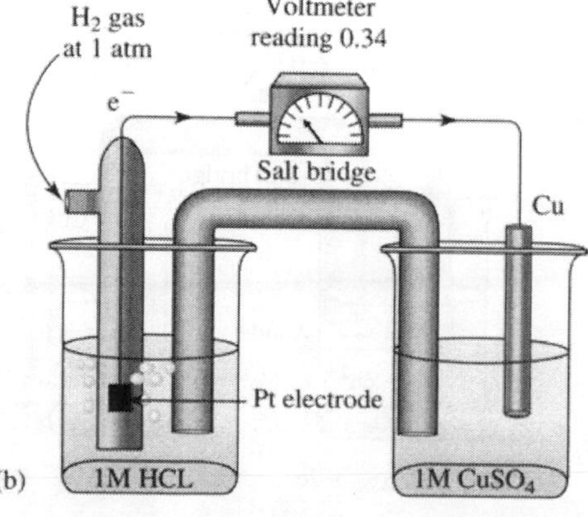

Figure 5.2
In order to rank the oxidation behavior of different metals, the potential difference for each metal is measured with respect to a standard hydrogen electrode. A hydrogen electrode is formed by bubbling hydrogen through a 1M solution of HCl containing a strip of platinum (an inert surface on which the hydrogen ions can be oxidized or reduced). From this particular setup, the standard reduction potential can be measured for zinc (a) and copper (b). (Adapted with permission from [2].)

TABLE 5.2

Standard Electromotive Force (EMF) Series

	Electrode Reaction	Standard Electrode Potential, E^0 (E)
↑	$Au^{3+} + 3e^- \rightarrow Au$	+1.420
	$O_2 + 4H^+ + 4e^- \rightarrow 2\,H_2O$	+1.229
	$Pt^{2+} + 2e^- \rightarrow Pt$	~+1.2
	$Ag^+ + e^- \rightarrow Ag$	+0.800
Increasingly inert	$Fe^{3+} + e^- \rightarrow Fe^{2+}$	+0.771
(cathodic)	$O_2 + 2\,H_2O + 4e^- \rightarrow 4(OH^-)$	+0.401
	$Cu^{2+} + 2e^- \rightarrow Cu$	+0.340
	$2H^+ + 2e^- \rightarrow H_2$	0.000
	$Pb^{2+} + 2e^- \rightarrow Pb$	−0.126
	$Sn^{2+} + 2e^- \rightarrow Sn$	−0.136
	$Ni^{2+} + 2e^- \rightarrow Ni$	−0.250
	$Co^{2+} + 2e^- \rightarrow Co$	−0.277
	$Cd^{2+} + 2e^- \rightarrow Cd$	−0.403
	$Fe^{2+} + 2e^- \rightarrow Fe$	−0.440
Increasingly active	$Cr^{3+} + 3e^- \rightarrow Cr$	−0.744
(anodic)	$Zn^{2+} + 2e^- \rightarrow Zn$	−0.763
	$Al^{3+} + 3e^- \rightarrow Al$	−1.662
	$Mg^{2+} + 2e^- \rightarrow Mg$	−2.363
↓	$Na^+ + e^- \rightarrow Na$	−2.714
	$K^+ + e^- \rightarrow K$	−2.924

(Adapted with permission from [3].)

Although standard reduction potentials are useful for comparing activities of various metals, in reality, it is rare to encounter pure metals in a 1M solution of their ions. While effects from changes in ion concentration can be taken into account using the Nernst equation (see below, equation 5.2), alterations in the nature of the solvent are more difficult to model. Therefore, the **galvanic series** has been developed from data collected on metal corrosion in seawater and provides a good indication of the relative activity of various metals in a salt solution, similar to that found in the human body. A summary of the galvanic series is found in Table 5.3. Although no exact potentials have been assigned, like the emf series, the metals towards the bottom of the list are more easily oxidized than those at the top.

5.2.1.3 Nernst Equation As mentioned above, the potential measured between the electrodes of an electrochemical cell depends in part on temperature and the concentration of the metal ions in each half-cell. Alterations in either of these parameters will affect the overall potential, as described by the Nernst equation.

For a generic two-metal cell, like the zinc-copper example given above, the reactions and corresponding measured potentials are as follows:

$$M_1 \longrightarrow M_1^{n+} + ne^- \qquad -E_1^0 \text{ (metal } M_1 \text{ is oxidized)}$$

$$M_2^{n+} + ne^- \longrightarrow M_2 \qquad E_2^0 \text{ (metal } M_2 \text{ is reduced)}$$

Here, the values for E_1^0 and E_2^0 are those from the standard reduction potential table (see Table 5.2). Because M_1 is oxidized, the sign of its reduction potential must be reversed ($-E_1^0$).

TABLE 5.3

Galvanic Series in Seawater	
Platinum	↑
Gold	Cathodic
Graphite	
Titanium	
Silver	
Stainless steel (passive)	
Nickel-base alloys (passive)	
Cu-30% Ni alloy	
Copper	
Aluminum bronze	
Cu-35% Zn brass	
Nickel-base alloys (active)	
Manganese bronze	
Cu-40% Zn brass	
Tin	
Lead	
316 stainless steel (active)	
50% Pb-50% Sn solder	
410 stainless steel (active)	
Cast iron	
Low carbon steel	
2024 aluminum	
2017 aluminum	
Cadmium	
Alclad	
1100 aluminum	
5052 aluminum	
Galvanized steel	
Zinc	
Magnesium alloys	Anodic
Magnesium	↓

(Adapted with permission from [4].)

The overall reaction is

$$M_1 + M_2^{n+} \longrightarrow M_1^{n+} + M_2$$

and, adding the standard half-cell potentials, the corresponding electrochemical potential for the entire cell is

$$\Delta E^0 = (E_2^0 - E_1^0) \tag{5.1}$$

In order to take into account deviations from the conditions in which the standard reduction potentials were measured (changes in temperature or ion concentration), the equation becomes

$$\Delta E^0 = (E_2^0 - E_1^0) - \frac{RT}{nF} \ln \frac{[M_1^{n+}]}{[M_2^{n+}]} \tag{5.2}$$

where R is the gas constant (8.314 J K^{-1} mol^{-1}), T is the absolute temperature (K), F is Faraday's constant (96,500 coulombs/mol), and n, E_1^0 and E_2^0 are as previously described. This is the **Nernst equation**.

EXAMPLE PROBLEM 5.1

Consider an electrochemical cell of zinc and copper as described in the text and illustrated in Fig. 5.1.

(a) Assuming that the concentrations of the solutions in each compartment are 1M and that the cell is tested at room temperature (standard conditions), show that the potential difference between the electrodes is 1.1V.

(b) Consider now that the conditions of the cell have changed as follows. The cell is tested at body temperature (37°C) and the concentrations of the zinc and copper solutions in each compartment are typical serum concentrations of these ions (107 μg/dL and 115 μg/dL, respectively). Calculate the potential difference between the electrodes under these conditions.

(c) Assuming the same ion concentrations as given in part (b), at what temperature would the system need to be tested for the potential difference between the electrodes to equal 1.15V?

Solution:

(a) In this electrochemical cell, the zinc is being oxidized and the copper is being reduced, as described in the text. Thus, the following chemical reactions are occurring:

$$\begin{array}{lr} & Zn \longrightarrow Zn^{2+} + 2e^- \\ & + \ Cu^{2+} + 2e^- \longrightarrow Cu \\ \hline \text{Net:} & Zn + Cu^{2+} \longrightarrow Zn^{2+} + Cu \end{array}$$

Looking up the standard electrode potentials from Table 5.2, we find that $E_1^o = -0.763V(Zn)$ and $E_2^o = +0.340V(Cu)$. Under standard conditions, the potential difference between the two electrodes is calculated by simply subtracting the standard emf of the anode from the cathode, as follows:

$$E^\circ = E_2{}^\circ - E_1{}^\circ = 0.340V - (-0.763V) = \underline{1.103V}$$

(b) In non-standard conditions, the potential difference between the electrodes should be calculated using the Nernst equation:

$$\Delta E^\circ = (E_2{}^\circ - E_1{}^\circ) - \frac{RT}{nF} \cdot \ln \frac{[M_1{}^{n+}]}{[M_2{}^{n+}]}$$

Here, the emf values are as before, R is the gas constant ($8.314\ J\ K^{-1}\ mol^{-1}$), F is Faraday's constant (96,500 C/mol), n is 2, and the absolute temperature T is given (37°C = 310K). The concentration of zinc can be calculated from the given information as follows:

$$(0.00107\ g/dL)(mole/65.39\ g\ Zn)(10\ dL/L) = 0.0164\ \mu M\ Zn$$

Similarly, the concentration of copper can be calculated as

$$(0.00115\ g/dL)(mole/63.55\ g\ Cu)(10\ dL/L) = 0.0181\ \mu M\ Cu$$

Plugging these values into the equation gives

$$\Delta E^\circ = (0.340V - (-0.763V)) - \frac{8.314\left(\frac{J}{K \cdot mol}\right)310K}{2 \cdot 96{,}500(C/mol)} \cdot \ln \frac{[.0164\ \mu M]}{[.0181\ \mu M]}$$

$$\underline{\Delta E^\circ = 1.104V}$$

(c) Using the same equation as in (b), and solving for $\Delta E^\circ = 1.15\text{V}$ yields

$$1.15\text{V} = (0.340\text{V} + 0.763\text{V}) - \frac{8.314\left(\frac{\text{J}}{\text{K}\cdot\text{mol}}\right)T}{2\cdot 96500(\text{C/mol})} \cdot \ln\frac{[.0164\ \mu M]}{[.0181\ \mu M]},$$

and solving for T, we find that the temperature must be approximately 11,061K for the potential difference between the electrodes to equal 1.15V! ■

5.2.1.4 Galvanic Corrosion One of the most common forms of corrosion corresponds well to the description of typical electrochemical cells, and thus is termed **galvanic corrosion.** In this case, two different types of metals are electrically coupled when placed in the body, like the wire connecting the two electrodes in Fig. 5.1. Physiological fluid becomes the salt bridge completing the circuit. In this situation, the more active metal will dissolve at an accelerated pace. For example, if stainless steel is used in conjunction with another alloy, it often undergoes anodic dissolution.

However, it is difficult to predict metal degradation in such a system solely based on the activities listed in the galvanic series (see Table 5.3) because corrosion is a very complex process. One important consideration is that the oxidation and reduction rates must be equal so that if localized changes reduce one reaction, then the overall corrosion may be significantly slowed. An example of this is metal *passivation*, discussed in the next section.

5.2.2 Pourbaix Diagrams and Passivation

In addition to the parameters discussed above, corrosion activity for a certain metal also depends on the pH of the solution in which it is immersed. In order to further refine predictions of corrosion in various environments, a Pourbaix diagram may be created. As shown in Fig. 5.3 for iron, a **Pourbaix diagram** for a

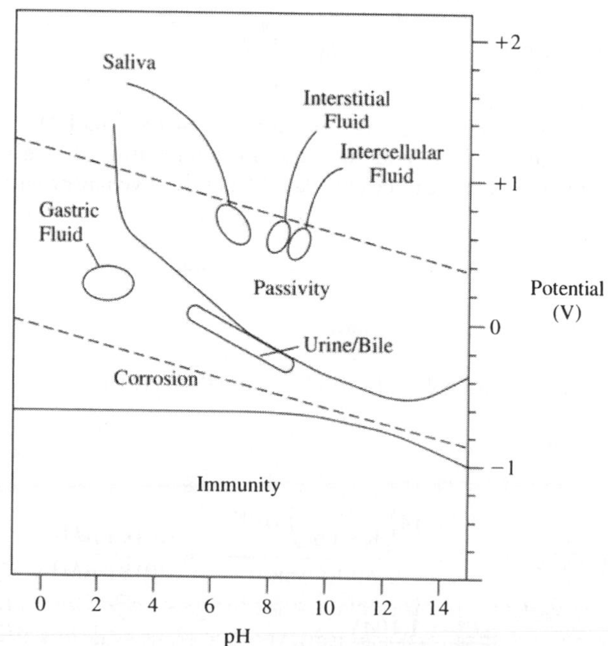

Figure 5.3
An example of a Pourbaix diagram for iron, depicting regions of corrosion and noncorrosion as a function of cell potential and pH. The regions depicted in this particular example assume that a surface film of lepidocrocite (an iron oxide-hydroxide mineral, γ FeOOH) forms under proper conditions and that this film is protective against corrosion. The stability of water is represented via the diagonal dashed lines. Aqueous corrosion, if it occurs, will take place in environments falling between these two lines. Sample physiological environments, such as saliva and gastric fluid, are also shown. (Adapted with permission from [5].)

given metal depicts regions of corrosion and non-corrosion as a function of cell potential and pH. Pourbaix diagrams are formed using results from the Nernst equation and the solubilities of possible degradation products, as well as other factors. The diagonal dashed lines in the figure represent the stability of water. Aqueous corrosion, if it occurs, will take place in environments falling between these two lines.

The Pourbaix diagram is divided into three main regions: corrosion, immunity, and passivation. Corrosion is arbitrarily defined as a region in which greater than 10^{-6} M of the metal's ions are found in solution at equilibrium. If less than this concentration is measured, the metal may fall into either of the other categories (immune or passive). In the **immune** region, it is not energetically favorable for the metal to corrode (dissolve). This phenomenon is also called **cathodic protection** because the metal cannot act as an anode under these conditions.

Passivation occurs when surface oxidation leads to the formation of a stable solid film (usually an oxide or hydroxide) that coats the surface of the metal. In this region, although it may be energetically favorable, corrosion can be slowed or stopped due to this thin, insulative barrier that prevents transfer of electrons in and out of the metal. In particular, metals such as chromium, iron, nickel, titanium, and aluminum have a tendency to form these coatings.

The diagram in Fig. 5.3 also includes areas representing the composition of different body fluids, so that it is possible to predict the response of a metal in various locations in the body. The regions found in Pourbaix diagrams give an idea of which reactions are possible *in vivo*, but cannot predict the rate of these reactions. This rate, which is often defined in terms of current flow per surface area, is dependent on other factors, such as possible depletion of ions around the cathode. A detailed discussion of corrosion rate calculation is beyond the scope of this text.

EXAMPLE PROBLEM 5.2

The pH of a wound site created through the implantation of a material can drop considerably to acidic values of 5 or lower. Imagine the hypothetical case of a surgeon implanting a bone plate composed of stainless steel with an iron coating. Assume that the pH of the tissue surrounding the implant drops to 5 during the wound healing response and that the surgical team did not notice an aluminum screw that was accidentally dropped into the patient near the implant. Assume also that an electrochemical cell is created through the interaction between the iron, aluminum and extracellular fluid. Using the Pourbaix diagram for iron given in Fig. 5.3, would you expect the iron coating to corrode with a cell potential of +0.10V? Would you expect the iron coating to corrode with a cell potential of −0.40V?

Solution: The dashed lines on the Pourbaix diagram indicate the range of conditions for which water is stable, with the conditions falling between these lines being conducive to the presence of water. Using the Pourbaix diagram for iron, at a pH of approximately 5, aqueous corrosion can occur when the cell potential lies between approximately +0.30V and −0.30V. Thus, at a cell potential of +0.10V, one would expect the iron to begin to corrode in the aqueous environment at a pH of 5. However, at a cell potential of −0.40V and a pH of 5, one would not expect aqueous corrosion of the iron to occur, as the conditions exceed the stability of water (as indicated by the dashed lines on the diagram). ■

5.2.3 Contribution of Processing Parameters

A number of additional factors besides metal composition can enhance corrosion *in vivo*. These include metal processing and handling techniques, discussed here, as well as mechanical loading and the presence of proteins, cells and bacteria, which are treated in subsequent sections. Anything that causes the presence of different microstructures within an implant can change localized ion concentrations and thus affect

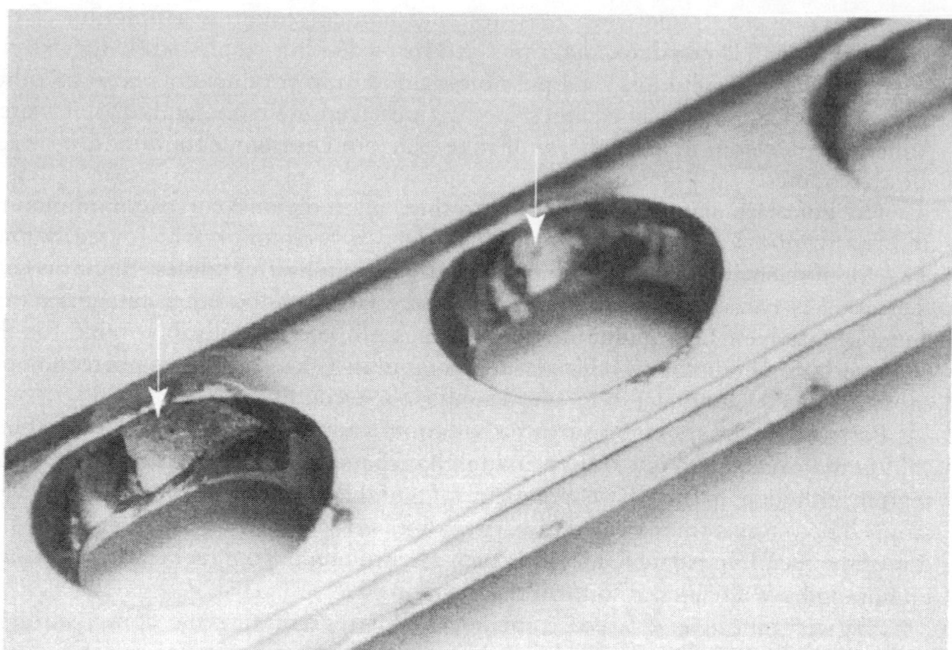

Figure 5.4
An example of crevice corrosion on the plate of a bone fixation device. Corrosion occurred in the narrow, deep crack between the screw (not shown) and plate. Arrows indicate where corrosion has occurred. (Reprinted with permission from [1].)

the corrosion rate. These can be the result of tiny flaws or cracks introduced during fabrication, or overall device design.

5.2.3.1 Crevice Corrosion As the name implies, **crevice corrosion** occurs in areas with a narrow, deep crack—for example, in between the screw and plate of a bone fixation device (Fig. 5.4). Certain metals commonly used in orthopedic applications, such as stainless steels, can exhibit this type of corrosion, while others, like titanium and cobalt-chromium alloys, are less susceptible. Although the exact mechanism of crevice corrosion is not fully understood, it is thought to begin with the depletion of oxygen within the crevice. At this point, only the anodic reaction is possible in the crevice, which results in oxidation of the metal in this area, while the remainder of the piece becomes the cathode. Outside the crevice, oxygen reduction results in an increase in pH. A diagram of this process is found in Fig. 5.5.

In the presence of sodium chloride solution, as found in the body, crevice corrosion is further accelerated by the diffusion of Cl^- ions into the crevice to balance the charge of the M^{n+} ions created. The compound formed can react further to produce an insoluble hydroxide and liberate H^+:

$$MCl_n + nH_2O \rightarrow M(OH)_n + nH^+Cl^-$$

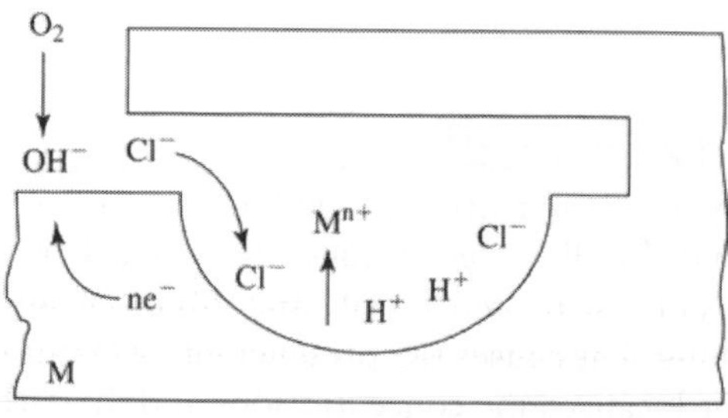

Figure 5.5
A theoretical mechanism of crevice corrosion. Depletion of oxygen occurs within the crevice, causing oxidation of the metal in that location, while the remainder of the piece becomes the cathode. (Adapted with permission from [6].)

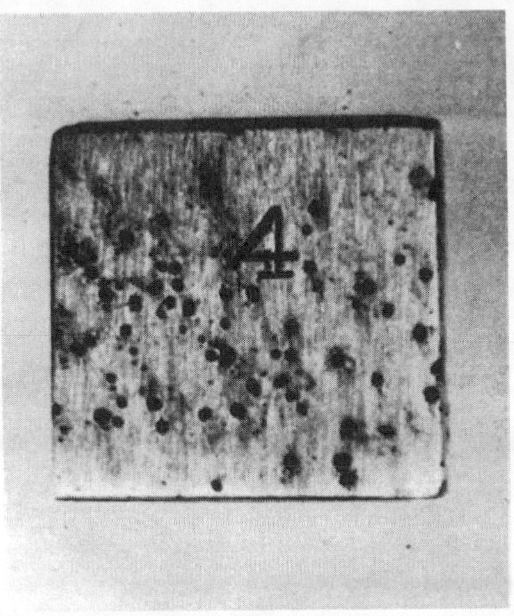

Figure 5.6
Pitting corrosion seen on a sample of stainless steel. Small defects on the surface of the material act as an anode, resulting in corrosion at that location. (Reprinted with permission from [7].)

This decreases the local pH and provides a more corrosive environment, thereby significantly increasing the rate of metal dissolution within the crevice.

5.2.3.2 Pitting Corrosion Pitting corrosion is caused by the same mechanism as crevice corrosion. As shown in Fig 5.6, stainless steels can also undergo this type of corrosion. In this case, processing or handling may lead to a small flaw or area in which the passivation film on the surface is disrupted, leading to the formation of a relatively small anode and large cathode. Because of this inequality in surface area and the fact that the rates of both reactions must be equal, the anodic regions undergo significant dissolution. This is a particularly dangerous type of corrosion because it can go undetected until device failure due to the small overall material loss.

5.2.3.3 Intergranular Corrosion Devices fabricated by casting (see Chapter 6) often have multiple grains and thus are particularly susceptible to **intergranular corrosion.** As discussed in Chapter 3, the grain boundaries are at a heightened energy state and therefore may represent more active (anodic) regions of the material. Particularly in alloys, this can lead to intergranular attack by a similar mechanism as that described for crevice corrosion (Fig. 5.7). A common example of this is corrosion of stainless steel at the grain boundaries due to depletion of chromium in the area. Chromium is required to form a passivating layer on the metal; if this is removed, the area quickly undergoes corrosion and, in the extreme case, may crumble into many tiny pieces.

5.2.4 Contribution of the Mechanical Environment

In addition to fabrication and handling parameters, the location of an implant has a large effect on the length of time elapsed before substantial corrosion occurs. If a device is used in a tissue that undergoes continued movement and is constantly under load, the corrosion rate can be significantly higher than for a similar device located in a less stressed environment. The presence of mechanical stress can potentiate corrosion by increasing the number of microcracks in a metal. Also, a material under stress is in a higher energy state, so it is more susceptible to the chemical reactions that produce corrosion.

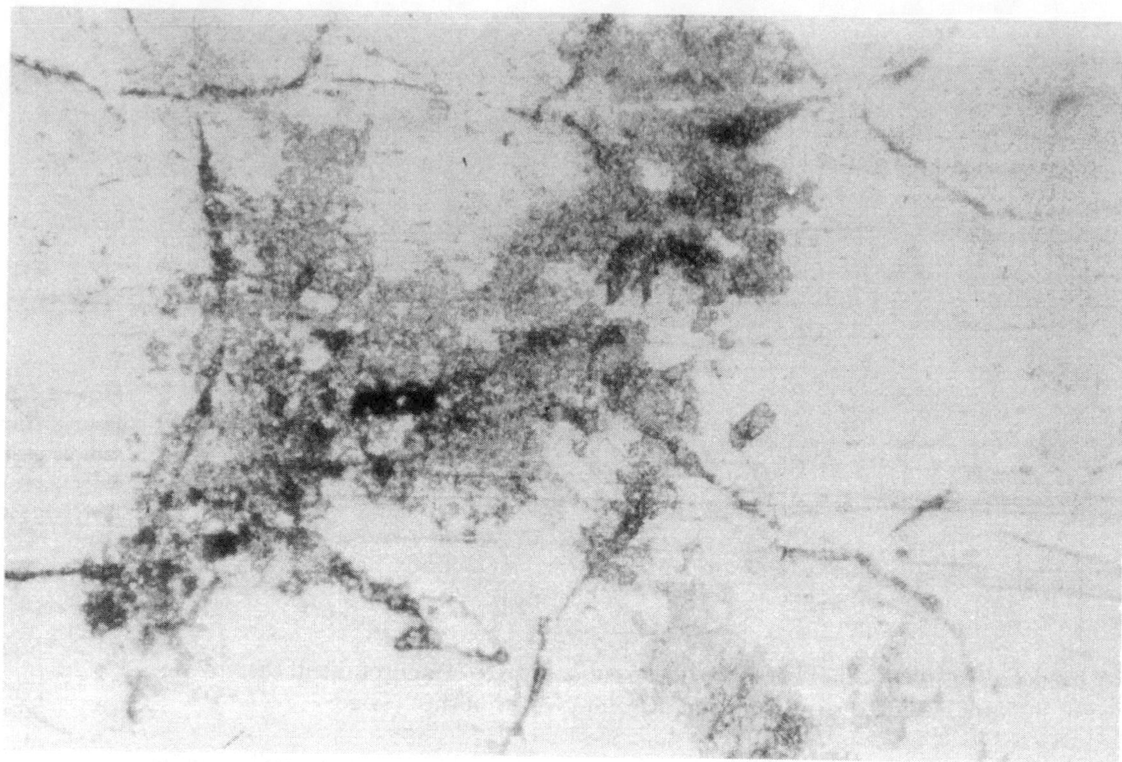

Figure 5.7
An example of intergranular corrosion. The same process seen in crevice corrosion occurs in this situation, with the grain boundaries acting as the anode. (Reprinted with permission from [8].)

5.2.4.1 Stress and Galvanic Corrosion Bending a metal rod or plate will cause the tensile side to be anodic compared to the side in compression. This encourages galvanic corrosion in a material that otherwise would have no difference in electrochemical potential between the two sides. This same effect can be observed near stress raisers (see Chapter 4) such as holes or sharp corners.

5.2.4.2 Stress Corrosion Cracking **Stress corrosion cracking** occurs to a metal that is both under tension and subjected to a corrosive environment. This combination results in small cracks that form perpendicular to the direction of applied stress, and is particularly dangerous because it can occur at relatively low loads (below the ultimate tensile strength) and in solutions that would normally be well tolerated by the material. Once formed, the cracks propagate and lead to brittle fracture, even though metals traditionally exhibit substantial ductility. Alloys, especially stainless steel, are susceptible to this type of degradation in the presence of saline solutions like that found *in vivo*.

5.2.4.3 Fatigue Corrosion In **fatigue corrosion**, continued bending, loading, or motion around the implant may disrupt the passivating film formed on the metal and expose the underlying surface, leading to corrosion of this area. As discussed in Chapter 4, fatigue properties are measured by recording how many cycles of loading a device can undergo at a certain stress without failure (fatigue life). In corrosion fatigue, the maximum stress at failure decreases continually as the number of loading cycles increases. Therefore, this type of corrosion may significantly shorten the fatigue life of the implant and result in premature device failure.

5.2.4.4 Fretting Corrosion Unlike the other types of corrosion listed in this section, **fretting corrosion** is not related to loading, but is dependent on motion near the implant. This type of corrosion involves removal of the metal's passivating layer by mechanical means. This can be the creation of a nick in the surface that does not repassivate, or a cyclic process in which the passive layer is formed and then destroyed repeatedly. It is thought that fretting corrosion plays a role in the degradation seen around connections between fixation plates and bone screws (Fig. 5.4).

5.2.5 Contribution of the Biological Environment

Besides the effects of mechanical factors, the implant's location in the body can influence corrosion in other ways. Chemical and cellular constituents of the biological milieu may affect the corrosion rate substantially. It is important to remember that the localized environment is rarely constant, with diffusion of ions, migration of cells, and chemical reactions taking place continuously, which adds yet another level of complexity to predicting corrosion rates *in vivo*.

The physiological fluids and tissues surrounding an implant are rich in proteins and cells. The recruitment of inflammatory cells to the area after biomaterial implantation can cause drastic changes in the chemistry surrounding the implant, including a drop in pH and release of strong oxidizing agents. Although it may seem that both of these responses would promote corrosion, it has been found for some metals that the oxidizing agents released during inflammation actually contribute to the growth of the passive layer on the surface, so the effects of surrounding cells on corrosion must be evaluated for the specific system of interest before use in the body.

The attachment of proteins to the metallic surface (see Chapters 7 and 8 for why this occurs) may also have a number of effects. Proteins can alter the nature of the passive layer on the metal by creating a barrier that reduces oxygen diffusion to the surface. This, in turn, reduces the stability of the oxide layer formed on the implant. Electrochemical potential can also be affected by proteins that act as electron carriers, thereby shifting cell parameters so that they fall outside the passive region on the Pourbaix diagram. Finally, certain proteins require metal ions to function, so they have a natural affinity to scavenge metals. If they consume a product of the corrosion reaction, their presence may alter the equilibrium and favor further dissolution.

As discussed further in Chapter 14, bacteria may attach to the implant during insertion or at some later point, leading to infection of the device. The by-products of bacterial metabolism can change the regional pH near the material, which affects the stability of the passive layer. Additionally, bacteria can consume hydrogen, an ion often found at the cathode. Like metal scavenging by proteins, this change in reaction equilibrium may encourage anodic dissolution.

5.2.6 Means of Corrosion Control

Although corrosive attack due to the nature of the biological environment cannot always be controlled, reduction of corrosion is possible via key decisions in the design and fabrication of the implant. For example, stress-induced corrosion can be mitigated by designing devices with few stress raisers. Similarly, galvanic corrosion may be prevented through selection of combinations of metals that are close together in the galvanic series. Ideally, the device would be fabricated from only non-reactive (cathodic) metals like gold, silver or platinum, but in many cases, the mechanical properties of these materials limit their usefulness. Therefore, as a compromise, metals known to form passive oxide coatings are often employed, either in their pure or alloyed form, to create implants with corrosion resistance as well as sufficient mechanical strength.

In addition, extra processing steps may be included to prevent specific types of corrosion. For instance, heat-treating stainless steels may reduce intergranular corrosion. Additionally, pre-treating a metal with nitric acid forms a passive surface layer before implantation (see Chapter 7 and ASTM standard F86 for more about these methods). This is one example of a protective layer that may be applied to metallic implants. Others, including metallic, ceramic, or polymeric coatings, are added on the surface via a variety of means (see Chapter 7) to provide a barrier between the active metal and its surroundings, thereby decreasing dissolution of the implant.

5.2.7 Ceramic Degradation

While the dissolution of metals is called corrosion, breakdown of ceramic materials is termed **degradation.** Passivating layers on metals are usually a form of ceramic material, so this indicates that ceramics are, in general, more stable than metals in the physiologic environment. This is because ceramics are composed of bonds with a largely ionic character, so much energy is required to break them.

However, some ceramic formulations are highly soluble in an aqueous environment. This has led to the classification of ceramics as either **inert, resorbable**, or having **controlled surface reactivity** in the body. Resorbable and surface reactive ceramics are treated in more detail in the section on biodegradable materials (see below).

Regardless of type, degradation of ceramics, like metals, depends on their mechanical environment, as well as the implant design. Stress-induced degradation can occur in ceramics under tension. If a crack is formed in these materials, the tensile stress may lead to further dissolution at the crack tip and, eventually, material fracture. Ceramic porosity also plays a large role in an implant's degradation characteristics. Pores are stress raisers, and thus may increase the formation of cracks or the rate of their propagation. Additionally, the presence of pores promotes degradation by creating more surface area for reaction with the environment (see Section 5.4 for further discussion of the effect of porosity on degradation).[1]

5.3 Degradation of Polymers

Like metals and ceramics, polymeric biomaterials may undergo unwanted degradation in the body due to interactions with surrounding fluids and tissues. Indications that this has occurred include discoloration of the implant, appearance of crazes, or a significant change in mechanical properties. These characteristics result from specific degradation mechanisms discussed in the following sections. As with other types of biomaterials, the implant location within the body, including access to water, proteins, inflammatory cells, and mechanical stress, plays a large role in the rate of polymer degradation.

5.3.1 Primary Means of Polymer Degradation

Polymers usually degrade by two main mechanisms: swelling/dissolution or chain scission. Many polymers with hydrophilic domains will **swell** in the physiologic environment. Here, the solvent (water) molecules are absorbed into the polymer and are small enough to occupy spaces between the macromolecular chains. In

---

[1]Although porosity in metals has the same effect on corrosion rate, the formation of pores in ceramic implants is more common and, therefore, plays a larger role in ceramic than metallic degradation.

this way, they act as plasticizers and make the material more ductile by reducing secondary bonding between chains. They may also affect the crystallinity of the polymer. Both mechanical and thermal properties (e.g. glass transition temperature) can be influenced by the presence of the absorbed solvent. In extreme cases, if the chains are soluble enough and there are few covalent bonds between chains, the polymer may **dissolve** completely in an aqueous environment.

In contrast, **chain scission** involves breaking primary, rather than secondary, bonds. There is a separation in chain segments at the point of bond rupture, which leads to an overall decrease in molecular weight. As discussed in previous chapters, this can have a significant impact on both the mechanical and thermal properties of the polymer. Chain scission may occur via hydrolysis or oxidation reactions, as described in the following sections.

5.3.2 Chain Scission by Hydrolysis

Depending on the susceptibility of chemical groups in the polymer, water molecules may facilitate the cleavage of certain bonds within a macromolecule. This process is called **hydrolysis**, and is a common degradation mechanism of condensation polymers. Many of the chemical moieties that can be cleaved in this manner are found in Fig. 5.8. There are a number of factors that affect the extent of polymer hydrolysis, including the following:

1. Reactivity of groups in the polymer backbone
2. Extent of interchain bonding
3. Amount of media (water) available to the polymer

As an example of how chemical and physical material properties affect hydrolysis rates, a polymeric implant that is highly susceptible to hydrolytic cleavage will contain a large number of cleavable groups like those shown in Fig. 5.8 as well as hydrophilic domains to allow the influx of water deep into the material. It will have a relatively low initial molecular weight and low crosslink density so there are fewer chain entanglements or covalent interactions between chains to be broken. It will possess low or no crystallinity and its T_g will be below body temperature, so the material is in an amorphous, rubbery state to encourage water penetration.

To further promote hydrolytic degradation, the polymer will be formed into an implant that has a high surface area to volume ratio so that the aqueous media reaches many areas of the implant simultaneously.

5.3.3 Chain Scission by Oxidation

In addition to hydrolysis, chain scission of polymers may occur via oxidation reactions. Here, **oxidation** means that highly reactive species (usually free radicals) attack and break covalent bonds in susceptible chemical groups within the macromolecule. Unlike hydrolysis, this reaction involves initiation, propagation and termination steps, similar to those described in Chapter 2 for addition polymerization. The initiation step can involve either homolysis or heterolysis of the polymer chain (Fig. 5.9).

As with hydrolysis, the extent of oxidative degradation depends, in part, on the number of susceptible chemical domains that the polymer contains. Examples of some of these groups are found in Fig. 5.10. Additionally, lower molecular weight polymers and those that are less tightly crosslinked will degrade more quickly because there are fewer primary and secondary interactions holding the material together.

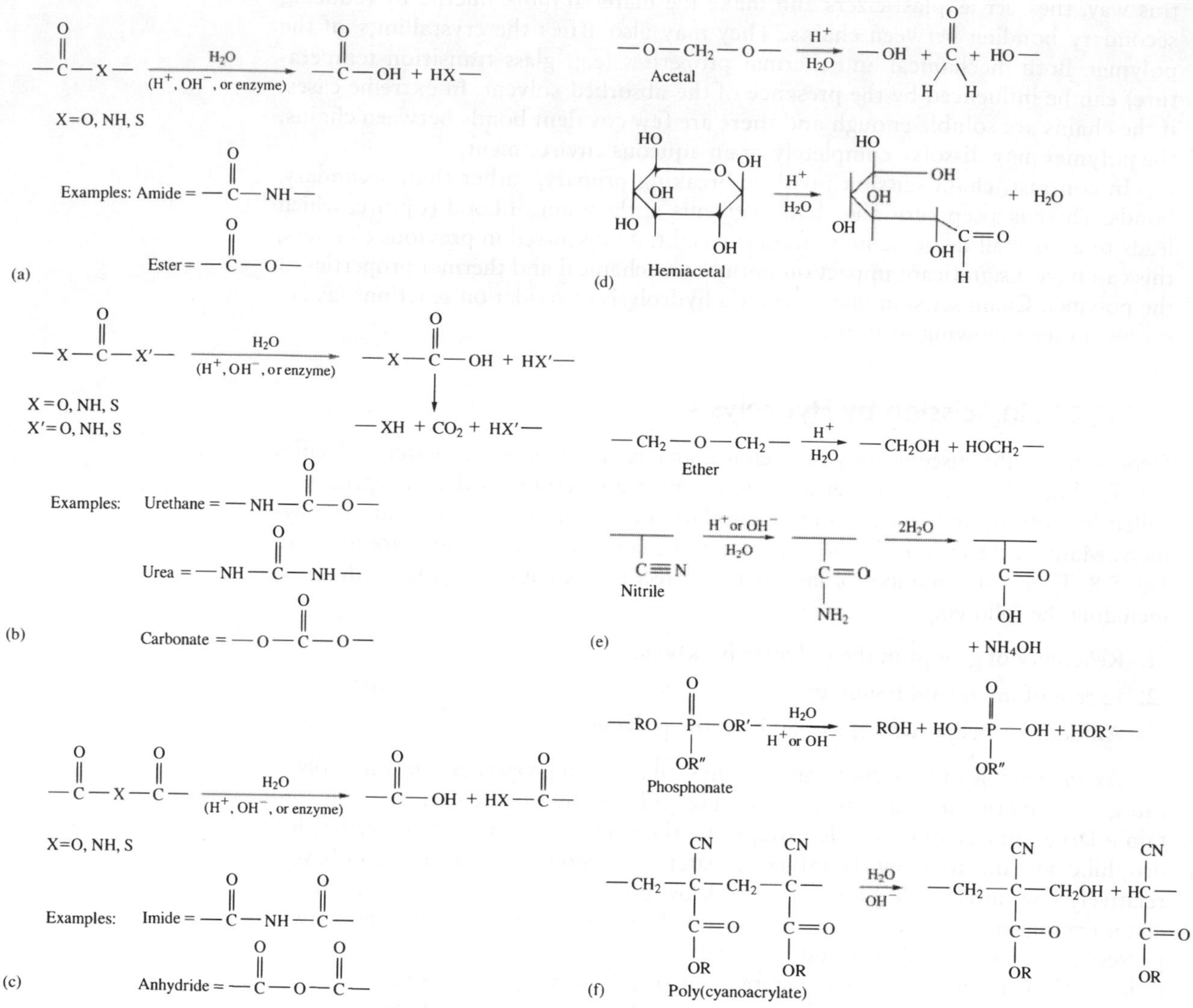

(a) H_2O (H^+, OH^-, or enzyme)

X=O, NH, S

Examples: Amide

Ester

(b) H_2O (H^+, OH^-, or enzyme)

X=O, NH, S
X′=O, NH, S

—XH + CO_2 + HX′—

Examples: Urethane

Urea

Carbonate

(c) H_2O (H^+, OH^-, or enzyme)

X=O, NH, S

Examples: Imide

Anhydride

(d) Acetal

Hemiacetal

(e) Ether

Nitrile

+ NH_4OH

Phosphonate

(f) Poly(cyanoacrylate)

Figure 5.8
Examples of chemical moieties susceptible to cleavage via hydrolysis. (Adapted with permission from [9].)

Homolysis

R–R ⟶ 2R·

Heterolysis

R–R ⟶ $R^+ + R^-$

Figure 5.9
The two different initiation steps (homolysis and heterolysis) that can lead to oxidation of a polymer chain. (Adapted with permission from [9].)

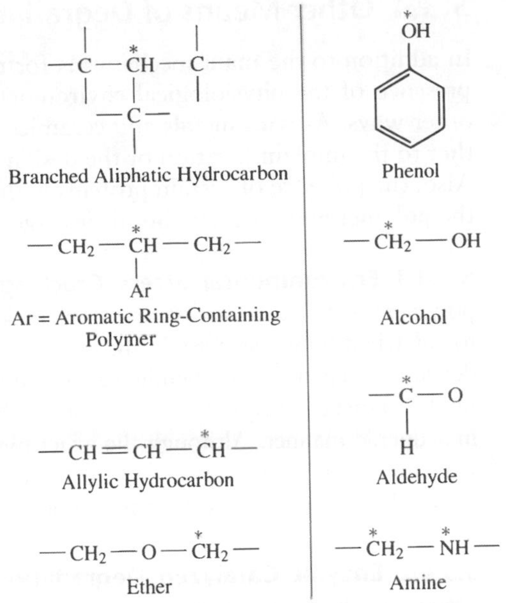

$$-\overset{|}{\underset{|}{C}}-\overset{*}{C}H-\overset{|}{\underset{|}{C}}-$$
$$-\overset{|}{\underset{|}{C}}-$$

Branched Aliphatic Hydrocarbon

$$-CH_2-\overset{*}{C}H-CH_2-$$
$$\quad\;|$$
$$\quad Ar$$

Ar = Aromatic Ring-Containing Polymer

$$-CH=CH-\overset{*}{C}H-$$

Allylic Hydrocarbon

$$-CH_2-O-\overset{*}{C}H_2-$$

Ether

$$\overset{*}{O}H$$ (on a benzene ring)

Phenol

$$-\overset{*}{C}H_2-OH$$

Alcohol

$$-\overset{*}{C}-O$$
$$\;\;|$$
$$\;\;H$$

Aldehyde

$$-\overset{*}{C}H_2-\overset{*}{N}H-$$

Amine

Figure 5.10
Examples of chemical domains that are susceptible to oxidative degradation. * denotes sites of homolysis or heterolysis. (Adapted with permission from [9].)

Oxidation occurs most often in the body due to active agents released during the inflammatory process, such as highly reactive oxygen radicals (see Chapter 10 for more on inflammation). However, **metal-catalyzed oxidation** is also found, particularly in the case of pacemaker leads. Unlike cracks induced by environmental stress (see the next section), which most often appear on the exterior of the implant, fissures resulting from metal-catalyzed oxidation are found on the interior of a polymer coating that is in contact with a metal wire. It is believed that this is caused by corrosion of the metal, which results in the formation of strong oxidizing agents that then, in turn, attack the polymer coating. This type of degradation is characterized by brittle fracture of the polymer, as seen in Fig. 5.11.

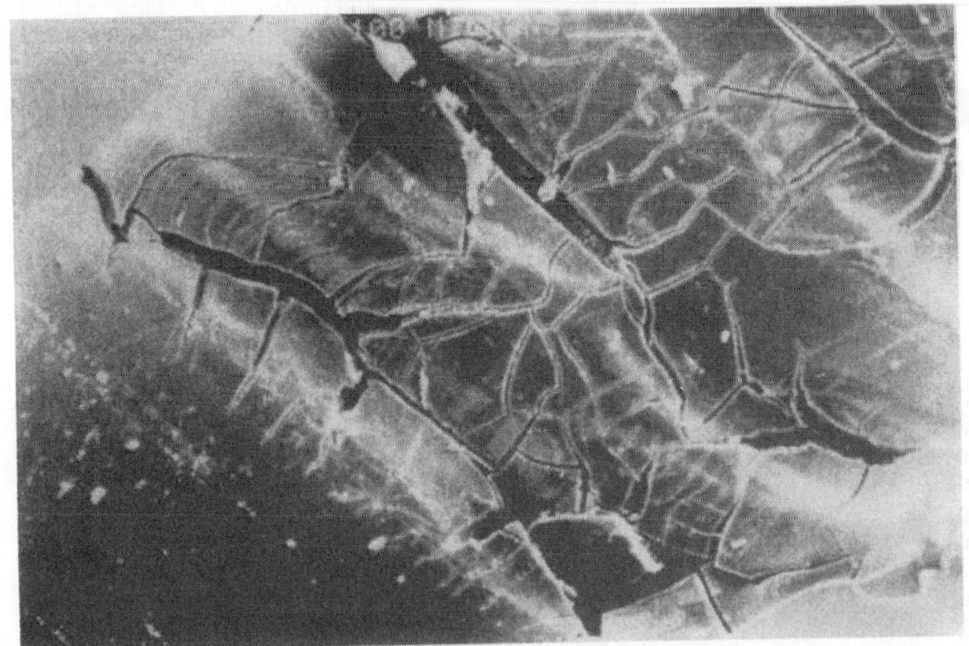

Figure 5.11
A brittle fracture is seen in the polymer, which is a sign of metal-catalyzed oxidation. In this case corrosion first occurs on the metal that the polymer is contacting, and the resultant strong oxidizing agents then attack the polymeric material. (Reprinted with permission from [9].)

5.3.4 Other Means of Degradation

In addition to the main mechanisms for polymer degradation described above, the presence of the physiological environment may encourage material dissolution in other ways. As with metals and ceramics, the addition of mechanical stress, due either to the implant location or the design of the device, can encourage degradation. Also, the presence of certain proteins with an affinity for chemical groups present in the polymer may facilitate bond cleavage.

5.3.4.1 Environmental Stress Cracking **Environmental stress cracking** seen in polymers is similar to stress corrosion cracking in metals. When a polymer is subjected to sufficient tensile stresses in the biological environment, the exterior of the implant develops deep cracks perpendicular to the primary loading axis (Fig. 5.12). However, unlike in metal-catalyzed oxidation, it is believed that in this case the material fractures in a ductile manner. Although the exact mechanism of this type of degradation is not well understood, it is known that the presence of inflammatory cells (or reactive species released from these cells) is required before environmental stress cracking will occur.

5.3.4.2 Enzyme-Catalyzed Degradation Of the many proteins present in the tissue and fluid surrounding a biomedical implant, **enzymes** have a particular affinity for certain chemical groups present in polymers. They then act as *catalysts*, lowering the required activation energy for specific reactions, usually involving those chemical groups. A variety of enzymes are used in the body to achieve efficient synthesis, as well as cleavage, of natural polymers (see Chapter 9 for more information on the structure and function of enzymes). However, in some cases, these same molecules can cause either hydrolytic or oxidative degradation of synthetic polymers, if the polymers possess chemical functional groups similar to the target moieties for the enzymes. Because each person produces different amounts of enzymes, it is difficult to predict to what extent enzyme-catalyzed degradation will affect polymeric materials in a given individual.

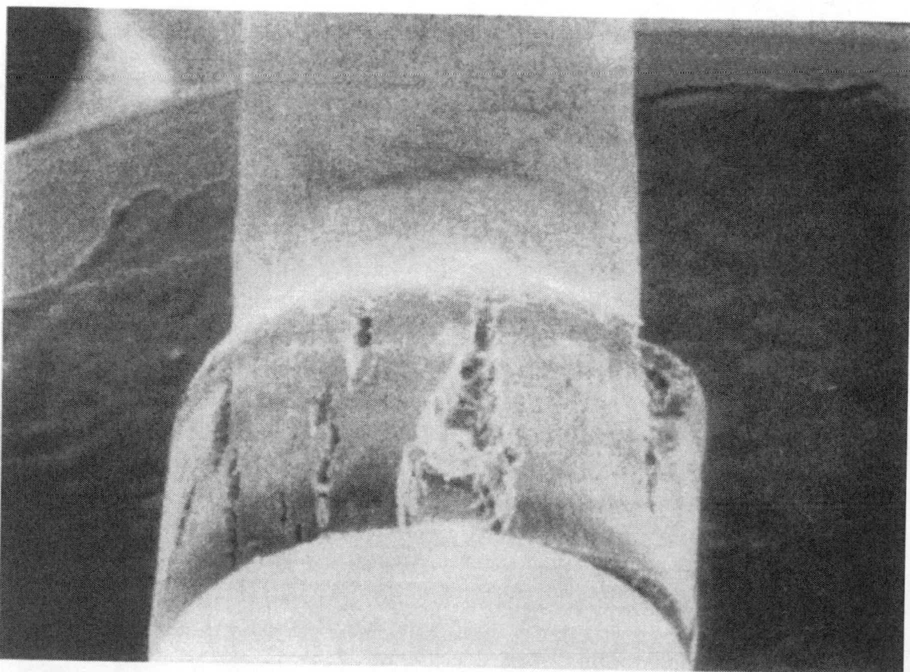

Figure 5.12
Environmental stress cracking seen in a polymer sample. This sample has undergone tensile loading in a biological environment, resulting in the development of deep cracks perpendicular to the primary loading axis. (Reprinted with permission from [9].)

5.3.5 Effects of Porosity

The effects of porosity on polymer degradation are similar to those for ceramic (and metallic) degradation. Because pores represent additional stress raisers, mechanically induced degradation may be increased in porous polymers. Also, porosity increases the surface area of the implant, thereby providing more space for cleavage by environmental factors such as water or oxidative species. Thus, in general, degradation occurs more quickly in porous than non-porous polymeric materials.

5.4 Biodegradable Materials

In contrast to the uncontrolled degradation discussed in the previous sections, which is generally undesirable, controlled biomaterial degradation can be used as an important part of tissue engineering and drug delivery therapies. For these applications, the temporary nature of the material is ideal to promote localized tissue healing or release of a bioactive agent without the need for a second surgery to remove the implant.

However, before materials with designed degradation properties can be described in detail, a few definitions should be clarified. Although international organizations have attempted to standardize the terminology associated with biodegradable implants, many expressions remain redundant and poorly defined. The following discussion is based, in part, on that presented by Kohn et al. [10]. In general, degradation refers to breaking chemical bonds within the material, while erosion involves a change in the size or shape of the material that may or may not be caused by degradation. Although the prefix "bio" was defined to mean that specific actions by a biological agent, such as an enzyme, cell, or bacterium, causes the material breakdown, often in the literature "biodegradation" or "bioerosion" are used simply to indicate that these processes are occurring in the body.

Therefore, in this book, we will refer to **biodegradation** as the chemical breakdown of a material mediated by any component of the physiological environment (such as water, ions, cells, proteins, and bacteria). **Bioerosion** is an even broader term indicating breakdown, including chemical degradation or other processes in which bond cleavage is not required (e.g. physical dissolution), of a material mediated by any component of the physiological environment.[2]

Although the use of biodegradable materials provides several advantages for the patient, particularly in the applications discussed above, degradables also exhibit more complex biocompatibility issues since not only the original materials, but also any degradation products, must be non-toxic. More information on *in vitro* and *in vivo* tests for biocompatibility of biodegradable materials can be found in Chapters 10 and 11. Biodegradable implants have, to date, been fabricated almost exclusively from specially formulated ceramics and polymers, and therefore these materials are the subject of the remainder of this section.

5.4.1 Biodegradable Ceramics

Biodegradable ceramics are usually a type of calcium phosphate, such as calcium hydroxyapatite (HA, $Ca_{10}(PO_4)_6(OH)_2$), or tricalcium phosphate (TCP, $Ca_3(PO_4)_2$),

[2]"Bioresorption" and "bioabsorption" are other terms commonly found in texts referring to biodegradable materials. These words are not well defined and, in general, can be considered to be synonyms of "biodegradation."

but they can be composed of hydrated calcium sulfate ($CaSO_4 \cdot 2H_2O$) or bioactive glasses. Biodegradable ceramics are often used in orthopedic applications due to their similarity to forms of calcium phosphate found naturally in bone tissue.

5.4.1.1 Erosion Mechanisms

Biodegradable ceramics actually erode under physiological conditions due to a combination of dissolution and physical disintegration. The extent of dissolution depends both on the solubility of the particular formulation in aqueous media and the local pH around the implant. Physical disintegration then occurs after preferential dissolution of the material at the grain boundaries.

5.4.1.2 Factors that Influence Degradation Rate

Because ceramic bioerosion occurs mainly due to interactions with water, the factors that control the erosion rate are similar to those discussed above for polymer hydrolysis and include the following:

1. Chemical susceptibility of the material
2. Amount of crystallinity
3. Amount of media (water) available
4. Material surface area to volume ratio

It has been found that the chemical composition of the ceramic can have a significant impact on the degradation rate, with hydrated forms such as hydrated calcium sulfate eroding faster than their nonhydrated counterparts. In addition, ionic substitutions of CO_3^{2-}, Mg^{2+}, or Sr^{2+} in HA decrease the overall degradation time, while F^- substitutions make this material less susceptible to dissolution.

Because ceramic degradation depends on water penetration, a more tightly packed crystalline material is less susceptible to dissolution than a ceramic that is mainly amorphous. Polycrystalline materials degrade more quickly than ceramics created from a single crystal due to the presence of grain boundaries. For the same reason, a material containing many smaller crystals is more susceptible to dissolution than one with fewer, larger crystals.

Degradation rates are also affected by the total amount of aqueous media available as well as the surface area of the implant. Therefore, highly porous materials will dissolve more quickly than the same ceramic with fewer pores due to the increase in area for interaction with the environment.

In addition to the factors listed above, ceramic bioerosion is encouraged in areas of high mechanical stress, either due to the implant site location or the presence of stress raisers in the device. As discussed in previous sections, dissolution can also be mediated by biological factors such as a pH drop caused by the presence of inflammatory cells.

5.4.2 Biodegradable Polymers

5.4.2.1 Introduction to Biodegradable Polymers and Definitions

A wide variety of biodegradable polymers have been synthesized, although only a few have been approved by the U.S. Food and Drug Administration for use in human applications. These include the common suture materials poly(lactic acid) and poly(glycolic acid), as well as poly(dioxanone) for fracture fixation. In addition, poly(ε-caprolactone) and a type of poly(anhydride) have been used in drug delivery devices. The chemical structure of the repeat unit for each of these polymers is found in Fig. 5.13.

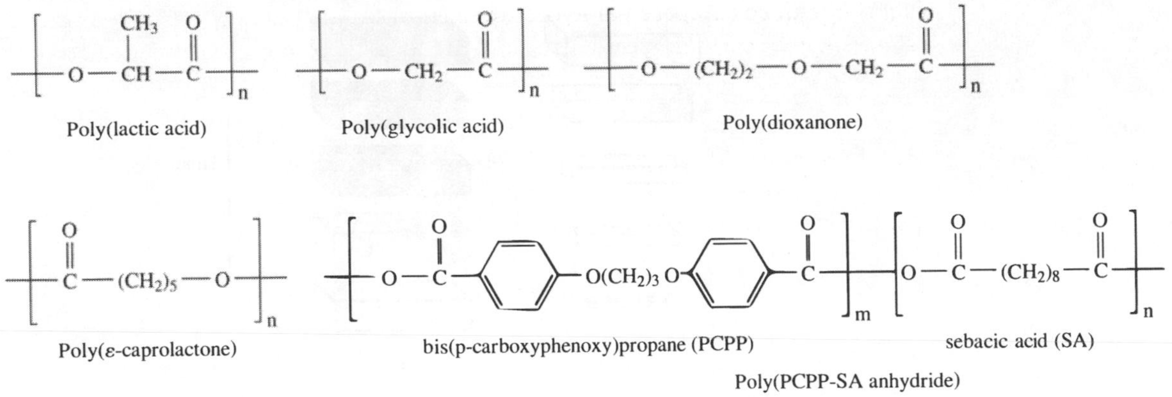

Poly(lactic acid)

Poly(glycolic acid)

Poly(dioxanone)

Poly(ε-caprolactone)

bis(p-carboxyphenoxy)propane (PCPP)

sebacic acid (SA)

Poly(PCPP-SA anhydride)

Figure 5.13
Biodegradable polymers used in medical devices approved by the U.S. Food and Drug Administration for use in human applications. (Adapted with permission from [10].)

Synthetic polymers can be designed to degrade in aqueous environments due to hydrolysis, as explained above, or in response to the actions of specific enzymes. In contrast, naturally derived materials usually undergo enzymatically induced cleavage. Hydrolytic degradation depends solely on the availability of water and is more consistent between patients. Enzyme levels may vary from patient to patient, creating potential problems in predicting material degradation rates for enzyme-responsive substances. However, because active enzymes are usually only found in particular tissues, enzymatically cleavable polymers allow for localized degradation, which may be an important advantage for applications like targeted drug delivery.

For polymers undergoing biodegradation via hydrolysis, two mechanisms can be distinguished: bulk and surface degradation. In **bulk degradation**, the rate of water ingress into the polymer is greater than the rate at which the polymer is converted into its (water-soluble) degradation products. Often, the implant will develop cracks and fissures before complete degradation occurs. Although most polymers degrade in this manner, the tendency of these materials to undergo a rapid decrease in mechanical properties leading to collapse of the implant in many small pieces may limit the potential applications of these polymers, particularly in load-bearing applications.

On the other hand, **surface degradation** occurs when the rate of water penetration into the material is less than the rate of polymer hydrolysis. In this case, the implant will decrease in thickness, but maintain much of its mechanical integrity during the degradation process. Surface-degrading materials represent a smaller subset of synthetic polymers. Of the biodegradable polymers mentioned above, only the poly(anhydrides) degrade via surface erosion. Such materials must possess highly hydrolytically labile bonds as well as hydrophobic moieties to prevent significant water penetration into the interior of the device. A potential disadvantage of surface-eroding polymers is that the continual turnover of the implant surface may make it difficult to establish good integration with the surrounding tissue *in vivo*.

EXAMPLE PROBLEM 5.3

Identify which of the following is representative of bulk polymer degradation and which is representative of polymer surface degradation. Which series of stress-strain curves best represents each of the degradation series shown?

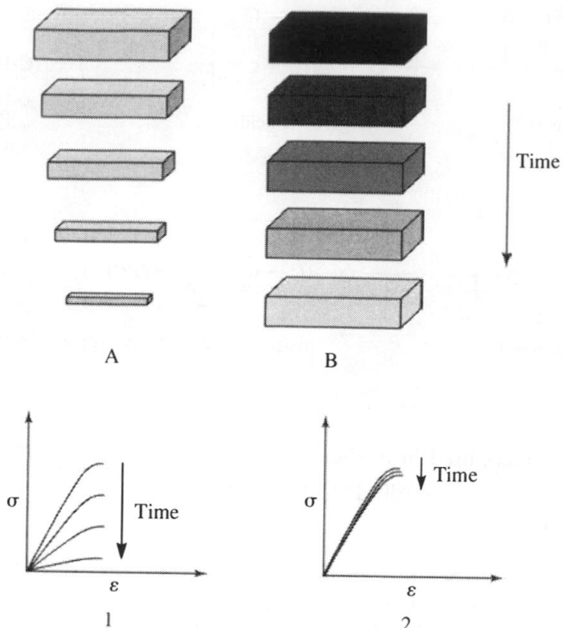

Solution: The series A is representative of surface degradation, as the dimensions of the polymer construct are decreasing with time as the surface of the material degrades. However, the structure of the material remains approximately the same with time; thus, the mechanical properties of the construct should change little with time, as illustrated in the stress-strain curve series 2. The degradation series B, however, represents bulk degradation, as the material maintains approximately the same gross dimensions, while polymer chains in the bulk of the material undergo increasing degradation with time. In this case, the mechanical properties of the bulk material would decrease substantially with time, as illustrated in the stress-strain curve series 1. ■

5.4.2.2 Degradation Mechanisms Three general mechanisms exist for polymer biodegradation, regardless of whether the polymer is degraded via hydrolysis or enzymatic means. This is because the goal of both types of degradation is usually to produce relatively low-molecular weight products that are water-soluble so that they may be cleared by the body's natural processes.

As depicted in Fig. 5.14, degradation can be achieved by breaking bonds in crosslinks between the polymer chains, which are water-soluble (Mechanism I). Alternatively, hydrophobic side chains may be cleaved to reveal hydrophilic groups, thus rendering the overall polymer water soluble (Mechanism II). In Mechanism III, there is attack of the polymer backbone itself, which is degraded into water-soluble monomers. In reality, two or more of these mechanisms often occur simultaneously during polymer biodegradation.

5.4.2.3 Factors that Influence Degradation Rate For enzymatically degradable materials, the rate of bioerosion depends most strongly on the amount of enzyme present at the implant site, as well as the number of cleavable moieties included in the polymer. Other types of polymers degrade via hydrolytic cleavage, so the factors governing degradation rate are the same as those discussed in the previous section on hydrolysis. These include the reactivity of the chemical groups in the polymer, the extent of primary and secondary bonding between chains, the amount of media available, and the surface area of the implant.

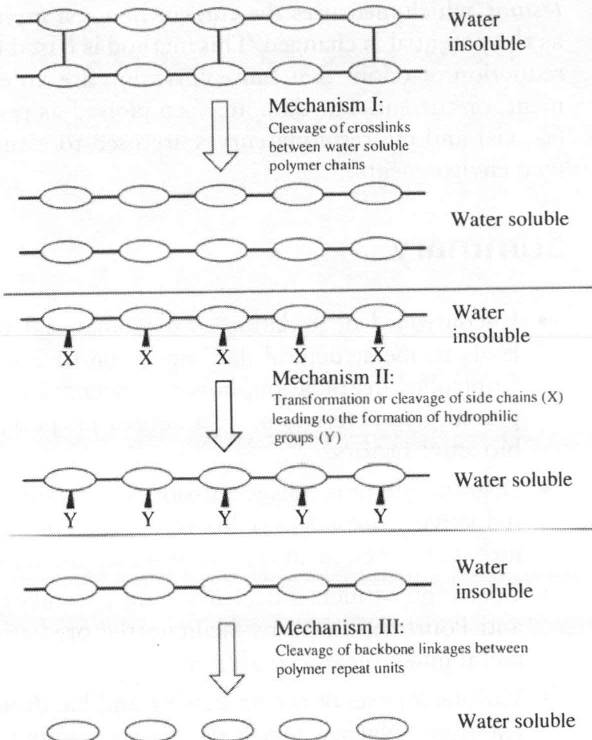

Figure 5.14
Three general mechanisms for polymer biodegradation. (Adapted with permission from [10].)

5.5 Techniques: Assays for Extent of Degradation

Quantification of biomaterial degradation (desired or undesired) can be carried out via either *in vitro* or *in vivo* testing. Often, *in vitro* experiments are first performed on new materials, and, if the degradation rate is acceptable, further *in vivo* assays are then undertaken. For *in vitro* testing, the material is cut to standard dimensions and then placed in vials containing a simulated body fluid with pH and ion content similar to what would be found *in vivo*.

In vivo experiments are more complicated and care must be taken to choose an animal model and an implantation site with characteristics similar to the intended location of final application in humans. This is extremely important, since, as discussed previously, implant-site parameters like pH and mechanical loading can have a large effect on the extent of material degradation during device function. More information on selection of appropriate animal models is found in Chapter 11.

For both *in vitro* and *in vivo* experiments, samples are taken at set time points during the course of the study and are then analyzed for signs of degradation. This includes weighing the sample to determine mass loss and measuring different physical and chemical properties, as well as visual inspection to appreciate changes in properties such as color and the appearance of cracks. Often, the material surface is further characterized using light or electron microscopy, as well as other surface analysis techniques like those described in Chapter 7.

To estimate corrosion of metallic implants *in vitro*, however, measuring changes in weight is often insufficient since the total amount of material lost in this process can be very small. A number of alternative methods for corrosion analysis have been developed (see [11, 12,]). One of the most common techniques involves *electrochemical testing*, which measures the current in a test metal resting in simulated body fluid as the potential is changed. This method is based on the concept that oxidation and reduction reactions that cause corrosion are, in essence, producing electron movement, or current. The data are then plotted as potential (y-axis) vs. current density (x-axis) and the resulting curves are used to estimate corrosion rates in various *in vivo* environments.

Summary

- Uncontrolled degradation of a biomaterial is usually undesirable, as it often leads to the structural decomposition of a material and failure of the device. Controlled degradation, however, occurs in accordance with designed and expected parameters to serve a desired purpose, such as the controlled release of bioactive factors.
- Degradation of metals (corrosion) occurs through the coupling of oxidative and reductive processes in redox reactions. These reactions result in the slow dissolution of the metal at the site at which oxidation occurs (anode).
- Corrosion of metals depends upon a number of factors. The Nernst equation and Pourbaix diagrams facilitate the prediction of the corrosion activity of a metal under certain conditions.
- Various aspects of the processing and handling of a metal can contribute to its corrosion. Narrow cracks or crevices within a metal or between two metal surfaces can lead to crevice corrosion, in which the metal in the crevice acts as an anode. Pitting corrosion occurs by the same process in small flaws or breaks in the passivation layer on the surface of a metal. Intergranular corrosion can occur as a result of the high energy at grain boundaries, which may serve as anodic regions.
- The mechanical environment can also contribute to the corrosion of a metal. The bending of a metal rod or plate will cause the side under tension to be anodic with respect to the side under compression, leading to galvanic corrosion. Small cracks can form and propagate in a metal under tension in a corrosive environment leading to brittle fracture (stress corrosion cracking). The passivating film on a metal implant may become disturbed through cyclic bending, loading or motion and lead to corrosion in the area (fatigue corrosion). Fretting corrosion, however, does not involve loading, but is dependent on the removal of the metal's passivating layer by mechanical means.
- The biological environment of a metal (e.g., presence of proteins, cells, or bacteria) can influence its corrosion rate.
- Ceramics degrade primarily via dissolution and are susceptible to failure via stress-induced degradation. Polymers typically degrade by either swelling/dissolution or chain scission. The chain scission mechanism of degradation can occur through hydrolysis (caused by presence of water) or oxidation (caused by presence of reactive free radical species).
- Biodegradable ceramics generally degrade by dissolution (influenced by the solubility of the ceramic formulation in the media and the pH of the media) coupled with physical disintegration. The rate of degradation of ceramics is controlled by the chemical susceptibility of the material, the degree of crystallinity, the amount of water available and the surface area to volume ratio of the material. Degradation can be additionally influenced by the mechanical environment.

- The degradation of enzymatically degradable polymers depends on the number of enzyme-cleavable groups and the concentration of available enzyme. Degradation of polymers by hydrolysis can be controlled through the reactivity of the chemical groups in the polymer, the extent of primary and secondary bonding between the polymer chains, the amount of available water and the surface area of the material.
- Bulk hydrolytic degradation occurs when the rate of water ingress into the polymer is greater than the rate at which the polymer is converted into its water-soluble degradation products. Surface degradation, however, takes place when the rate of water ingress into the material is less than the rate of polymer hydrolysis.

Problems

5.1 You are examining a hip implant with a stem made of Ti6Al4V and a femoral head made of CoCr.

(a) Select two of the following corrosion mechanisms and describe why/how these could be a problem for this application: galvanic corrosion, crevice corrosion, pitting, stress corrosion, fatigue corrosion.

(b) Of the tests described in Section 5.5, which would you select to examine the potential occurrence of these corrosive events?

5.2 You want to compare the degradation susceptibility of two polymeric materials used in vascular grafts.

Poly(ethylene terephthalate):

$$\left[-O-\overset{O}{\overset{\|}{C}}-C_6H_4-\overset{O}{\overset{\|}{C}}-O-CH_2-CH_2- \right]_n$$

Poly(tetrafluoroethylene):

$$\left(-\underset{F}{\overset{F}{C}}-\underset{F}{\overset{F}{C}}- \right)_n$$

(a) Which of these materials is more susceptible to hydrolytic cleavage (chain scission)? Why?

(b) If these materials were manufactured into a tubular shape and used to replace a section of the vascular system, would degradation be more likely to affect the inner surface or outer surface of the graft?

5.3 You need to determine which degradable material to use as a tissue engineering scaffold for repair of a critical-sized bone defect. (A critical-size defect is one that will not heal unaided.) You are planning to seed the scaffold with cells then implant it into the defect. While the cells proliferate and generate bone, the scaffold will degrade and create void space into which the new tissue may grow. What degradation method would you prefer for this scaffold material and why? (hydrolytic vs. enzymatic degradation, bulk vs. surface degradation)

5.4 You examine the degradation of poly(DL-lactic-co-glycolic acid) foams both *in vitro* and *in vivo* and obtain the following results:

In Vitro		*In Vivo*	
Weeks	Molecular Weight	Weeks	Molecular Weight
0	104300	0	101800
1	82539	1	74070
2	65318	2	53894
3	51690	3	39213
4	40906	4	28532
5	32371	6	15105
6	25617		
8	16043		
10	10047		
12	6292		

What is the molecular weight half-life for each case? Why does this variation occur?

5.5 You have developed two hydrogel systems for controlled release of a therapeutic growth factor (GF). In one system the GF is dispersed throughout a synthetic polymer hydrogel material that degrades by hydrolysis. In the second system, the GF is loaded into gelatin microspheres, which are subsequently dispersed throughout the same synthetic hydrogel material used in the first system (in this case the GF is only loaded into the microspheres). You measure the release *in vitro* of the GF from each system in both (1) phosphate buffered saline (PBS) and (2) PBS containing collagenase (an enzyme that degrades gelatin). The graphs below illustrate the results of the study. What do the results suggest regarding the GF release mechanism from each system?

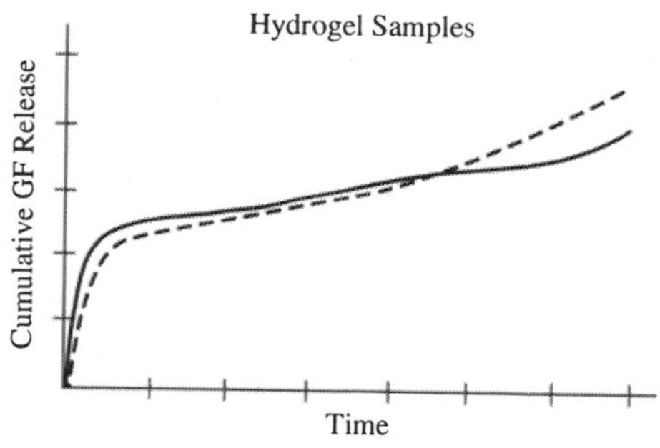

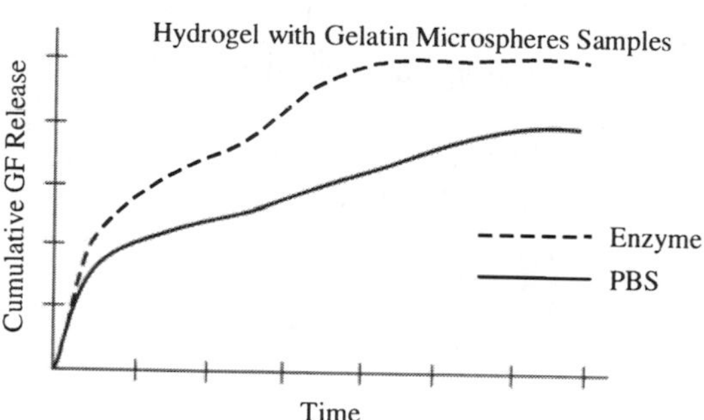

5.6 You are comparing two different processing methods used for forming Ti6Al4V into a femoral hip stem. The following diagram shows the structures that result from the two methods.

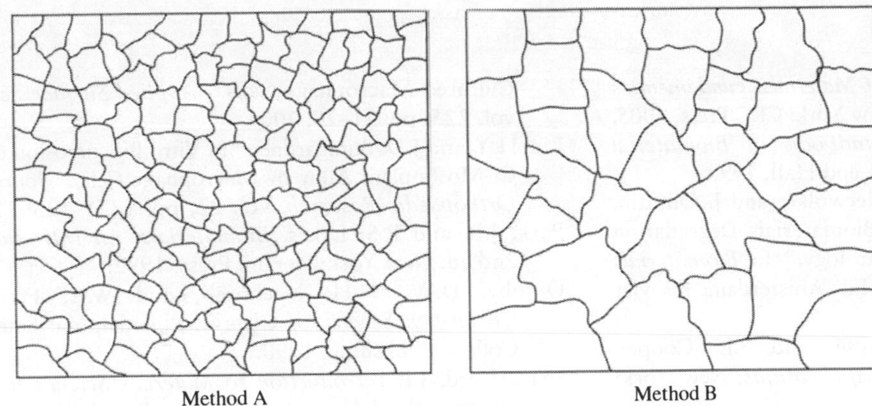

Which of the two processing methods would result in a material that is more susceptible to corrosion? Why?

References

1. Williams, D.F. and R.L. Williams. "Degradative Effects of the Biological Environment on Metals and Ceramics." In *Biomaterials Science: An Introduction to Materials in Medicine*, B.D. Ratner, A.S. Hoffman, F.J. Schoen, and J.E. Lemons, Eds., 2nd ed. San Diego: Elsevier Academic Press, pp. 430–439, 2004.
2. Myers, R. *The Basics of Chemistry*. Westport: Greenwood Press, 2003.
3. Callister, Jr., W.D. *Materials Science and Engineering: An Introduction*, 3rd ed. New York: John Wiley and Sons, 1994.
4. *Metals Handbook*, 8th ed., Vol. 1, "Properties and Selection of Metal", Materials Park, OH: ASM International, 1961.
5. Pourbaix M., "Electrochemical Corrosion of Metallic Biomaterials" *Biomaterials*, vol.5, pp. 122–134, 1984.
6. Angelini, E., A. Caputo, and F. Zucchi. "Degradation Process on Metallic Surfaces." In *Integrated Biomaterials Science*, R. Barbucci, Ed. New York: Kluwer, pp. 297–324, 2002.
7. Fontana, M.G., *Corrosion Engineering*, 3rd ed. New York: McGraw-Hill, 1986.
8. Williams, D.F. and R.L. Williams. "Degradative Effects of the Biological Environment on Metals and Ceramics." In *Biomaterials Science: An Introduction to Materials in Medicine*, B.D. Ratner, A.S. Hoffman, F.J. Schoen, and J.E. Lemons, Eds., 1st ed. San Diego: Elsevier Academic Press, pp. 260–267, 1996.
9. Coury, A.J. "Chemical and Biochemical Degradation of Polymers." In *Biomaterials Science: An Introduction to Materials in Medicine*, B.D. Ratner, A.S. Hoffman, F.J. Schoen, and J.E. Lemons, Eds., 2nd ed. San Diego: Elsevier Academic Press, pp. 411–430, 2004.
10. Kohn, J., S. Abramson, and R. Langer. "Bioresorbable and Bioerodible Materials." In *Biomaterials Science: An Introduction to Materials in Medicine*, B.D. Ratner, A.S. Hoffman, F.J. Schoen, and J.E. Lemons, Eds., 2nd ed. San Diego: Elsevier Academic Press, pp. 115–127, 2004.
11. Bundy, K.J. "Corrosion and Other Electrochemical Aspects of Biomaterials." *Critical Reviews in Biomedical Engineering*, vol. 22, pp. 139–251, 1994.
12. Lemons, J.E., R. Venugopalan, and L.C. Lucs. "Corrosion and Biodegradation." In *Handbook of Biomaterials Evaluation*, A. von Recum, Ed., 2nd ed: Taylor Francis Inc., pp. 155–170, 1999.

Additional Reading

Black, J. *Biological Performance of Materials: Fundamentals of Biocompatibility*, 4th ed. New York: CRC Press, 2005.

Black, J. and G. Hastings. *Handbook of Biomaterial Properties*. London: Chapman and Hall, 1998.

Burny, F., Y. Andrianne, M. Donkerwolke, and J. Quintin. "Clinical Manifestations of Biomaterials Degradation in Orthopaedics and Traumatology." In *Biomaterials Degradation*, M.A. Barbosa, Ed. Amsterdam: Elsevier Science, pp. 291–326, 1991.

Lamba, N.M.K., K.A. Woodhouse, and S.L. Cooper. *Polyurethanes in Biomedical Applications*. New York: CRC Press, 1998.

Lin, H.Y. and J.D. Bumgardner. "Changes in Surface Composition of the Ti–6Al–4V Implant Alloy by Cultured Macrophage Cells." *Applied Surface Science*, vol. 225, pp. 21–28, 2004.

Lin, H.Y. and J.D. Bumgardner. "In Vitro Biocorrosion of Co-Cr-Mo Implant Alloy by Macrophage Cells." *Journal of Orthopaedic Research*, vol. 22, pp. 1231–1236, 2004.

Park, J.B. and R.S. Lakes. *Biomaterials: An Introduction*, 2nd ed. New York: Plenum Press, 1992.

Oxtoby, D.W., N.H. Nachtrieb, and W.A. Freeman. *Chemistry: Science of Change*. Philadelphia: Saunders College Publishing, 1990.

Shackelford, J.F. *Introduction to Materials Science for Engineers*, 6th ed. Upper Saddle River: Prentice Hall, 2004.

Biomaterial Processing

CHAPTER 6

Main Objective

To understand the need and techniques for processing to improve strength, form desired shapes, and sterilize all classes of biomaterials.

Specific Objectives

1. To understand the molecular mechanisms behind strengthening techniques for metals and polymers.
2. To understand how thermal processing affects microstructure and bulk properties of metals and polymers.
3. To compare and contrast types of forming techniques for metals, ceramics and polymers.
4. To understand the need for, killing mechanisms of, and limitations of various sterilization techniques.

6.1 Introduction: Importance of Biomaterials Processing

In previous chapters, chemical principles underlying both the creation and degradation of metallic, ceramic, and polymeric biomaterials were explained. This chapter concentrates on the practical processes relating to the formation of these materials into shapes, and how these processes affect their chemical compositions.

Processing of biomaterials is usually undertaken to change the bulk or surface properties of the material, obtain a desired shape, or sterilize or otherwise improve the biocompatibility of the material. This chapter will describe mechanisms for altering bulk properties and then discuss shaping techniques and processing for biocompatibility. Methods for altering surface properties of biomaterials are the subject of the following chapter.

6.2 Processing to Improve Bulk Properties

Most often, the bulk property targeted in material processing is mechanical strength. A number of methods for improving the strength of various classes of

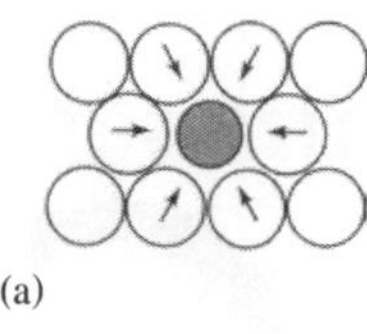
(a)

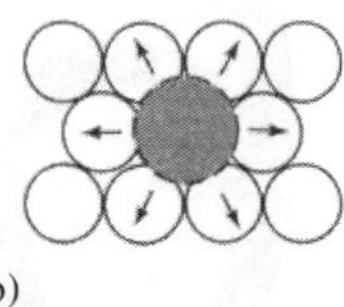
(b)

Figure 6.1
Localized lattice strain caused by alloying. (a) If the impurity atom is smaller than those in the base metal, a tensile strain will be created on the surrounding environment. (b) Conversely, a substitute atom that is larger than the host atoms will cause localized compressive strains. (Adapted with permission from [1].)

biomaterials have been developed. As mentioned in Chapter 4, in order to create stronger or harder materials, dislocation motion should be reduced so that more energy is needed before plastic deformation can occur. Methods to prevent dislocation movement, as well as the reasons they are effective, are outlined in the following paragraphs.

6.2.1 Metals

Processing is a very efficient means to affect mechanical properties in metals. In these materials, defects can be added to the crystal structure to prevent dislocation motion. These can be in the form of point, line, planar or volume defects and are introduced via the mechanisms described below. A summary of how different processes detailed here and in section 6.3 affect the strength of metals is found in Table 6.1.

6.2.1.1 Alloying In addition to having greater corrosion resistance, alloys are almost always stronger than pure metals. This is because alloys are a type of solid solution, and thus, alloying is like adding many substitutional point defects to the base metal. These point defects cause localized lattice strain, as seen in Fig. 6.1. If the impurity atom is smaller than those in the base metal, a tensile strain will be created locally [see Fig. 6.1(a)]. Similarly, a substitute atom that is larger than the host atoms will cause localized compressive strain [Fig. 6.1(b)].

At the same time, there is crystal distortion around a dislocation, of either a tensile or compressive nature, depending on which side of the dislocation the atoms are located. Therefore, as depicted in Fig. 6.2, impurity atoms can cluster around the area of a dislocation to help cancel the lattice strains imposed by both of these phenomena. For example, it would be more stable for large atoms to lie on the "tensile side" of an edge dislocation where the atoms are already slightly farther apart due to the presence of the dislocation. If the dislocation is moved away from the impurity, the overall lattice strain in the system would increase. This must be overcome by increasing the shear stress required to cause dislocation movement, thus strengthening the material.

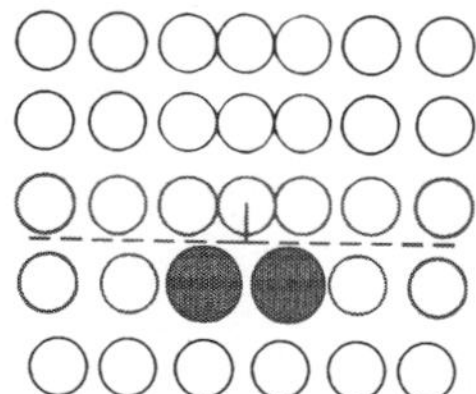
(a)

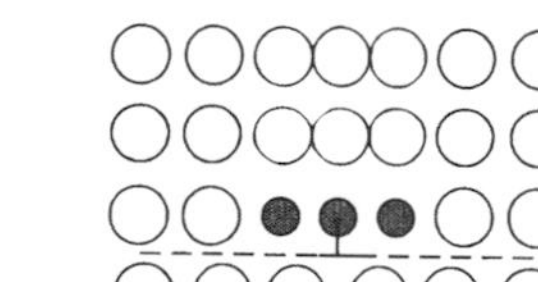
(b)

Figure 6.2
Crystal distortion around a dislocation. Any impurity atoms will cluster around the area of a dislocation to help cancel the lattice strains. (a) Larger atoms will cluster on the tensile side of a dislocation, whereas (b) smaller atoms will cluster on the compressive side. (Adapted with permission from [1].)

EXAMPLE PROBLEM 6.1

316L stainless steel is an alloy containing about 70% iron with 30% other metals, usually chromium and nickel. Consider an alloy of about 70% iron, 18% chromium, and 12% nickel.

(a) Would the alloy be mechanically weaker or stronger than pure iron? Why?
(b) Given that the atomic radius of an iron atom is 1.24Å, the radius of a chromium atom is 1.25Å, and the radius of a nickel atom is 1.25Å, will the chromium and nickel atoms in the lattice cause localized tensile or compressive strain? Why?
(c) Name the type of defect created by the addition of copper atoms.

TABLE 6.1

Processing Methods and their Effect on the Properties of Metals

Strengthens	Weakens
Alloying	Annealing
Cold working	Hot working
Precipitation hardening	Porosity (due to casting and powder processing)

(Adapted with permission from [2].)

Solution:

(a) The alloy would be mechanically stronger than the pure iron, as the other atoms serve as point defects in the lattice, introducing lattice strains and increasing the energy needed for dislocation motion.
(b) As the chromium and nickel (impurity) radii are slightly larger than that of the iron, the presence of the impurity atoms in the material will cause localized compressive strain.
(c) The impurity atoms serve as substitutional point defects. ■

6.2.1.2 Strain Hardening Just as adding point defects improves the strength of a metal, additional line defects also create a stronger material. The phenomenon in which a metal becomes stronger as it is plastically deformed is known as **strain hardening**, and is due to an increase in the number of dislocations (line defects) during this process. As mentioned above, there is lattice strain associated with each dislocation, and it requires more energy to move the stress field of a dislocation through the combined localized strains resulting from other dislocations. Because during plastic deformation there is a continual increase in the number of dislocations, it is logical that higher and higher forces will be required to continue deformation.

Strain hardening is also called **cold working** since it is carried out at low temperatures relative to the melting point of metals. Although this process improves the strength of the material, there is a concomitant reduction in ductility. If the ductility of the cold-worked metal is not sufficient for the intended application, the effects of strain hardening can be reduced by annealing procedures (discussed below).

6.2.1.3 Grain Size Refinement Most commonly used metals are polycrystalline, consisting of grains with different orientations sharing a common boundary. In order for plastic deformation to occur, dislocations must cross between grains. However, if the orientations of the neighboring grains are not the same, the direction of dislocation motion must be altered at the grain boundary. This becomes more difficult with increasing misalignment between grains. Additionally, this mismatch will result in a discontinuity of slip planes between grains, further discouraging dislocation motion.

For these reasons, a material with many smaller grains is usually stronger than the same material with larger grains. In essence, planar defects have been added to the smaller-grained material in the form of grain boundaries. Grain size can be affected by thermal processing, as described in the following section. However, as discussed above, not only the size, but also the relative orientations of the grains are important to the overall mechanical properties of the material, since small angle grain boundaries are not as effective in preventing dislocation motion as larger-angle boundaries.

6.2.1.4 Annealing Cold working improves the strength of metals, but decreases material ductility and can negatively affect corrosion resistance. Therefore, heat treatment may be employed to recover some of these properties. **Annealing** is a form of heat treatment in which the material is exposed to high temperatures for relatively long periods of time in order to increase the ductility or toughness of the material, reduce internal stresses (these often promote corrosive attack, see Chapter 5), or produce a specific grain structure.

Although there are a number of means by which heat treatment affects grain size, one of the most important is that, due to the excess energy associated with the grain boundary, reduction in the total amount of these boundaries is favored thermodynamically. Thus, at high temperatures where atomic diffusion is encouraged, larger grains will spontaneously grow while the smaller ones shrink, leading to an overall increase in the size of the grains and concomitant decrease in area of the grain boundaries.

Annealing occurs in three distinct stages: heating to the required temperature, maintaining or "soaking" the material at that temperature, and controlled cooling (**quenching**). Parameters that affect the product resulting from the annealing process include the material composition and the quenching rate. The quenching rate actually refers to the rate of heat extraction from the material, which is important because the outside of the specimen will always cool more quickly than the inside. This leads to the formation of a temperature gradient that can affect the final grain structure and thus the overall properties of the metal.

Heat extraction depends on the media in which the material is quenched—water causes a faster cooling rate than oil, which is faster than air. Movement of the quenching media over the surface also increases heat extraction and causes a more rapid quench. Similarly, because cooling occurs primarily at the surface, pieces with a higher surface area to volume ratio will experience faster quenching.

EXAMPLE PROBLEM 6.2

Imagine a material scientist (in this case a blacksmith) in late Medieval Europe trying to fashion a metallic hip implant. The blacksmith was able to cast a femoral stem-shaped implant from steel, but has hypothesized that the mechanical properties are not sufficient for use in a hip application. After some thought, the blacksmith grips the implant with tongs, submerges it among blazing hot coals for several minutes, then removes it and strikes it repeatedly with a hammer against an anvil. When the red glow of the implant begins to dim, the smithy replaces it in the coals and repeats the hammering process for several cycles.

(a) Will the cycles of hammering the hot implant increase the mechanical strength of the implant? Why or why not?
(b) If the strength of the implant increases with the hammering cycles, would the ductility of the material potentially be affected? Why or why not?
(c) Name the processing technique that the blacksmith has employed.
(d) The smithy thinks that the material has become too strong and brittle after his hammering cycles. He has decided to place the implant in hot coals overnight then remove it to cool in the air in the morning. Could this process increase the ductility of the implant? How?
(e) After heating the implant in coals overnight, the blacksmith realizes that he has several options for cooling the glowing hot implant. He can (1) submerge it in a bucket of water from the stream behind his shack, (2) submerge it in the flowing stream behind his shack, (3) submerge it in a bucket of oil, or (4) stick with the original plan of letting it cool in the air. Rank the methods of cooling the implant in order from the slowest to the quickest.

Solution:

(a) The cycles of hammering the hot implant will increase the strength of the implant through introduction of line defects into the crystal structure of the metal. As the number of dislocations increases with increasing hammering, they begin to interact on an increased basis. The increased number of dislocations and the lattice strains that they create result in an increase in the energy or force required to deform the material plastically. Thus, the material becomes stronger through the introduction and interaction of dislocations.
(b) The increase in strength introduced through the hammering cycles comes at the potential cost of a loss in ductility. As more energy is required to plastically deform the metal, the metal does not yield as easily with applied forces, making it less ductile.
(c) The smithy employed the process of strain hardening or cold working. Interestingly, the term "smithy" (one who works in metal) is derived from the word "smite" (to hit or strike).
(d) The proposed process of heating the implant to a high temperature below the melting point of the metal for an extended time, then cooling it could increase the ductility of the implant

through reducing some of the internal stresses in the metal. The energy associated with the high temperature facilitates the diffusion of atoms in the lattice to form larger grains (decrease in the area of the grain boundaries). The decrease in grain boundaries increases the ductility of the material by lowering the energy required to plastically deform the implant.

(e) Cooling in air < cooling in bucket of oil < cooling in bucket of water < cooling in running stream of water. ■

6.2.1.5 Precipitation Hardening In the previous sections, means to insert point, linear and planar defects into metals to reduce dislocation motion have been reviewed. In the same vein, volume defects may be added to a material via **precipitation hardening.** Here, precipitates are included within the host crystal, which causes local lattice strains. These strains then provide a barrier to dislocation motion in the area, thereby strengthening the material.

6.2.2 Ceramics

Due to the nature of the ionic bonds involved, dislocation motion in ceramics is difficult, and therefore there is little use for techniques to further reduce dislocation movement. On the contrary, a large problem in ceramics processing is how to increase the number of slip systems to improve ductility of this class of materials. Descriptions of these techniques are beyond the scope of this text.

6.2.3 Polymers

As with ionic materials, dislocation motion is difficult in covalent crystals, but many polymers are semicrystalline, so it is possible to improve the strength of polymeric materials by increasing their percent crystallinity. One way to achieve this is through thermal processing methods. If the polymer is cooled slowly after being heated, this will allow time for the chains to become more fully aligned, thus increasing the crystallinity of the material. This increase in crystallinity is described by the Avrami equation discussed in Chapter 3 (equation 3.3).

Another means to improve the strength of polymers is to use pre-drawing procedures, which are analogous to strain hardening in metals. As mentioned in Chapter 4, polymer chains become aligned in response to deformation, such as in the necked region of a sample undergoing tensile testing. If such a method is applied to a material during or after fabrication (such as may occur with polymer fibers, see below), this can increase the overall strength along the axis of loading.

The strength and hardness of polymeric materials can also be augmented with additional crosslinking, which reduces the ability of chains to slide past each other. This can be accomplished by exposing the polymer to either chemical initiators or high-energy radiation after it has been formed into the desired geometry.

EXAMPLE PROBLEM 6.3

A graduate student finished a six-pack of soda and decided to pull on the polymer rings that formerly held the cans together. The student placed the index and middle finger of each hand through opposite sides of one of the rings and moved her hands outward in opposite directions, stretching the polymer ring. The student found that pulling the ring required a lot of force initially, then less force, and finally a great deal more force just before the ring broke. Draw a generalized stress-strain curve that could be used to describe the mechanical behavior of the polymer ring (no numerical values needed). Explain the observed behavior on a molecular level. How did the tensile force likely affect the crystallinity of the polymer in the area of greatest stress?

Solution: The polymer sample underwent necking during the tensile testing by hand. A general stress-strain curve for what was described is as follows:

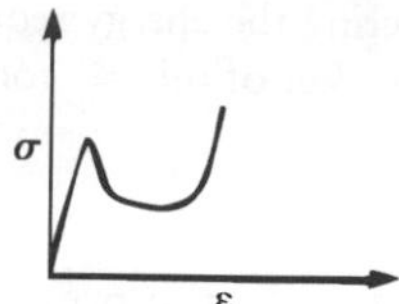

It can be assumed that the polymer is a semicrystalline material. As the polymer is initially pulled with tensile force, the polymer chains (lamellae and tie molecules) begin to align along the axis of the applied force. This process of chain alignment along the axis of force is represented in the initial slope of the curve. The next region of the curve illustrating great increases in strain with little stress represents blocks of crystalline phases separating from each other and aligning along the axis of force. Once the polymer chains are aligned and extended, more force is needed for further strains to disrupt primary interactions in the polymer backbone, leading to breakage of the soda can ring. The alignment of the polymer chains along the axis of force in the area of greatest stress resulted in an increased percent crystallinity of the polymer in that region. ■

6.3 Processing to Form Desired Shapes

Although strengthening mechanisms that involve the reduction of plastic deformation can be very useful to improve the final properties of biomaterials, it should be noted that plastic deformation is crucial to the utility of many materials because it allows for fabrication of complex shapes. Processing methods to produce implants with desired geometries include forming, casting, powder processing, machining, and joining operations. In addition, the past decade has brought significant development of rapid manufacturing (also called rapid prototyping) technologies. Examples of these techniques as applied to processing of each class of biomaterials are discussed in the following sections.

6.4 Processing of Metals

6.4.1 Forming Metals

Forming operations are those in which the shape of a metal is altered via plastic deformation. Forging, rolling, extrusion, and drawing are all common forming techniques. If these processes are conducted at temperatures at or above about $0.3T_m$ (the recrystallization temperature), this is termed **hot working**. If the deformation occurs at a lower temperature, this is cold working, which was discussed previously. The advantages of hot working are that large deformations are possible and the energy required for these deformations is less than would be needed in cold working. However, during this process, materials often undergo surface oxidation, which results in a poor finish.

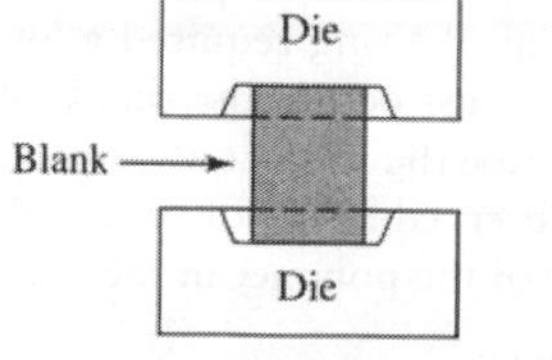

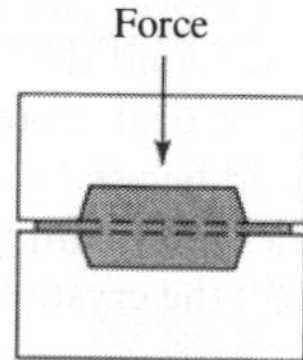

Figure 6.3
Diagram of closed-die forging process. In this manufacturing technique, a force is exerted on two die halves, which causes the deformation of the stock material (blank) into the desired shape. (Adapted with permission from [1].)

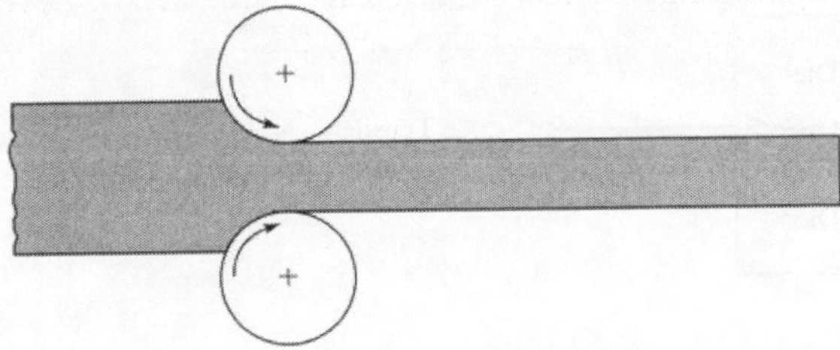

Figure 6.4
Schematic of rolling process. Here, the metal is placed between two rollers that exert compressive forces on the material and cause a reduction in thickness as the material is fed through the rollers. This process can be performed at room temperature or higher. (Adapted with permission from [1].)

In contrast, cold-worked metals are stronger and have a more appealing surface finish. Additionally, there is better control of the dimensions of the final product if the forming procedure is carried out at lower temperatures. Disadvantages of cold working include that smaller amounts of deformation may be possible than in hot working and that materials often experience a decrease in ductility and corrosion resistance after undergoing this process.

6.4.1.1 Forging Metals **Forging** has been used for centuries by blacksmiths in order to create items such as tools, horseshoes, and jewelry. A common type of modern forging, closed-die forging, is depicted in Fig. 6.3. In this procedure, a force is exerted on the two die halves so that the stock metal is deformed and takes the shape of the cavity between them. This method is one of those commonly used for forming orthopedic implants from a variety of metals, including titanium and stainless steel.

6.4.1.2 Rolling Metals As the name implies, **rolling** involves moving a metal between two rollers, which exert compressive forces on the material and cause a reduction in thickness. An illustration of this process can be found in Fig. 6.4. Rolling is employed to form stock shapes (bars, rods, etc.) for further processing to create orthopedic and dental implants.

6.4.1.3 Extrusion of Metals As shown in Fig. 6.5, in **extrusion**, the stock metal is pushed through a die containing an orifice via forces generated by the ram. The final piece that emerges has the required shape and a smaller cross-sectional area than the stock. This technique can be used to form wires, such as those utilized in orthodontics.

6.4.1.4 Drawing Metals **Drawing** is similar to extrusion, but rather than pushing on the entrance side, the metal is pulled from the exit side through a die having a tapered

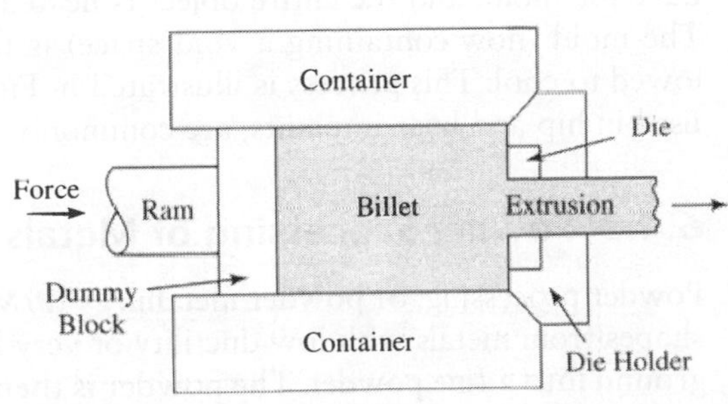

Figure 6.5
Schematic of extrusion process. The stock metal is pushed (via the forces generated by a ram) through a die containing an orifice of the desired shape. Altering the die can allow the piece that emerges to have a variety of cross-sectional shapes. (Adapted with permission from [1].)

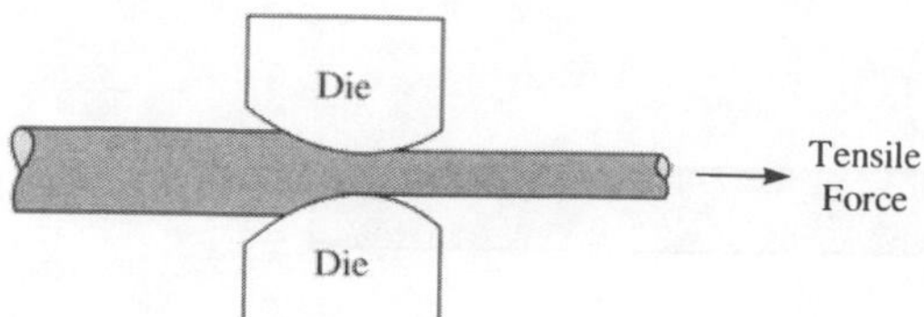

Figure 6.6
Schematic of drawing process. This is similar to extrusion, except that the stock material is pulled through the die, not pushed through. (Adapted with permission from [1].)

orifice (see Fig. 6.6). The result is a product with a smaller cross-sectional area and greater length than the original. Drawing devices can be used in series to obtain final pieces with a variety of dimensions. Metal wire and tubing are often manufactured in this manner. Drawing is also used to form stock shapes for orthopedic and dental applications.

As mentioned in Chapter 3, after extrusion or drawing, fine metal fibers may be fabricated into three-dimensional meshes, which have been explored recently as substrate materials for tissue engineering applications. Although a variety of techniques exist for mesh formation, often non-woven meshes are created from metals. In this case, the fibers are aligned and then bonded together in a specific structure using thermal or mechanical means (e.g. sintering/pressing techniques described below). However, it must be kept in mind that metal meshes have limited use in the tissue engineering field because they are not intrinsically biodegradable.

6.4.2 Casting Metals

Casting is another means of forming complex shapes from metallic materials. In this procedure, molten metal is poured into a mold and cooled. When it solidifies, it retains the shape of the mold, although some shrinkage occurs. The advantage of this fabrication technique is that complicated shapes can be easily created, even with less ductile metals than those that are commonly used in forming. In addition, it is relatively inexpensive. However, internal defects (such as pores) and less desirable grain structures are found more often in cast products than in pieces produced by other methods. Two of the many types of casting, sand and investment casting, are described below.

6.4.2.1 Sand Casting of Metals One of the most simple and commonly used casting methods is **sand casting.** In this procedure, sand is packed around an object that has the shape of the intended piece (the pattern) to make a two-piece mold. The pattern is then removed and the molten metal is poured into the mold. After cooling, the mold is removed, as shown in Fig. 6.7.

6.4.2.2 Investment Casting of Metals **Investment**, or lost-wax, **casting,** is similar to sand casting, but, here, the pattern is created from a wax or polymer with a low melting point. The pattern is encased in a slurry (usually plaster of Paris) to produce the mold, and the entire object is heated to melt and/or burn out the pattern. The mold (now containing a void space) is then filled with molten metal and allowed to cool. This process is illustrated in Fig. 6.8. Cobalt-chromium alloys, often used in hip and knee implants, are commonly investment cast.

6.4.3 Powder Processing of Metals

Powder processing, or **powder metallurgy (P/M)**, techniques are often used to create shapes from metals with low ductility or very high melting points. First the metal is ground into a fine powder. The powder is then placed in a mold and compressed to

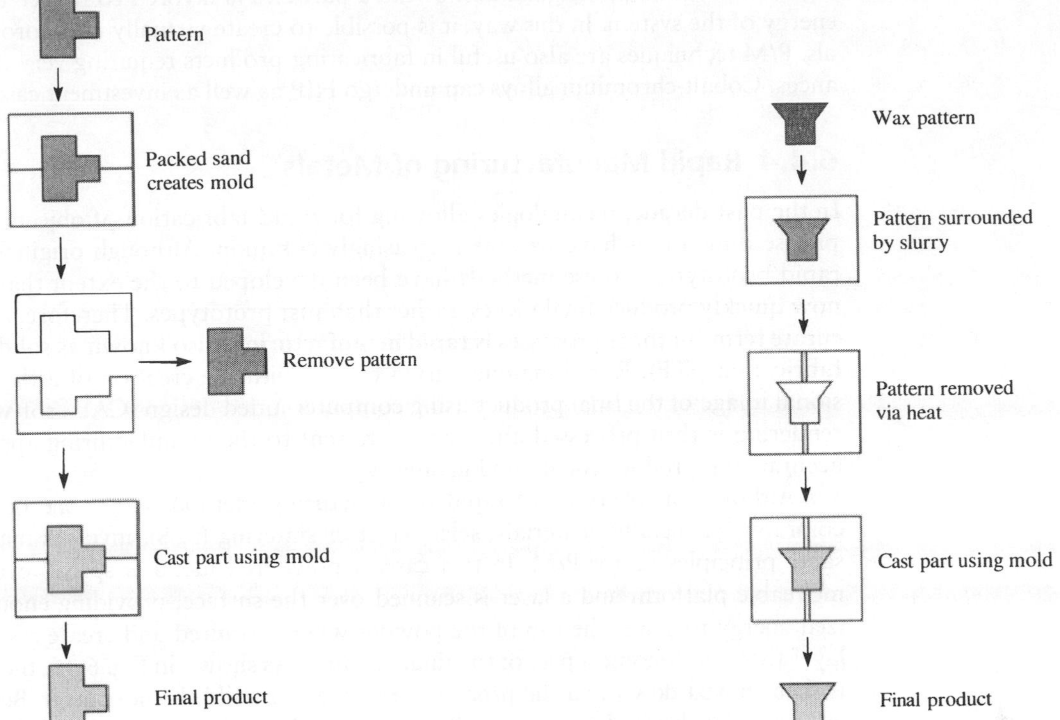

Figure 6.7
Diagram of sand casting process. First, sand is packed around an object that has the shape of the intended piece (the pattern) to make a two-piece mold. The pattern is removed and the molten metal is poured into the mold. After cooling, the mold is separated, resulting in the final product.

Figure 6.8
Diagram of investment casting process. A pattern is first created from a wax or polymer with a low melting point. The pattern is encased in a slurry to produce the mold, and the entire object is heated to melt and/or burn out the pattern. The empty mold is then filled with molten metal and allowed to cool, resulting in the final piece when the mold is separated.

create a denser material with good particle-to-particle contact. After this stage, the piece is termed a green compact.

The green compact then usually undergoes further compaction at elevated temperatures, known as **hot isostatic pressing (HIP)**. Pressures of up to 100 MPa and temperatures up to 1100°C are typically used for this process. During HIP, the metal powder is **sintered**, or densified by removal of small voids between particles, as shown in Fig. 6.9. The driving force for sintering is the high energy associated with the many surfaces present due to the small size of the metal particles. Therefore, at

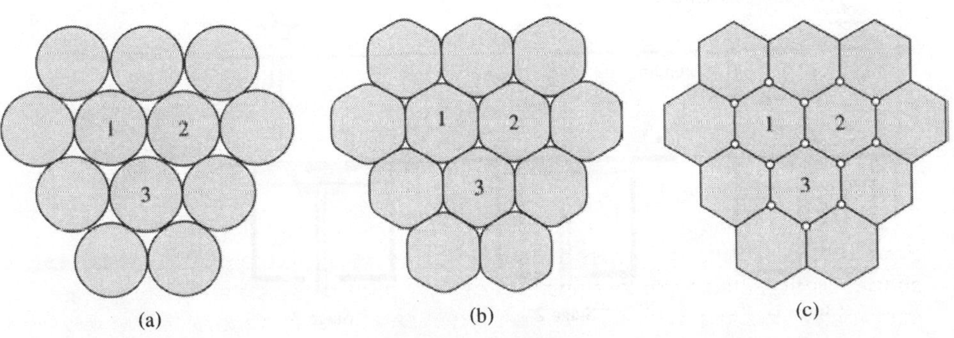

Figure 6.9
Diagram of sintering process used in powder metallurgy. The green compact (a) is compressed and heated (b) until the small pores between the particles have been removed (c). (Adapted with permission from [3].)

high temperatures, amalgamation of these particles is favored to reduce the overall energy of the system. In this way, it is possible to create virtually non-porous materials. P/M techniques are also useful in fabricating products requiring very close tolerances. Cobalt-chromium alloys can undergo HIP as well as investment casing.

6.4.4 Rapid Manufacturing of Metals

In the past decade, technologies allowing for rapid fabrication of objects with very precise dimensions have become increasingly common. Although originally named rapid prototyping, these methods have been developed to the extent that they can now quickly produce final pieces, rather than just prototypes. Therefore, a more accurate term for these processes is **rapid manufacturing,** also known as **solid freeform fabrication (SFF).** Rapid manufacturing begins with the creation of a three-dimensional image of the final product using computer-aided design (CAD) software. This rendering is then processed and signals are sent to the manufacturing apparatus to accurately reproduce the desired geometry.

Although many types of rapid manufacturing methods exist, one of the most common for metallic materials, **selective laser sintering** (SLS), involves many of the same principles as for P/M. In this case, a powdered metal is spread evenly on a moveable platform and a laser is scanned over the surface, providing enough localized energy to sinter the top of the powder where required and create a small solid layer that will become a part of the final product. As shown in Fig. 6.10, the platform is then moved down and the process is repeated to build the next layer. Because the laser can be directed at very small areas, complicated geometries including fibers, channels or interconnected pores can be produced during the fabrication process.

6.4.5 Welding Metals

Welding is a process used to join two materials together. During welding, the contact location of the metals are heated to their melting point, a metallic filler is added, and the connection is allowed to cool, resulting in a solid bridge of metal between the two materials. Welding is a technique that is used after the above mentioned manufacturing techniques to allow for the formation of more complex shapes.

6.4.6 Machining of Metals

During machining, a cutting implement (such as a blade rotated at high speeds or a laser) is used to remove material from a stock piece, resulting in shapes that are too complex or costly to construct using one of the aforementioned techniques.

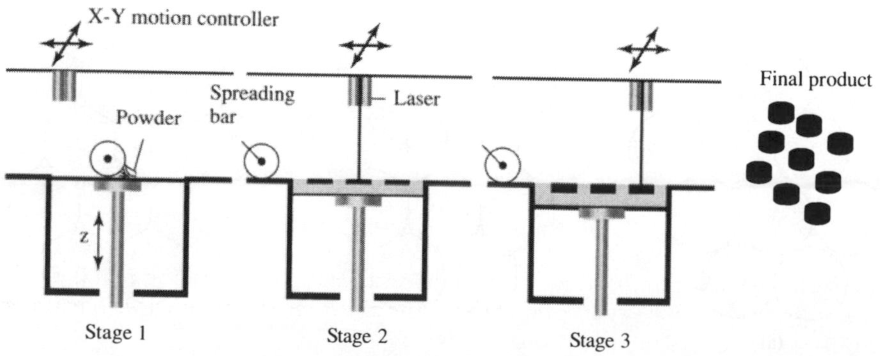

X-Y motion controller
Spreading bar
Laser
Powder
Final product
z
Stage 1
Stage 2
Stage 3

Figure 6.10
Diagram of selective laser sintering (SLS) process. In stage 1, a powdered metal is spread evenly on a moveable platform and, in stage 2, a laser is scanned over the surface, providing enough localized energy to sinter the top of the powder where required and create a small solid layer that will become part of the final product. The platform is then moved down and the process is repeated to build the next layer (Stage 3). In this way, products with complex shapes can be created. (Adapted with permission from [4].)

Machining is commonly performed on metals and polymers (ceramics are generally too brittle) as a second step after one of the other manufacturing techniques.

6.5 Processing of Ceramics

There are several types of ceramic biomaterials, including glasses, crystalline ceramics and glass-ceramics. Each has different processing methods as well as distinct final properties. Although many variants exist, the most common procedures for creating specific shapes from each type of ceramic are discussed below. Layering of ceramics on top of preshaped materials is also possible through plasma spray coating techniques, which are discussed in Chapter 7.

6.5.1 Glass Forming Techniques

Because glasses are completely amorphous (no grains present), heat treatment is required to form them into shapes, but it does not significantly affect their mechanical properties. The **softening point** for a glass is arbitrarily defined as the temperature when its viscosity is 4×10^7 P. This is the maximum temperature at which the piece can be handled without significant changes in shape. At higher temperatures, such as the **working point** (the temperature when its viscosity is 10^4 P), the glass is easily deformed. Therefore, the glass is usually shaped between these two temperatures.

In this temperature range, the glass may be formed via several methods, including pressing, blowing, and drawing. **Pressing** is similar to forging for metals and involves applying an even pressure to a softened glass placed in a heated mold. Upon cooling, the glass will retain the shape of the mold. In modern commercial glass **blowing** operations, pressing techniques are first used to form the stock glass into a shape generally similar to the final product, called a **parison** (see Fig. 6.11). The parison is then placed into a more detailed mold (a finishing mold) and a jet of air forces the soft glass to conform to the shape of the mold.

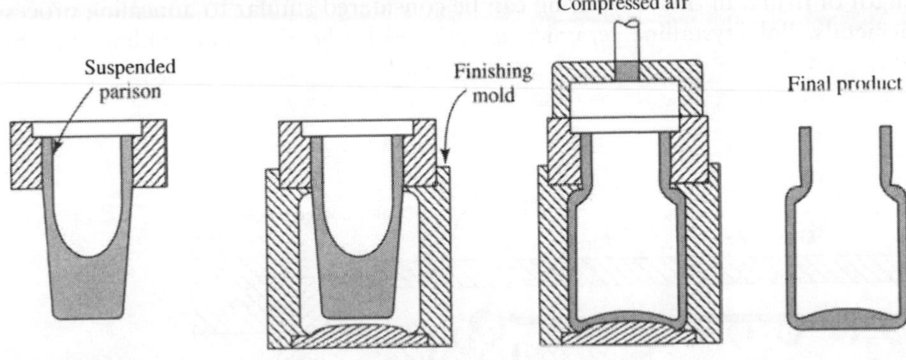

Figure 6.11
In modern commercial glass blowing operations, pressing techniques are first used to form the stock glass into a shape called a parison, which is of similar shape to the final product. The parison is then placed into a more detailed mold (finishing mold) and a jet of air forces the soft glass to conform to the shape of the mold. (Adapted with permission from [5].)

Drawing processes in glasses are analogous to those for metals. Here, molten glass can be pulled over rollers to form long pieces such as sheets or tubing (see Fig. 6.12). Alternatively, the glass may be drawn though small orifices at the bottom of a heating tank to form fibers. As discussed above for metals, it is possible to use glass fibers to form three-dimensional scaffolds for tissue engineering applications, but glass-based scaffolds have not been widely explored due to their lack of biodegradability. (However, certain bioactive glasses have been used to improve bone bonding in orthopedics; see Chapter 7.)

6.5.2 Casting and Firing of Ceramics

6.5.2.1 Casting Ceramics As with metals, *casting* can also be used for ceramics to produce specific geometries. This method is preferred for work with crystalline ceramic materials and glass-ceramics rather than with amorphous glasses. After the formation of a relatively non-porous mold via a variety of means, small ceramic particles are mixed with water and an organic binder material and then are poured/pressed into the mold.

After molding, the piece is left to dry and, as the water evaporates, the ceramic shrinks away from the walls of the mold, which aids in mold removal. At this point, the cast object is considered green ware because it still contains water and binding agents, and is more porous (and thus weaker) than the final piece. Further drying will remove additional water; however, this process must be monitored because if the surface of the object dries more quickly than the internal portions, shrinkage and cracking can result.

6.5.2.2 Firing Ceramics Once dried, the cast piece is then fired, or exposed to temperatures between 900–1400°C. This is done to burn out the binding agent, as well as increase the density and mechanical properties of the final object. As mentioned in Chapter 3, porous ceramic materials may be created during this process by including a second ceramic type that is burnt out at a lower temperature than that at which densification occurs, leaving voids within the sample. Casting and firing is the most common way to make ceramic implants for both orthopedic and dental applications.

Different classes of ceramics may be formed depending on the temperature and length of firing. In this way, firing can be considered similar to annealing processes in metals. Polycrystalline ceramics are created by heating and holding the object

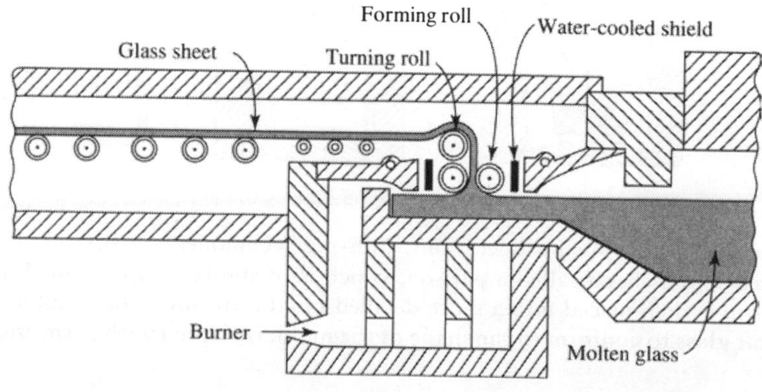

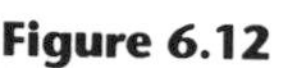
Figure 6.12
The drawing processes in glasses are analogous to those for metals. Here, molten glass is pulled over a series of rollers to form long pieces such as sheets or tubing. (Adapted with permission from W.D. Kingery, *Introduction to Ceramics,* 2nd ed. as appears in [1].)

above the melting temperature of the ceramic, followed by rather rapid cooling. This allows time for crystal growth, but produces large-grained materials that are not often used commercially due to their inferior mechanical properties.

Vitrified materials are created when powdered ceramics are fired and held at a temperature below the melting point. **Vitrification** is the gradual formation of soft glass that flows around the particulates to fill some of the void areas. After cooling, this results in a solid comprised of glassy areas surrounding unreacted particles and any residual pores. The amount of vitrification depends both on the firing time and temperature.

Glass-ceramics are so named because the materials begin as glasses, but become polycrystalline ceramics during processing. To accomplish this, the original, glassy material is first heat treated at 500–700°C to form a large concentration of crystal nuclei. Then, like with grain growth in metals, the temperature of the ceramic is increased to promote enlargement of these crystals. The final material is fine-grained and contains randomly oriented crystals.

6.5.3 Powder Processing of Ceramics

Although casting also begins with a ceramic powder/water mixture, powder processing in ceramics usually refers to a technique similar to that described above for metals (P/M) that is most often used for crystalline materials. In this procedure, a powdered ceramic and small amount of water and/or a binding agent is pressed into the desired shape and the object is then subjected to sintering. High temperatures are required to allow sufficient atomic diffusion to reduce to the overall surface area present in the material. However, this process occurs well below the melting point of the ceramic. Like with metals, this technique results in a significant reduction in material porosity (see Fig. 6.9), with individual crystals ionically bonded to each other. Also analogous to P/M, pressing and sintering can take place simultaneously with hot pressing procedures.

6.5.4 Rapid Manufacturing of Ceramics

As with metals, rapid manufacturing techniques using powdered ceramics have been developed to efficiently create products with complicated geometries. Sintering techniques like those described in section 6.4.4 can be employed for ceramics. However, a wide variety of other processes are also common, including a binder-based method called **three-dimensional printing** (3DP).

3DP is similar to selective laser sintering, but in this case, instead of a laser, a printhead is scanned over the top of the platform containing the powder (see Fig. 6.10). As directed by the computer, the printhead drops small amounts of liquid binder in certain regions. For ceramics, this is often a type of silica binder, which encourages the aggregation of the particles into a solid. As for other SFF techniques, the platform is then lowered, more powder is spread, and the process is repeated until the entire object has been fabricated.

Although rapid manufacturing of ceramic pieces is often achieved in this manner, it is also possible to use SFF to produce a mold, rather than the final object itself. Additional material is then cast into this mold in a traditional fashion. As shown in Fig. 6.13, this method has been used to create ceramic molds for metallic orthopedic implants having a textured surface (this is used to improve implant integration with the surrounding bone). It must be remembered that, for such applications, the object created in the rapid manufacturing procedure should have void space in the shape of the final object.

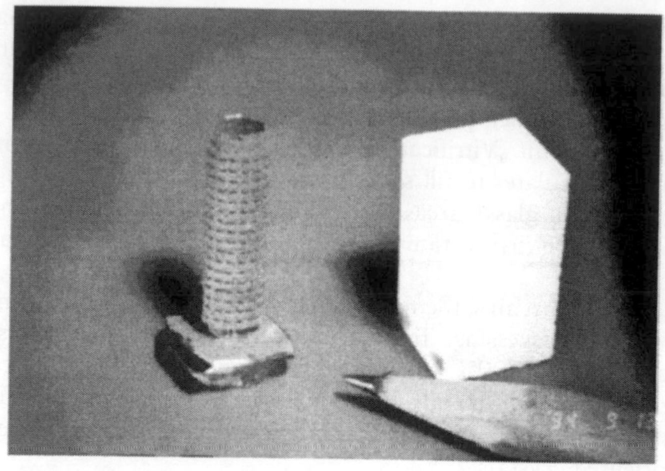

Figure 6.13
Rapid prototyping can be used to create a mold for a metallic object. The figure shows a ceramic mold on the right that was created via rapid prototyping, which was then used to create a textured bone screw on the left (pencil is used to indicate relative scale). The formation of complex shapes is possible with this manufacturing method. (Adapted with permission from [6].)

6.6 Processing of Polymers

6.6.1 Thermoplasts vs. Thermosets

Similar to ceramics, transition temperatures such as T_g and T_m are important in selecting appropriate processing methods for polymers. Another key parameter is whether a particular polymer is a thermoplast or a thermoset. **Thermoplastic polymers** soften (liquify) when heated and harden when cooled. This is due to a reduction in secondary bonding between chains at higher temperatures, allowing the macromolecules to slide past each other. Most linear polymers are thermoplastic. During processing, it should be remembered that these polymers can be heated and cooled repeatedly, but that degradation occurs at temperatures where there is enough molecular motion to break the covalent bonds in the backbone.

In contrast, **thermosetting polymers** become permanently hard when heated to a high temperature and do not subsequently soften. This is because, as the temperature is increased, covalent crosslinks are created between polymer chains. These highly crosslinked macromolecules are then unable to slide past each other and deform plastically. Thermosetting polymers include vulcanized rubbers, epoxies and resins. As in thermoplastic materials, heating these polymers excessively will cause degradation due to cleavage of the crosslinks.

Complex shapes can be produced from either of these types of polymers. The most common technique to form shapes from thermosets is casting, especially compression molding, whereas all of the following forming and casting methods are employed for creation of objects from thermoplastic polymers. In addition, as discussed in Chapter 3, gases may be bubbled through the molten thermoplast during these procedures to produce porous foams. During processing, it should be kept in mind that thermosets can be removed from the mold at high temperatures, while pressure must be maintained as thermoplastic polymers are cooled below their T_g to assure that the proper shape is maintained before removal from the mold.

EXAMPLE PROBLEM 6.4

A production manager at a biomaterials plant made 40,000 artificial heart valve leaflets out of a proprietary thermosetting polymer resin. The fabrication process involved heat treatment of the leaflets at a high temperature to cure them. Unfortunately, it was discovered after the production run that a calculation error was made, resulting in all of the artificial heart valve leaflets being too large to be used. Interested in lessening the economic impact of the mistake,

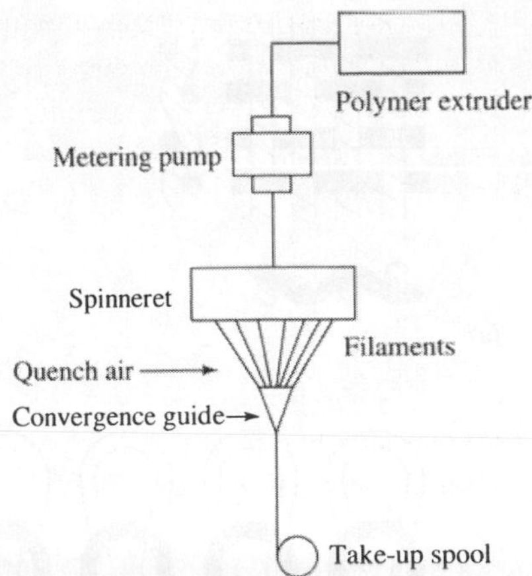

Figure 6.14 Schematic of fiber spinning process. A molten polymer is pumped through a plate (spinneret) containing many small holes. The polymer exiting from each hole forms a single fiber, which cools upon contact with air. These filaments are then packaged on spools for storage and shipping. (Adapted with permission from [7].)

the production manager asks you (the resident biomaterials expert) if the leaflets can be melted to recycle the polymer resin in order to produce a new batch of leaflets of the proper dimensions. How would you respond (justify your answer)?

Solution: Since a thermosetting polymer resin was used to fabricate the leaflets, and a high temperature treatment was applied to cure the resin, the material cannot be recycled. The setting of the polymer resin resulted in the formation of covalent crosslinks between the polymer chains. Thus, the material cannot be melted and reused, as any heat applied to the polymer sufficient to break the crosslinks would be sufficient to break the bonds in the backbones of the polymer chains as well, thereby decomposing the polymer. ■

6.6.2 Forming Polymers

6.6.2.1 Extrusion of Polymers Polymer extrusion is similar to extrusion of metals and is based on plastic deformation of the material. A screw moves within a heated chamber filled with polymer pellets, causing them to melt and form a continuous feed stock. This viscous fluid is then forced through an orifice, while jets of air or water on the exterior cool and solidify the polymer into its final shape. As with metals, this method is often used to produce lengths of polymeric rods or tubing. In the biomedical field, extrusion is commonly employed in the fabrication of expanded PTFE (GORE-TEX®) vascular grafts.

6.6.2.2 Fiber Spinning of Polymers A variant of extrusion for polymers is **fiber spinning.** In this procedure, a molten polymer is pumped through a plate (spinneret) that has many small holes (see Fig. 6.14). The polymer exiting from each hole forms a single fiber, which cools upon contact with air. As mentioned in Section 6.2.3, the strength of the polymer along the main fiber axis can be improved after formation by applying tension along this axis (called drawing[1] or pre-drawing).

As with metal and ceramic fibers, meshes may be produced from polymeric fibers. Because many polymers can be degraded *in vivo*, polymer meshes are popular as carriers for cells or bioactive agents in tissue engineering applications. Several methods for organizing these fibers in three dimensions have been developed, and some of these are illustrated in Fig. 6.15. They include weaving, knitting and braiding the fibers into specific structures. In these meshes, the porosity is dependent on the diameter as well as the packing density of the fibers. Braided, woven,

[1]This is similar, but not identical, to drawing of metals and glasses, a type of forming procedure described in sections 6.4.1.4 and 6.5.1

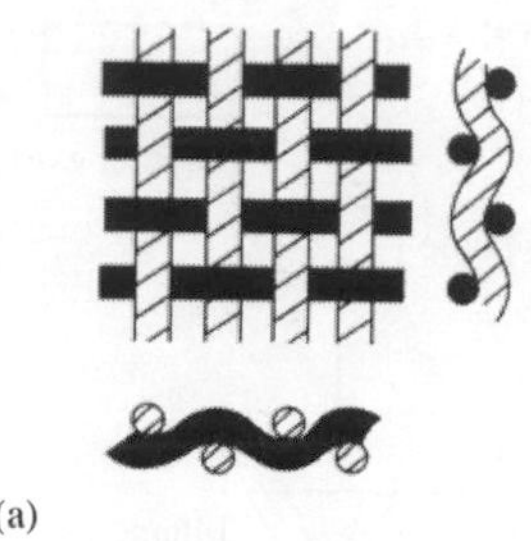

(a)

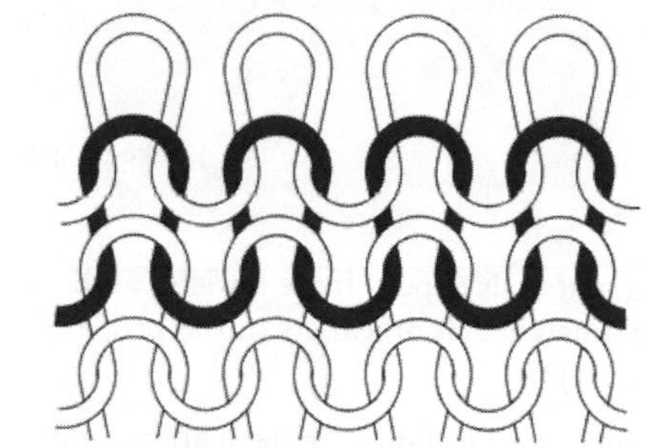

(b)

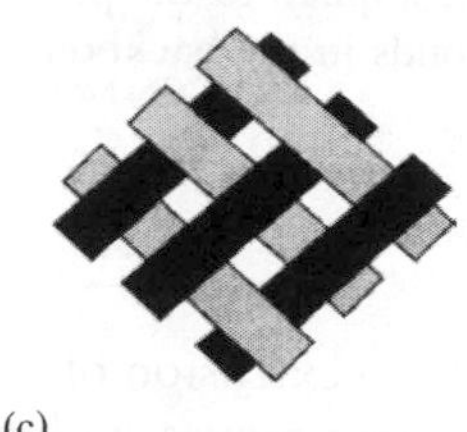

(c)

Figure 6.15
Several methods for organizing fibers into three dimensions have been developed. Some examples include (a) weaving, (b) weft knit, and (c) regular braid. These different structures can affect the porosity and mechanical properties of the material. (Adapted with permission from [7].)

and knitted materials have been used in artificial blood vessels as well as replacement tendon/ligaments.

If fiber diameters less than about 10 μm are required, it is necessary to employ alternative spinning procedures to those described above. One such method that is currently under investigation is **electrospinning**, depicted in Fig. 6.16. In this case, the molten polymer is extruded from a nozzle into a strong electrostatic field (voltages of

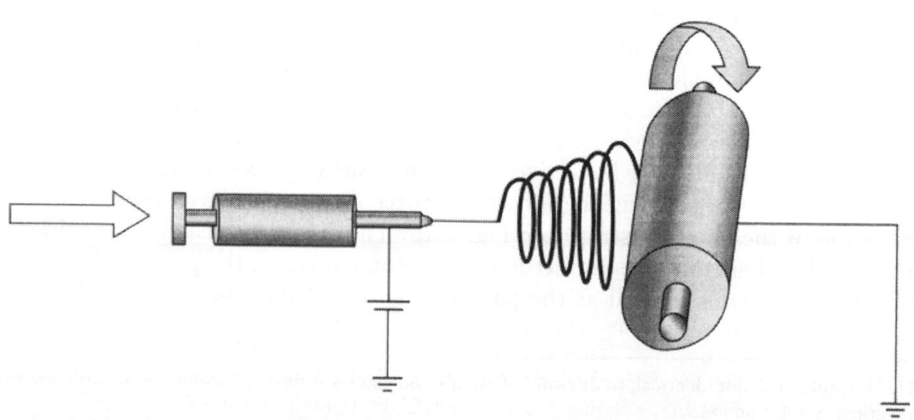

Figure 6.16
In electrospinning, molten polymer is extruded from a nozzle into a strong electrostatic field, which acts to overcome the surface tension of the liquid and accelerates parts of this liquid in the general direction of a (grounded) target, in this case a rotating spool. Each part of the liquid cools upon contact with air, forming fine, looping fibers. (Adapted with permission from [8].)

5–30 kV). This field acts to overcome the surface tension of the liquid and accelerates parts of this liquid in the general direction of a (grounded) target. Each part of the liquid cools upon contact with air, forming fine, looping fibers that can be collected. However, because of the looping nature of the fibers, the collected material is usually formed into a three-dimensional nonwoven mesh, rather than one of the woven or knitted structures illustrated in Fig. 6.15.

6.6.3 Casting Polymers

Like metals and ceramics, polymers can be cast into a mold and allowed to solidify. However, for polymeric materials, this process is usually called *molding*. Three of the most common types of molding are described in this section.

6.6.3.1 Compression Molding of Polymers In **compression molding,** the stock polymer is placed in a heated mold (die). One half of the mold is then moved down to come in contact with the stock material. This applies pressure and forces the polymer into the desired shape (see Fig. 6.17). As mentioned previously, this is a common shaping method for thermosets, but is also used with thermoplastic polymers. For example, high-molecular weight poly(ethylene) can be processed in this manner to form orthopedic implants.

6.6.3.2 Injection Molding of Polymers Injection molding requires first melting the stock polymer in a heated chamber. As depicted in Fig. 6.18, the viscous liquid polymer is then forced through the nozzle due to pressure applied by the ram. After the correct amount of polymer has exited the nozzle to fill the die, the pressure is maintained until the polymer has cooled and solidified, when it is removed from the mold. A main advantage of injection molding is its speed—a new piece may be fabricated every few seconds using this method.

6.6.3.3 Blow Molding of Polymers Blow molding is very similar to glass blowing operations and is used to make hollow objects. The molten polymeric parison is placed in a heated mold, and then blowing air or steam forces the polymer to conform to the shape of the mold.

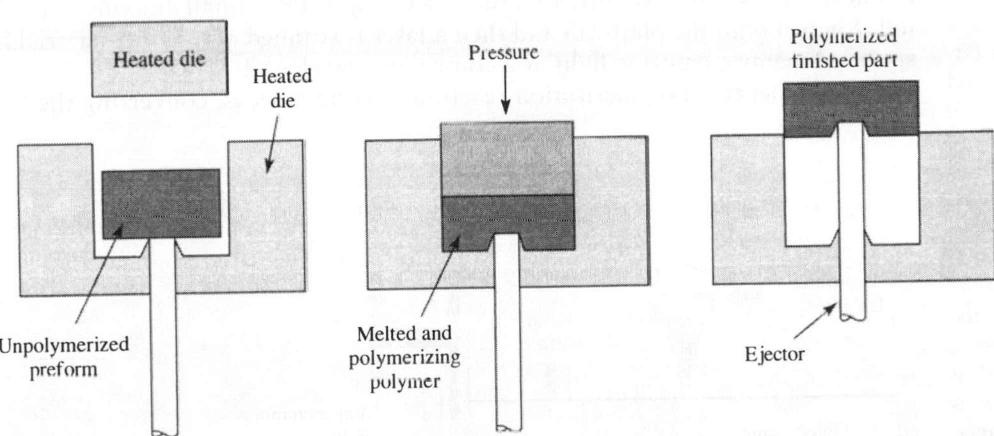

Figure 6.17
In compression molding, the stock polymer (preform) is placed in a heated die (mold). Part of the mold is then moved down to come in contact with the stock material, applying pressure and forcing the polymer into the desired shape. An ejector pin is manufactured into the mold to facilitate rapid removal of the final, polymerized product. (Adapted with permission from [9].)

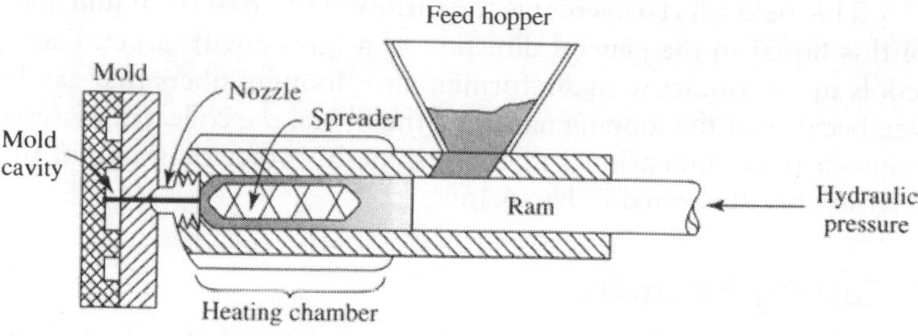

Figure 6.18
Schematic of injection molding process. First, polymer (in pellet form) is added to the feed hopper, where it is carried to the heating chamber. After it is melted, the viscous liquid polymer is forced through a nozzle due to pressure applied by a ram. After a measured amount of polymer has exited the nozzle and filled the die, the pressure is maintained until the polymer has cooled and solidified. At this point the final product is removed via ejector pins, similar to the compression molding process. (Adapted with permission from [10].)

6.6.4 Rapid Manufacturing of Polymers

Although many rapid manufacturing techniques are currently being investigated for biomedical polymers, we provide descriptions of two, 3DP and stereolithography, as examples of the type of technology available for polymeric SFF. Powder processing is less common for polymeric materials than for metals or ceramics. However, SFF techniques like 3DP do employ finely ground polymers as a starting material. 3DP of polymeric implants is identical to that described for ceramics (see Fig. 6.10), although, in this case, the binder is an organic solvent (often chloroform) that is used to partially dissolve the polymer particles in localized areas. As the solvent evaporates, the particles remain adherent and form a solid. The platform is then lowered and more polymer powder is placed on top to fabricate the final piece layer by layer.

Stereolithography is an analogous procedure using liquid stock. In this process, the moveable platform is located in a pool containing a polymeric precursor (usually monomers or low-molecular weight polymers) and a light-responsive initiator molecule (photoinitiator). As seen in Fig. 6.19, a small amount of the liquid is wiped onto the platform and then a laser is scanned across the material in a specified manner, emitting light at a controlled wavelength. This causes the initiator to commence a polymerization reaction in certain areas, converting the stock

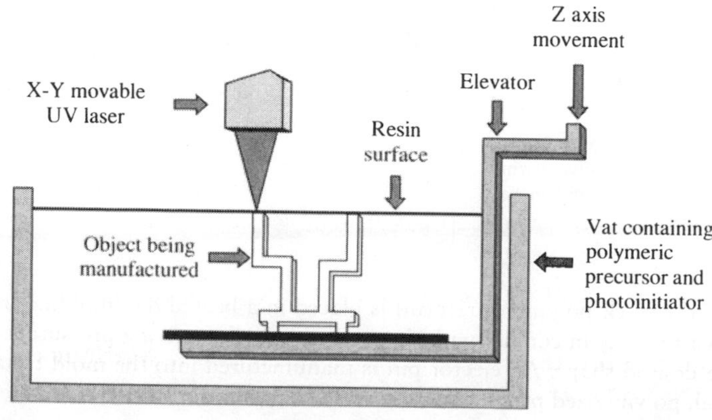

Figure 6.19
Schematic of stereolithography process. This is a rapid manufacturing method that uses a liquid stock. In this process, the moveable platform is located in a pool containing a polymeric precursor (usually monomers or low-molecular weight polymers) and a light-responsive initiator molecule (photoinitiator). A small amount of the liquid is wiped onto the platform (attached to the elevator) and then a laser emitting light at a controlled wavelength is scanned across the material to create a particular profile. This causes the initiator to commence a polymerization reaction in certain areas on the resin surface, converting the stock from a liquid into a solid. The platform is then lowered and the next layer is formed in the same manner. This process is repeated until the final desired three-dimensional shape is produced. (Adapted with permission from [11].)

from a liquid into a solid. The platform is then lowered and the next layer is formed in the same manner.

6.7 Processing to Improve Biocompatibility

As introduced in Chapter 1, biocompatibility is a broad term suggesting that a material produces an acceptable host response in a given application. Although there are many aspects to biocompatibility, many of which are governed by biomaterial surface properties, as described in the next chapter, two important considerations are that the material does not induce infection or a deleterious immune response (rejection). Postfabrication processing can play a significant role in reducing both of these responses. Techniques for sterilization of both synthetic and naturally derived materials are outlined in this section, followed by a discussion of methods for reducing the immune response to natural materials.

6.7.1 Sterilization

Sterilization of biomedical implants prior to implantation is extremely important because the presence of a biomaterial may promote serious infection from even normally innocuous pathogens (see Chapter 14 for further discussion of biomaterials-related infections). In addition, pre-sterilization decreases the possibility of the transfer of viruses associated with naturally derived materials. This section, based on a discussion by Kowalski and Morrissey [12], will focus on the most common sterilization/decontamination methods. More information on other sterilization methods, such as dry heat sterilization and UV sterilization, can be found in the references mentioned at the end of this chapter. Depending on key properties of the material (such as the melting point), these methods can be used for both natural and synthetic biomaterials.

Because it is virtually impossible to remove all pathogens from an implant, the concept of a **sterility assurance level (SAL)** was developed. The SAL for a given device is measured by culturing implants in nutrient media after various sterilization times and determining how many bacterial colonies remain. From these data, manufacturers can choose the time and dose of sterilization to maintain a certain SAL (probability that the implant will remain sterile). Therefore, in selecting from the sterilization methods described below, biomaterialists must consider both the ability of the technique to achieve a desired SAL and the compatibility of the process with the material and packaging material, so that the biomaterial is not degraded or deformed during the sterilization procedure.

6.7.1.1 Steam Sterilization As the name indicates, biomaterials can be sterilized by exposure to high pressure at a temperature of at least 121°C. Also known as autoclaving, this technique denatures protein and lipid constituents important to microorganism survival. Advantages of this method include that it is effective, relatively quick and simple, and leaves no toxic residues within the sample. However, the high temperatures employed limit its use with materials having low melting points. Additionally, hydrolytically cleavable materials are particularly susceptible to degradation in such an environment, so this technique is not suitable for sterilization of this class of polymers.

6.7.1.2 Ethylene Oxide Sterilization A specialized sterilization apparatus is required to expose implants to ethylene oxide (EtO) gas. Because EtO is toxic, may cause cancer and is potentially flammable, it is often mixed with an inert gas within the machine. Sterilization occurs when a chamber holding the implants at 30 to 50°C is first evacuated, then flooded with EtO, and finally purged several times with air. Following this, further aeration outside the sterilizer aids in removal of any remaining EtO.

EtO causes pathogen death primarily through permanent, chemical alteration of nucleic acids (DNA, RNA). This sterilization method is effective, even deep within crevices or pores, and, because it is carried out at a low temperature, it is can be used for a wide variety of materials. However, toxic resides of EtO that may be left in the device are of great concern. In addition, due to the reactivity and possible carcinogenic nature of the gas, personnel must be properly protected while performing the sterilization procedure.

6.7.1.3 Radiation Sterilization The radiation used in radiation sterilization can be provided in the form of gamma rays or an electron beam. In both cases, the samples are placed in an irradiator and monitored to assure they have received the proper dosage of radiation. The gamma ray source is a ^{60}Co isotope, while an accelerator creates the electron beam. The advantage to the electron beam method is that when the accelerator is turned off, no radiation is produced, while the ^{60}Co source is constantly decaying and releasing radiation, which can be detrimental to the operator's health.

Radiation acts by ionizing important cellular elements, including nucleic acids, thus killing adherent microorganisms. Advantages of radiation sterilization are that it is rapid, effective and compatible with many materials. Disadvantages are that it requires a large capital investment to install an irradiator and that certain polymers, such as poly(tetrafluoroethylene) or hydrolytically cleavable polymers like poly(lactic acid), are susceptible to radiation degradation. Additionally, the electron beam method has a very small penetration depth, so only thin devices may be sterilized in this manner.

EXAMPLE PROBLEM 6.5

Consider a novel vascular stent made from a surgical grade steel. The stent has been coated with a novel polymer to help integration with native tissue and prevent further narrowing of the vessel. Would steam sterilization, ethylene oxide sterilization, or radiation sterilization be preferred for this device? Why?

Solution: Ethylene oxide would generally be preferred for sterilization of the coated stent. Recalling that polymers have lower melting temperatures than metals, steam sterilization would not be appropriate because it may melt the polymer coating. Although both radiation and EtO treatment may damage polymeric materials, this is often more of a concern with radiation. Therefore, the recommended method would be to sterilize the device with EtO and characterize both the metal and polymer components post-treatment to assure that no degradation has occurred.

■

6.7.2 Fixation of Natural Materials

In addition to harboring potential pathogens, naturally derived materials can evoke an immune response (be immunogenic) because certain areas of the material may be recognized as "foreign" by the body. If this occurs, a cascade of events (see Chapter 11–12) is initiated that may lead to degradation or walling off of the implant, thus reducing the efficacy of the device.

In order to decrease immunogenicity, particularly in collagen-derived materials, the implants are often crosslinked with fixatives such as gluteraldehyde after fabrication into the appropriate shape. Although the exact reason for the efficacy of this treatment has not been elucidated, it is thought that the crosslinking process alters the chemical structure of the regions in the material that are recognized as foreign to the body, thus reducing any unwanted immune response.

Summary

- Metals can be strengthened by a number of techniques whereby defects are added to the crystal structure to prevent dislocation motion. Alloying strengthens a metal by introducing point defects that increase the shear stress required for dislocation motion. Strain hardening introduces line defects into a metal that increase the energy needed to move the stress field through the combined localized strains from other dislocations. Precipitation hardening occurs through the introduction of precipitates in a metal, which create local strains that inhibit dislocation motion in the area.
- Strengthening techniques for polymers include heat treatment; predrawing procedures, in which the polymer chains become aligned along the axis of loading; and additional crosslinking, in which the ability of chains to slide past one another is reduced.
- Annealing generally results in an increase in grain size, decrease in grain boundaries, reduction of internal stresses and an increase in the ductility of a metal. The rate of heat extraction strongly influences the resulting grain structure of an annealed metal. The percent crystallinity of semicrystalline polymers can be increased through heat treatment during which polymer chains are free to align with the increased energy. As with the annealing of metals, the rate of cooling strongly influences the final structure of the annealed polymer.
- Metals can be formed into desired shapes through a number of processes. The application of force to the metal to achieve the desired form is required with forming methods, which include forging, rolling, extrusion and drawing. Casting methods involve filling a mold with molten metal and can typically result in more ductile, intricately shaped materials than forming techniques. Powder processing involves filling a mold with a fine powder of the metal of choice, condensing it with high pressure, and then sintering it at high temperature.
- Glasses can be formed into desired shapes through pressing, blowing and drawing, all of which require the application of mechanical force. Casting techniques can be used with crystalline ceramics and glass-ceramics. Ceramic casting involves filling a mold with small ceramic particles mixed with water and an organic binder, drying the ceramic, and firing it to burn out remaining water and binding agent. Powder processing techniques can be used with ceramic materials and, although conducted at high temperatures, occur well below the melting point of the ceramic.
- Certain parameters of a polymer material, including T_g, T_m, and whether a polymer is a thermoplast or a thermoset, must be considered before identifying an appropriate processing technique. As with metals and ceramics, forming techniques, including extrusion, fiber spinning, and electrospinning, and casting techniques, including compression, injection, and blow molding, can be used to produce products of desired form.
- It is important that biomaterials be sterile prior to contact with the recipient to ensure prevention of pathogen and/or other biological contaminant transmission. Biomaterial sterilization via autoclaving involves treatment with high pressure

steam to denature proteins and lipid constituents necessary to the survival of microorganisms. Ethylene oxide exposure under controlled conditions sterilizes the material by chemically altering nucleic acids of microorganisms. Biomaterials can also be sterilized through radiation exposure techniques, including gamma ray sterilization and electron beam sterilization.

Problems

6.1 Compare and contrast casting methods for metals, ceramics, and polymers. Also compare the effect of cooling rate (quenching) between metals and polymers.

6.2 Which fabrication methods lend themselves to the creation of porous metals, ceramics, and polymers? For each of the three material classes, which method would you choose to make a porous structure out of each type of material, and why?

6.3 When a hip stem is implanted in the femur it is sometimes held in place with a bone cement, made out of poly(methyl methacrylate). During implantation, the ingredients for the bone cement (consisting mainly of the monomer methyl methacrylate and an initiator) are mixed in the surgical suite and packed into the femur, prior to the insertion of the hip stem of the prosthesis. At this point, the mixture polymerizes *in situ*. Using this information, and what is provided in the book, is this material a thermoplastic or thermoset? Why?

6.4 Create a table showing two advantages and two disadvantages of each of the three main sterilization methods (steam, ethylene oxide, and radiation).

References

1. Callister, Jr., W.D. *Materials Science and Engineering: An Introduction*, 3rd ed. New York: John Wiley and Sons, 1994.
2. Shackelford, J.F. *Introduction to Materials Science for Engineers*, 5th ed. Upper Saddle River: Prentice Hall, 2000.
3. Ashby M.F. and D.R.H. Jones, *Engineering Materials 2: An Introduction to Microstructures, Processing and Design*, Oxford: Elsevier Science Ltd., Pergamon Imprint, 1986.
4. Sherwood, J.K., S.L. Riley, R. Palazzolo, S.C. Brown, D.C. Monkhouse, M. Coates, L.G. Griffith, L.K. Landeen, and A. Ratcliffe. "A Three-Dimensional Osteochondral Composite Scaffold for Articular Cartilage Repair." *Biomaterials*, vol. 23, pp. 4739–4751, 2002.
5. Pfaender, H., *Schott Guide to Glass*, London: Chapman and Hall, 1996.
6. Melican, M.C., M.C. Zimmerman, M.S. Dhillon, A.R. Ponnambalam, A. Curodeau, and J.R. Parsons. "Three-Dimensional Printing and Porous Metallic Surfaces: A New Orthopedic Application." *Journal of Biomedical Materials Research*, vol. 55, pp. 194–202, 2001.
7. Weinberg, S. and M.W. King. "Medical Fibers and Biotextiles." In *Biomaterials Science: An Introduction to Materials in Medicine*, B.D. Ratner, A.S. Hoffman, F.J. Schoen, and J.E. Lemons, Eds., 2nd ed. San Diego: Elsevier Academic Press, pp. 86–100, 2004.
8. Pham, Q.P., U. Sharma, and A.G. Mikos. "Electrospinning of Polymeric Nanofibers for Tissue Engineering Applications: A Review." *Tissue Engineering*, vol. 12, pp. 1197–1211, 2006.
9. Askeland, D.R. *The Science and Engineering of Materials*, 2nd ed. Boston: PWS-KENT Publishing Company, 1989.
10. Allcock, H.R. and F.W. Lampe, *Contemporary Polymer Chemistry*, Englewood Cliffs, NJ: Prentice Hall, 1981.
11. Cooke, M.N., J.P. Fisher, D. Dean, C. Rimnac, and A.G. Mikos. "Use of Stereolithography to Manufacture Critical-Sized 3D Biodegradable Scaffolds for Bone Ingrowth." *Journal of Biomedical Materials Research*, vol. 64B, pp. 65–69, 2003.
12. Kowalski, J.B. and R.F. Morrissey. "Sterilization of Implants and Devices." In *Biomaterials Science: An Introduction to Materials in Medicine*, B.D. Ratner, A.S. Hoffman, F.J. Schoen, and J.E. Lemons, Eds., 2nd ed. San Diego: Elsevier Academic Press, pp. 754–760, 2004.

Additional Reading

Black, J. and G. Hastings. *Handbook of Biomaterial Properties*. London: Chapman and Hall, 1998.

Brunski, J.B. "Metals." In *Biomaterials Science: An Introduction to Materials in Medicine*, B.D. Ratner, A.S. Hoffman, F.J. Schoen, and J.E. Lemons, Eds., 2nd ed. San Diego: Elsevier Academic Press, pp. 137–153, 2004.

Cooper, K.P. "Layered Manufacturing: Challenges and Opportunities." *Material Research Society Symposium Proceedings*, vol. 758, pp. 23–34, 2003.

Fisher, J.P. and D.M. Yoon. "Polymeric Scaffolds for Tissue Engineering Applications." In *Tissue Engineering and Artificial Organs*, J.D. Bronzino, Ed., 3rd ed. New York: Taylor and Francis, pp. 1–18, 2006.

Hench, L.L. "Ceramics, Glasses, and Glass-Ceramics." In *Biomaterials Science: An Introduction to Materials in Medicine*, B.D. Ratner, A.S. Hoffman, F.J. Schoen, and J.E. Lemons, Eds., 1st ed. San Diego: Elsevier Academic Press, pp. 73–84, 1996.

Murphy, M.B. and A.G. Mikos. "Porous Scaffold Fabrication for Tissue Engineering." In *Principles of Tissue Engineering*, R.P. Lanza, R. Langer, and J.P. Vacanti, Eds., In press.

Park, A., B. Wu, and L.G. Griffith. "Integration of Surface Modification and 3D Fabrication Techniques to Prepare Patterned Poly(L-Lactide) Substrates Allowing Regionally Selective Cell Adhesion." *Journal of Biomaterials Science Polymer Edition*, vol. 9, pp. 89–110, 1998.

Park, J.B. and R.S. Lakes. *Biomaterials: An Introduction*, 2nd ed. New York: Plenum Press, 1992.

Schaffer, J.P., A. Saxena, S.D. Antolovich, T.H. Sanders, Jr., and S.B. Warner. *The Science and Design of Engineering Materials*, 2nd ed. Boston: McGraw-Hill, 1999.

Yannas, I.V. "Natural Materials." In *Biomaterials Science: An Introduction to Materials in Medicine*, B.D. Ratner, A.S. Hoffman, F.J. Schoen, and J.E. Lemons, Eds., 2nd ed. San Diego: Elsevier Academic Press, pp. 127–137, 2004.

CHAPTER 7 Surface Properties of Biomaterials

Main Objective

To understand how biomaterial surface properties affect thermodynamics of protein adsorption and how different surface treatments can affect these properties.

Specific Objectives

1. To understand basic thermodynamic principles and how thermodynamics relates to protein adsorption to biomaterial surfaces.
2. To understand how physical and chemical properties of the biomaterial surface affect protein adsorption and why protein adsorption is important to the biological response.
3. To distinguish between physicochemical and biological surface modification techniques.
4. To compare and contrast various physicochemical surface modification methods and to understand which are appropriate for each class of biomaterial.
5. To distinguish among covalent coatings, noncovalent coatings, and physicochemical surface modification with no overcoat.
6. To compare and contrast various biological surface modification methods and to understand which are appropriate for each class of biomaterial.
7. To understand how surface characteristics differ on degradable vs. nondegradable materials over time.
8. To distinguish between two types of processing for substrate surface patterning.
9. To understand the theory behind and possible limitations to the characterization techniques presented.

7.1 Introduction: Concepts in Surface Chemistry and Biology

Chapters 1 to 6 have discussed bulk properties of biomaterials, such as their thermal, mechanical, and degradative characteristics, and the corresponding atomic causes. However, since the biomaterial surface is extremely important in determining the biological response and thus implant success, this chapter will focus solely on surface properties of biomaterials. This includes a description of both physicochemical and biological means to modify solid surfaces, as well as processing techniques to form patterned biomaterial surfaces.

7.1.1 Protein Adsorption and Biocompatibility

As described in Chapter 3, the surface of a material can be considered a type of planar defect. Because the atoms at the surface are not bonded on all sides to other atoms, there is extra energy associated with this region due to unfilled valence shells. This excess energy is often called (due to historical reasons) the **surface tension** (**γ**). Because this state is thermodynamically unstable, there is a driving force to minimize the surface tension by the adsorption of atoms or molecules, which satisfy the unfilled bonds at the material surface. **Adsorption** is the adhesion of molecules to a solid surface. This can be distinguished from **absorption**, which is the penetration of molecules into the bulk of another material, such as water is absorbed by a sponge. We focus in the next few chapters on protein adsorption to biomaterials.

At physiological conditions, the **adsorbate** on the biomaterial surface is composed primarily of ions, water, and proteins. It is to this coated surface, rather than to the "pure" biomaterial, that the body reacts. Therefore, controlling protein adsorption to biomaterial surfaces is a key aspect to assuring biocompatibility. We begin this chapter with a discussion of the impact of the biomaterial surface on the thermodynamics of protein adsorption.

7.1.2 Surface Properties Governing Protein Adsorption

Although a driving force exists at the biomaterial surface in the form of surface tension, in order to predict the adsorption of proteins or other molecules, one must examine the entire system, which includes the material surface (discussed in this chapter), the proteins, and the solvent (discussed in more detail in Chapter 8). In particular, the system before and after prospective adsorption must be analyzed from a thermodynamic standpoint to see if it is energetically favorable for the adsorption to occur. The following section discusses the contribution of the biomaterial surface to protein adsorption, while the contributions of the other components will be addressed in Chapter 8.

Using thermodynamic principles[1] to examine the system before adsorption occurs, we see that two surface properties have the largest effect on the favorability of adsorption:

1. Surface hydrophobicity
2. Surface charge

As discussed previously, the **hydrophobicity** of a material describes how it responds to the presence of water. To quantify hydrophobicity, a biomaterial surface is subjected to contact angle analysis, which is described later in the chapter. An example of a **hydrophobic** (water-fearing, or water-repelling) surface is a freshly-waxed car—water forms small balls ("beads up") on this surface. In contrast, after the wax coating has worn away, water drops spread on the more **hydrophilic** (water-loving) metallic painted surface. Examples of hydrophobic biomaterials include most of the synthetic polymers listed in Table 2.5, particularly those containing pendant methyl [e.g., poly(methyl

[1]It should be noted that these thermodynamic models can be most directly used to explain only nonspecific adsorption to surfaces, not protein-receptor interactions, which are discussed later in this chapter and again in Chapter 9.

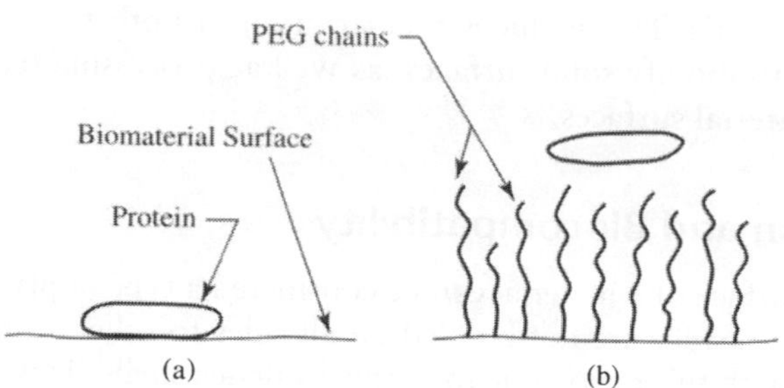

Figure 7.1
Schematic of steric hindrance due to PEG chains. a) On a material without steric hindrance proteins have free access to adhere to the material surface. b) PEG chains inhibit the attachment of proteins by physically blocking access to the surface.

methacrylate)] or styrene [e.g., poly(styrene)] groups. Ceramic and metallic biomaterials are often more hydrophilic than these polymers in their unmodified state. Although it is difficult to predict exactly how surface hydrophobicity affects protein adsorption for a specific system, it has been found that protein adsorption generally increases with increasing hydrophobicity of the surface and the protein.

The effects of surface charge cannot be completely separated from the effects of hydrophobicity, especially when using contact angle methods to determine hydrophobicity, since contact angle is also sensitive to surface charge. However, a significant surface charge can have the additional effect of attracting or repelling charged areas of proteins. Surface charge occurs via dissociation of ionizable surface groups or though specific adsorption of ions from the solution. Again, how this property affects protein adsorption depends on both the charge of the surface and that of the protein.

In addition to the properties above that affect the thermodynamics of protein adsorption to biomaterials, the physical characteristics of the biomaterial surface are also important. These include **steric concerns** and **surface roughness.** For example, adding large, flexible hydrophilic polymer chains such as poly(ethylene glycol) (PEG) to a biomaterial surface will result in a decrease in protein adsorption (Fig. 7.1). This is due to the fact that a large volume at the surface is taken up by these bulky chains that are in constant motion. Since they move too quickly to allow the proteins to adsorb to them and are too large for the proteins to move through, they form a type of wall, using **steric repulsion** to prevent adsorption to the surface. In contrast, a surface with a high degree of roughness may promote protein adsorption in certain areas by physically "trapping" the proteins in the valleys on the surface.

Thus, the hydrophobicity, charge, steric hindrance and/or roughness of a biomaterial surface can be altered during formation or processing to change the protein adsorption profile of the final material. Because this is the most accessible control point to influence the final biocompatibility of the material, many methods have been developed to modify biomaterial surfaces. In some cases, these were designed to impart surface properties other than those directly relating to protein adsorption (such as increased hardness or reduced friction), but it is important to remember that any changes in surface chemistry will affect the type and/or amount of protein on the surface. An overview of the means to effect surface modifications for various classes of biomedical materials is the subject of the remainder of this chapter.

EXAMPLE PROBLEM 7.1

Consider the following hypothetical protein and two materials (A) and (B). Assume that in this case the water contact angle correlates directly with the hydrophobicity of the material surface. To which material would greater adsorption of the given protein be expected? Why?

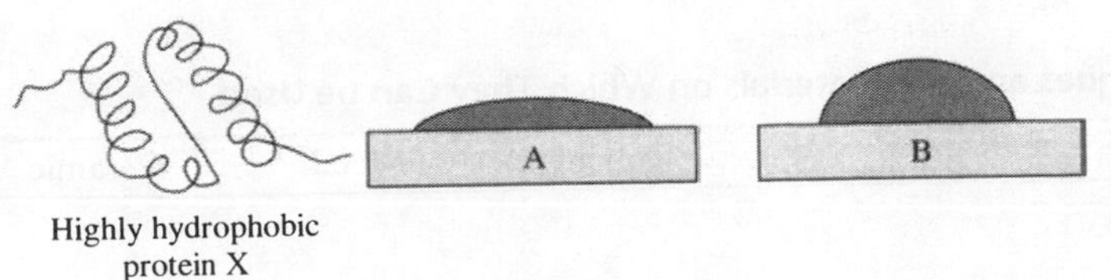

Solution: Although the contact angles for the materials are not given directly, it can be deduced through visual examination of the figure that Material B has a greater contact angle than A. Given that in this case we are to assume that the contact angle corresponds directly with the hydrophobicity of the material, it can be concluded that Material B is more hydrophobic than Material A. Consequently, one would expect greater adsorption of the highly hydrophobic protein X to the surface of Material B, through hydrophobic interaction, assuming that the surface charges of Materials A and B are comparable. ■

7.2 Physicochemical Surface Modification Techniques

7.2.1 Introduction to Surface Modification Techniques

There are a wide variety of surface modification techniques designed to treat all types of biomaterials, including naturally based and synthetic polymers, metals, and ceramics (see Table 7.1). Many of these can be considered as postfabrication processing techniques, similar to those discussed in Chapter 6, while in other cases, final surface modification is designed into the chemical nature of the biomaterial (e.g. surface-modifying additives, discussed below). Surface modification possesses the advantage that bulk characteristics such as mechanical properties are not altered. However, the possibility of delamination *in vivo* is a serious concern.

Therefore, an ideal technique would produce a surface treatment with the following characteristics:

1. Thin (to minimize effects on bulk properties)
2. Resistant to delamination
3. Simple and robust (to promote commercialization)

In addition, a means to discourage surface rearrangement, which happens continually due to the free energy at the surface (see Section 7.1) and can destroy the modification, should be included. A number of methods have been developed to produce surface treatments that meet these criteria. They are generally grouped into **physicochemical** and **biological** modifications, and each type is discussed in more detail in the following sections.

7.2.2 Physicochemical Surface Coatings: Covalent Surface Coatings

As summarized in Table 7.2, **physicochemical** surface treatments use physical principles or chemical reactions to alter the surface composition of the sample. However, in contrast to biological methods, none of these modifications involves the attachment of active biological molecules. Physicochemical modifications can involve the formation of a coating or can include no overcoat, but only those using coating methods will be described in this section (see next section for discussion of other physicochemical methods). Surface coatings can be covalently or non-covalently attached.

TABLE 7.1

Various Surface Modification Techniques and the Materials on Which They Can be Used

	Polymer	Metal	Ceramic	Glass
Non-covalent				
Solvent coating	√	√	√	√
Langmuir–Blodgett film deposition	√	√	√	√
Surface-active additives	√	√	√	√
Vapor deposition of carbons and metals[a]	√	√	√	√
Vapor deposition of parylene (*p*-xylylene)	√	√	√	√
Covalently attached coatings				
Radiation grafting (electron accelerator and gamma)	√	—	—	—
Photografting (UV and visible sources)	√	—	—	√
Plasma (gas discharge) (RF, microwave, acoustic)	√	√	√	√
Gas-phase deposition				
• Ion beam sputtering	√	√	√	√
• Chemical vapor deposition (CVD)	—	√	√	√
• Flame spray deposition	—	√	√	√
Chemical grafting (e.g., ozonation + grafting)	√	√	√	√
Silanization	√	√	√	√
Biological modification (biomolecule immobilization)	√	√	√	√
Modifications of the original surface				
Ion beam etching (e.g., argon, xenon)	√	√	√	√
Ion beam implantation (e.g., nitrogen)	—	√	√	√
Plasma etching (e.g., nitrogen, argon, oxygen, water vapor)	√	√	√	√
Corona discharge (in air)	√	√	√	√
Ion exchange	√[b]	√	√	√
UV irradiation	√	√	√	√
Chemical reaction				
• Nonspecific oxidation (e.g., ozone)	√	√	√	√
• Functional group modifications (oxidation, reduction)	√	—	—	—
• Addition reactions (e.g., acetylation, chlorination)	√	—	—	—
Conversion coatings (phosphating, anodization)	—	√	—	—
Mechanical roughening and polishing	√	√	√	√

[a] Some covalent reaction may occur.
[b] For polymers with ionic groups.
(Adapted with permission from [1].)

We begin our discussion with coatings that are covalently bonded to the surface. The methods described below do not represent an exhaustive list, but are included as examples to demonstrate the variety of techniques that result in covalent coatings. Some of these methods, which include plasma discharge, chemical or physical vapor deposition, radiation or photografting, and self-assembled monolayers, have been used to create biological coatings as well (see Section 7.3).

7.2.2.1 Plasma Treatment **Plasma discharge** is a broad term that encompasses several methods of physicochemical surface modification, some of which result in surface coatings, while others do not. Additionally, exposure to a plasma environment can also be used as a pretreatment to other surface modification techniques. **Plasma** refers to an assembly of species in an atomically/molecularly dissociated gaseous environment. The

TABLE 7.2

Summary of Physicochemical Surface Modification Methods

General Surface Modification Method	Examples
Covalent coatings	Plasma treatment Chemical vapor deposition Physical vapor deposition Radiation grafting / photografting Self-assembled monolayers
Noncovalent coatings	Solution coatings Langmuir-Blodgett films Surface-modifying additives
Surface modification methods with no overcoat	Ion beam implantation Plasma treatment Conversion coatings Bioactive glasses
Laser methods for surface modification	Paterning

gaseous species present can include positive and negative ions, free radicals, electrons, atoms, molecules, and photons. Plasma discharge can occur at a range of temperatures (usually 25°C and higher) and is most often created under vacuum.

A plasma environment is obtained by applying an electric potential across a gas. A simplified depiction of one of the means to achieve plasma discharge treatment is found in Fig. 7.2. As shown in the figure, the cathode is the surface to be

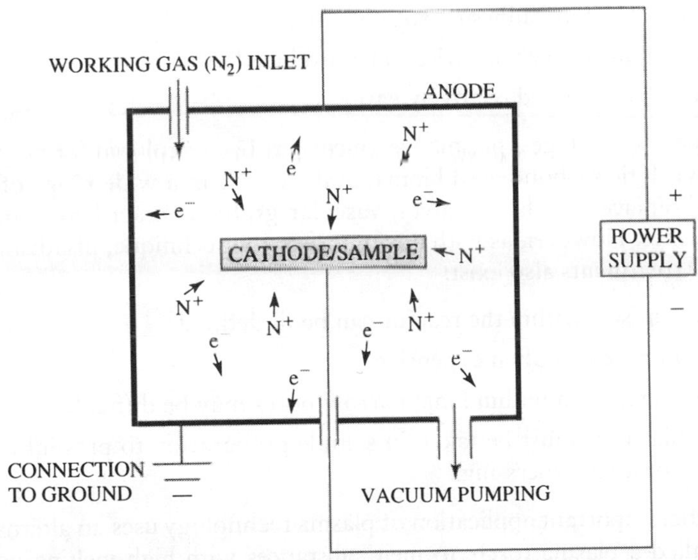

Figure 7.2
Schematic of plasma discharge treatment. The cathode is the surface to be treated and has a negative potential relative to the anode. Electrons must traverse the gas in the chamber to travel from the cathode to the anode. During this stage, they collide with molecules in the gaseous environment to form gaseous ions and radicals. These species can then interact with the sample and cause a variety of surface reactions. The plasma is sustained because electrons flow from the sample while positive ions flow toward the sample.

treated and has a negative potential relative to the anode. To travel from the cathode to the anode, electrons must traverse the gas in the chamber and collide with the molecules to form gaseous ions and radicals. These species can then interact with the sample and cause a variety of surface reactions. The plasma is sustained because electrons flow from the sample while positive ions flow toward the sample.

At the sample surface, there is competition between deposition and ablation/etching. Since the formed species are very energetic, they can result in significant changes to surface chemistry simply through etching. If this process is very rapid, no deposition will be observed. However, in many instances, a mixed process takes place. For these cases, deposition can occur via at least two possible methods. For example, free radicals may polymerize other molecules from the gas phase onto the surface, or small molecules may combine into larger particulates that settle on the surface.

Plasma discharge is often used for cleaning or addition of hydroxyl (OH) or amine (NH_2) groups to biomaterials as a precursor to further modification (see the self assembled monolayer and the biological modification sections later in this chapter). As mentioned above, the energetic plasma may also be employed to directly polymerize molecules on the sample. For example, a copolymer can be placed on the surface of another polymer and exposed to plasma to crosslink the copolymer to the surface.

Plasma discharge treatments possess several advantages. According to Ratner and Hoffman [1], they

1. are conformal.
2. are free of voids/pinhole defects.
3. are easily prepared.
4. are sterile when removed from the reactor.
5. produce a low amount of leachable substances.
6. demonstrate good adhesion to substrate.
7. allow unique film chemistries to be produced.
8. can be characterized relatively easily.

Due to these advantages, plasma treatment has been explored for polymeric, metallic and pyrolytic carbon-based biomaterials for use in a wide range of applications, including replacement heart valves, vascular grafts, contact lenses and even tissue culture dishes. However, as with any modification technique, disadvantages of plasma-based treatments also exist:

1. The chemistry within the reactor can be ill defined.
2. The equipment is often expensive.
3. Uniform reaction within long, narrow pores may be difficult.
4. Particular care must be taken in sample preparation to prevent contamination during or after processing.

Another important application of plasma technology uses an alternative configuration, called a plasma torch, to melt substances with high melting points, such as ceramics, and accelerate the molten particulates to a high velocity. Using this method, the torch can produce **plasma spray coatings**. This technique is commonly used in biomaterials to add ceramic coatings to metallic orthopedic or dental implants to improve their integration with the surrounding bone.

7.2.2.2 Chemical Vapor Deposition **Chemical vapor deposition** (CVD) is a surface treatment in which a mixture of gases is exposed to a sample at a high temperature.

This environment causes a variety of reactions resulting in the decomposition of one or more components of the gas mixture and subsequent deposition on the substrate. To form these coatings, equipment providing control of the gas sources, heating of the coating chamber, and means to dispose of waste gases is required. In order to reduce the reaction temperature, plasma environments are often used to increase the reactivity of the gaseous species. This is termed **plasma-assisted chemical vapor deposition.**

CVD techniques are most commonly used in biomaterials applications to deposit **pyrolytic carbon** coatings on substrates such as tantalum, molybdenum/rhenium or graphite. In this case, the gases are hydrocarbons and they undergo thermal decomposition, or **pyrolysis**, within the reaction chamber, allowing carbon deposition on the surface of the material.

7.2.2.3 Physical Vapor Deposition **Physical vapor deposition** (PVD) results in surface coating via deposition of atoms generated through physical processes onto the sample. PVD techniques have been employed successfully for applications such as orthopedic implants, surgical tools, and orthodontic appliances. For example, metal alloy coatings have been deposited using this method to increase wear resistance of metallic hip implants.

This class of techniques includes sputtering and thermal evaporation, among others. We will focus in this section on sputtering techniques since they can be used for biomaterials surface modification, and are often employed to coat nonconductive samples with a thin layer of metal before imaging with an electron microscope (see Section 7.6.6. for a further description of electron microscopy).

Sputter deposition is a two-step process. First, energetic ions or atoms bombard a target material and transfer their momentum to atoms within the target. This causes the ejection of a certain number of target surface atoms. In the second step, the released target atoms strike the sample surface and condense to form a thin film. Both covalent and non-covalent coatings are possible via this method.

Like for CVD, there are also **plasma-assisted PVD** techniques in which the formation of plasma is used to create high-energy species to collide with the target. An example of such a process is shown in Fig. 7.3. Here, the target is held at a large negative potential compared to the sample to be coated. Under sufficient vacuum, this environment will initiate formation of plasma near the target, much like that which was described in Section 7.2.2.1. Species from the plasma then strike the target to release atoms that can be deposited on the substrate surface.

7.2.2.4 Radiation Grafting/Photografting Both **radiation grafting** and **photografting** form well-bonded surface coatings via similar mechanisms. The substrate is exposed to a radiation source of high energy, which forms reactive species at the surface to create covalent bonding of the coating to the underlying material. These methods are often employed to bind hydrogels to hydrophobic substrates. This technique also provides a means to easily tailor the properties of the coating since a mixture of monomers or other precursors can be used.

In one type of radiation grafting (**mutual irradiation**), the biomaterial substrate is placed in a monomer solution and then irradiated by electrons or gamma rays to produce the polymerized coating. Alternatively, the substrate may be irradiated at low temperature or in an inert atmosphere to stabilize the surface free radicals and then the sample is exposed to the coating precursors in a separate step. Another type of radiation grafting occurs in air rather than in an inert environment. In this case, reactive oxygen species such as peroxides are formed on the substrate surface as a result of the interaction between the radiating species and oxygen. Heating the

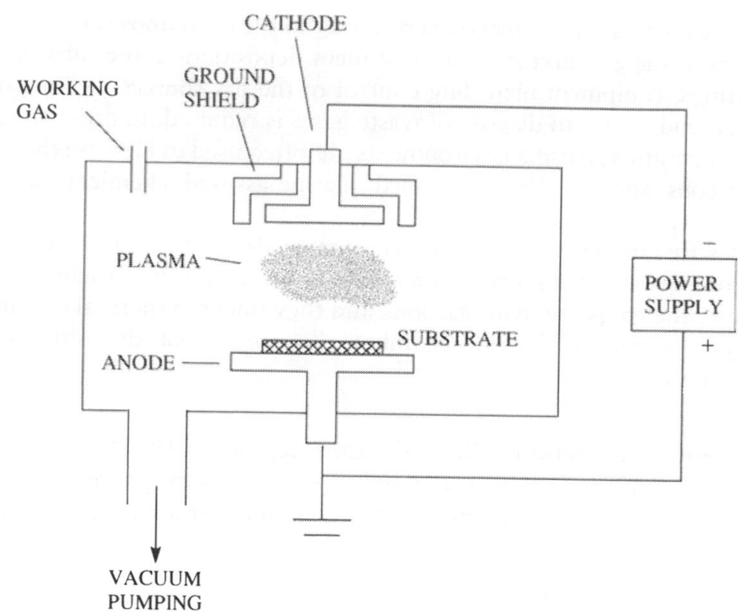

Figure 7.3 Schematic of a type of physical vapor deposition. The formation of plasma is used to create high-energy species which collide with the target in plasma-assisted physical vapor deposition. The target is held at a large negative potential compared to the sample to be coated. An environment of sufficient vacuum will initiate formation of plasma near the target. Species from the plasma then strike the target to release atoms that can be deposited on the substrate surface. (Adapted with permission from [2].)

substrate will further decompose the peroxides, leaving free radicals to initiate polymerization of the coating on the biomaterial.

Photografting is similar to radiation grafting, but, here, the radiation is UV or visible light. A number of photoresponsive chemical moieties have been developed to facilitate this type of surface modification. Two common methods involve either phenyl azide or benzophenone chemistry. If these functional groups are present in the coating precursor, they will be excited by exposure to the light and form free radicals or other reactive species. The activated molecules can then participate in reactions at the substrate surface resulting in covalent linkage of the coating to the underlying biomaterial.

7.2.2.5 Self-Assembled Monolayers Surface treatment using **self-assembled monolayers (SAMs)** is based on different principles than those coating methods described previously. In this technique, the molecules composing the coating are designed so that it is thermodynamically favorable for them to align on and form covalent bonds with the surface of the biomaterial. Therefore, in contrast to the previous treatment methods, no specialized equipment is required, and the modification can be carried out at room temperature and under normal atmospheric pressure.

Self-assembling molecules are **amphiphilic**, meaning they have both hydrophilic (polar) and hydrophobic (nonpolar) areas. These molecules possess three key regions, as depicted in Fig. 7.4:

1. Attachment group
2. Long hydrocarbon (alkyl) chain
3. Functional (polar) head group

Of these, both the attachment group and the nonpolar hydrocarbon chains play a large role in self-assembly. The functional group can be used to alter the hydrophobicity of the substrate material, or it can be a point of further chemical reaction to attach biologically active molecules, for example.

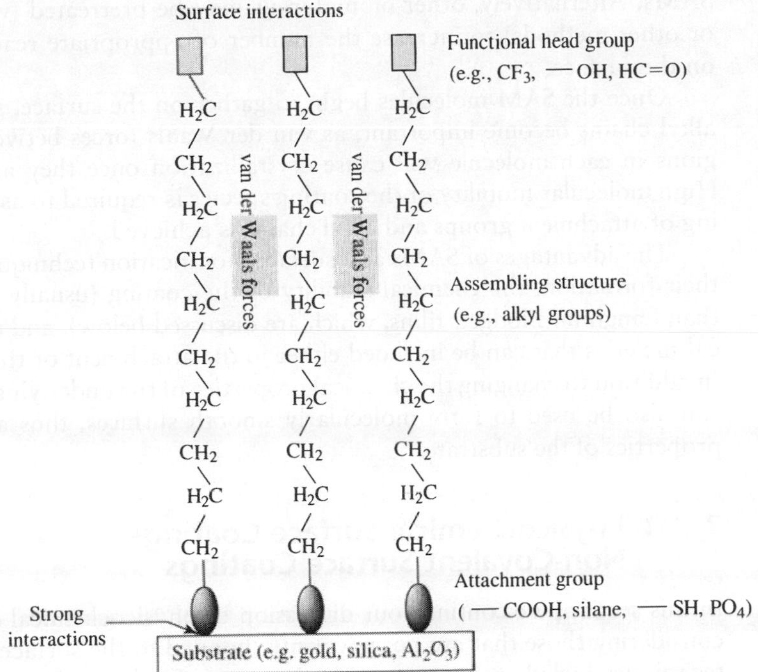

Figure 7.4
The three key regions of amphiphilic self-assembling molecules: the attachment group, a long hydrocarbon (alkyl) chain, and a functional (polar) head group. (Adapted with permission from [1].)

A strong, exothermic reaction between the substrate and the attachment group is the driving force for assembly. For example, silanes are commonly used attachment groups (Fig. 7.5) because they react readily with amine (NH_2) or hydroxyl (OH) groups. Therefore, materials containing large amounts of hydroxyl groups, such as glass and metal oxides, are preferred substrates for these types of

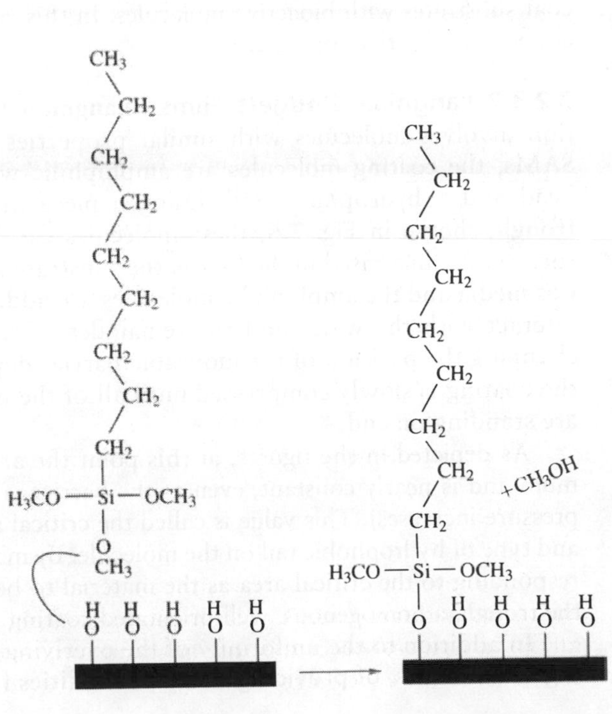

Figure 7.5
Self-assembly of alkyl silanes on substrates containing hydroxyl groups. A strong, exothermic reaction between the hydroxyl groups on the substrate and the silane attachment group is the driving force for self-assembly. (Adapted with permission from [1].)

SAMs. Alternatively, other biomaterials may be pretreated (via plasma discharge or other methods) to increase the number of appropriate reactive groups present on the surface.

Once the SAM molecules begin to gather on the surface, the properties of the alkyl chains become important, as van der Waals forces between the nonpolar regions in each molecule will cause crystallization once they are sufficiently close. High molecular mobility of the coating species is required to assure that tight packing of attachment groups and alkyl chains is achieved.

The advantages of SAMs as a surface modification technique include the ease of their formation, the chemical stability of the coating (usually significantly greater than Langmuir-Blodgett films, which are discussed below), and the variety of chemical moieties that can be included either in the attachment or the functional groups. In addition to changing the chemical properties of the underlying biomaterial, SAMs can also be used to form molecularly smooth surfaces, thus altering the physical properties of the substrate.

7.2.3 Physicochemical Surface Coatings: Non-Covalent Surface Coatings

In this section, we continue our discussion of physicochemical coating methods by considering those that are not covalently bonded to the surface. Examples of these techniques include solution coating, Langmuir-Blodgett films, and surface-modifying additives. Such procedures have also been employed to coat biologically active molecules on biomaterials (see Section 7.3 of this chapter).

7.2.3.1 Solution Coatings The least complex of the surface modification procedures producing coatings that are not covalently bound to the biomaterial surface are **solution coating** methods. In this technique, the substrate is dipped in a solution containing the dissolved coating material (usually a polymer dissolved in an organic solvent). The substrate is then left to dry and, as the solvent evaporates, the coating is deposited on the surface. This method can also be employed as a simple means to coat substrates with bioactive molecules. In this case, however, the solvent is often aqueous rather than organic.

7.2.3.2 Langmuir-Blodgett Films **Langmuir-Blodgett film (LB film)** deposition involves molecules with similar properties as those used for SAMs. Like SAMs, the coating molecules are amphiphilic with two regions—a hydrophilic head and a hydrophobic tail. Using a piece of equipment called a **Langmuir trough**, shown in Fig. 7.6, these molecules can be transferred to a biomaterial surface. As illustrated in the figure, the substrate to be coated is placed into aqueous media and the amphiphilic molecules are added so that the polar head groups interact with the water and the remainder of the molecule rests in the air. By changing the position of the moveable barrier depicted in the right of the figure, the coating is slowly compressed until all of the molecules are orientated so they are standing on end.

As depicted in the figures, at this point the area per molecule reaches a minimum and is nearly constant, even as the barrier is further compressed (the surface pressure increases). This value is called the **critical area** and is a function of the size and type of hydrophobic tail on the molecule. By maintaining a surface pressure corresponding to the critical area as the material to be coated is slowly removed from the trough, a homogenous, well-orientated coating can be deposited.

In addition to the uniformity of the overlying layer, LB films have the advantage, like SAMs, of providing many possibilities for altering the chemistry of the

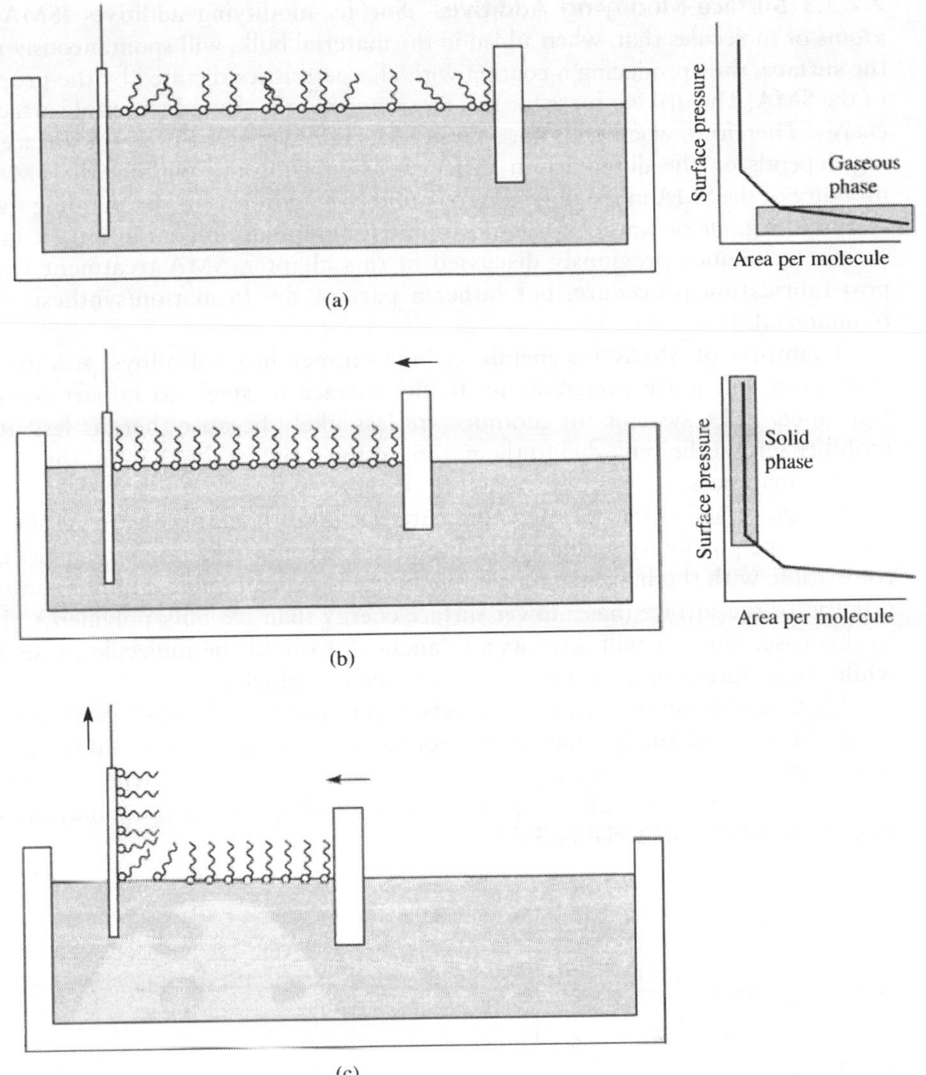

Figure 7.6
A Langmuir trough, used for Langmuir-Blodgett film deposition. In this process, coating molecules that are amphiphilic (have a hydrophilic head and a hydrophobic tail) are transferred to a biomaterial surface using a Langmuir trough. (a) As illustrated in the figure, the substrate to be coated is placed into aqueous media and the amphiphilic molecules are added so that the polar head groups interact with the water and the remainder of the molecule rests in the air. (b) By changing the position of the moveable barrier, the coating is slowly compressed until all of the molecules are orientated so they are standing on end. (c) At this point, the area per molecule reaches a minimum and is nearly constant, even as the barrier is further compressed (the surface pressure increases). This value is called the critical area and is a function of the size and type of hydrophobic tail on the molecule. By maintaining a surface pressure corresponding to the critical area as the material to be coated is slowly removed from the trough, a homogenous, well orientated coating can be deposited. (Adapted with permission from [1].)

coating molecules. A major disadvantage is the relative instability of the coating, due in large part to the fact that it is not chemically bonded to the surface. The addition of moieties on the head groups of the LB coatings to allow for crosslinking to other coating molecules or to the biomaterial surface is one way to overcome this limitation.

7.2.3.3 Surface-Modifying Additives Surface-modifying additives (SMAs) are atoms or molecules that, when added in the material bulk, will spontaneously rise to the surface, thus producing a coating with characteristics dictated by the properties of the SMA. The driving force for this rearrangement is the reduction of surface free energy. Therefore, whether or not a given SMA is effective at forming a surface coating depends on the difference in surface tension with and without the SMA, the mobility of the SMA in the bulk material, and the environment surrounding the biomaterial (e.g. air or water). It should be noted here that, unlike the surface modification techniques previously discussed in this chapter, SMA treatment is not a post-fabrication procedure, but rather a part of the formation/synthesis of the biomaterial.

Examples of SMAs for metals include copper in gold alloys. Additionally, chromium will move preferentially to the surface of steels to impart corrosion resistance. SMA systems for ceramics are less likely because there is less atomic mobility within the bulk due to the nature of the ionic bonds that are found within these materials.

Design of SMAs for polymeric biomaterials is considerably easier. As shown in Fig. 7.7, one possibility would be the use of a block copolymer in which block A is compatible with the bulk polymer, while block B is incompatible and possesses an affinity for the surface (has a lower surface energy than the bulk polymer/A block). In this case, block A will serve as an "anchor" to hold the molecule in the bulk, while the surface characteristics will be provided by block B.

With all of these systems, care must be taken to design the SMAs with consideration of the final (usually aqueous) environment of biomaterials. An additive with a large hydrophobic group may spontaneously move to the surface when the material is in contact with air, but after implantation in a hydrophilic milieu, it may favor the more hydrophobic material bulk.

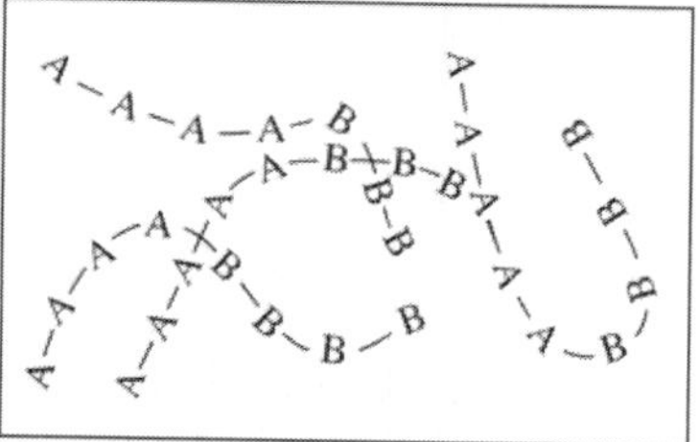

During fabrication

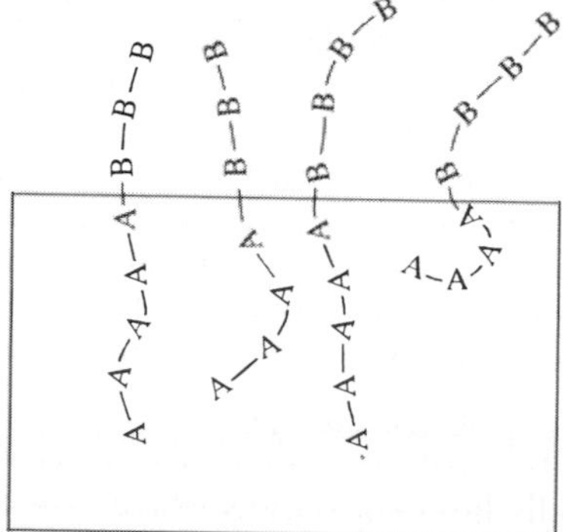

Post-fabrication

Figure 7.7
A depiction of the use of surface-modifying additives in a polymeric material. In this example the additive is a block copolymer in which block A is compatible with the bulk polymer, while block B is incompatible and possesses an affinity for the surface (has a lower surface energy than the bulk polymer/A block). Block A then serves as an "anchor" to hold the molecule in the bulk, while the surface characteristics will be provided by block B, as seen in the post-fabrication diagram. (Adapted with permission from [1].)

7.2.4 Physicochemical Surface Modification Methods with No Overcoat

This section addresses physicochemical modification methods that alter the surface properties of biomaterials without the formation of a separate coating. These techniques are designed to modify existing atoms at the surface, but not attach a distinct coating layer. However, similar results (changes in surface hydrophobicity, protein affinity, or wear resistance, for example) may be obtained though various types of physicochemical modification methods, with some techniques performing more optimally in certain types of material systems.

7.2.4.1 Ion Beam Implantation **Ion beam implantation** is a process whereby accelerated ions with high energies are directed at the surface of a biomaterial. This method is usually employed for metals and ceramics, although some work with polymers has been undertaken. Because the ions are very energetic, there is a high probability that they will penetrate into the surface (Fig. 7.8).

As the ion interacts with the material surface, there are many possible results. Formation of a cascade of vacancies and interstitials is triggered, with each atom

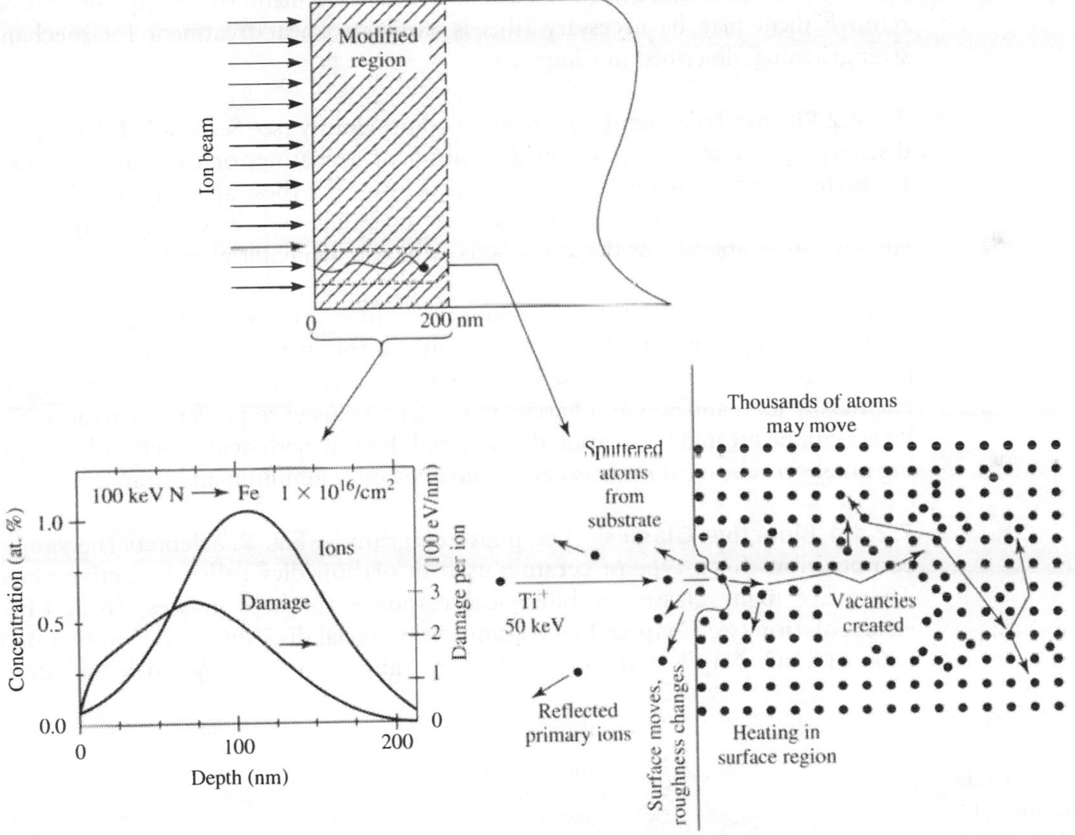

Figure 7.8
Schematic representation of ion beam implantation. Ions with high energy states are projected at the surface of the material at high speed, where they break the surface. Once within the material, some atoms from the material are ejected, while others collide with each other and create vacancies and changes within the crystal structure. Using different ions at various concentrations can alter the degree of modification. (Adapted with permission from [1] and [3].)

usually displaced several times before slowing to rest in a new location. At the same time, atoms may be sputtered from the substrate due to the high energy of the bombarding ions. Such changes can affect the overall surface roughness of the sample. Localized heating at the surface also occurs, which can alter crystal structure or kinetics of defect formation in this area.

Although specifics regarding equipment for ion beam implantation are beyond the scope of this text, the procedure usually occurs through the formation of plasma from which the ion beam is extracted and focused on the sample. Examples of ion beam implantation for biomaterial applications include the addition of nitrogen to titanium to increase wear resistance and the implantation of boron and carbon into stainless steel to improve fatigue life. Since all of these materials are used in orthopedic implants, good wear and fatigue properties are crucial to success in their final applications.

One of the main advantages to ion beam implantation is that, because almost all elements can be subjected to ionization, there exists a variety of possibilities to affect properties such as hardness, wear, corrosion, and biocompatibility. However, much of what occurs in the sample during this procedure must be more fully understood before surfaces with very well controlled characteristics can be created. Additionally, vacancy and interstitial defects often remain after treatment, so subsequent heating to remove them may be necessary (this is similar to heat treatment for mechanical strengthening, described in Chapter 6).

7.2.4.2 Plasma Treatment As mentioned previously (see Section 7.2.2.1.), plasma discharge processes can result in deposition of a coating, or can alter the surface properties through etching and cleaning processes. For these applications, the plasma is created as described previously using an inert gas and the energy of the plasma species causes ablation as the atoms/ions strike the biomaterial surface.

7.2.4.3 Conversion Coatings Despite its name, a **conversion coating** is not an overlay coating, but a modification of atoms at the surface of a metallic implant to form an oxide layer. As discussed in Chapter 5, this very thin (5–500 nm) region is chemically inert and acts as a barrier to electron transfer to prevent corrosion. These layers can be created by treating the material directly with acid (steel) or by employing an electrochemical process called *anodization* (aluminum and titanium).

7.2.4.4 Bioactive Glasses The phase diagram in Fig. 7.9 depicts the range of compositions for a type of ceramic used in orthopedics called **bioactive glasses.** There are many classes of biological response to these glasses, from fibrous encapsulation (see Chapter 11) to complete material dissolution, depending on the ratio of CaO, Na_2O, and SiO_2 used in the fabrication. The I_B index included on

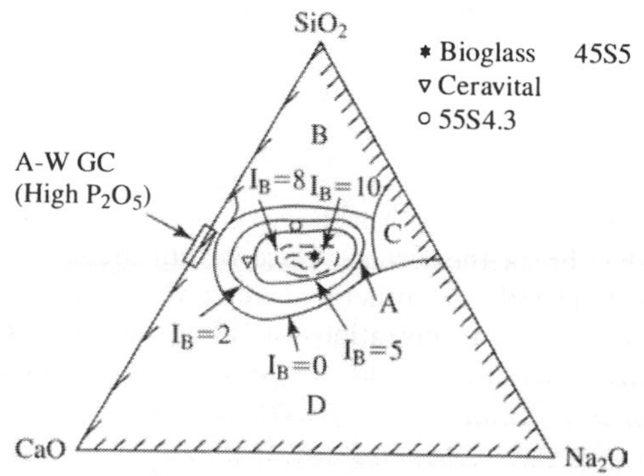

Figure 7.9
A phase diagram depicting the range of compositions for bioactive glasses, often used as orthopedic biomaterials. The I_B index is a measurement of the bioactivity of these materials, with a higher number indicating that the material integrates with the surrounding bone more quickly. (Adapted with permission from [4].)

the diagram is a measurement of the bioactivity of these materials, with a higher number indicating that the material is integrated with the surrounding bone more quickly.

Certain compositions of bioactive glasses cause coating of the surfaces with layers of CaO/P_2O_5 and SiO_2 under physiological conditions. This protective layer allows calcium-phosphate films to precipitate on the material and promote bonding with the native bone, thus increasing the I_B of that formulation. Therefore, this is an example of another surface treatment strategy: *in vivo* modification of a bulk material to produce a surface-active layer.

7.2.5 Laser Methods for Surface Modification

In many cases, *lasers* can be used to carry out the previously mentioned surface modifications. By focusing a high-powered light beam at the sample, a large amount of energy can be quickly deposited in a small area, which facilitates reactions such as annealing/alloying, etching, film deposition and polymerization at the surface.

When deciding on the laser source or treatment regime to perform a particular modification, one must consider whether a pulsed or continuous wave beam would be more appropriate, as well as the effects of possible surface heating by the laser. Much of this depends on the degree of laser energy absorption by the substrate and the amount of interfacial reflection and scattering.

The use of lasers in surface modification technology presents the advantages that treatment can often be performed at atmospheric conditions and with a wide range of very precise wavelengths. In addition, with this equipment there is specific control of reaction time as well as the spatial location of the excitation beam. Lasers also allow the use of a combination of heat and light-induced excitation to initiate the desired reaction.

7.3 Biological Surface Modification Techniques

Biological surface modification techniques involve attachment of biologically active molecules to a substrate through a variety of means, including many of the physicochemical methods described in the previous sections. The attached molecules are then free to interact with specific target areas on cells or other tissue components (these interactions are explained in detail in Chapter 9). Therefore, a primary concern with these techniques is that the molecule of interest remain attached while maintaining its biological activity. Since many biologically based molecules are sensitive to changes in conformation, particular attention must be paid to the orientation and rotational ability of individual molecules after coating.

A list of the types of biomolecules used in surface modifications and their potential applications is found in Table 7.3. Although the specifics of many of these will be discussed in future chapters, biomolecules for surface treatment are often either proteins or carbohydrates derived from various tissues and are attached to facilitate interactions with certain cell types. Other major categories include nucleic acid derivatives (DNA or RNA) or drugs, which are added to the surface in order to alter specific cellular functions in a controlled manner.

Although biological modification of all types of biomaterials is possible, most of the work in this area has centered on polymeric substrates. Biomolecule attachment has been successfully achieved on soluble polymers, solid polymers, solid polymers containing pores to form three-dimensional scaffolds, and hydrogels.

TABLE 7.3

Types of Biomolecules Used in Surface Modifications and Applications

Enzymes	Bioreactors (industrial, bio-medical) Bioseparations Biosensors Diagnostic assays Biocompatible surfaces
Antibodies, peptides, and other affinity molecules	Biosensors Diagnostic assays Affinity separations Targeted drug delivery Cell culture
Drugs	Thrombo-resistant surfaccs Drug delivery systems
Lipids	Thrombo-resistant surfaces Albuminated surfaces
Nucleic acid derivatives and nucleotides	DNA probes Gene therapy

(Adapted with permission from [5].)

7.3.1 Covalent Biological Coatings

A range of immobilization technologies exist, including both covalent and non-covalent means to link the biomolecule and the substrate. A few of these techniques will be discussed here to provide an overview of the types of reactions commonly employed for immobilization. Like physicochemical techniques, covalently linked coatings may impart additional stability and thus are preferred in many applications. However, they require the presence of a reactive substrate surface, often containing hydroxyl (OH), carboxyl (COOH), or amine (NH_2) groups. If these are not found on the chosen biomaterial surface, it may be modified (via plasma discharge, for example) to add appropriate functionality before proceeding with the reaction.

Figure 7.10 depicts several schemes for covalent attachment of biomolecules. In any of these, the molecule can be bound to the substrate directly or by a **spacer arm**, which is an inert molecule that provides physical space between the biomolecule and the substrate. The spacer arm may allow for greater rotational freedom and thus improve the activity of the biological molecule. In addition, it is possible to design biodegradable spacer arms to release the biomolecule in a localized region after biomaterial implantation.

Biomolecules may be attached to a substrate surface using post-fabrication reactions, as shown in Fig. 7.10(a–c), or may be included as part of the material synthesis [Fig. 7.10(d–e)]. In the former case, a type of binding agent is often used to facilitate interaction of the molecule with the surface. The binding agent can then remain as “glue” or catalyze the reaction and be released. For combined conjugation/synthesis reactions, there are two main methods: (1) The biomolecule may be bound to a precursor (monomer) that is then polymerized in three dimensions or as a surface coating [Fig. 7.10(d)]. (2) An activated precursor containing groups

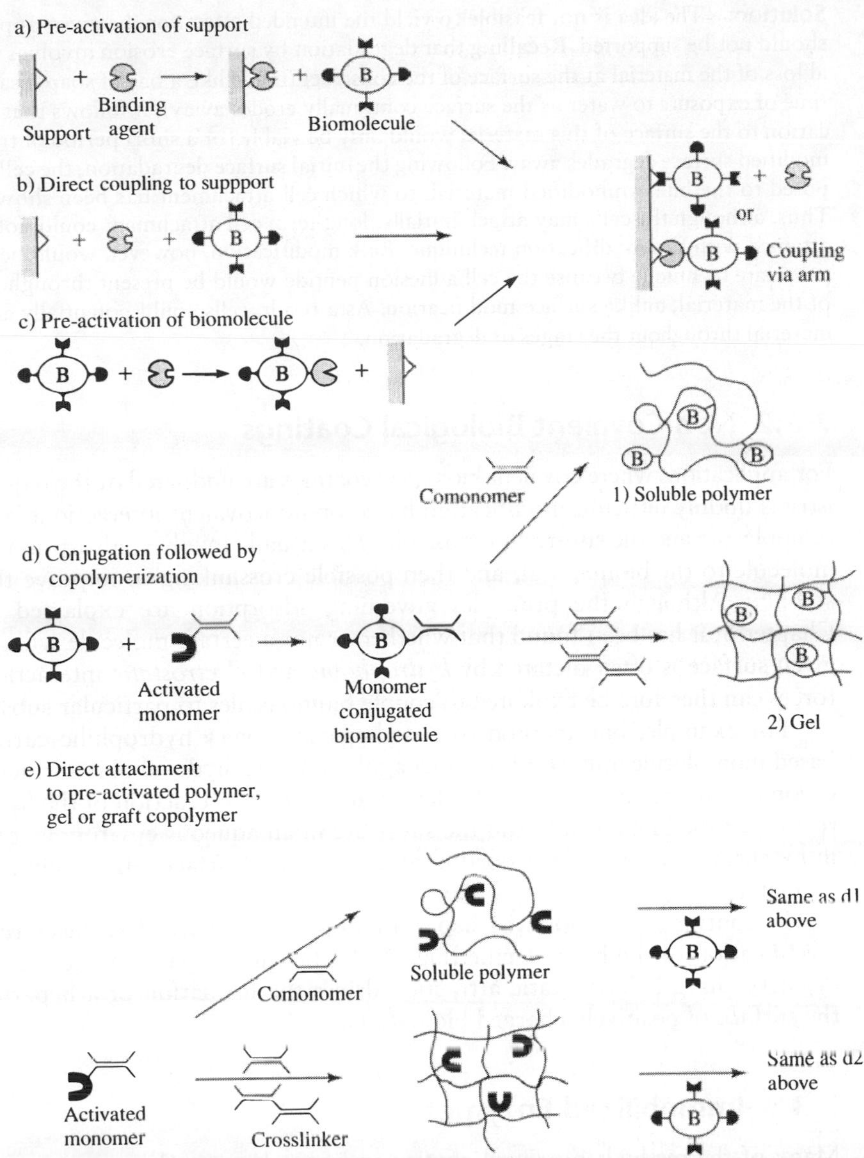

Figure 7.10 Methods for the covalent attachment of biomolecules to a biomaterial surface. (a–c) attachment via postfabrication methods, (d–e) attachment during synthesis. The biomolecule (B) may be attached with or without a spacer arm in any of these methods. (Adapted with permission from [5].)

with affinity for the biomolecule is polymerized and the formed biomaterial is subsequently exposed to the molecule of interest [Fig. 7.10(e)].

EXAMPLE PROBLEM 7.2

A researcher has created a biodegradable polymeric implant material that degrades through a surface erosion mechanism. The material is intended to serve as a tissue engineering scaffold, in which long-term cell adhesion to the material is important. Initial studies have found that cells will not adhere to the surface of the material. The researcher is considering covalent attachment [with a poly(ethylene glycol) spacer of 3400 Da] of a peptide sequence known to improve cell attachment to other materials to the surface of this material. The researcher asks if you support the idea. Will you support the idea? Why or why not? Would bulk modification with the peptide sequence be a more or less appropriate method of modification for the intended result?

Solution: The idea is not feasible to yield the intended effect for the given application and should not be supported. Recalling that degradation by surface erosion involves the continual loss of the material at the surface of the construct (much like a bar of soap disappears with time of exposure to water as the surface continually erodes away), it follows that any modification to the surface of this material would only be viable for a short period of time until the modified surface degrades away. Following the initial surface degradation, the cells will be exposed to the bulk unmodified material, to which cell attachment has been shown to be nil. Thus, although the cells may attach initially, long-term cell attachment could not feasibly be attained with this modification technique. Bulk modification, however, would be a more appropriate technique because the cell adhesion peptide would be present throughout the bulk of the material, unlike surface modification. As a result, cells could potentially attach to the material throughout the stages of degradation. ■

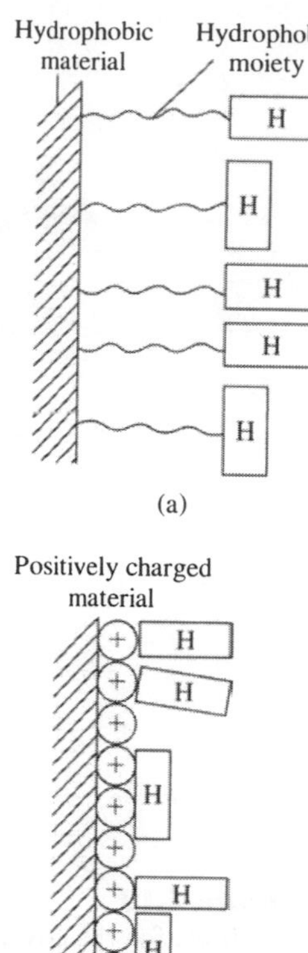

Figure 7.11
Two methods for coating a surface with heparin, a hydrophilic biomolecule. (a) A hydrophobic region is added to the heparin. Thus, interaction of the hydrophobic regions of the biomolecule and the substrate in an aqueous environment will result in extension of the heparin portion away from the surface, effectively coating the biomaterial. (b) The adsorption of heparin to positively charged surfaces requires no modification of the biomolecule. Because heparin possesses significant negative charge, electrostatic attraction drives the formation of a heparin layer at the surface of positively charged biomaterials. (Adapted with permission from [5] and [6].)

7.3.2 Non-Covalent Biological Coatings

For applications where covalent biological coatings are undesired or the required chemistry is unduly difficult, modification based on noncovalent interactions between the biomolecule and the substrate is possible. This usually involves adsorption of the biomolecule to the biomaterial, and then possible crosslinking to improve the coating stability. Although the principles governing adsorption are explained further in Chapter 8, it has been found that whether or not a certain molecule will gather at a given surface is often dictated by *hydrophobic* and *electrostatic* interactions. These forces can therefore be exploited to couple biomolecules to particular substrates.

For example, one method to coat heparin, a very hydrophilic carbohydrate-based biomolecule important in anticoagulation, on a hydrophobic surface is the addition of a hydrophobic region to the heparin. Thus, interaction of the hydrophobic regions of the biomolecule and the substrate in an aqueous environment will result in extension of the heparin portion away from the surface, effectively coating the biomaterial (Fig. 7.11).

In contrast, adsorption of heparin to positively charged surfaces requires no modification of the biomolecule (Fig. 7.11). Because heparin possesses significant negative charge, electrostatic attraction drives the formation of a heparin layer at the surface of positively charged biomaterials.

7.3.3 Immobilized Enzymes

Many of the methods discussed above can be used to attach enzymes to solid substrates (carriers). This process, called **enzyme immobilization**, has been highly developed over the past 50 years and now has a variety of applications in such areas as biosensors, controlled release devices, and protein analysis. As discussed further in Chapter 9, enzymes are a subclass of proteins that act to promote specific chemical reactions involving other biomolecules. Regardless of the application, because the function of the device depends on the action of the enzyme, the bioactivity of this molecule is of utmost importance. Thus, much research has been devoted to immobilization techniques, which range from simple adsorption to more complex mechanisms involving covalent linkages with spacer arms. Both hydrophilic hydrogel carriers, such as poly(acrylamide) or poly(ethylene glycol), and hydrophobic carriers, such as nylon or poly(styrene), have been explored, with optimal results dependent on the properties of the enzyme of interest.

An additional concern for these devices is that the biomolecule that the enzyme targets (its **substrate**) must be able to diffuse into the area to physically interact with the immobilized enzyme. Thus, the geometry of the carrier is crucial to allow a sufficiently large surface area for enzyme contact. Both parameters relating to the chemical activity of the enzyme and to the availability of substrate continue to be optimized to produce more efficient biomedical devices, such as glucose sensors, that depend on the actions of these immobilized enzymes to produce reliable readings.

7.4 Surface Properties and Degradation

Surface treatments are particularly susceptible to alteration caused by degradation, either of the surface coating itself, or of the underlying substrate. In some cases, such as conversion coatings, the surface treatment is designed as a method to decrease unwanted degradation (corrosion) of the underlying material. However, even in cases where controlled degradation of the bulk material is desired, such as for biodegradable polymers, the removal of the supporting material or actions of degradation reaction by-products may have significant deleterious effects on the surface coating. In extreme cases, such as surface-eroding materials, it may be impossible to find an effective, lasting surface treatment method.

7.5 Patterning Techniques for Surfaces

Surface or **substrate patterning** is a term that encompasses several methods developed to alter the surface properties of biomaterials in a controlled manner, resulting in a geometric design of well-defined regions with very different characteristics (Fig. 7.12). Surface patterning can be used with a variety of surface-active molecules, and common substrates include both metals and polymers. Two of the most widely used patterning techniques are microcontact printing and microfluidics.

In **microcontact printing**, a mold of the desired pattern is first created, often via photolithographic techniques on a silicon wafer (Fig. 7.13). A silicone rubber material [poly(dimethylsiloxane), PDMS] is then polymerized in the mold to make a positive "stamp." The stamp is "inked" with the surface-modifying substance by dipping it into a solution containing the molecule of interest, and the inked stamp is then pressed onto the substrate. After carefully removing the stamp, the biomaterialist can repeat the process to modify the portion of the substrate that was not stamped the first time, thus creating multifunctional surfaces

This technique has been employed successfully with physicochemical approaches such as SAMs to modify the hydrophilicity of portions of a surface, and it is

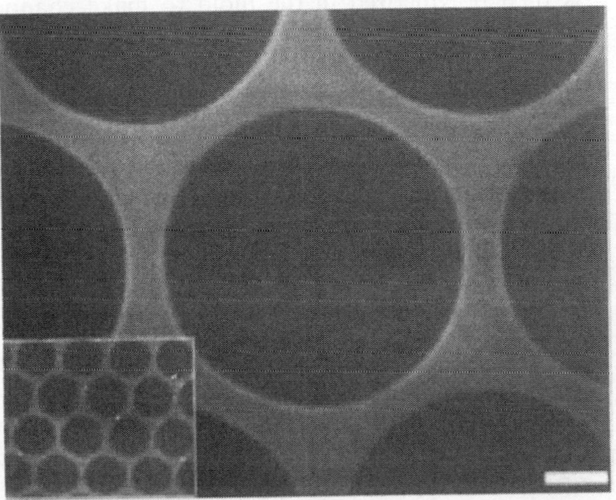

Figure 7.12
Surface substrate patterning can be used to alter the surface properties of a material in controlled, well-defined areas, as seen in the circular pattern in the photo. The inset presents a lower magnification view of the same surface. (Reprinted with permission from [7].)

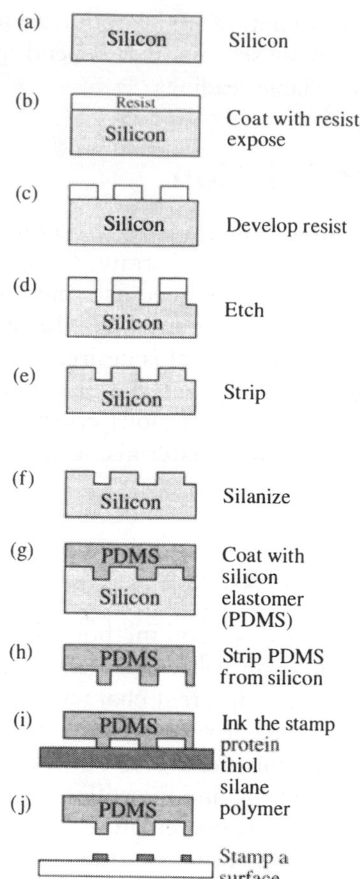

Figure 7.13
In microcontact printing, a mold of the desired pattern is first created, often via photolithographic techniques on a silicon wafer (a–e). A silicone rubber material (PDMS) is then polymerized in the mold to make a positive "stamp" (f–h). The stamp is "inked" with the surface-modifying substance by dipping it into a solution containing the molecule of interest (i) and the inked stamp is then pressed onto the substrate (j). After carefully removing the stamp, the process can be repeated to modify the portion of the substrate that was not stamped the first time, thus creating multifunctional surfaces. (Adapted with permission from [1].)

equally useful for biological modification methods. In this case, a biomaterial could be modified to expose one or more proteins with a well-controlled spatial orientation, thus potentially modulating cell attachment and improving interaction of the implant with the native tissue.

As depicted in Fig. 7.14, **microfluidics** employs many of the same materials as microcontact printing. For this technique, the mold is fabricated as described above, but the mold is a positive, rather than a negative, image of the desired design. PDMS is then polymerized in the mold to make channels where required. The formed PDMS is pressed against a glass slide and plasma-treated to increase the hydrophilicity of inner areas of the channels only, while the regions between channels remain hydrophobic to maintain the integrity of each channel.

Like for microcontact printing, the PDMS form is then pressed against the substrate and a small amount of a solution containing the molecule of interest is injected or placed near the opening of a channel. Capillary action pulls liquid through all the channels and the areas of the substrate under the channels are appropriately modified. After the molecule has reacted with the surface, the PDMS form is removed and the surface is rinsed.

As described above, it may be possible to produce multi-functional surfaces using this method by a series of treatments including different surface-active molecules. Similar to microcontact printing, this technique has been employed with a variety of both physicochemical and biological coating methods. A distinct advantage of this process is that it takes very little fluid volume, so it can be easily used with expensive or difficult-to-produce biologic reagents.

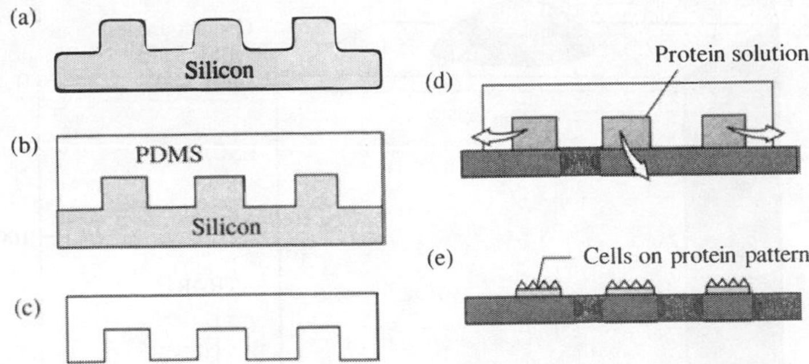

Figure 7.14
For the microfluidics technique, (a) the mold is fabricated as described in microcontact printing, but the mold is a positive, rather than a negative, image of the desired design. (b) PDMS is then polymerized in the mold. (c) The formed PDMS is then removed from the mold and pressed against a glass slide. This setup is then plasma-treated to increase the hydrophilicity of inner areas of the channels only, while the regions between channels remain hydrophobic to maintain the integrity of each channel. Like for microcontact printing, (d) the PDMS form is then pressed against the substrate and a small amount of a solution containing the molecule of interest is injected or placed near the opening of a channel, where capillary action pulls the liquid throughout the channels. The areas of the substrate under the channels are appropriately modified. (e) After the molecule has reacted with the surface, the PDMS form is removed and the surface is rinsed. (Adapted with permission from [7] and [8].)

7.6 Techniques: Introduction to Surface Characterization

Surface characterization of biomaterials is important, both to determine the quality of the surface treatments described in this chapter and also to provide information about the extent of protein adsorption to a material. Because surfaces are chemically active, many surface techniques require special preparation equipment or conditions such as high vacuum to prevent contamination.

As depicted in Fig. 7.15, there are surface characterization methods that record data from various depths. We begin our discussion in this section with the simplest, least expensive techniques for general surface analysis, including contact angle analysis and light microscopy. Surface spectroscopic techniques, which involve the absorption of electromagnetic radiation by the material, are then treated in order of descending energy (electron spectroscopy for chemical analysis and attenuated total internal reflectance Fourier-transform infrared spectroscopy). A modification of mass spectrometry for surface analysis (secondary ion mass spectrometry) and, finally, more advanced methods for obtaining topographical information (electron microscopy and scanning probe microscopy) are also described. A summary of each of these surface analysis methods is found in Table 7.4.

7.6.1 Contact Angle Analysis

7.6.1.1 Basic Principles Contact angle analysis is often used to provide overall information about the hydrophobicity of a surface. The surface free energy or surface tension (γ) of a material can be defined thermodynamically as the work of making a unit area of new surface. In most contact angle experiments, a system with three interfaces (and corresponding γ values) is created (Fig. 7.16)—the liquid-vapor surface (γ_{LV}), the solid-liquid surface (γ_{SL}), and the solid-vapor surface (γ_{SV}). In most cases, the liquid chosen for testing of biomedical materials is water. The energetics at each

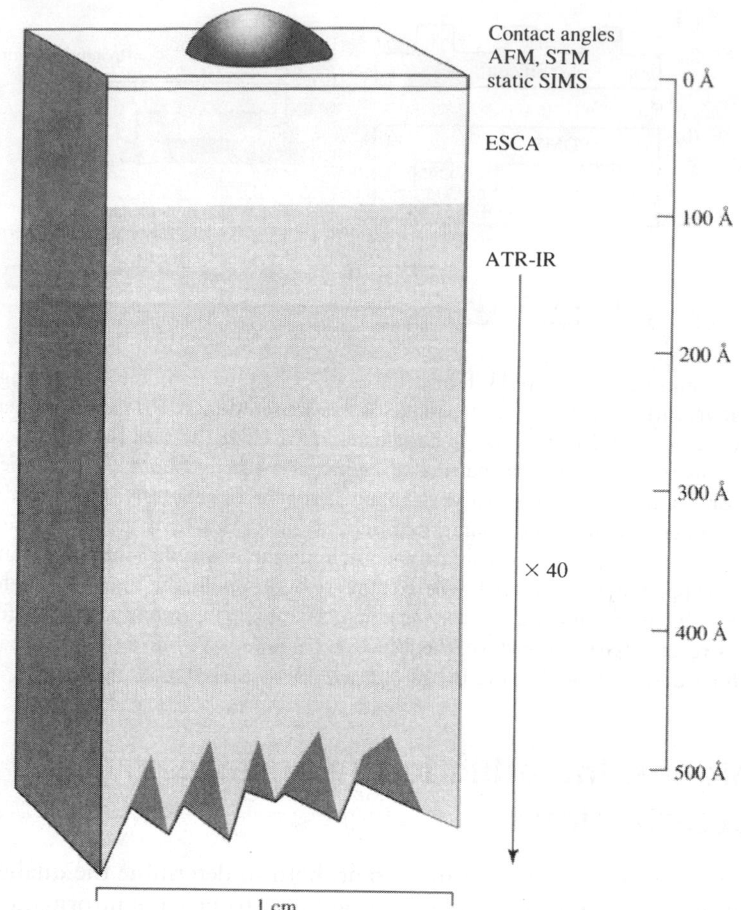

Figure 7.15
Surface penetration of various surface analysis methods. Some surface analysis techniques actually penetrate relatively deeply into the bulk of the material. (Adapted with permission from [9].)

TABLE 7.4

Characterization Methods for Biomaterial Surfaces

Method	Principle	Depth Analyzed	Spatial Resolution	Analytical Sensitivity	Cost[c]
Contact angles	Liquid wetting of surfaces is used to estimate the energy of surfaces	3–20 Å	1 mm	Low or high depending on the chemistry	$
ESCA (XPS)	X-rays induce the emission of electrons of characteristic energy	10–250 Å	10–150 μm	0.1 atom %	$$$
Auger electron spectroscopy[a]	A focused electron beam stimulates the emission of Auger electrons	50–100 Å	100 Å	0.1 atom %	$$$
SIMS	Ion bombardment sputters secondary ions from the surface	10 Å–1 μm[b]	100 Å	Very high	$$$
FTIR-ATR	IR radiation is adsorbed and excites molecular vibrations	1–5 μm	10 μm	1 mol %	$$
STM	Measurement of the quantum tunneling current between a metal tip and a conductive surface	5 Å	1 Å	Single atoms	$$
SEM	Secondary electron emission induced by a focused electron beam is spatially imaged	5 Å	40 Å, typically	High, but not quantitative	$$

[a] Auger electron spectroscopy is damaging to organic materials and is best used for inorganics.
[b] Static SIMS ≈ 10 Å, dynamic SIMS to 1 μm
[c] $, up to $5000; $$, $5000–$100,000; $$$, >$100,000.
(Adapted with permission from [10].)

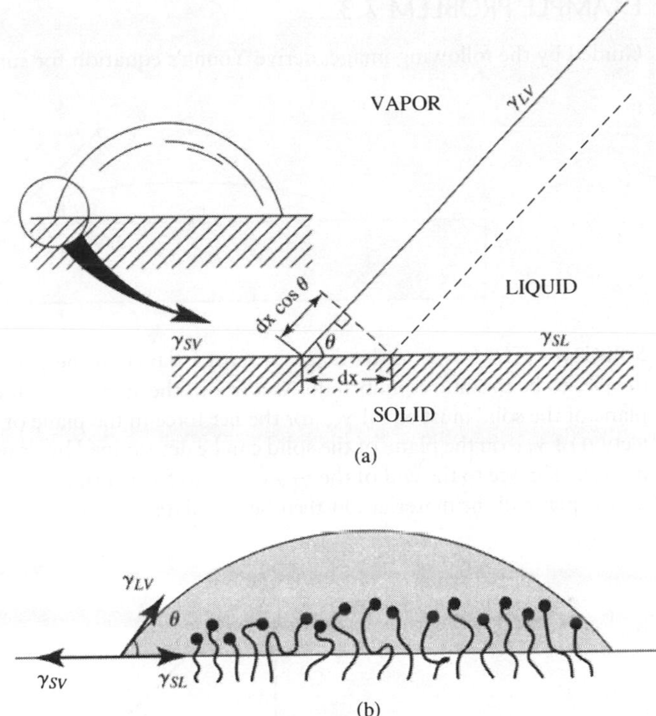

Figure 7.16
(a) Schematic of contact angle testing. Around the water droplet, there are three important interfaces: liquid-vapor (γ_{LV}), solid-liquid (γ_{SL}), and solid-vapor (γ_{SV}). (Adapted with permission from [11].) (b) Change in wettability via surface modification. The water droplet spreads more on the modified surface because the modification decreases the surface tension of the liquid/solid interface, thus reducing the contact angle as calculated using Young's equation (7.1). (Adapted with permission from [12].)

of the interfaces causes the water droplet to assume a particular shape (different degree of spreading). Therefore, by accurately measuring the angle between the drop and the solid surface (the **contact angle, θ**), the surface tension can be calculated using the following equation, which represents a force balance between the horizontal components of three surface tensions (Young's equation, see Fig. 7.16):

$$\gamma_{SV} - \gamma_{SL} - \gamma_{LV} \cos \theta = 0 \tag{7.1}$$

This equation contains two unknowns, γ_{SV} and γ_{SL}. γ_{SV} is often approximated using the critical surface tension (γ_c), as developed by **Zisman**. γ_c is determined by testing the material using various liquids with a range of γ_{LV} values. A plot of contact angle vs. γ_{LV} is generated and extrapolated to $\theta = 0$ (complete spreading on the surface). The value of γ_{LV} at this point is called γ_c. This is illustrated pictorially in Fig. 7.17.

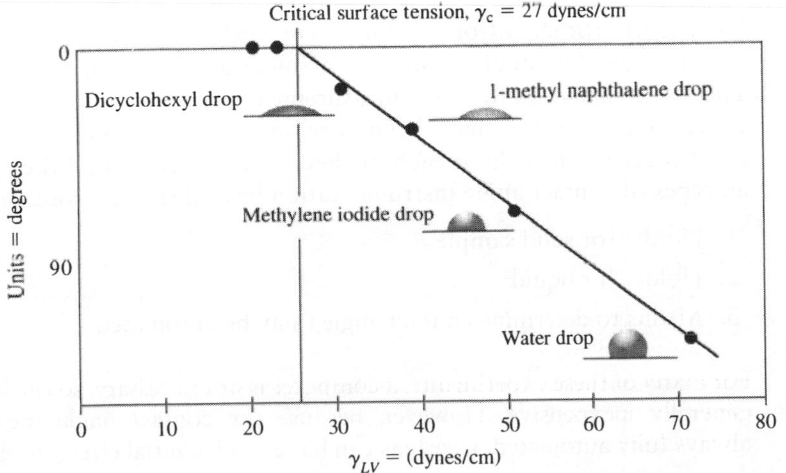

Figure 7.17
Diagram showing how the critical surface tension (γ_c) is determined. The contact angle of various liquids is measured for a specific material, and a plot of contact angle versus γ_{LV} is generated. The extrapolated value of γ_{LV} at $\theta = 0$ is γ_c. (Adapted with permission from [10].)

EXAMPLE PROBLEM 7.3

Guided by the following image, derive Young's equation for surface tension:

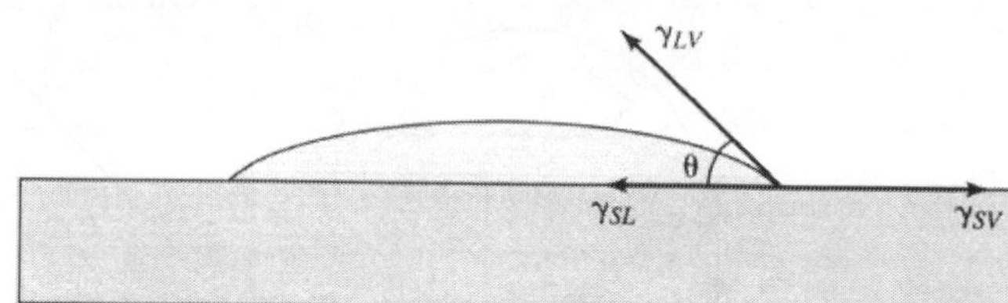

Solution: The forces in the diagram must balance in the plane of the solid material for the droplet to be in static equilibrium. As a result, the sum of γ_{SL} and the projection of γ_{LV} on the plane of the solid must equal γ_{SV} for the net force in the plane of the material to be 0. The projection of γ_{LV} on the plane of the solid can be determined by drawing a perpendicular from the material surface to the end of the γ_{LV} vector to form a right triangle. The projection (p) of γ_{LV} on the plane of the material can then be calculated as follows:

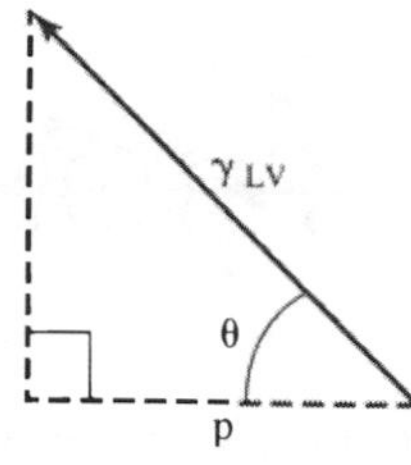

$$\cos = \frac{\text{adjacent}}{\text{hypotenuse}}$$

$$\cos\theta = \frac{p}{\gamma_{LV}}$$

$$p = \gamma_{LV}\cos\theta$$

Consequently, the vectors can be balanced as follows to yield Young's equation:

$$\gamma_{SL} + \gamma_{LV}\cos\theta = \gamma_{SV}$$

$$\underline{\gamma_{SV} - \gamma_{SL} - \gamma_{LV}\cos\theta = 0}$$

■

7.6.1.2 Instrumentation Unlike many other characterization techniques, the output of contact angle analysis is a single number (θ or γ_c), rather than a plot. The instrumentation for these measurements is fairly straight-forward, but several experimental methods have been developed, as shown in Fig. 7.18. Although the exact mechanisms behind each of these methods is beyond the scope of this text, all types of contact angle instrumentation have these components in common:

1. Holder for solid sample
2. Holder for liquid
3. Means to determine contact angle (may be automated)

For many of these experiments, a computer is not necessary, so the instrumentation is generally inexpensive. However, because the contact angle measurement is not always fully automated, user bias can have a substantial effect on the results.

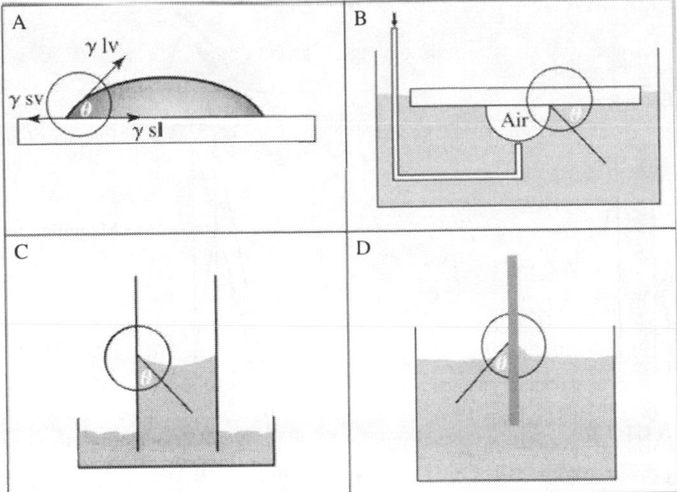

Figure 7.18
Different experimental setups for determining the contact angle: (a) sessile drop, (b) captive air bubble, (c) capillary rise method, and (d) Wilhelmy plate method. The circles indicate where the contact angle is measured. (Adapted with permission from [10].)

7.6.1.3 Information Provided Although contact angle data is widely available for most biomedical materials, this technique cannot provide detailed information about the chemical composition of the surface, so it is often used as a first step in surface characterization. **Dynamic contact angle measurements** are also used to measure **contact angle hysteresis.** In the most common of these measurements, water is slowly added to an area of the surface with a syringe and the **advancing contact angle** is measured. The water is then removed via the same mechanism and the **receding contact angle** is recorded. The difference between these two values represents the contact angle hysteresis for that material and describes how the surface tension of the material changes before and after it has been exposed to an aqueous environment. Hysteresis can occur for a variety of reasons. For example, hydrophilic domains within the material may become reorientated outward from the surface after contact with water, whereas they may be "hidden" within the bulk when exposed to hydrophobic environments such as air.

7.6.2 Light Microscopy

7.6.2.1 Basic Principles Light microscopy is a relatively simple technique that is used as a first approach to gain primarily qualitative information about surface topography, or to view thin sections of a sample. In one type of light microscope, the **compound microscope,** a white light source is projected through the sample, where the combination of ocular (in the eyepiece) and objective lenses reflect the light in such a manner as to magnify the sample many times, providing a detailed image of features usually undetectable to the naked eye. A diagram of the light path in such a microscope is found in Fig. 7.19.

For opaque samples, the light source can be located above rather than below the sample. The **resolution** of such instruments (distance under which two objects will appear as one) is limited by the wavelength of white light, and in most cases is around 0.2 μm. Therefore, features that are smaller than this, or that are more closely spaced than this, cannot be distinguished using this method.

7.6.2.2 Instrumentation Light microscopy images, like that found in Fig. 7.20, are widespread and have a variety of uses. Of particular interest in this chapter, surface topographical features on the order of microns can be imaged via this

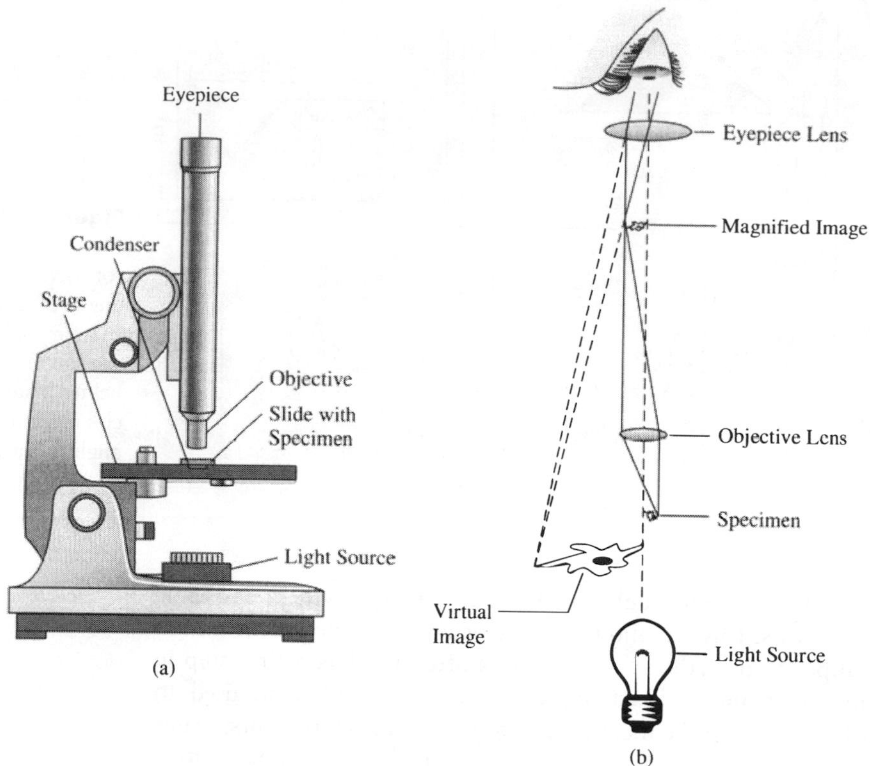

Figure 7.19
(a) Gross image of a compound microscope. On a compound microscope, the light source is placed below the specimen and the specimen is viewed from above. (b) Light path of a compound microscope. The objective forms a magnified image of the object that is larger than the original object. This image is then magnified many times by the eyepiece to form the large (inverted) virtual image.

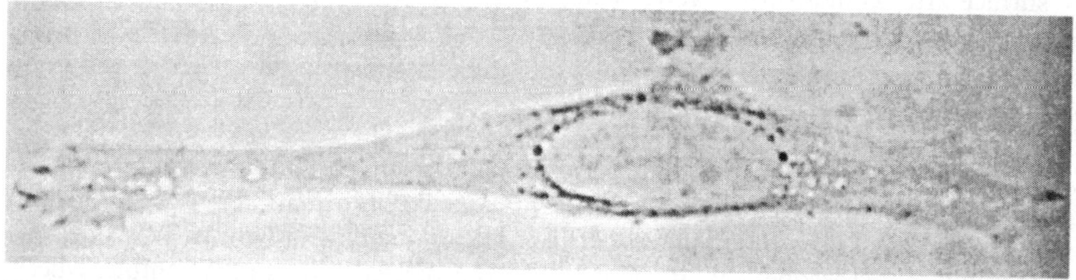

Figure 7.20
Sample of a light microscopy image, in this case, a fibroblast attached to a substrate. (Reprinted with permission from [13].)

technique (Fig. 7.21). As shown in Fig. 7.22, there are four basic components to a light microscope:

1. Source—produces white light.
2. Lenses—glass lenses focus light beam and/or magnify image of sample.
3. Sample stage—holds sample securely.
4. Detector (camera or human eye)—views and captures resulting image.

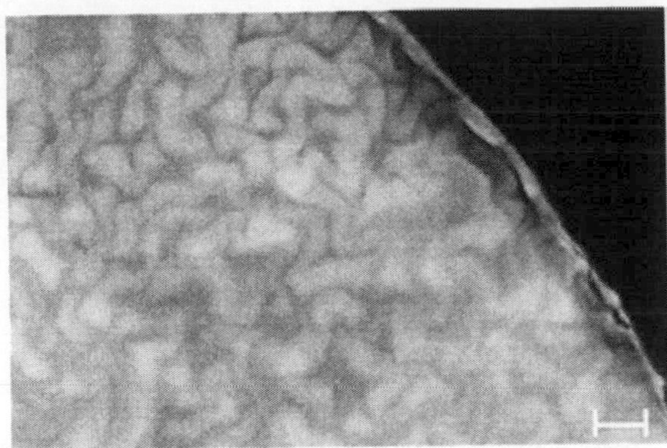

Figure 7.21
Surface topographical ridges as seen on a polymer surface. The sample is viewed via a particular type of light microscopy called *fluorescence microscopy*. Scale bar is 200 μm. (Reprinted with permission from [14].)

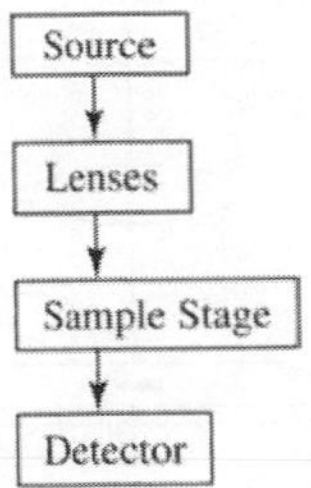

Figure 7.22
Block diagram of the components of a light microscope, which include the source, lenses, sample stage, and detector (camera or human eye).

If a camera is used as the detector, the image can be stored on a computer for further image analysis.

As illustrated in Fig. 7.23, the sample surface (or a thin section from the bulk) is placed on the stage. The condenser lens focuses the light beam before it passes through the sample. After the light exits the specimen, the objective and ocular lenses act in concert to magnify the sample image. The image can then be either directed to a camera or viewed directly through the eyepiece.

7.6.2.3 Information Provided Light microscopy is used exclusively for imaging, and provides in itself only qualitative assessment. Images can be further analyzed using specialized software to obtain semi-quantitative measures of certain colors or other user-defined parameters. In addition to imaging surface topography, this instrument is extremely important in histological analysis for biocompatibility assessment (discussed further in the second half of this text). Briefly, serial sections of a sample containing, for example, both the biomaterial and surrounding tissue after *in vivo* implantation, are taken, stained, and viewed through a light microscope to determine the extent of the inflammatory response to the implant.

While light microscopy has the advantage that vacuum is not required to view samples, it remains difficult to see thick or hydrated samples, so relating images directly to what would be seen *in vivo* is not possible. In addition, light microscopy remains a first approach to imaging, particularly for sample surface features, due to its limited spatial resolution.

7.6.3 Electron Spectroscopy for Chemical Analysis (ESCA) or X-ray Photoelectron Spectroscopy (XPS)

7.6.3.1 Basic Principles As mentioned in Chapter 2, X-rays are a type of very high energy electromagnetic radiation used as a source in ESCA (also called XPS) analysis of material surfaces. In this type of spectroscopy, X-ray absorption causes the removal of an electron from one of the innermost atomic orbitals (not the valence shell). The kinetic energy of the emitted electron is then recorded. Measurement of the kinetic energy of this ejected electron separates this technique

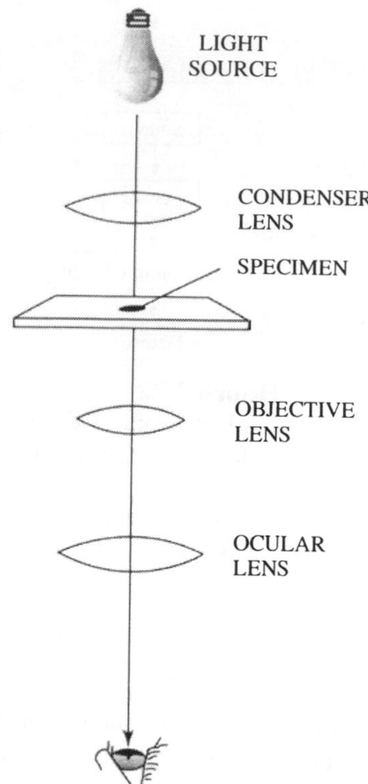

Figure 7.23
Light path through a light microscope. The sample surface (or a thin section from the bulk) is placed on the stage. The condenser lens focuses the light beam before it passes through the sample. The objective and ocular lenses act in concert to magnify the sample image from the light that exits the specimen. The image can then be viewed directly through the eyepiece or directed to a camera. (Adapted with permission from [13].)

from other types of X-ray spectroscopy, such as X-ray fluorescence, which is discussed later in the section on electron microscopy, and Auger electron spectroscopy, which is beyond the scope of this book. Table 7.5 summarizes the distinctions between X-ray methods.

From the kinetic energy (E_k), the binding energy (E_b) of the electron can be calculated as

$$E_b = h\nu - E_k \tag{7.2}$$

where ν is the frequency and h is the Planck's constant (6.6×10^{-34} J-s). Since the electrons are attracted to and held in place by the positively-charged nucleus, the more they can feel the effects of the positive charge [either because they are located closer to the nucleus or because there are more positive charges in the nucleus (higher atomic number)], the larger their binding energy. Therefore, the binding energy gives an idea of how tightly bound the electron is to the nucleus, and it changes in accordance with the type of atom as well as interactions with the nuclei of neighboring atoms.

ESCA is often used to identify elements present at the surface of a material. Its analytical capabilities are limited to the uppermost ~100 Å of a sample because the energy of the emitted electrons allows escape from only the first few atomic layers.

7.6.3.2 Instrumentation A typical ESCA spectrum of poly(dimethyl siloxane) is found in Fig. 7.24. ESCA spectra are generally plotted as electron count (y-axis) as a function of binding energy (x-axis). As shown in Fig. 7.25, there are four basic components to an electron spectrometer:

TABLE 7.5

Summary of the Differences Between X-ray Techniques

X-ray diffraction	Interaction between X-rays and electrons of the sample material causes X-ray scattering. The angle of scattering gives information about the crystal structure of the material.
Electron spectroscopy for chemical analysis (ESCA)	Exposure of a sample to X-rays causes the removal of core electrons with a certain kinetic energy. From this, the binding energy, which gives information about the chemical composition of the material, can be calculated. The kinetic energy of ejected Auger electrons maybe detected as an artifact.
X-ray fluorescence	Exposure of the sample to an electron beam or X-ray causes the removal of a core electron and formation of an ion. The ion can return to its ground state as one of the outer electrons falls into the vacancy, and, in the process, X-rays of a certain wavelength that is characteristic for that atom are emitted. It is often used in biomaterial analysis as an addition to electron microscopy to determine the composition of a sample that has been imaged.
Auger electron spectroscopy	Exposure of the sample to an electron beam or X-ray causes the removal of a core electron and formation of an ion. The ion can return to its ground state as one of the outer electrons falls into the vacancy, and, in the process, a second electron (Auger electron) with a kinetic energy characteristic for that atom is emitted. Auger emission and X-ray fluorescence are competing events, with atoms of higher atomic number favoring relaxation through X-ray fluorescence.

1. Source—produces X-rays with known wavelength.
2. Electron analyzer—uses an electrostatic field to separate electrons based on kinetic energy[2].
3. Detector—converts impact by separated electrons into an electrical signal.
4. Processor (computer)—translates the signal from the detector into the appropriate spectrum.

As illustrated in Fig. 7.26, the sample is first bombarded with X-rays. The resulting emitted electrons then enter the analyzer chamber. Because of the geometry of the analyzer and the difference in voltage between the two walls, only electrons with a certain kinetic energy can be collected by the detector, while all the others strike non-detectable areas. (This is similar to the operation of mass analyzers in mass spectroscopy, as described in Chapter 2). By altering the voltage difference between the walls in a controlled manner, the electrostatic field is altered to permit the detector to record the amount of electrons having various kinetic energies. At the end of the voltage sweep, the entire spectrum is plotted for that sample. As indicated in Fig. 7.26, ESCA analysis is performed under vacuum to prevent unwanted interactions of emitted electrons with gas molecules in the air.

[2]Although there are other means to determine kinetic energy of electrons, this method, called a *dispersive analyzer*, is the most common and therefore is the focus of this discussion.

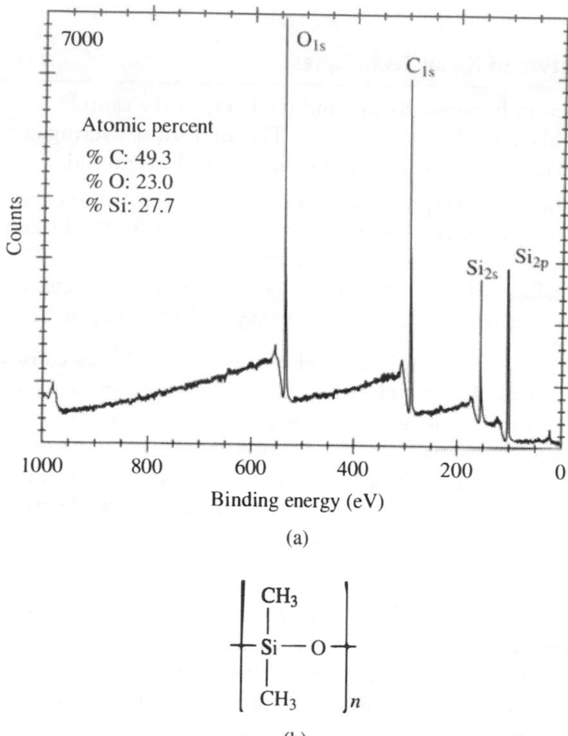

Figure 7.24
(a) A typical ESCA spectrum of poly(dimethyl siloxane) (PDMS), plotted as electron count (y-axis) as a function of binding energy (x-axis). (b) Chemical structure of PDMS. (Adapted with permission from [9].)

7.6.3.3 Information Provided ESCA methods are extremely sensitive and can detect all elements except hydrogen and helium in the outermost ~100 Å of an organic or inorganic material at concentrations down to 0.1 atomic percent. At the same time, the ESCA spectrum also provides information about neighboring atoms to which an element is bonded. For example, as shown in Fig. 7.27 for ethyl trifluoroacetate, binding energies can be distinguished for the various carbons in this molecule. Of the atoms depicted, fluorine has the most ability to withdraw valence electron density from carbon (it is the most electronegative). Therefore, the positive nuclear charge is less shielded, and the core carbon electrons are held more tightly. This results in a higher binding energy for this carbon atom than for others in the molecule.

7.6.4 Attenuated Total Internal Reflectance Fourier Transform—Infrared Spectroscopy (ATR-FTIR)

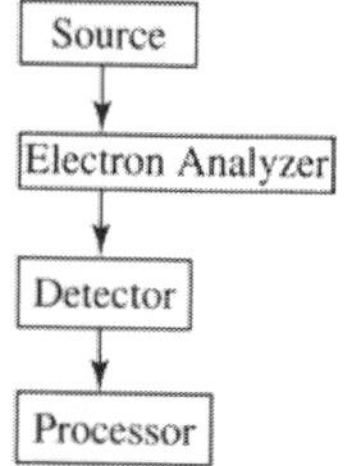

Figure 7.25
Block diagram of the components of an ESCA instrument. The four main components are an X-ray source, an electron analyzer, a detector, and a processor (computer).

7.6.4.1 Basic Principles ATR-FTIR is an analysis technique that has developed through modification of a bulk characterization method to probe particular parameters at the material surface. The theory behind IR excitation of molecules has been described previously in Chapter 2. The major distinguishing characteristic of ATR-FTIR is the addition of a specialized probe made of a high-refractive index crystal that intimately contacts the sample surface and through which the IR beam is transmitted.

When a beam of electromagnetic radiation passes from a medium that is more dense to one that is less dense, reflection occurs. Upon reflection, the beam penetrates a small distance into the less dense medium and this penetrating radiation is called an **evanescent wave**. Like for other IR methods, the sample may absorb the evanescent beam due to the vibration frequency of bonds found within

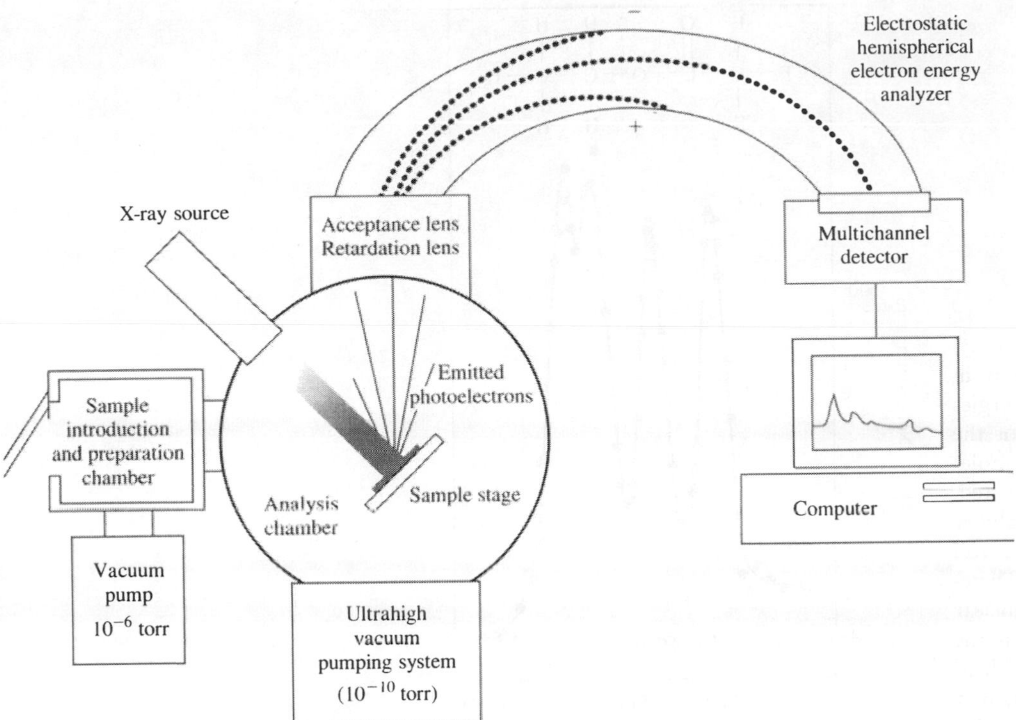

Figure 7.26
Schematic of ESCA equipment. First, the sample is bombarded with X-rays. The resulting emitted electrons then enter the analyzer chamber. Because of the difference in voltage between the two walls and the geometry of the analyzer, only electrons with a certain kinetic energy can be collected by the detector, with the remaining electrons striking non-detectable areas. By altering the voltage difference between the walls in a controlled manner, the electrostatic field is altered to permit the detector to record the amount of electrons having various kinetic energies. At the end of the voltage sweep, the entire spectrum is plotted for that sample. (Adapted with permission from [10].)

the material. Absorption of certain wavelengths causes their attenuation (thus giving the method its name) and provides information about the chemical structure of the material.

In order to increase the level of absorption to detectable values, the probe is designed so that, at certain angles of incident radiation, reflection of the IR beam is complete. Therefore, multiple reflection processes and multiple attenuations occur as the beam passes close to the sample (Fig. 7.28), thereby increasing the signal. By placing the probe in contact with the material, ATR-FTIR is thought to record only surface characteristics, but it should be noted that a signal can be obtained from relatively deep within the sample by surface analysis standards (1–5 μm).

7.6.4.2 Instrumentation A typical IR spectrum of poly(dimethyl siloxane) is found in Fig. 7.29. Like other IR spectra, ATR-FTIR data are generally plotted by transmittance (or absorbance) (y-axis) as a function of wavelength (or wavenumber) (x-axis). The basic instrumentation for ATR-FTIR spectroscopy is very similar to that described preciously for other FTIR methods and includes an IR source, an interferometer, a detector and a processor. Fourier-transform techniques are required for this application because they significantly increase the signal strength

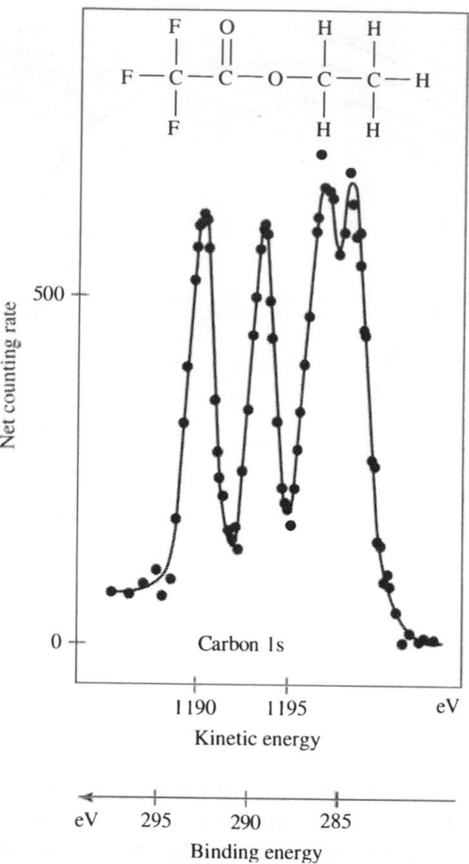

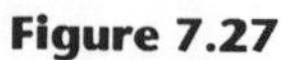

Figure 7.27
An ESCA spectrum for ethyl trifluoroacetate. As seen in the graph, binding energies can be distinguished for the various carbons in this molecule. Of the atoms depicted, fluorine has the most ability to withdraw valence electron density from carbon. Therefore, the positive nuclear charge is less shielded, and the core carbon electrons are held more tightly. This results in a higher binding energy for this carbon atom than for others in the molecule. (Adapted with permission from [15] and [16].)

(signal to noise ratio), which, as mentioned previously, is weak due to the small mass at the material surface. Two types of ATR sample cells, one for solids and one for the solid/liquid interface, are shown in Fig. 7.30. Cells allowing for the presence of liquid have particular application in the study of protein adsorption via ATR-FTIR techniques (see below).

7.6.4.3 Information Provided Although ATR-FTIR spectra are similar, they are not identical to regular IR spectra. While absorbance occurs at the same wavelengths, the intensity of the peak may be altered with respect to the spectra described in Chapter 2. Many of the applications for ATR-FTIR are identical to those of its

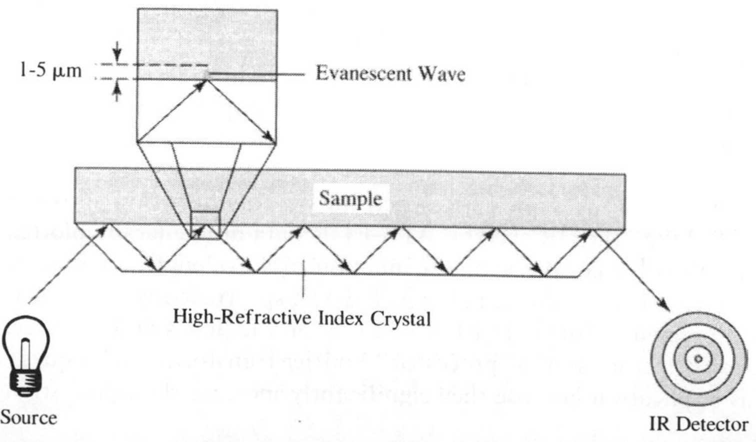

Figure 7.28
Schematic of the light path within an ATR-FTIR probe. In order to increase the level of absorption, the probe is designed so that, at certain angles of incident radiation, reflection of the IR beam is complete. Therefore, multiple reflection processes and multiple attenuations occur as the beam passes close to the sample, increasing the signal.

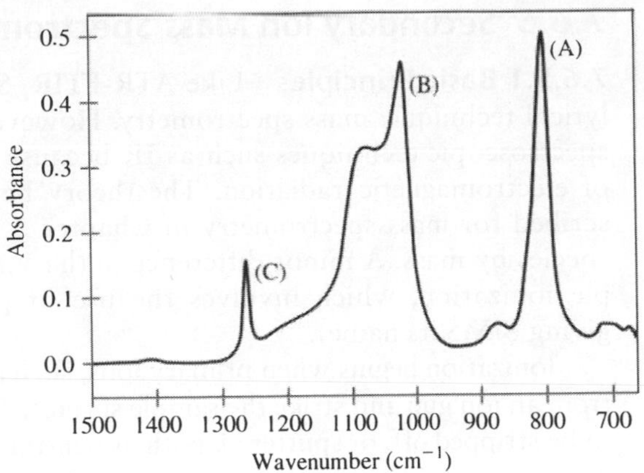

$$\left[-\underset{\displaystyle CH_3}{\overset{\displaystyle CH_3}{\mathrm{Si}}}-O- \right]$$

Poly(dimethyl siloxane)

Figure 7.29
Typical ATR-FTIR spectrum of poly(dimethyl siloxane). Characteristic peaks include the C–H bond in Si–CH_3 at 800 cm^{-1}(A), the Si-O-Si bonds at 1020 cm^{-1}(B), and the C–H bond in Si–CH_3 at 1260 cm^{-1}(C).

bulk counterpart, including recording spectra to gain insight into chemical composition of the biomaterial surface.

Another common use for this technique is to follow the relative change over time of certain peaks that correspond to a specific type of bond. Examining the appearance of amide bonds, for example, allows the kinetics of protein adsorption to a biomaterial to be sensitively monitored. The development of sample cells that permit the introduction of a liquid/water interface [Fig. 7.30(b)] has greatly facilitated these types of experiments.

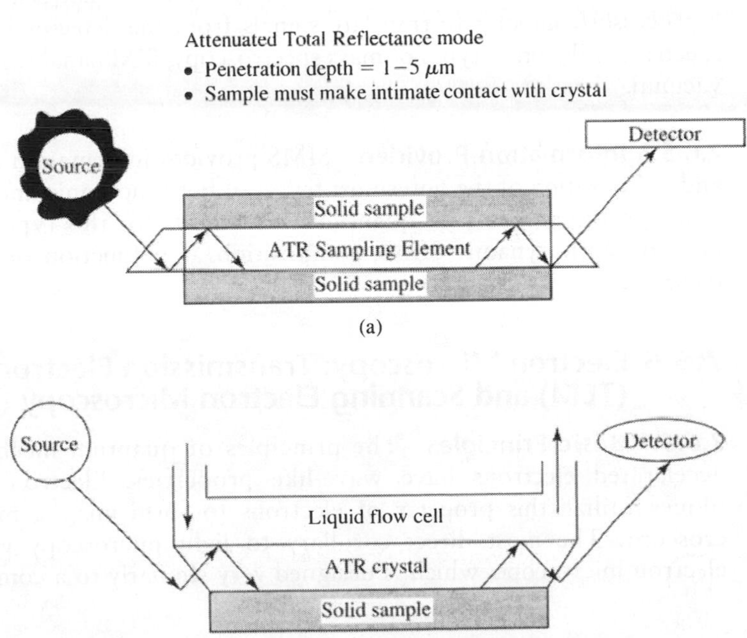

Figure 7.30
Two types of ATR sample cells, (a) one for solids and (b) one for the solid/liquid interface. (Adapted with permission from [9] and [10].)

7.6.5 Secondary Ion Mass Spectrometry (SIMS)

7.6.5.1 Basic Principles Like ATR-FTIR, SIMS is a derivation of a bulk analytical technique: mass spectrometry. However, SIMS can be distinguished from spectroscopic techniques such as IR because it does not involve the absorption of electromagnetic radiation. The theory behind SIMS is identical to that described for mass spectrometry in Chapter 2 and centers on separation of ionic species by mass. A minor difference in the surface version is the method of sample ionization, which involves the use of primary and secondary ions (thus giving SIMS its name).

Ionization begins when primary ions, such as O_2^+, Ar^+, Xe^+, or Cs^+, are ejected from an ion gun and strike the sample surface. This causes the surface layer of atoms to be stripped off, or **sputtered**, both as neutral species and as ions. (This is a similar process to the sputtering of atoms from the target in sputter coating or removal of atoms from the sample surface during ion beam implantation.) These emitted ions are called **secondary ions** and are drawn into the analyzer for separation by mass in a similar manner to bulk mass spectroscopy.

SIMS is considered a surface analysis technique since the energy of the incident ions generates collision cascades only in the surface region of the sample, and, of these collisions, only those that occur in the outermost layers produce secondary ions with sufficient energy to escape from the surface. Both static and dynamic SIMS methods have been developed. **Static SIMS** uses a relatively low ion dose (less than 10^{13} ions/cm^2) and induces minimal surface damage. In contrast, **dynamic SIMS** bombards the sample with a much larger ion dose. In this case, so much material is sputtered that the surface erodes while the experiment is being performed. This allows **depth profiling** of specimens (monitoring the intensity of a peak of interest as the surface erodes).

7.6.5.2 Instrumentation As demonstrated in Fig. 7.31, like bulk mass spectra, SIMS spectra are plotted as relative intensity (y-axis) as a function of mass (x-axis). Figure 7.32 reveals that the instrumentation required for SIMS is very similar to that for bulk mass spectroscopy, and includes the four main components: an ionization chamber containing the sample, a mass analyzer, an ion detector, and a processor/computer to translate signals from the detector into the appropriate spectrum. Like other types of mass spectroscopy, SIMS analysis is completed under vacuum.

7.6.5.3 Information Provided SIMS provides information about the structure and composition of the outermost few Å of both inorganic and organic materials, although the accuracy of quantitative methods for this type of spectroscopy is limited. With dynamic SIMS, composition as a function of depth can also be recorded.

7.6.6 Electron Microscopy: Transmission Electron Microscopy (TEM) and Scanning Electron Microscopy (SEM)

7.6.6.1 Basic Principles The principles of quantum mechanics predict that accelerated electrons have wave-like properties. Electron microscopy techniques utilize this property of electrons to form images, much like light microscopy. The most direct corollary to light microscopy is the transmission electron microscope, which is designed very similarly to a compound microscope

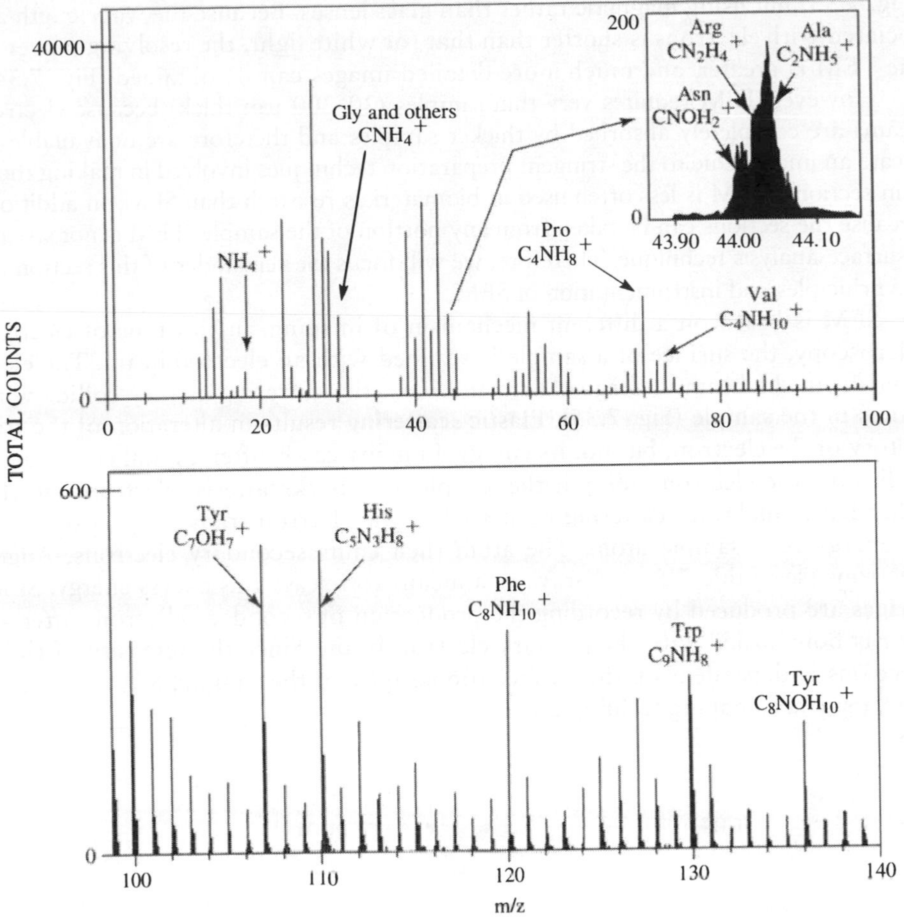

Figure 7.31
A spectrum produced by a type of SIMS (Time of Flight SIMS recording only positive ions) for fibronectin adsorbed on a poly(styrene) surface. The various peaks correspond to different amino acids found in the fibronectin protein. By comparing the relative intensities of certain peaks as the protein is adsorbed on different surfaces, the biomaterialist can obtain information about the orientation of the protein on each surface. (Adapted with permission from [17].)

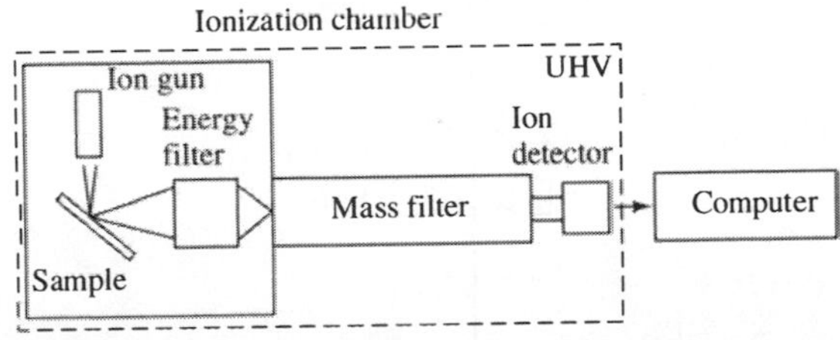

Figure 7.32
Block diagram of instrumentation for SIMS, which includes four main components: an ionization chamber containing the sample and ion gun, a mass analyzer (mass filter), an ion detector, and a processor/computer to translate signals from the detector into the appropriate spectrum. SIMS analysis is conducted under ultra-high vacuum (UHV). (Adapted with permission from [18] and [19].)

(Fig. 7.33) but using magnetic rather than glass lenses. Because the wavelength associated with electrons is shorter than that for white light, the resolving power of the TEM is greater, and much more detailed images can be obtained (Fig. 7.34).

However, TEM requires very thin samples (20–200 μm thick) because electron beams are completely absorbed by thicker samples and therefore are unavailable to create an image. Due to the stringent preparation techniques involved in making these thin sections, TEM is less often used in biomaterials research than SEM. In addition, because the sections can be taken from any portion of the sample, TEM is not strictly a surface analysis technique. Therefore, we will focus the remainder of this section on the principles and instrumentation of SEM.

SEM is based on a different mechanism of imaging. In this type of electron microscopy, the surface of a sample is scanned with an electron beam. The electrons from the beam undergo elastic and inelastic scattering as they collide with atoms in the sample (Fig. 7.35). **Elastic scattering** results in alteration of the trajectory of the electron, but not its energy. In many cases, after a number of elastic collisions, the electron will exit the sample as a **backscattered electron.** On the other hand, **inelastic scattering** occurs when the electron transfers part or all of its energy to a sample atom. The atom then emits secondary electrons, Auger electrons (see Table 7.5) or X-rays as a means to release this excess energy. SEM images are produced by recording the production of secondary electrons after an area is bombarded with the primary electron beam. Since the intensity of these electrons is dependent on the surface topography of the sample, SEM is considered a surface imaging technique.

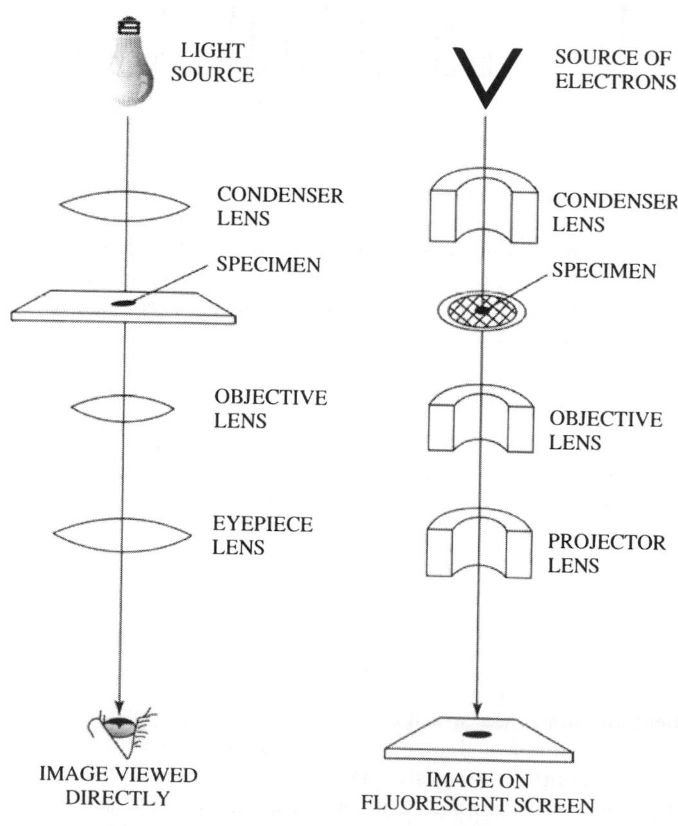

Figure 7.33
Comparison of Energy path in (a) light microscopy and (b) transmission electron microscopy, which is designed very similarly to a compound microscope but uses magnetic lenses, as opposed to glass. (Adapted with permission from [13].)

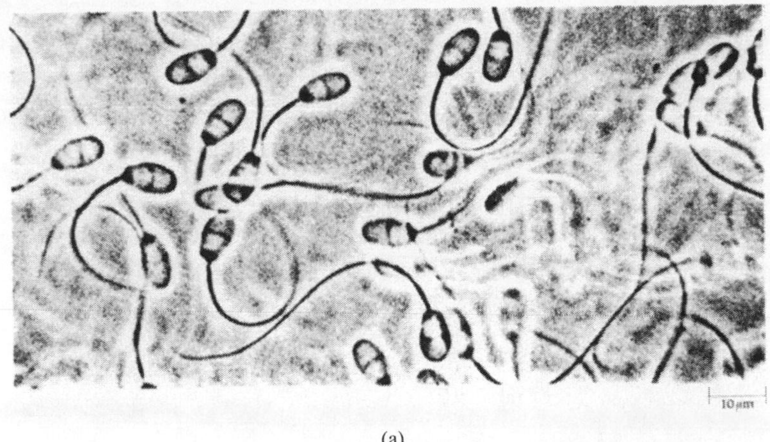

(a)

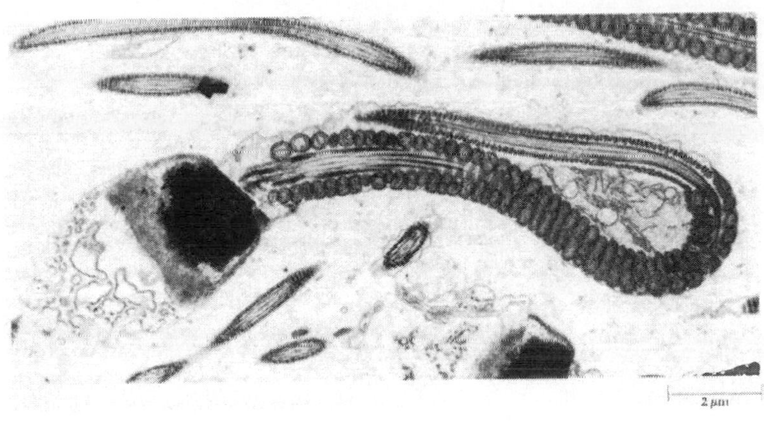

(b)

Figure 7.34
(a) Image of sperm cells under a white light microscope (scale bar 10 μm). (b) Image of a sperm cell under transmission electron microscopy (scale bar 2 μm). Because the wavelength associated with electrons is shorter than that for white light, the resolving power of the TEM is greater, and much more detailed images can be obtained. (Reprinted with permission from [13].)

SEM also provides the possibility of gaining information about the chemical composition of the imaged sample by analyzing the X-rays emitted, rather than the secondary electrons, after bombardment by the primary electron beam. As summarized in Table 7.5, X-ray fluorescence occurs if exposure to an electron beam causes removal of a core electron from an atom in the sample. To return to its ground state, one of the outer electrons falls into the vacancy, producing an X-ray of a certain wavelength that is characteristic for that atom. Therefore, recording the wavelength of the emitted X-rays provides an idea of the elemental composition of the sample. However, since the X-rays formed via this means can be produced from atoms deeper (1 μm or more) within the sample, this method does not provide information about the chemical nature of the surface.

7.6.6.2 Instrumentation A typical SEM image of osteoblasts on a titanium mesh is found in Fig. 7.36. This image shows the interaction of cells and a biomaterial scaffold for bone tissue engineering. As shown in Fig. 7.37, there are five basic components to a SEM:

1. Source—produces accelerated electrons.
2. Lenses—magnetic coils focus electron beam and reduce spot size.
3. Sample holder—holds sample securely.

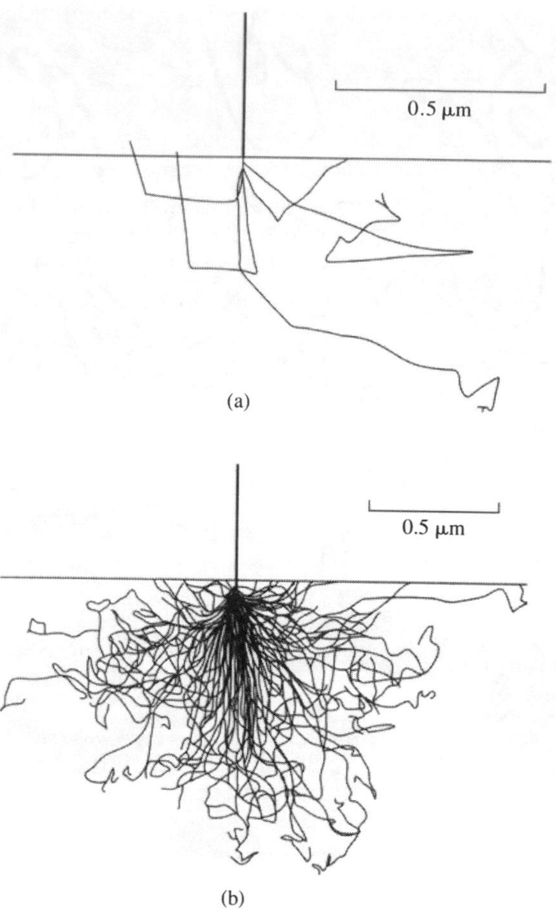

Figure 7.35
Examples of an electron beam hitting an iron surface in SEM. (a) shows the path of 5 electrons scattering within the sample and (b) shows 100 electrons. The electrons from the beam undergo elastic and inelastic scattering as they collide with atoms in the sample. Elastic scattering results in alteration of the trajectory of the electron, but not its energy. In many cases, after a number of elastic collisions, the electron will exit the sample as a backscattered electron. On the other hand, inelastic scattering occurs when the electron transfers part or all of its energy to a sample atom. The atom then emits secondary electrons, Auger electrons or X-rays as a means to release this excess energy. (Adapted with permission from [20].)

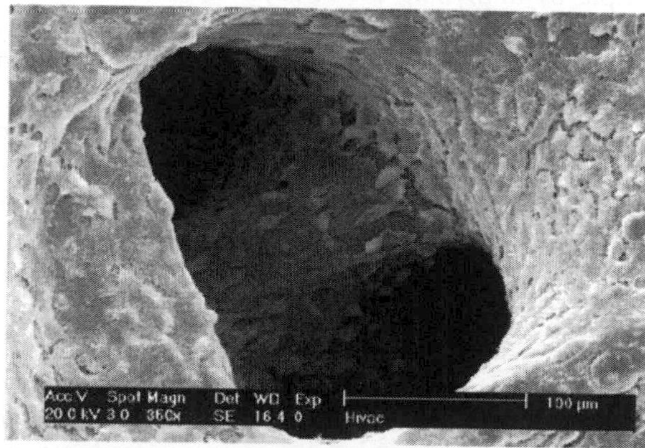

Figure 7.36
SEM image of osteoblasts cultured on a titanium mesh. The individual cells can be seen, particularly on the fiber in the back of the pore (in the center of the image). Scale bar 100 μm. (Reprinted with permission from [21].)

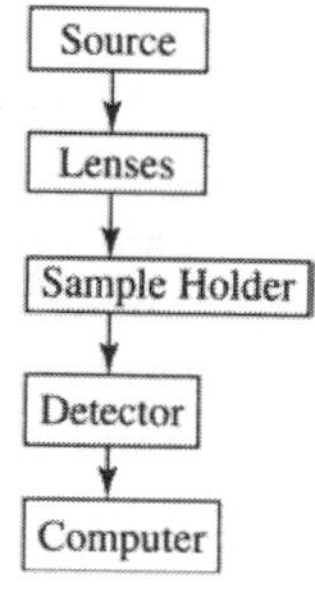

Figure 7.37
Block diagram of the components of a SEM. There are five basic components to a SEM: the accelerated electron source, lenses, the sample holder, the detector, and a computer, which produces the final image.

4. Detector—records the spatial position of secondary electron impact and converts this information into an electrical signal.
5. Computer—translates the signal from the detector to produce an image.

For optimal imaging, nonconductive samples, such as polymers, must be precoated with a thin layer of conductive material (metal) to reduce charge build-up during scanning. This is accomplished via physical sputtering from a metallic target (see previous sections of this chapter) onto the sample before imaging. In reality, the secondary electrons are produced from the coating only, so a high-fidelity image of the surface topography is produced only if the coating is sufficiently thin and conformational.

As illustrated in Fig. 7.38, the (coated) sample is placed into the holder and the electron beam is scanned over the surface in a raster motion. (The beam scans each line from side to side and all the lines from top to bottom.) The secondary electron detector is positioned so that the locations of the emitted electrons are recorded. The signal from the detector (indicating electron impact intensity and position) is then processed using appropriate software to produce a three-dimensional image. If emitted X-rays are also to be examined, a specialized detector system called **energy-dispersive X-ray analysis (EDXA)** is included to collect and analyze this radiation (Fig. 7.38).

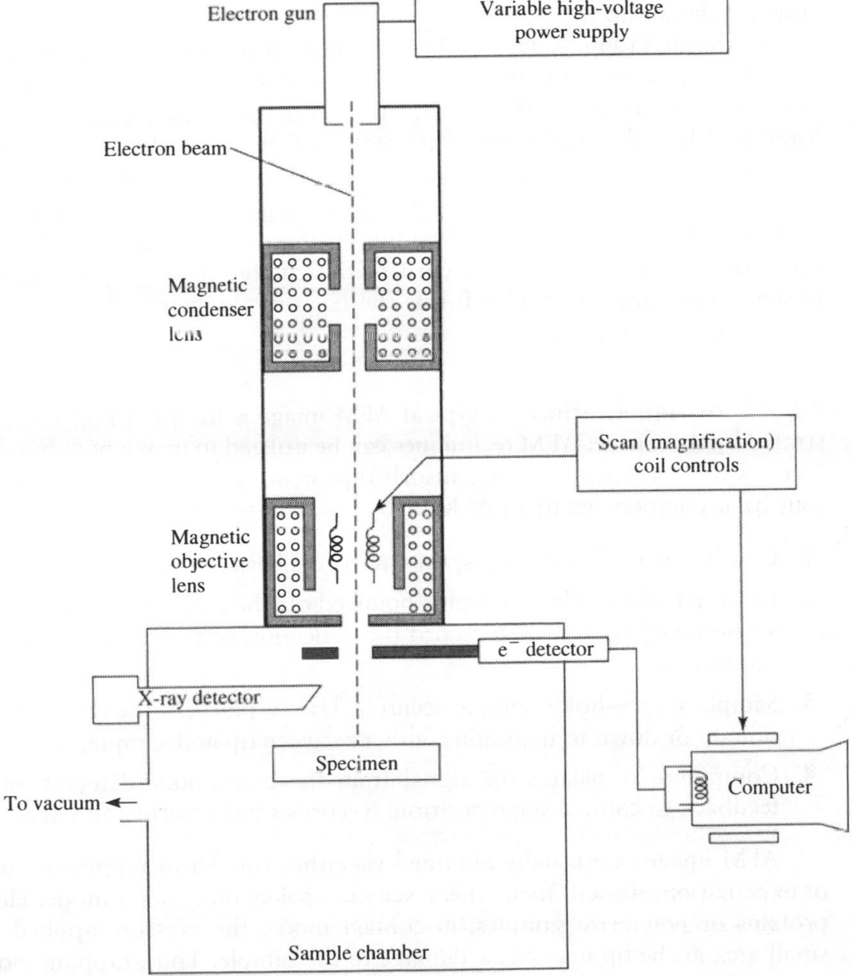

Figure 7.38
Schematic of a SEM. First, the specimen is placed into the sample chamber and the electron beam is scanned over the surface. The secondary electron detector is positioned so that the locations of the emitted electrons are recorded. The signal from the detector is then processed using appropriate software to produce a three-dimensional image. If emitted X-rays are also examined, a specialized detector system called energy-dispersive X-ray analysis (EDXA) is included to collect and analyze this radiation. (Adapted with permission from [15].)

Because electrons readily interact with atoms in the air, all electron microscopy must be completed under vacuum.

7.6.6.3 Information Provided SEM is commonly used to visualize the surface topography of a biomaterial, or a biomaterial with attached tissue or cells. Although the requirement of imaging in vacuum prevents full analysis of biomaterials as they would be found *in vivo*, recent development of the environmental SEM allows imaging of partially hydrated samples. The combination of SEM and EDXA provides information about chemical composition of the sample, although the ability to distinguish surface chemistry is limited.

7.6.7 Scanning Probe Microscopy (SPM): Atomic Force Microscopy (AFM)

7.6.7.1 Basic Principles **Scanning probe microscopy** is a general term that refers to any number of techniques producing a three-dimensional image due to the interactions between a small probe and atomic constituents of the sample surface. Of these, we will confine our discussion to *atomic force microscopy* (AFM). Like SEM, AFM can provide three-dimensional images of material surfaces with Å to nm spatial resolution. The analytical capabilities of AFM are limited to the uppermost atomic layer of a sample because its operation is based on interactions with the electron clouds of atoms at the surface.

As shown in Fig. 7.39, in AFM, a small tip is attached to a cantilever. When the tip encounters the material surface, van der Waals and electrostatic interactions between atoms in the tip and those on the surface create a characteristic force profile and cause eventual attraction of the tip to the surface, thus bending the cantilever. To obtain an image, the cantilever/tip assembly is rastered across the material in a controlled manner and the stage containing the sample is moved up or down in response to the bending of the cantilever so that the tip contacts the surface at all times. The record of the change in stage position required to achieve this constant contact forms the basis of the height data displayed in the three-dimensional image.

7.6.7.2 Instrumentation A typical AFM image is found in Fig. 7.40. As demonstrated by this figure, AFM techniques can be utilized to image pure biomaterial surfaces as well as those including adsorbed proteins. As shown in Fig. 7.41, there are four basic components to an AFM:

1. Cantilever/tip—bends in response to forces between tip and sample.
2. Laser/detector—a laser beam is bounced off the cantilever and directed toward a photodiode detector to record the deflection of the cantilever in response to the surface.
3. Sample stage—holds sample securely. Uses a piezoelectric driver to alter position up or down to maintain contact between tip and sample.
4. Computer—translates the signal from the photodiode detector and provides feedback to control stage position. Records stage position and produces image.

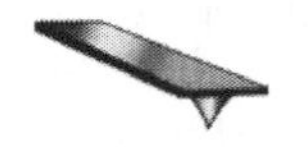

Figure 7.39
Tip used for atomic force microscopy. The tip is attached to the end of a cantilever beam. (Adapted with permission from [10].)

AFM images are usually obtained via either contact or tapping mode. For ease of explanation, we will focus this discussion solely on contact mode. However, for proteins or polymeric samples, in contact mode, the pressure applied due to the small area at the tip may cause damage to the sample. Thus, tapping mode is more

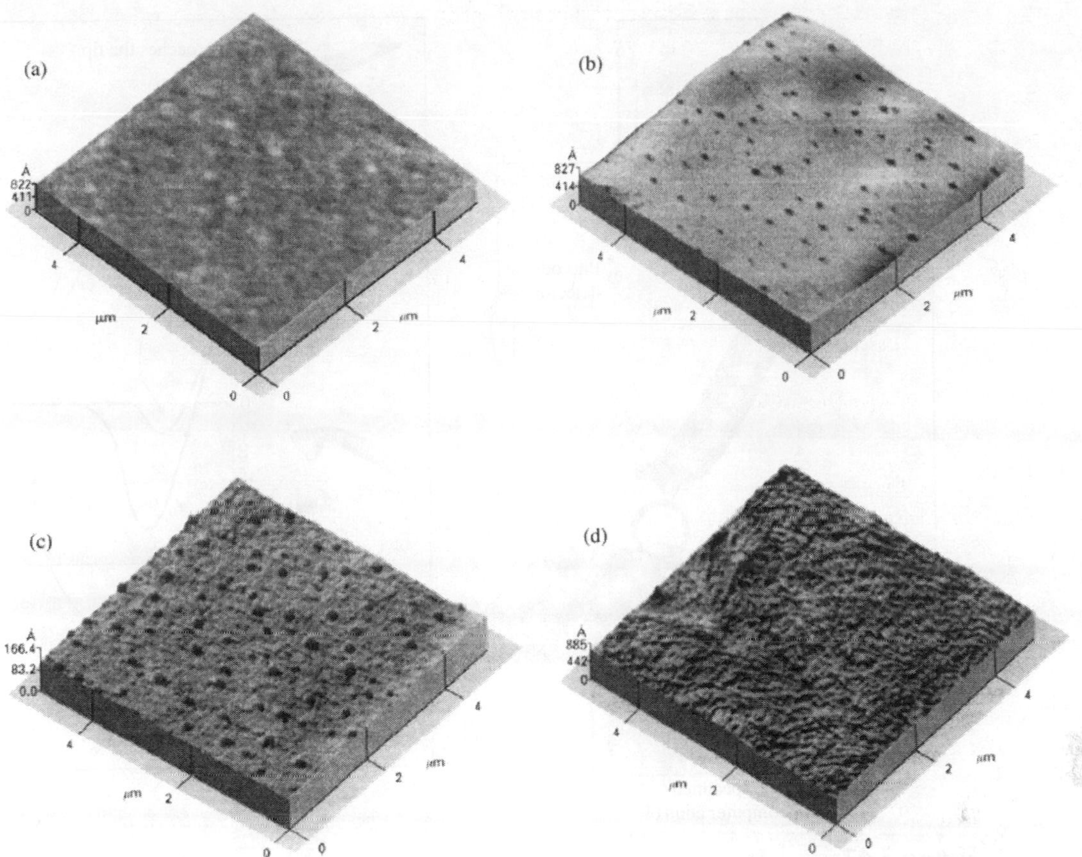

Figure 7.40
Surface topography (via AFM) of poly(D,L-lactic acid)-poly(ethylene glycol)-monomethyl ether diblock copolymer (Me.PEG-PLAs—numbers indicate the weight of the corresponding polymer blocks in kDa) films compared to a PLA film: (a) PLA, (b) Me.PEG5-PLA45, (c) Me.PEG5-PLA20, (d) Me.PEG5-PLA10 as observed by AFM. The PLA film has an almost smooth, nonstructured surface. With increasing Me.PEG content of the polymers, the density of particulate structures (predominantly crystallized PEG) increases tremendously. (Reprinted with permission from [22].)

often employed for more delicate specimens. Both modes can be used with a specially designed fluid cell to allow imaging of biomaterials in aqueous conditions like those found *in vivo*.

As illustrated in Fig. 7.42, imaging begins when the sample is placed on the stage and the tip is lowered until it contacts the surface. When this occurs, reflection of the laser off the cantilever indicates that the cantilever is bent toward the sample (Fig. 7.42). The tip/cantilever are then moved across the sample surface in a controlled manner and the cantilever deflection is monitored. In response to changes in deflection, the stage is moved up and down to maintain contact between the sample and the tip. Alterations in stage position are recorded and processed by the appropriate software to form a three-dimensional image.

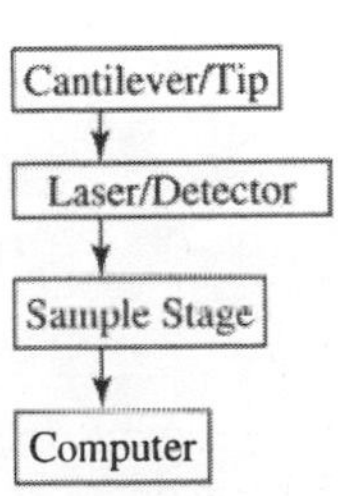

Figure 7.41
Block diagram of an AFM setup.

7.6.7.3 Information Provided AFM is most often used to visualize surface topography, either of a biomaterial or a layer of adsorbed proteins. As illustrated in Fig. 7.43, the number of interacting atoms increases as the width of the tip increases,

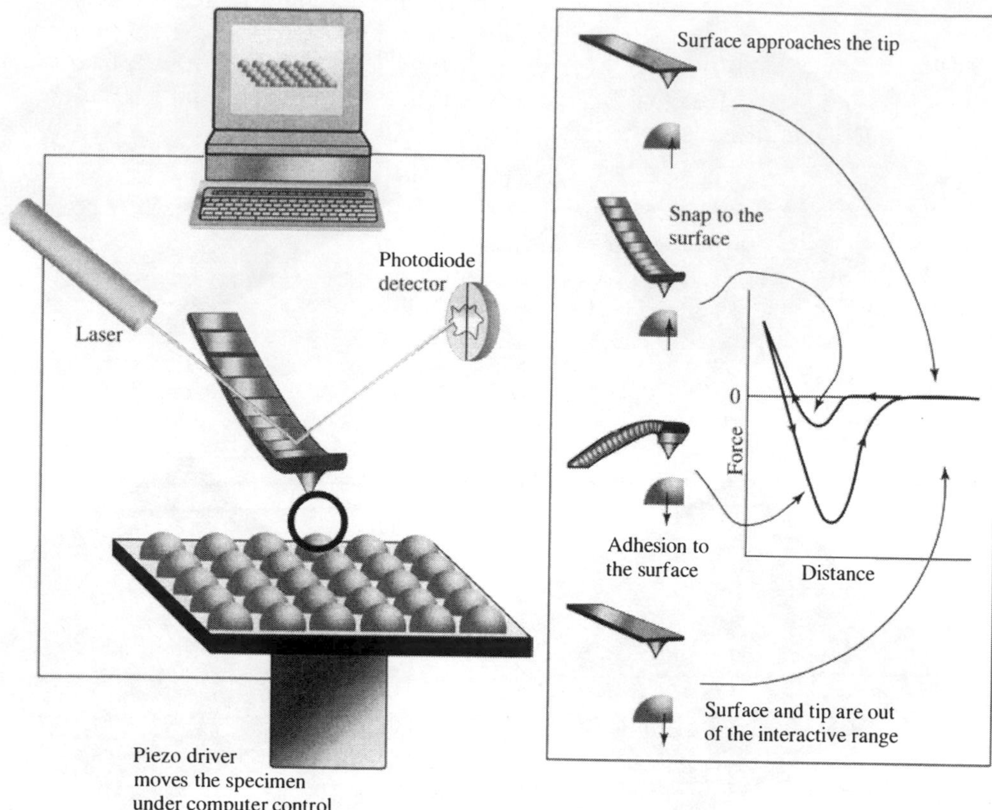

Figure 7.42
Schematic of AFM instrumentation. Imaging begins when the sample is placed on a stage and the tip is lowered until it contacts the surface. When this occurs, reflection of a laser off the cantilever indicates that the cantilever is bent toward the sample. The tip/cantilever are then moved across the sample surface and the cantilever deflection is monitored. In response to changes in defection, the stage is moved up and down to maintain contact between the sample and the tip. Alterations in stage position are recorded and processed by the appropriate software to form a three-dimensional image. (Adapted with permission from [10].)

thus decreasing the spatial resolution. Therefore, for optimal results, the width of the end of the tip should be smaller than the smallest feature to be imaged.

AFM can also be employed for quantitative force measures using a variant of Hooke's law (see Chapter 4) to relate the deflection of the cantilever to the force

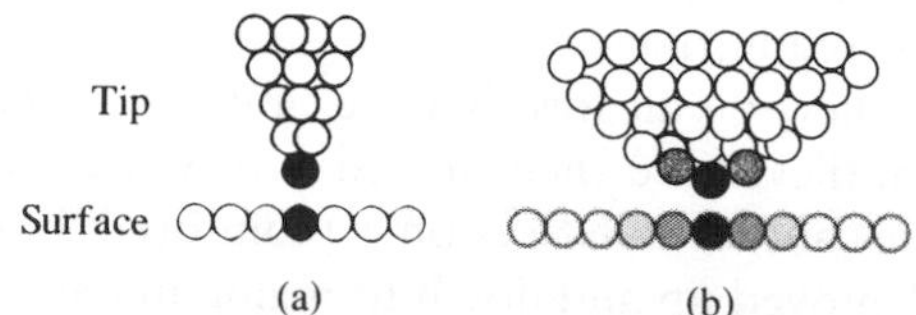

Figure 7.43
Two sample tips for use with AFM. The number of interacting atoms increases as the width of the tip increases, thus decreasing the spatial resolution. Due to this characteristic it is desirable to have the width of the end of the tip smaller than the smallest feature to be imaged (a). If the tip is too wide, then artifacts in the imaging can occur (b). (Adapted with permission from [23].)

between the tip and the surface (to do this, the spring constant of the cantilever, E, must be known). This modality has been exploited to determine binding forces between biological molecules. In these experiments, a molecule is covalently bonded to the tip and the adhesive force is recorded between the tip and a second molecule of interest that is attached to the sample surface.

EXAMPLE PROBLEM 7.4

The following graph illustrates the roughness profile from the surface scan of a pyrolitic carbon artificial heart valve leaflet using an atomic force microscope. The graph represents the surface profile of a 5-μm stretch of the surface of the carbon material. The table gives the distances between several of the landmarks indicated on the graph. In the host environment, the leaflet could encounter bacteria (~10 μm in diameter when modeled as spheres), fibrils made of the protein fibrin (~1 μm in length), red blood cells (~2.5 μm across), platelets (~1 μm across and 1μm tall when in blood) and other similar cells and molecules. Considering only the surface roughness information and the sizes of the listed blood elements, would the material be expected to result in much interaction with the blood elements listed? Why or why not?

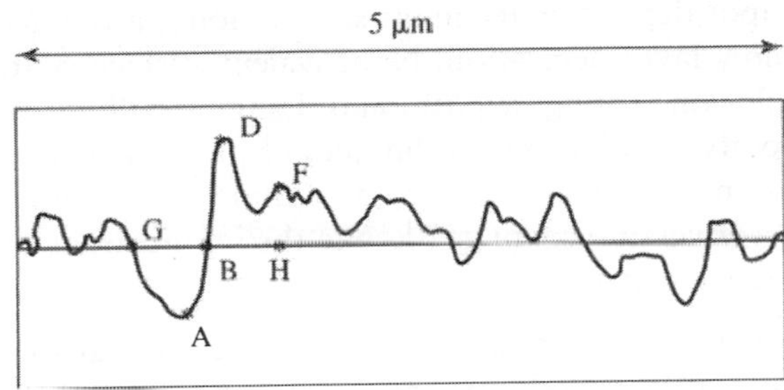

Points	Horizontal Distance (nm)	Vertical Distance (nm)
G&B	312.5	0
B&D	0	98.561
A&B	0	55.423
H&F	0	57.313

Solution: Although the surface appears to be quite rough upon initial visual examination of the AFM scan, the scale of these surface features must be compared with the size of the elements with which the surface could potentially interact. Examination of the data in the table reveals that the vertical distances between peaks is typically on the order of 100 nm or less. Considering that the listed elements of the blood with which the material could interact range from approximately 1 to 10 μm, these surface features are significantly smaller (one to two orders of magnitude smaller). Thus, the surface of the material appears rather smooth in this reference frame and minimal interactions between the material and the listed elements of the blood would be expected based on surface roughness. It should be noted that, in relation to the size of many proteins in the blood, the surface would be rough. It is possible that the surface roughness could promote protein adsorption that could, in turn, affect cell adhesion. However, the blood proteins were not included in the list of elements to be considered in this problem. ■

Summary

- The adsorption of proteins onto a biomaterial surface is governed by thermodynamic principles that are strongly influenced by two surface properties: surface hydrophobicity and surface charge. Other physical properties of the material surface, such as surface roughness and steric hindrance, influence protein adsorption, as well.
- Controlling protein adsorption to the biomaterial surface is extremely important because it is to this coated surface, rather than the original implant, that the body reacts.
- Physicochemical surface treatments of biomaterials entail alteration of the surface composition of the material through use of physical principles or chemical reactions, but they do not involve the attachment of biological molecules to the material. Biological surface modification techniques, however, are used to attach biologically active molecules to a material surface.
- Physicochemical methods of surface modification can either involve a coating of the surface or not. Surface modifications that result in surface coatings can involve covalent or noncovalent bonding to the surface. Covalent surface coatings can be achieved through plasma discharge, chemical vapor deposition, physical vapor deposition techniques, radiation grafting techniques, or self-assembled monolayer deposition. Noncovalent surface coatings can be formed through solution coating, deposition of Langmuir-Blodgett films, or the use of surface-modifying additives. Techniques of physicochemical surface modification that do not produce an overcoat include ion beam implantation, plasma treatment, conversion coatings (despite the implications of the name) and the use of bioactive glasses.
- Biological surface modifications can be either covalent or non-covalent in nature. For covalent modifications, biomolecules may be attached to reactive material surfaces through a number of reaction schemes. Biomolecules can modify a material surface through forming noncovalent coatings by such mechanisms as hydrophobic or electrostatic interactions between the material and the biomolecules.
- Surface characteristics of a material can change with time. They are particularly susceptible to alteration caused by degradation, either of the surface coating itself or of the underlying substrate.
- Patterning techniques for altering the surface properties of biomaterials in a controlled manner, resulting in a geometric design of well-defined dimensions, include microcontact printing and microfluidics.
- A number of techniques for the characterization of biomaterial surfaces exist. Contact angle analysis provides information related to the hydrophobicity of the material, and is typically an initial step in material surface characterization. Microscopy techniques, including light microscopy, electron microscopy, and scanning probe microscopy, primarily provide information about the appearance and topology of the biomaterial. Like for bulk materials, surface

spectroscopic techniques, which involve the absorption of electromagnetic radiation by the material, include electron spectroscopy for chemical analysis (ESCA) and attenuated total internal reflectance Fourier-transform infrared spectroscopy (ATR-FTIR). These methods, along with a modification of mass spectrometry for surface analysis, secondary ion mass spectrometry (SIMS), record information about the structure and composition of the outermost few layers of both organic and inorganic materials.

Problems

7.1 You are given a relatively hydrophobic material with PEG chains covalently attached to its surface (with the attachment occurring at one end of each chain). What do you expect to be the effect of PEG attachment on protein adsorption to the material surface?

7.2 You have designed a bone plate that is manufactured via rolling under cold working conditions, and tests show good biocompatibility results for the device. The Manufacturing Department has put in a request to change the processing method to rolling under hot working conditions in an effort to reduce the total manufacturing cost. Since the material from which the device is fabricated will not change, do you need to rerun the biocompatibility tests? Why or why not?

7.3 Someone in your company has developed a material that closely matches the native mechanical properties of bone, and would be an ideal femoral stem of a hip joint prosthesis. Unfortunately, the material is cytotoxic. Another engineer in the company has developed a coating that can be applied to the material, sealing the cytotoxic material away from the body. Is this a viable option?

7.4 A coworker wants to use titanium as the head for a femoral stem of a hip implant. She has asked you to determine a way to improve the wear resistance of this material. What would you do?

7.5 You are considering two different surface modification techniques (Langmuir-Blodgett films and self-assembled monolayers) to control protein adsorption to the interior surface of an artificial vascular graft material. Which method would be better suited for this particular application? Why?

7.6 You are considering two biomaterials for a vascular graft application. One has a large quantity of hydroxyl groups exposed on its surface, while the other has fluorine groups exposed. Which material would be more appropriate for this application in terms of protein adsorption?

7.7 Given that a water-based liquid has γ_{LV} of ~72 dynes/cm, which of the two materials depicted below is more hydrophobic? Explain how the Zisman method is used to determine critical surface tension and how the critical surface tension relates to the surface properties of the material. (Figure adapted with permission from [23].)

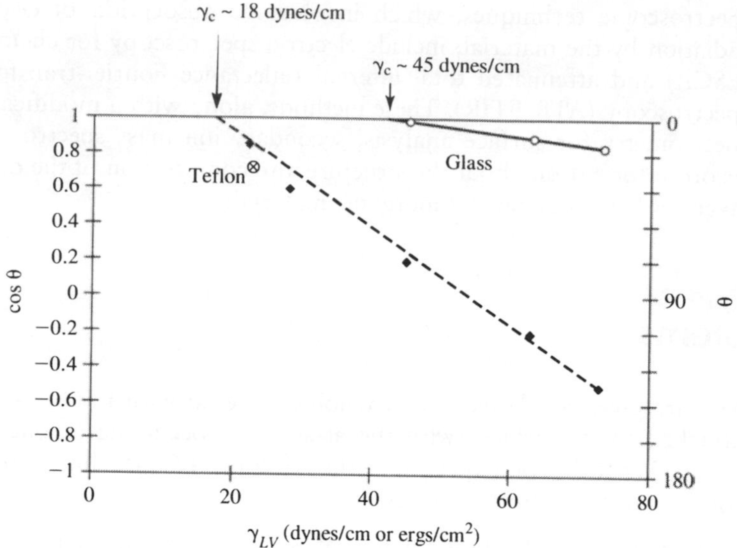

7.8 One potential problem associated with the long-term release of a drug from an implanted material is the initial burst release of significant amounts of the drug. One approach to reduce this burst release is to apply a coating to the material in an attempt to modulate the diffusion of the drug. In a study performed by Kwok *et al.* [24] the effectiveness of butyl methacrylate as a coating material was tested. Figure 1 below shows the chemical structure and a ESCA scan of the surface of this coating material. Plasma treatment of its surface was also performed in an attempt to increase its hydrophilicity. Part of the study explored how the power of the plasma-generating equipment affects the surface chemistry (Fig. 2 below). At high power, some of the polymer begins to degrade. Which of the bonds in the polymer is subject to degradation at high power? Explain in terms of the results in Fig. 2. Which power setting would you recommend for surface treating this polymer and why? (Figures adapted with permission from [24].)

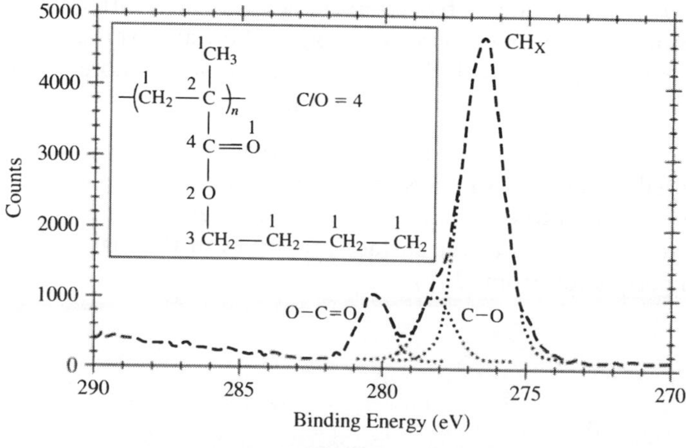

Figure 1

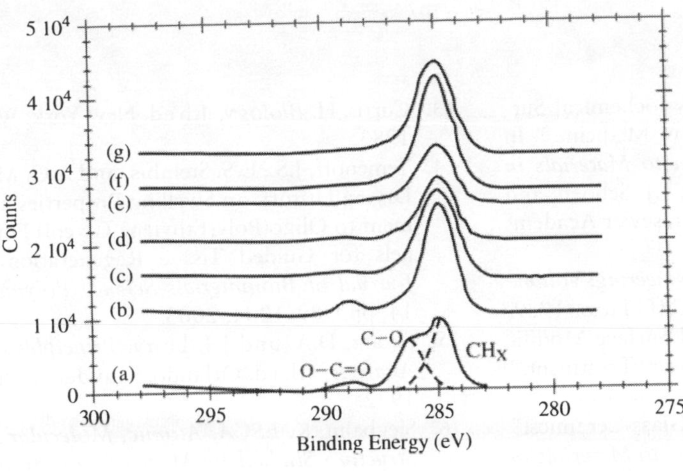

Figure 2

Legend:
(a) untreated polymer
(b–g) plasma-treated polymer: (b) 5W, (c) 10W, (d) 20W,
(e) 40W, (f) 50W, (g) 60W

7.9 Of the surface analysis methods discussed in this chapter, which require physical contact with the material surface? Which do not?

7.10 Self-assembled monolayers (SAMs), a type of surface coating, are composed of three key regions. You have just created a SAM to interact with a glass substrate that you intend to use for protein attachment. Explain the purpose of each region in the molecule and give specific examples of the chemical groups you would expect to find in each region. Would the use of SAMs produce a smooth or rough surface on your substrate, as characterized by atomic force microscopy? Why?

7.11 The graph below represents the ESCA peak from the 1*s* carbon of a poly(methyl methacrylate) bone cement. On the graph, draw the 2*s* carbon peak from the same material and explain why the peak is located in that position.

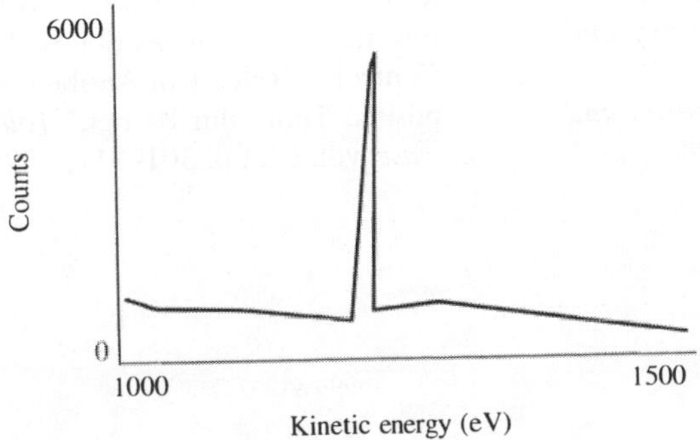

References

1. Ratner, B.D. and A.S. Hoffman. "Physiochemical Surface Modification of Materials Used in Medicine," In *Biomaterials Science: An Introduction to Materials in Medicine*, B.D. Ratner, A.S. Hoffman, F.J. Schoen, and J.E. Lemons, Eds., 2nd ed. San Diego: Elsevier Academic Press, pp. 201–218, 2004.
2. Kossowsky, R. *Surface Modification Engineering: Volume I: Fundamental Aspects.* Boca Raton: CRC Press, 1989.
3. Picraux, S.T. and L.E. Pope. "Tailored Surface Modification by Ion Implantation and Laser Treatment." *Science*, vol. 226, pp. 615–622, 1984.
4. Hench, L.L. "Ceramics, Glasses, and Glass-Ceramics." In *Biomaterials Science: An Introduction to Materials in Medicine*, B.D. Ratner, A.S. Hoffman, F.J. Schoen, and J.E. Lemons, Eds., 1st ed. San Diego: Elsevier Academic Press, pp. 73–84, 1996.
5. Hoffman, A.S. and J.A. Hubbell. "Surface-Immobilized Biomolecules." In *Biomaterials Science: An Introduction to Materials in Medicine*, B.D. Ratner, A.S. Hoffman, F.J. Schoen, and J.E. Lemons, Eds., 2nd ed. San Diego: Elsevier Academic Press, pp. 225–233, 2004.
6. Kim, S.W. and J. Feijen. "Surface Modification of Polymers for Improved Blood Compatibility," In *CRC Critical Reviews in Biocompatibility*, D.F. Williams, Ed., vol. 1, Boca Raton: CRC Press, pp. 229–260, 1985.
7. Folch, A. and M. Toner. "Cellular Micropatterns on Biocompatible Materials." *Biotechnology Progress*, vol. 14, pp. 388–392, 1998.
8. Patel, N., R. Padera, G.H. Sanders, S.M. Cannizzaro, M.C. Davies, R. Langer, C.J. Roberts, S.J. Tendler, P.M. Williams, and K.M. Shakesheff. "Spatially Controlled Cell Engineering on Biodegradable Polymer Surfaces." *FASEB Journal*, vol. 12, pp. 1447–1454, 1998.
9. Ratner, B.D. "Characterization of Biomaterial Surfaces" *Cardiovascular Pathology*, vol. 2, pp. 87S–100S, 1993.
10. Ratner, B.D. "Surface Properties and Surface Characterization of Materials." In *Biomaterials Science: An Introduction to Materials in Medicine*, B.D. Ratner, A.S. Hoffman, F.J. Schoen, and J.E. Lemons, Eds., 2nd ed. San Diego: Elsevier Academic Press, pp. 40–59, 2004.
11. Andrade, J.D. *Surface and Interfacial Aspects of Biomedical Polymers: Volume 1: Surface Chemistry and Physics.* New York: Plenum Press, 1985.
12. Tsujii, K. *Surface Activity: Principles, Phenomena and Applications.* San Diego: Academic Press, 1998.
13. Curtis, H. *Biology*, 4th ed. New York: Worth Publishers, 1983.
14. Temenoff, J.S., E.S. Steinbis, and A.G. Mikos. "Effect of Drying History on Swelling Properties and Cell Attachment to Oligo(Poly(Ethylene Glycol) Fumarate) Hydrogels for Guided Tissue Regeneration Applications." *Journal of Biomaterials Science Polymer Edition*, vol. 14, pp. 989–1004, 2003.
15. Skoog, D.A. and J.J. Leary. *Principles of Instrumental Analysis*, 4th ed. Orlando: Saunders College Publishing, 1992.
16. Siegbahn, K. *ESCA, Atomic, Molecular and Solid State Structure Studied by Means of Electron Spectroscopy.* Uppsala: Almquist and Wiksells, 1967.
17. Lhoest, J.B., E. Detrait, P. van den Bosch de Aguilar, and P. Bertrand. "Fibronectin Adsorption, Conformation, and Orientation on Polystyrene Substrates Studied by Radiolabeling, XPS, and ToF SIMS." *Journal of Biomedical Materials Research*, vol. 41, pp. 95–103, 1998.
18. Vickerman, J.C. *Surface Analysis: The Principal Techniques.* New York: John Wiley and Sons, 1997.
19. Vickerman, J.C. "Secondary Ion Mass Spectroscopy." *Chemistry in Britain*, vol. 23, pp. 969–971, 973–974, 1987.
20. Goldstein, J.I., Newbury, D.E., Echlin, P., Joy, D.C., Fiori, C.E. and E. Lifshin. *Scanning Electron Microscopy and X-Ray Microanalysis: A Text for Biologists, Scientists and Geologists*, New York: Plenum Press, 1981.
21. Bancroft, G.N., V.I. Sikavitsas, J. van den Dolder, T.L. Sheffield, C.G. Ambrose, J.A. Jansen, and A.G. Mikos. "Fluid Flow Increases Mineralized Matrix Deposition in 3D Perfusion Culture of Marrow Stromal Osteoblasts in a Dose-Dependent Manner." *Proceedings of the National Academy of Sciences*, vol. 99, pp. 12600–12605, 2002.
22. Lucke, A., J. Tessmar, E. Schnell, G. Schmeer, and A. Gopferich. "Biodegradable Poly(D,L-Lactic Acid)-Poly (Ethylene Glycol)-Monomethyl Ether Diblock Copolymers: Structures and Surface Properties Relevant to Their Use as Biomaterials." *Biomaterials*, vol. 21, pp. 2361–2370, 2000.
23. Dee, K.C., D.A. Puleo, and R. Bizios. *An Introduction to Tissue-Biomaterial Interactions.* Hoboken: Wiley-Liss, 2002.
24. Kwok, C.S., T.A. Horbett, and B.D. Ratner. "Design of Infection-Resistant Antibiotic-Releasing Polymers: II. Controlled Release of Antibiotics through a Plasma-Deposited Thin Film Barrier," *Journal of Controlled Release*, vol. 62, pp. 301–311, 1999.

Additional Reading

Andrade, J.D. *Surface and Interfacial Aspects of Biomedical Polymers: Volume 2: Protein Adsorption*. New York: Plenum Press, 1985.

Andrade, J.D. and V. Hlady. "Protein Adsorption and Materials Biocompatibility: A Tutorial Review and Suggested Hypotheses." In *Biopolymers/Non-Exclusion HPLC*, K. Dusek, C.G. Overberger, and G. Heublein, Eds. New York: Springer-Verlag, pp. 1–63, 1986.

Burdick, J.A., A. Khademhosseini, and R. Langer. "Fabrication of Gradient Hydrogels Using a Microfluidics/Photopolymerization Process." *Langmuir*, vol. 20, pp. 5153–5156, 2004.

Callister, Jr., W.D. *Materials Science and Engineering: An Introduction*, 7th ed. New York: John Wiley and Sons, 2006.

Cao, L. *Carrier Bound Immobilized Enzymes: Principles, Application and Design*. Weinheim, Germany: Wiley-VCH, 2006.

Chen, C.S., M. Mrksich, S. Huang, G.M. Whitesides, and D.E. Ingber. "Micropatterned Surfaces for Control of Cell Shape, Position, and Function." *Biotechnology Progress*, vol. 14, pp. 356–363, 1998.

Chu, P.K., J.Y. Chen, L.P. Wang, and N. Huang. "Plasma-Surface Modification of Biomaterials." *Material Science and Engineering R*, vol. 36, pp. 143–206, 2002.

Cullity, B.D. *Elements of X-Ray Diffraction*, 2nd ed. Reading: Addison Wesley Publishing, 1978.

Davies, J. *Surface Analytical Techniques for Probing Biomaterial Processes*. New York: CRC Press, 1996.

Ewing, G.W. *Analytical Instrumentation Handbook*, 2nd ed. New York: Marcel Dekker, 1997.

Horbett, T.A. "Principles Underlying the Role of Adsorbed Plasma Proteins in Blood Interactions with Foreign Materials." *Cardiovascular Pathology*, vol. 2, pp. 137S–148S, 1993.

Hubbell, J.A. "Matrix Effects." In *Principles of Tissue Engineering*, R.P. Lanza, R. Langer, and J. Vacanti, Eds., 2nd ed. Austin: Academic Press, pp. 237–250, 2000.

Laidler, K.J. *Physical Chemistry*, 4th ed. Princeton: Houghton Mifflin, 2003.

Lloyd, A.W., R.G. Faragher, and S.P. Denyer. "Ocular Biomaterials and Implants." *Biomaterials*, vol. 22, pp. 769–785, 2001.

More, R.B., A.D. Haubold, and J.C. Bokros. "Pyrolytic Carbon for Long-Term Medical Implants." In *Biomaterials Science: An Introduction to Materials in Medicine*, B.D. Ratner, A.S. Hoffman, F.J. Schoen, and J.E. Lemons, Eds., 2nd ed. San Diego: Elsevier Academic Press, pp. 170–181, 2004.

Norde, W. and J. Lyklema. "Why Proteins Prefer Interfaces." *Journal of Biomaterials Science Polymer Edition*, vol. 2, pp. 183–202, 1991.

O'Connor, D.J., B.A. Sexton, and R.S.C. Smart. *Surface Analysis Methods in Material Science*. 2nd ed. New York: Springer-Verlag, 2003.

Park, J.B. and J.D. Bronzino. *Biomaterials: Principles and Applications*. Boca Raton: CRC Press, 2003.

Rouessac, F. and A. Rouessac. *Chemical Analysis: Modern Instrumental Methods and Techniques*. New York: John Wiley and Sons, 2000.

Saltzman, W.M. "Cell Interactions with Polymers." In *Principles of Tissue Engineering*, R.P. Lanza, R. Langer, and J. Vacanti, Eds., 2nd ed. Austin: Academic Press, pp. 221–235, 2000.

Schaffer, J.P., A. Saxena, S.D. Antolovich, T.H. Sanders Jr., and S.B. Warner. *The Science and Design of Engineering Materials*, 2nd ed. Boston: McGraw-Hill, 1999.

Sudarshan, T.S. *Surface Modification Technologies*. New York: Marcel Dekker, 1989.

Tarcha, P.J. and T.E. Rohr. "Diagnostics and Biomaterials." In *Biomaterials Science: An Introduction to Materials in Medicine*, B.D. Ratner, A.S. Hoffman, F.J. Schoen, and J.E. Lemons, Eds., 2nd ed. San Diego: Elsevier Academic Press, pp. 684–697, 2004.

Tran, H., M. Puc, F. Chrzanowski, C. Hewitt, D. Soll, B. Singh, N. Kumar, S. Marra, V. Simonetti, J. Cilley, and A. Del Rossi. "Surface Modifications of Mechanical Heart Valves," In *Biomaterials Engineering and Devices: Human Applications*, vol. 1, D.L. Wise, Ed. Totowa: Humana Press, pp. 137–144, 2000.

Vaidya, R., L.M. Tender, G. Bradley, M.J. O'Brien, 2nd, M. Cone, and G.P. Lopez. "Computer-Controlled Laser Ablation: A Convenient and Versatile Tool for Micropatterning Biofunctional Synthetic Surfaces for Applications in Biosensing and Tissue Engineering." *Biotechnology Progress*, vol. 14, pp. 371–377, 1998.

Voet, D. and J.G. Voet. *Biochemistry*, 3rd ed. New York: John Wiley and Sons, 2004.

Whitesides, G.M. "The 'Right' Size in Nanobiotechnology." *Nature Biotechnology*, vol. 21, pp. 1161–1165, 2003.

Whitesides, G.M., J.P. Mathias, and C.T. Seto. "Molecular Self-Assembly and Nanochemistry: A Chemical Strategy for the Synthesis of Nanostructures." *Science*, vol. 254, pp. 1312–1319, 1991.

Yager, P. "Biomedical Sensors and Biosensors." In *Biomaterials Science: An Introduction to Materials and Medicine*, B.D. Ratner, A.S. Hoffman, F.J. Schoen, and J.E. Lemons, Eds., 2nd ed. San Diego: Elsevier Academic Press, pp. 669–684, 2004.

CHAPTER 8

Protein Interactions with Biomaterials

Main Objective

To understand thermodynamic principles governing protein adsorption to biomaterial surfaces and relate protein structure and transport properties to kinetics and reversibility of adsorption.

Specific Objectives

1. To understand basic thermodynamic equations for protein-substrate systems.
2. To compare and contrast the three major factors that govern protein adsorption.
3. To understand basic protein chemistry and hierarchy of organization.
4. To understand how structure of proteins affects folding and adsorption.
5. To use equations to model protein transport to surfaces.
6. To compare and contrast reversible and irreversible protein binding, including molecular reasons behind these phenomena.
7. To understand how adsorption may be altered in solution with the presence of many protein types.
8. To understand the theory behind and possible limitations to the characterization techniques presented.

8.1 Introduction: Thermodynamics of Protein Adsorption

As discussed previously, since the body reacts to the layer of adsorbed proteins on a biomaterial surface rather than the surface itself, by changing the protein adsorption profile, one can affect the overall biological response to an implant. In Chapter 7, various means to modify biomaterial surfaces and the potential impact on protein adsorption were described. In this chapter, we will address the issue from a different perspective: the composition of proteins and how it affects their ability to bind to material surfaces.

Usually, protein attachment to biomaterials involves noncovalent interactions with the surface, and these types of interactions are the focus of this chapter. Occasionally, however, such as in the case of complement (see Chapter 12), covalent bonding to the biomaterial is possible. Further examples of protein-biomaterial interactions and their biological sequelae are found in later chapters of this text.

8.1.1 Gibbs Free Energy and Protein Adsorption

In order to understand the adsorption process, the system (protein, solvent, and surface) before and after the event must be analyzed to see if it is thermodynamically favorable for adsorption to occur. In order to do this, we must employ the basic thermodynamic quantity of **Gibbs free energy** (G).

The Gibbs free energy includes contributions from entropy (S), but there is also an enthalpic (H) component. Briefly, **enthalpy** is a measure of the amount of energy in a system available for mechanical work. **Entropy**, on the other hand, is a measure of the disorder of the system. The second law of thermodynamics states that spontaneous processes occur to increase the disorder of the universe (increase entropy). The Gibbs free energy,

$$G = H - TS \tag{8.1}$$

where T is the temperature of the system, relates these two concepts and can be used to determine whether it is favorable for a given reaction to proceed.

In general, the Gibbs free energy cannot be measured, but changes in free energy (ΔG) can be quantified for a system before and after a reaction. The previous equation then becomes (at constant temperature and pressure)

$$\Delta G = \Delta H - T\,\Delta S \tag{8.2}$$

where Δ in each case is the value for the products minus the value for the reactants. Due to the constraints imposed by the second law of thermodynamics, $\Delta G \leq 0$ indicates a spontaneous reaction and anything that lowers ΔG is energetically favorable.

These equations for a chemical reaction are applicable to adsorption processes since the adsorption of a protein (P) to an empty site on a surface (*) can be modeled as a reversible chemical reaction; that is,

$$P + {*} \longleftrightarrow P^*$$

where P^* denotes a surface site that has a protein adsorbed to it. Then, the change in G for the entire adsorption process (ΔG_{ads}) can be represented as

$$\Delta G_{ads} = \Delta H_{ads} - T\,\Delta S_{ads} \tag{8.3}$$

However, this equation is a generalization—it is important to remember that it includes calculation of ΔG for each component of the system before and after the adsorption event. These individual calculations include those

1. For the protein(s):

$$\Delta G_{prot} = \Delta H_{prot} - T\,\Delta S_{prot} \tag{8.4}$$

2. For the solvent (such as water and ions) near the adsorption surface:

$$\Delta G_{sol} = \Delta H_{sol} - T\,\Delta S_{sol} \tag{8.5}$$

3. For the biomaterial surface:

$$\Delta G_{surf} = \Delta H_{surf} - T\,\Delta S_{surf} \tag{8.6}$$

In each case, Δ is the value after adsorption minus the value before adsorption. These ΔG values are combined to get an overall ΔG for the adsorption reaction:

$$\Delta G_{ads} = \Delta G_{prot} + \Delta G_{sol} + \Delta G_{surf} \tag{8.7}$$

Therefore, if the adsorption event reduces ΔG for one or more components of the system with minimal concurrent increase in ΔG for another component, protein adsorption will be thermodynamically favored.

EXAMPLE PROBLEM 8.1

Consider the equation for changes in Gibbs free energy in terms of the following cases of ΔH and ΔS:

Case 1: $\Delta H < 0$ and $\Delta S < 0$
Case 2: $\Delta H > 0$ and $\Delta S < 0$
Case 3: $\Delta H < 0$ and $\Delta S > 0$
Case 4: $\Delta H > 0$ and $\Delta S > 0$

For each case, indicate what conditions would lead to positive values of ΔG. Also, indicate the temperatures for which the process or reaction is spontaneous.

Solution: Recall the equation for changes in Gibbs free energy:

$$\Delta G = \Delta H - T\,\Delta S$$

For Case 1, where $\Delta H < 0$ and $\Delta S < 0$, ΔG will be positive when $T\,\Delta S > \Delta H$. Recalling that reactions or processes are spontaneous when $\Delta G < 0$, it follows that the process for Case 1 is spontaneous when $T\,\Delta S < \Delta H$, or rearranged, $T < \Delta H/\Delta S$. For Case 2, where $\Delta H > 0$ and $\Delta S < 0$, ΔG will always be positive. Consequently, the process for Case 2 is nonspontaneous at all temperatures. For Case 3, where $\Delta H < 0$ and $\Delta S > 0$, ΔG will always be negative. As a result, the process for Case 3 is spontaneous at all temperatures. For Case 4, where $\Delta H > 0$ and $\Delta S > 0$, ΔG will be positive when $T\,\Delta S < \Delta H$. It follows that the process for Case 4 is spontaneous when $T\,\Delta S > \Delta H$, or rearranged, $T > \Delta H/\Delta S$.

Summary of Cases:

Case 1: $\Delta H < 0$ and $\Delta S < 0 \rightarrow \Delta G < 0$ when $T < \Delta H/\Delta S$
Case 2: $\Delta H > 0$ and $\Delta S < 0 \rightarrow \Delta G > 0$ for all T
Case 3: $\Delta H < 0$ and $\Delta S > 0 \rightarrow \Delta G < 0$ for all T
Case 4: $\Delta H > 0$ and $\Delta S > 0 \rightarrow \Delta G < 0$ when $T > \Delta H/\Delta S$ ■

8.1.2 System Properties Governing Protein Adsorption

In the previous chapter, it was found that the following surface attributes most affect protein adsorption:

1. Surface hydrophobicity
2. Surface charge

When these concepts are generalized to the entire system, the factors that have the largest impact on protein adsorption are as follows:

1. Dehydration of the surface and protein (contribution of hydrophobicity)
2. Redistribution of charged groups (contribution of charge)
3. Structural rearrangement of the protein

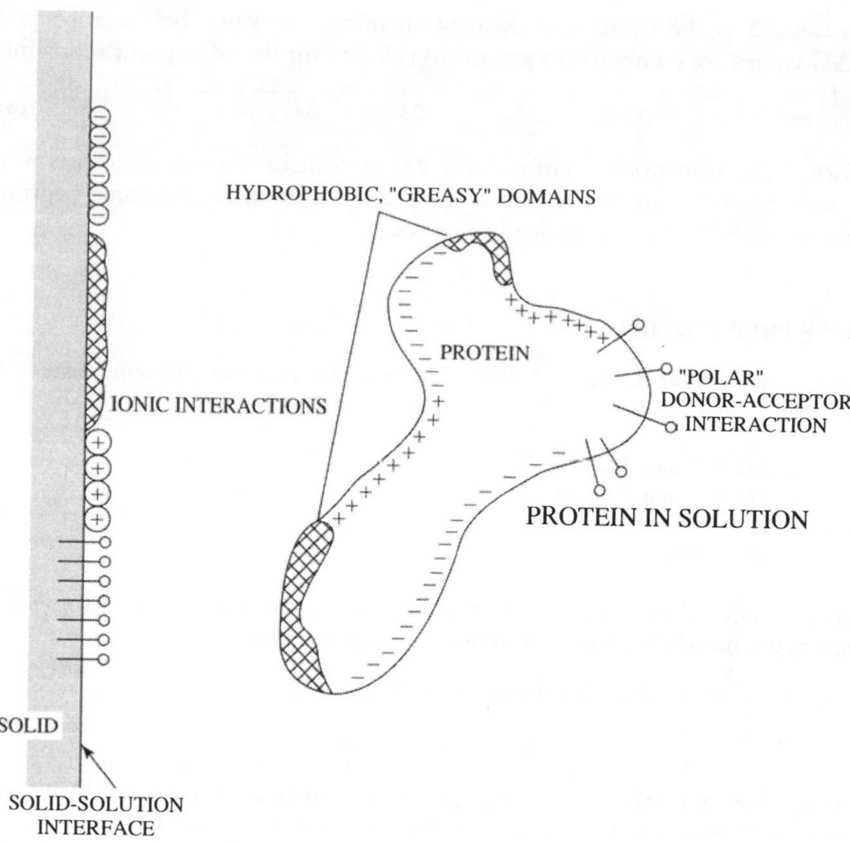

Figure 8.1
Schematic showing the interaction between a biomaterial surface and a protein. The surface of a protein can have multiple locations that interact with the material surface. (Adapted with permission from [1].)

When analyzing the system before and after adsorption, it is useful to think of interactions between domains on the biomaterial surface and the protein, rather than the entire surface or the protein as a whole. This concept is illustrated in Fig. 8.1. An overview of various properties of proteins and surfaces, and how they affect their interactions, is found in Tables 8.1 and 8.2.

TABLE 8.1

Protein Properties that Affect Surface Interactions

Property	Effect
Size	Larger molecules have more sites for surface contact.
Charge	Molecules near their isoelectric point* generally adsorb more readily.
Hydrophobicity	More hydrophobic molecules generally adsorb more readily on hydrophobic surfaces.
Structure:	
Stability	Less stable proteins (such as those with less intramolecular crosslinking) can unfold to a greater extent and form more surface contact points.
Unfolding Rate	Molecules that rapidly unfold can form surface contacts more quickly.

*Isoelectric point: The pH at which the electrolyte concentration of an amphoteric substance such as protein is electrically zero because the concentration of its cation form equals the concentration of its anion form. (Adapted with permission from [2].)

TABLE 8.2

Surface Properties that Affect Interactions with Proteins

Feature	Effect
Topography	Greater texture exposes more surface area for interaction with proteins.
Composition	Chemical makeup of a surface will determine the types of intermolecular forces governing interaction with proteins.
Hydrophobicity	Hydrophobic surfaces tend to bind more protein.
Heterogeneity	Nonuniformity of surface characteristics results in domains that can interact differently with proteins.
Potential	Surface potential will influence the distribution of ions in solution and interaction with proteins.

(Adapted with permission from [2].)

Dehydration is a major driving force in protein adsorption. Water molecules become more ordered at hydrophobic surfaces (either biomaterial surfaces or protein surfaces). Therefore, if hydrophobic areas are able to come together through adsorption to reduce the overall hydrophobic surface area, disordering of the water (solvent) in the region and an increase in the entropy of the system results. From the second law of thermodynamics, this increase in entropy is highly desirable.

Charge can also play a significant role in determining if protein adsorption to a given surface is thermodynamically favorable. For example, if a protein and surface both have the same charge, a repulsive force will develop that reduces protein attachment. Since this process occurs in aqueous conditions, charge repulsion between the surface and the protein can be overcome through adsorption of ions with opposite charge from the media (Fig. 8.2). However, this involves an expenditure of energy to transfer the ions in the solvent to the adsorbed layer. Therefore, adsorption is

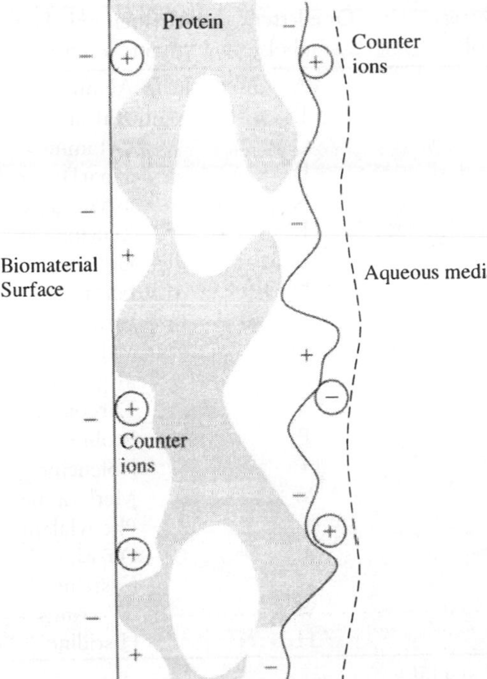

Figure 8.2 Schematic of protein adsorbed to surface. Charge can play a significant role in determining if protein adsorption to a given surface is thermodynamically favorable. For example, if the same charge is found on a protein and the surface, then a repulsive force will develop that reduces protein attachment. This repulsion between the surface and the protein can be overcome through adsorption of ions with opposite charge from the surrounding aqueous media (depicted here by charge signs surrounded by circles). Shading indicates hydrophobic regions. (Adapted with permission from [3].)

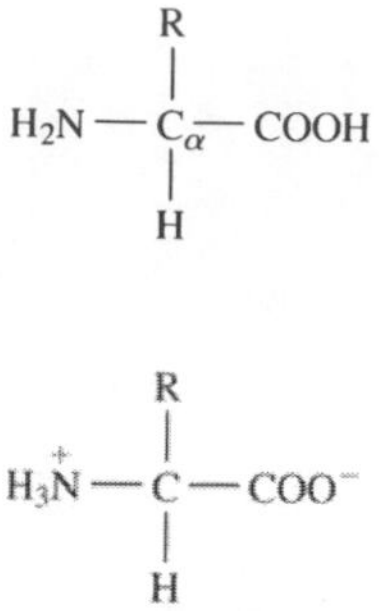

$$H_2N-C_\alpha(R)(H)-COOH$$

(a)

$$H_3\overset{+}{N}-C(R)(H)-COO^-$$

(b)

Figure 8.3
(a) Amino acids have a central carbon atom attached to a hydrogen atom, a carboxyl group (COOH), an amine group (NH_2), and a R group. Differences in R groups are what distinguish amino acids from one another. (b) At physiological pH, the amino and carboxyl groups carry equal but opposite charges.

preferred when many areas of the protein have opposite charge to regions of the biomaterial surface, because, in this instance, the transfer of fewer ions from the solvent is required.

Finally, structural rearrangement of the protein molecule during the adsorption process is extremely important to both the extent of the protein coat on the material surface and its resistance to delamination. If a protein is less structurally stable, it may preferentially adsorb to a biomaterial surface, since conformational rearrangement is easier. This rearrangement allows for an optimal conformation so that hydrophobic and charged regions of the protein can be placed to best fulfill the above two criteria.

A protein's stability is primarily determined by intramolecular bonds, which are directly related to its chemical composition. The following sections describe the chemical subunits found in proteins and how they dictate protein structure and stability.

8.2 Protein Structure

8.2.1 Amino Acid Chemistry

Amino acids are the basic subunits of protein structure. As depicted in Fig. 8.3, these molecules have a central carbon atom attached to a hydrogen atom, an amine group (NH_2), a carboxyl group (COOH), and an R group. Differences in R groups distinguish amino acids from one another. At physiological pH, the amino and carboxyl groups carry equal but opposite charges (Fig. 8.3) so amino acids are considered **zwitterions** and can act as either acids or bases.

There are 20 standard amino acids, as shown in Table 8.3. They are represented in shorthand form by either a three-letter or one-letter code. Each amino acid is

TABLE 8.3

The Amino Acid Residues of Proteins

Amino acid residue	Three-letter symbol	One-letter symbol	Mnemonic help for one-letter symbol	MW of residue at pH 7.0 (daltons)*	pK value of side chain
Alanine	Ala	A	Alanine	71	
Glutamate	Glu	E	gluEtamic acid	128	4.3
Glutamine	Gln	Q	Q-tamine	128	
Aspartate	Asp	D	asparDic acid	114	3.9
Asparagine	Asn	N	asparagiNe	114	
Leucine	Leu	L	Leucine	113	
Glycine	Gly	G	Glycine	57	
Lysine	Lys	K	before L	129	10.5
Serine	Ser	S	Serine	87	
Valine	Val	V	Valine	99	
Arginine	Arg	R	aRginine	157	12.5
Threonine	Thr	T	Threonine	101	
Proline	Pro	P	Proline	97	
Isoleucine	Ile	I	Isoleucine	113	
Methionine	Met	M	Methionine	131	
Phenylalanine	Phe	F	Phenylalanine	147	
Tyrosine	Tyr	Y	tYrosine	163	10.1
Cysteine	Cys	C	Cysteine	103	
Tryptophan	Trp	W	tWo rings	186	
Histidine	His	H	Histidine	137	6.0

(Adapted with permission from [4] and [5].)

designated genetically by a **codon,** a set of three sequential bases in the DNA strand. Each amino acid has one or more unique codons.

The properties of the individual amino acids vary greatly and are most affected by the size and composition of the R group. As illustrated in Fig. 8.4, under physiological conditions, the R groups can be nonpolar, polar, positively charged or negatively charged. Charge interactions between amino acids have a significant impact on the final protein structure, as discussed in the following sections.

Two non-charged amino acids that play a large role in determining the secondary, tertiary and even quaternary structure of a protein are proline and cysteine. Proline, because it contains a ring structure as part of its backbone, has fewer degrees of rotational freedom than the other amino acids and therefore can limit protein folding in three dimensions. Cysteine contains a sulfide (SH) moiety in its R group and thus provides the possibility of forming disulfide (S-S) bonds with other cysteine residues (see below for further discussion).

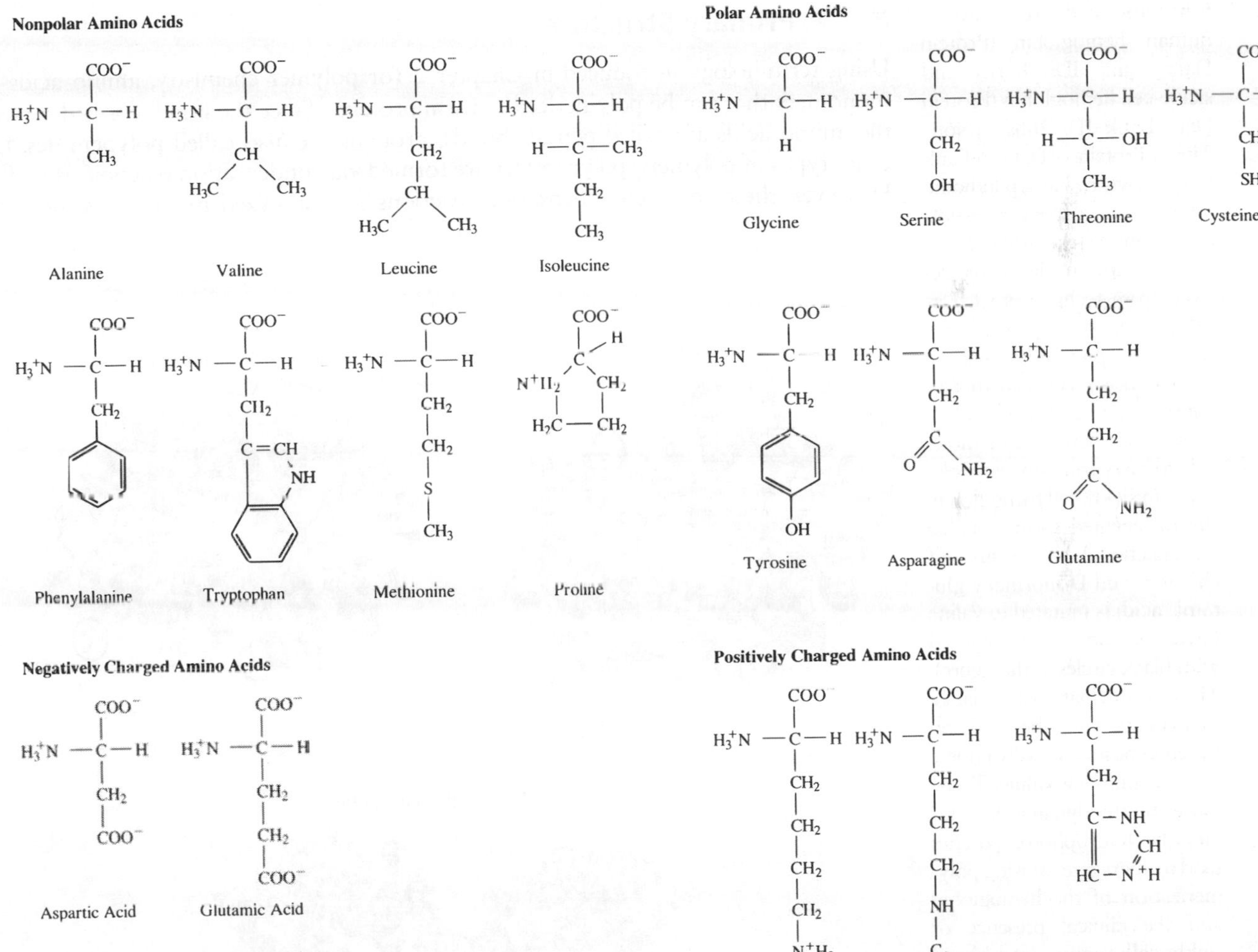

Figure 8.4
The various R groups of amino acids, which can be nonpolar, polar, positively charged, or negatively charged.

$$H_3\overset{+}{N}-CH(R_1)-COO^- + H-\overset{+}{N}H_2-CH(R_2)-COO^- \xrightarrow{-H_2O} H_3\overset{+}{N}-CH(R_1)-C(=O)-NH-CH(R_2)-COO^-$$

Figure 8.5
Schematic of a condensation reaction. As shown here, this type of reaction can result in the formation of polypeptides and always releases water.

8.2.2 Primary Structure

Using terminology introduced in Chapter 2 for polymer chemistry, amino acids are monomers that can be polymerized to form proteins. Since the bonds formed between the amino acids are called **peptide bonds**, proteins are also called **polypeptides.** Like other types of polymers, polypeptides are formed via condensation reactions (Fig. 8.5). However, these specific condensation reactions are catalyzed by enzymes inside the

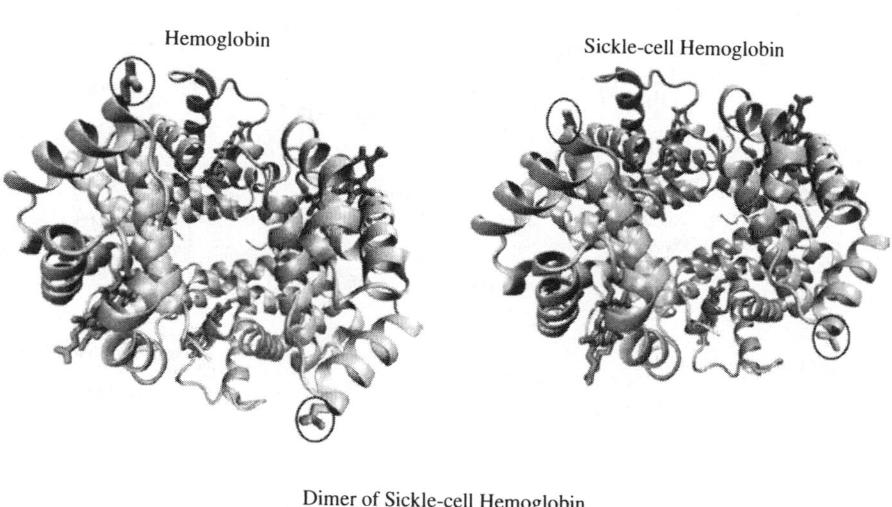

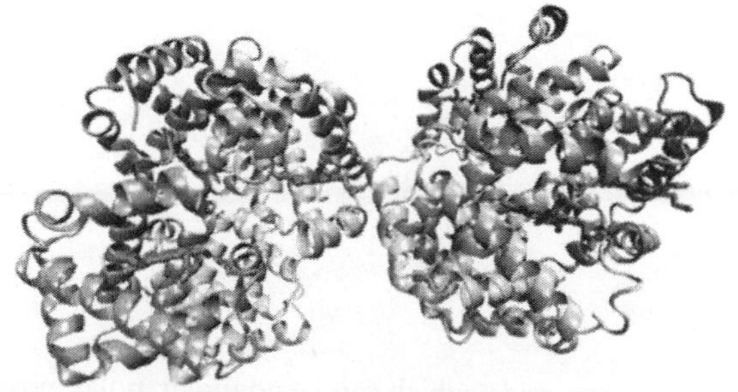

Figure 8.6
Schematic of the structures of human hemoglobin (Protein Data Bank ID: 1o1n) and sickle-cell hemoglobin (Protein Data Bank ID: 2hbs). [Note: The Protein Data Bank (http://www.resb.org/pdb/home/home.do) is a freely accessible collection of structural data for proteins and nuclic acids derived from techniques such as NMR spectroscopy and X-ray crystallography and submitted by scientists.] The structure of the four chains of hemoglobin, allows one hemoglobin molecule to carry four oxygen molecules. In sickle-cell hemoglobin, the oxygenated form is stable and functional, but residue 6 of chains B and D (normally glutamic acid) is mutated to valine (areas of mutation marked with black circles in the figure). The conformational change that occurs when the O_2 is released exposes the hydrophobic patch containing valine. To be more thermodynamically stable, the hydrophobic patches tend to aggregate, causing polymerization of the hemoglobin and the clinical presence of sickle-cell anemia (red blood cells containing the polymerized hemoglobin take on an elongated shape). (Image courtesy of N. Haspel and L.E. Kavraki, Rice University.)

cells in response to the template provided by the codons found in the cellular DNA. Protein production is described further in Chapter 9.

A protein's **primary structure** is the linear order of its amino acids as dictated by the codons. The primary structure is extremely important as it directs all of the other levels of structure, and thus the final functionality of the protein. For example, substitution of a single amino acid (valine instead of glutamate) in the polypeptide chain that composes hemoglobin, the protein that carries oxygen in the blood, changes its overall folded shape and results in the disease known as sickle cell anemia (see Fig. 8.6).

8.2.3 Secondary Structure

As depicted in Fig. 8.7, there are multiple levels of protein structure, which ultimately result in the final conformation, or three-dimensional arrangement, of the molecule. While the primary structure addresses only the linear order of the amino acids, the **secondary structure** is caused by localized interactions between these amino acid residues. The formation of hydrogen bonds between the carboxyl and amino groups of amino acids lying closely together creates twists and folds in the polypeptide chain.

Primary Structure (E-helix)

SAQVKGHGKKVADALTNAV

Secondary Structure (E-helix)

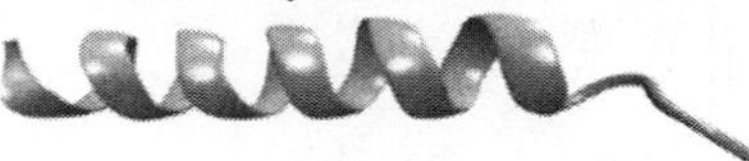

Tertiary Structure (α subunit)

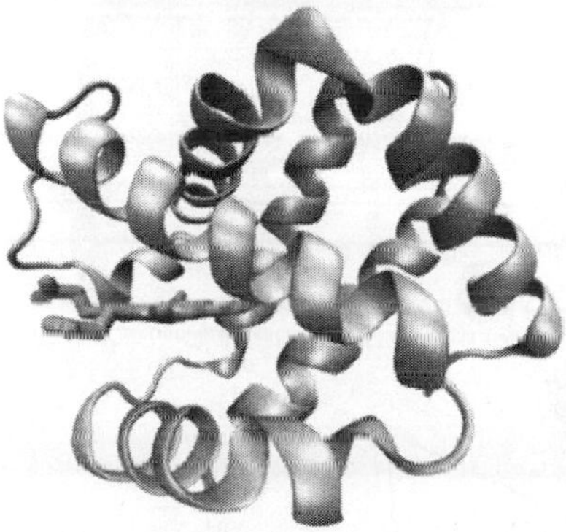

Quaternary Structure (Human hemoglobin)

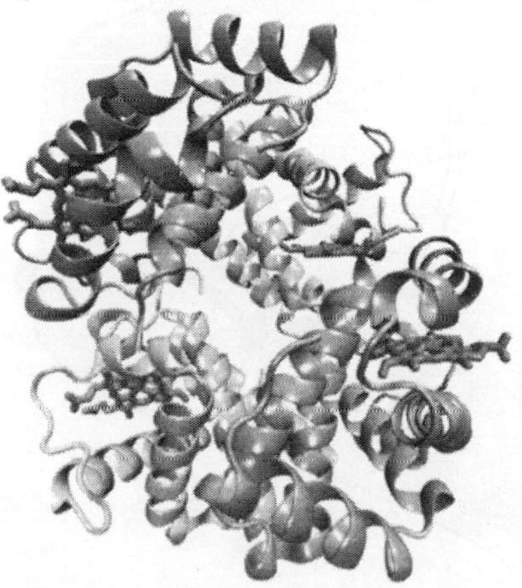

Figure 8.7
An example of the multiple levels of protein structure, which ultimately result in the final conformation, or three-dimensional arrangement, of the molecule (in this case human hemoglobin). While the primary structure addresses only the linear order of the amino acids, the secondary structure is caused by localized interactions between these amino acid residues. The formation of hydrogen bonds between the carboxyl and amino groups of amino acids lying close together creates twists and folds in the polypeptide chain, as seen in the E helix of this example. Further folding of these secondary structures in three dimensions forms the tertiary structure, as depicted in the α subunit of this example. Quaternary structure describes the orientation of multiple polypeptide chains and is caused by interactions between side groups belonging to different chains. In this example different subunits, such as α subunit, interact to form the quaternary structure of human hemoglobin. (Image courtesy of N. Haspel, L.E Kavraki, J.S. Olson, and J. Soman, Rice University.)

The two most common types of secondary structures (because they are the most thermodynamically favorable) are the **α-helix** and the **β-pleated sheet**. Either left- or right-handed α-helices can be formed, but right-handed are more stable. As shown in Fig. 8.8, there are 3.6 amino acids per turn to allow for hydrogen bonding between an amino acid and one that lies four residues behind it. The amino acids are oriented with the side chains of their R groups toward the outside of the helix. An example of a protein

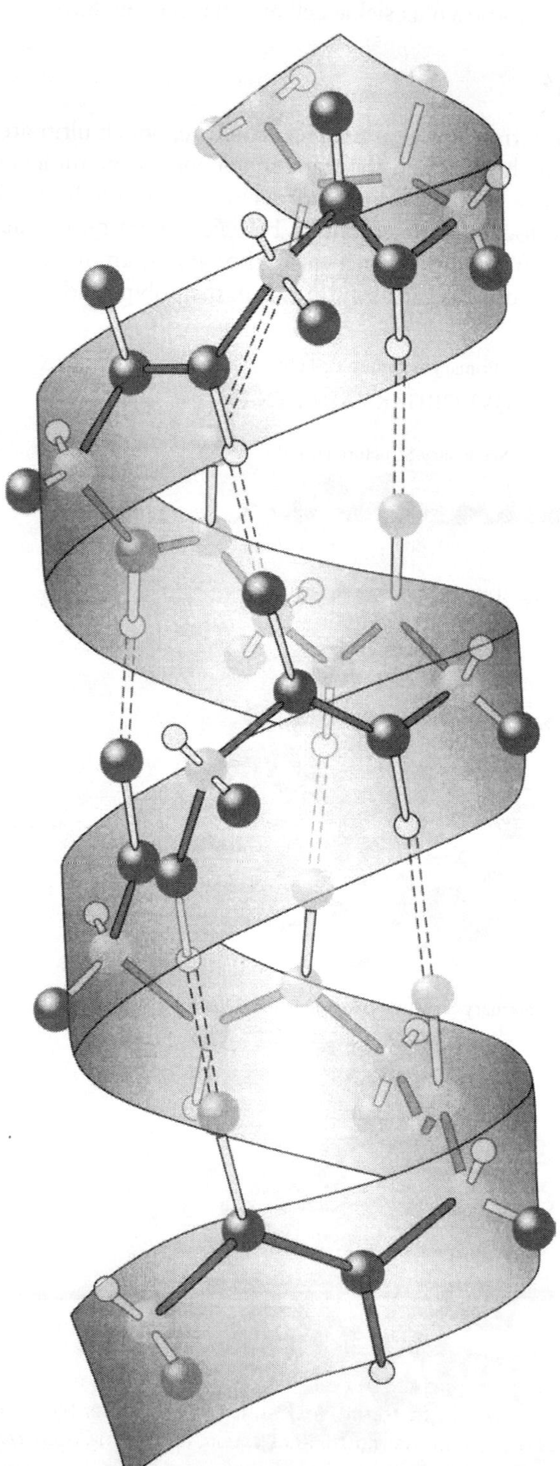

Figure 8.8
An α-helix structure. The amino acids are oriented with the side chains of their R groups toward the outside of the helix. There are 3.6 amino acids per turn to allow for hydrogen bonding between an amino acid and one that lies four residues behind it. Hydrogen bonds are depicted here as dashed lines. (Illustration, Irving Geis. Rights owned by Howard Hughes Medical Institute. Not to be used without permission.)

with an α-helical secondary structure is collagen (see Fig. 9.15), which is found in a number of human tissues. The collagen helix contains many proline resides. As mentioned in the previous section, there is less possibility for movement around the backbone of proline, which, in combination with the other amino acids in the primary structure of collagen, acts to stabilize the helical structure. However, in other cases (different primary structures), proline may disrupt the helix because it is difficult for sections of the chain containing this amino acid to twist and allow the correct positioning of the amino groups for the formation of stabilizing hydrogen bonds.

In contrast to the α-helix, the β-pleated sheet structure is stabilized by hydrogen bonds between two chains or portions of a chain. In this case, each of the neighboring chains adopts an extended linear zigzag conformation, as illustrated in Fig. 8.9. In this figure, the side chains project above and below the plane of the

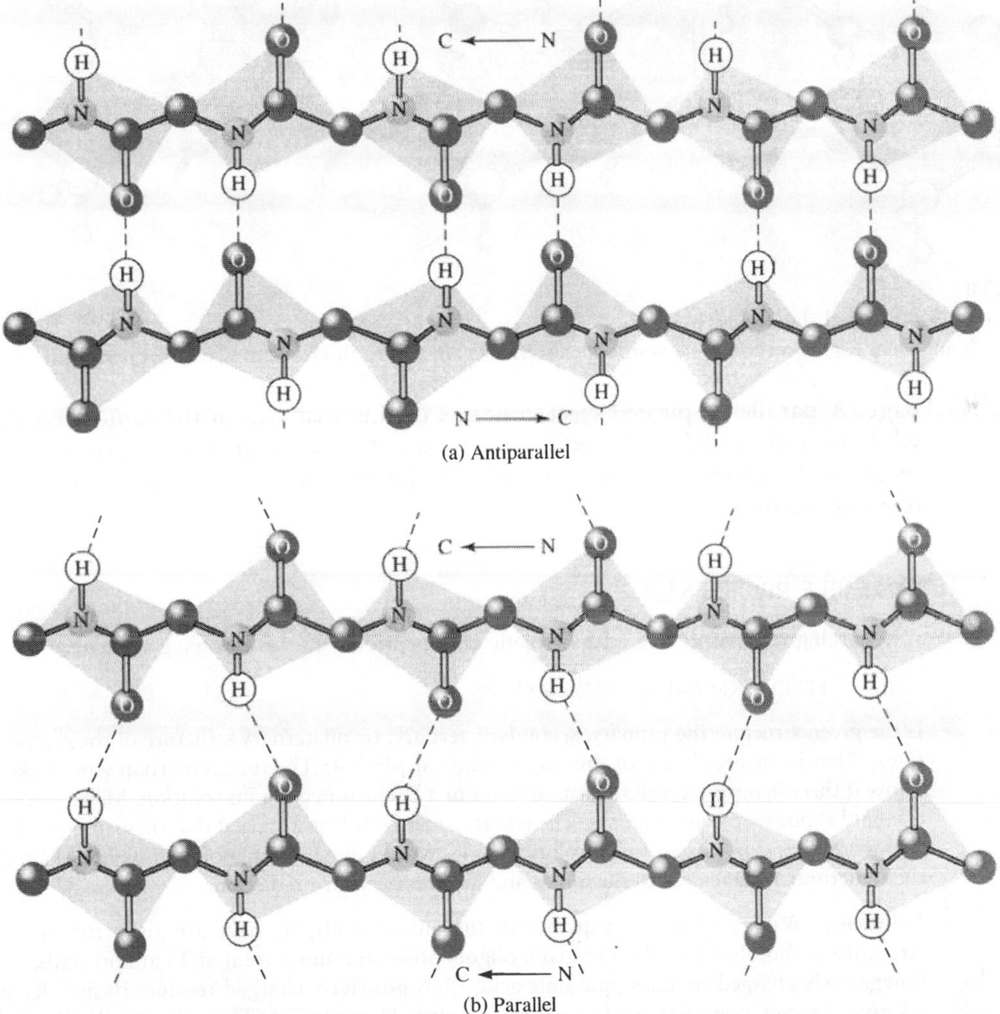

Figure 8.9
The β-pleated sheet structure, which is stabilized by hydrogen bonds between portions within a chain or between chains. In this case, each of the neighboring chains adopts an extended linear zigzag conformation. The side chains project above and below the plane of the page. An **antiparallel β-pleated sheet** (a) consists of chains that extend in opposite directions, while a **parallel β-pleated sheet** (b) contains chains that run in the same direction. "H" indicates hydrogen, "N" indicates nitrogen, and "O" indicates oxygen in the figure. (Illustration, Irving Geis. Rights owned by Howard Hughes Medical Institute. Not to be used without permission.)

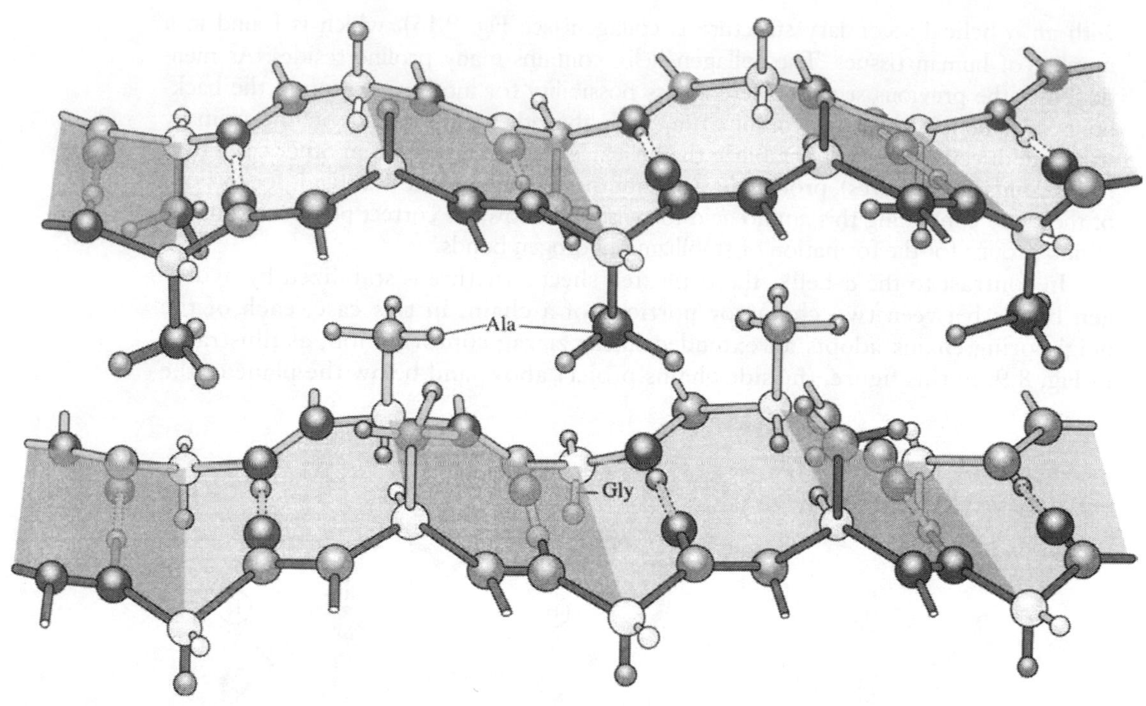

Figure 8.10
Schematic of the β-pleated sheet structure of silk.
(Illustration, Irving Geis. Rights owned by Howard Hughes Medical Institute. Not to be used without permission.)

page. A **parallel β-pleated sheet** contains chains that run in the same direction, while an **antiparallel β-pleated sheet** consists of chains that extend in opposite directions. A natural polymer that contains this type of secondary structure is silk (see Fig. 8.10).

EXAMPLE PROBLEM 8.2

A research group has generated a synthetic oligopeptide with the following sequence:

FEFEFEFKFKFKFEFEFEFKFKFKF

Is the given structure the primary, secondary, tertiary, or quaternary structure of the oligopeptide? What is the net charge of this oligopeptide at pH 7.4? The research group would like to know if this oligopeptide will form an α-helix or a β-sheet in aqueous solution. Make a prediction and rationalize your response. The research team has hypothesized that these oligopeptides will form dimers in physiological solution. Why would dimer formation be favorable? Predict the structural arrangement of the dimer and rationalize your prediction.

Solution: We are given the sequence of the amino acids, thus we are given the primary structure of this oligopeptide. The given oligopeptide contains a total of 25 amino acids, with 6 negatively charged residues (glutamic acid, E), 6 positively charged residues (lysine, K) and 13 non-charged, nonpolar residues (phenylalanine, F) at pH 7.4. Thus, the net charge of the oligopeptide at pH 7.4 is zero. The oligopeptide would likely form a β-sheet in aqueous solution, as a result of the regular pattern between non-polar residues and charged residues and consideration of the amino acids themselves. The regular repetition of the large aromatic R group of phenylalanine would likely present a steric barrier to the formation of an α-helix structure. Additionally, steric repulsion between the charged R groups of glutamic acid and lysine could strain an α-helix. A β-sheet structure, however, schematically indicated as follows, allows for the side groups of the phenylalanine to be on one side of the sheet, while the charged groups are on the other side of the sheet.

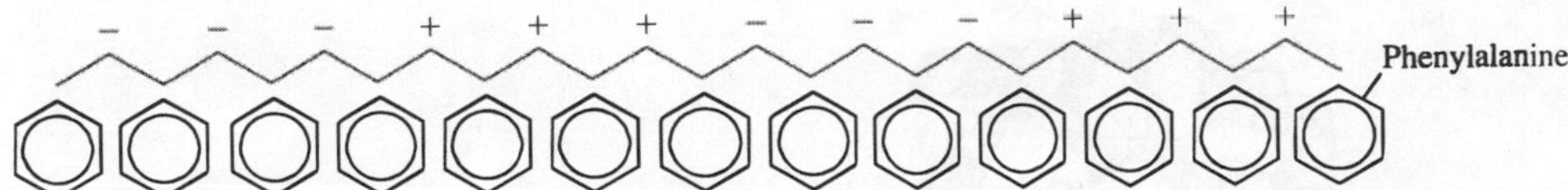

It is reasonable to hypothesize that the sheets would dimerize or form other assemblies of multiple sheets, as hydrogen bonding and charge interactions between the sheets stabilize the structures. The dimers would likely form as schematically illustrated below; however, the manner in which the sheets associate depends upon the conditions of the solution (ionic strength, temperature, presence, concentrations and charges of other solutes, etc.). The proposed dimerization shown below allows for interaction of the non-polar phenylalanine groups on the interior of the dimer, with the charged residues exposed to the aqueous solvent. From a thermodynamics point of view, it is favorable to have the charged groups exposed to the media, as exposure of the non-polar groups would increase local order of the water molecules, and decrease entropy. ■

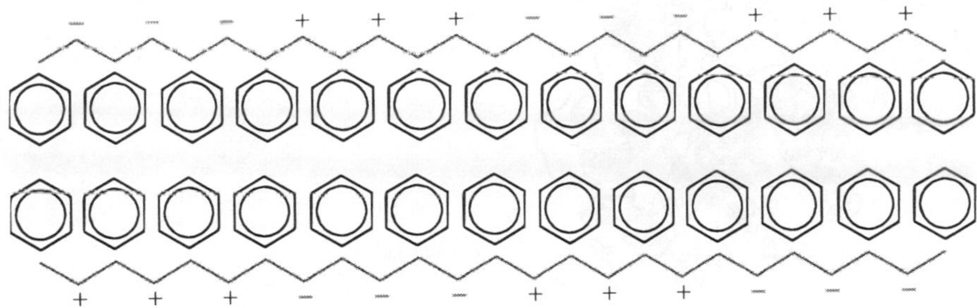

8.2.4 Tertiary Structure

The **tertiary structure** of a protein is the three-dimensional arrangement of an entire polypeptide chain (how the secondary structural elements are folded, see Fig. 8.7). This is caused by interactions between distant amino acids on the same chain. Unlike the secondary structure, which is mainly dictated by bonding between groups in the backbone of the chain, interactions between R group side chains play a large role in determining the tertiary structure of a protein. A common example of a unique tertiary structure is the so called **TIM-barrel fold**, shown in Fig. 8.11, named because it was first identified in triosephosphate isomerase (TIM), a protein involved in energy production in cells. This distinctive structure has eight parallel β-strands surrounded by eight α-helices on the outside.

A number of types of interactions between side chains can occur to influence the folding of a protein in three dimensions, including the following:

1. Covalent bonding
2. Ionic interactions
3. Hydrogen bonding
4. Hydrophobic interactions

Covalent bonds are most commonly found between sulfur atoms on cysteine residues, as discussed above. Since covalent bonds are quite strong, disulfide bonds impart a great deal of stability to protein conformation. Although ionic interactions are weaker, they are also important in the final protein arrangement. These occur between positively and negatively charged side groups on the amino acids. Similarly, hydrogen bonds can be formed between polar amino acids. Folding due to hydrophobicity is caused by the mutual benefit of removing ordered water from near nonpolar residues through the interaction of the hydrophobic (nonpolar) residues with each other. This "hydrophobic effect" is based on the

(a)

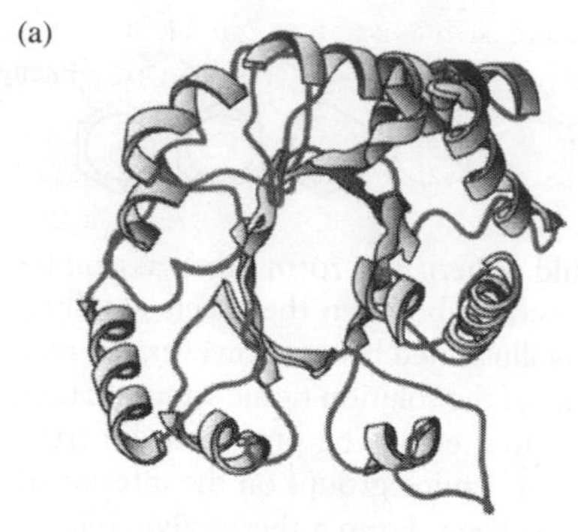

(b)

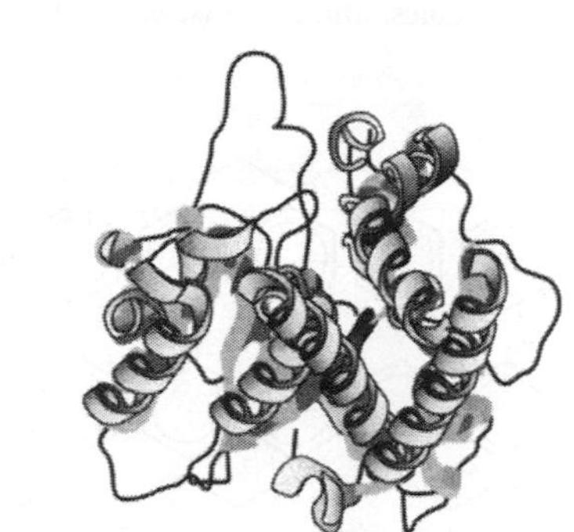

Figure 8.11
Schematic of the TIM-barrel fold structure viewed from (a) above, and (b) the side. This distinctive structure has eight parallel β-strands surrounded by eight α-helices on the outside. (Adapted with permission from [6].)

same entropic arguments as presented earlier for protein adsorption on hydrophobic biomaterial surfaces.

Because of thermodynamic concerns similar to those discussed above for protein adsorption to surfaces, the most stable protein structures place most of the hydrophobic residues on the interior and most of the polar or charged residues on the exterior of the molecule to interact with the aqueous environment. In spite of these general rules, hydrophobic amino acids can occasionally be found on the external surface of a molecule and vice versa for charged residues. However, the energy cost in allowing this to occur indicates that there is a specific reason for such a structure. For example, external hydrophobic areas may provide binding sites for other proteins or cells. Similarly, charged residues found deep within the protein core may help stabilize a particular three-dimensional conformation.

8.2.5 Quaternary Structure

Most proteins are actually composed of several polypeptide chains, each with their own primary through tertiary structure. Each of these chains is referred to as a protein subunit, and the **quaternary structure** of a protein describes the three-dimensional arrangement of these subunits (Fig. 8.7). In this nomenclature, a single subunit is called a monomer, two subunits is a dimer, three is a trimer, etc.

As with tertiary structure, quaternary structure is a result of the interactions between side chains of the R groups of the amino acids, but in this case, the amino acids are on different peptide chains. The types of interactions that stabilize the structure are identical to those described above. Quaternary structure is usually very important to the overall activity of the protein. For example, it is the interactions of four separate polypeptide chains that allow the hemoglobin molecule to carry oxygen molecules in the blood (see Fig. 8.6).

Because the charge of both the peptide backbone and especially the side groups is pH dependent, pH changes may greatly affect both the tertiary and quaternary structures of proteins, which, in turn, could impact their adsorption profiles. The hierarchy presented here suggests that protein conformation is rigidly dictated by the order of amino acids and their subsequent interactions, but it is important to keep in mind that protein folding is a dynamic event. In reality, a protein's "structure" may refer to an equilibrium between several different conformations caused by thermodynamic fluctuations in bonds holding the protein in a certain arrangement. Although this dynamic folding and unfolding process is constantly occurring, the general idea holds that certain proteins are more stable than others (for example, because of a larger number of covalent or hydrogen bonds per volume), which, as described above, will affect their ability to adsorb to solid surfaces.

EXAMPLE PROBLEM 8.3

Some individuals with naturally straight hair choose to "perm" their hair to add long-lasting waves. The permanent or perm procedure typically involves the wrapping of hair around curlers, followed by treatment of the hair with a reducing agent for a period of time and subsequent treatment with an oxidizing agent to set the form of the curl into the hair. Given the fact that a major structural component of human hair is keratin, a protein rich in the amino acid cysteine, explain in terms of protein chemistry how this method of curling hair works.

Solution: The amino acid cysteine contains a sulfide moiety in its R residue. Disulfide bonds formed between cysteine residues in the keratin proteins contribute to the structural stability and elasticity of hair by serving as crosslinks between the protein chains. When hair that is naturally straight is wrapped around a curler, the protein components of the hair are subjected to tensile forces. The addition of a reducing agent results in the breaking of the naturally occurring disulfide bonds between and within the keratin proteins in the hair. The subsequent addition of an oxiding agent to the hair facilitates the reformation of disulfide bonds. However, the bonds are now able to form in a configuration that stabilizes the curled structure that has been imparted to the hair by the curler. Thus, when the chemicals and the curlers are removed, the hair will have waves that are maintained by the new disulfide bonds between and within the keratin proteins of the hair. ■

8.3 Protein Transport and Adsorption Kinetics

The previous sections have revealed that hydrophobicity and charge of both the protein and surface, as well as the structural stability of the protein, can affect adsorption to biomaterials. For proteins, these characteristics are dictated by their primary through quaternary structure. However, before adsorption can occur, the proteins must be transported to the solid surface, and the rate of this transport can affect the kinetics of adsorption.

8.3.1 Transport to the Surface

Equations modeling protein transport generally include factors for the four main types of transport:

1. Diffusion
2. Thermal convection
3. Flow (also called convective transport)
4. Coupled transport (combinations of others, such as convection and diffusion)

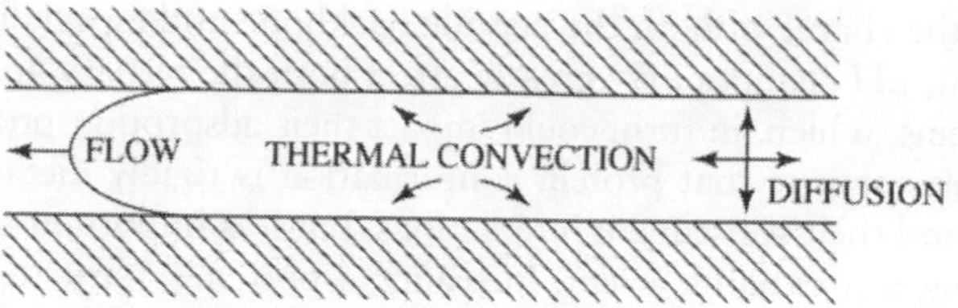

Figure 8.12
Three types of transport phenomena seen in protein adsorption: flow, thermal convection, and diffusion. A concentration gradient drives diffusion, whereas a temperature gradient is responsible for thermal convection. (Adapted with permission from [1].)

Although an in-depth treatment of transport phenomena is beyond the scope of this text, a short discussion of basic transport principles as they relate to protein adsorption is included here. Of the types of transport listed above and depicted in Fig. 8.12, we will focus on the effects of diffusion and flow on protein movement toward a solid surface.

Since transport properties are dependent on geometry, for the sake of the following discussion, we will define a system involving flow inside a cylinder as shown in Fig. 8.13. This would be a simplified model of conditions that are found in blood vessels away from branch points, for example. In this case, the diagram would represent a cross-sectional view of the vessel and the fluid flowing through would be blood, with all its constituent proteins.

Due to interactions with the walls, liquids move more slowly near the sides of a channel, forming a parabolic velocity profile, as illustrated in Fig. 8.13. For this type of geometry, the velocity profile can be represented by

$$V = \frac{2Q}{\mu R^2}\left(1 - \left(\frac{r}{R}\right)^2\right) \tag{8.8}$$

where V is the velocity, μ is the viscosity, r and R are defined in Fig. 8.13, and Q is the volumetric flow rate of liquid through the cylinder. An interesting characteristic of this equation is that at $r = R$ (the wall), $V = 0$. Because of the nature of this parabolic

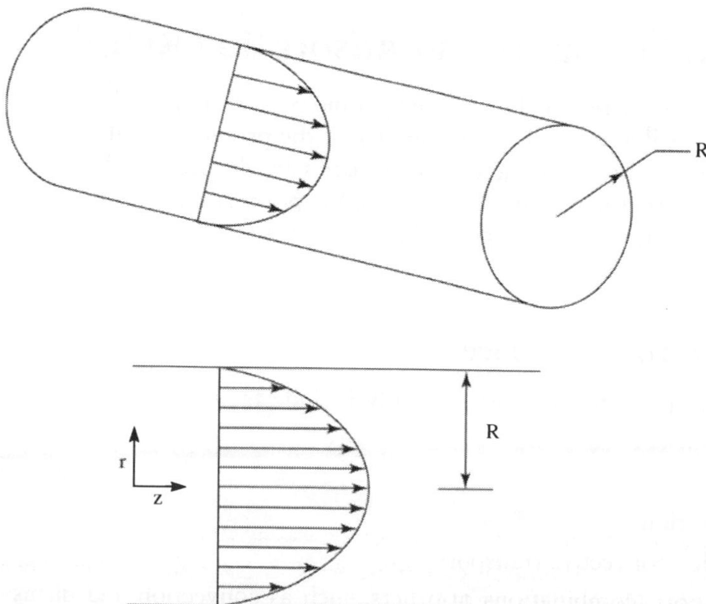

Figure 8.13
Velocity distribution for flow in a cylinder of radius R.

profile, there is no flow at the surface and therefore proteins cannot reach the interface by flow (convection) alone. Thus, diffusion plays a large role in protein transport to solid surfaces even in the presence of flow. In turn, however, the concentrations of proteins close to the surface, which affect the diffusion rate, are influenced by flow conditions.

In light of this, an equation is needed that considers both the convective and diffusional contributions to overall protein transport. This transport equation for the above-defined system is

$$\frac{\partial C}{\partial t} + V\frac{\partial C}{\partial z} = D\frac{1}{r}\frac{\partial}{\partial r}\left(r\frac{\partial C}{\partial r}\right) \tag{8.9}$$

where C stands for the concentration of a protein at time t and position (z,r). In this equation, which considers radial but not axial diffusion, the term including V represents the flow contribution, while the term including D takes into account diffusional contributions. Here, D (diffusion coefficient) is a constant related to the size of the protein and its surrounding medium. The first term in the equation represents the unsteady state term: the change in the concentration with time.

The convective diffusion equation only describes the transport of the protein through a solution. Adsorption of the protein onto the surface can be incorporated using a boundary condition for the solution of this equation, which states that the rate of protein adsorption at the surface ($r = R$) is equal to the rate of transport of protein to the surface. Solutions of this and similar equations are left for more advanced texts on transport phenomena [7].

8.3.2 Adsorption Kinetics

As indicated above, due to their velocity profiles, all flowing fluids contain a layer of undisturbed solution (of varying thickness) near the walls of a vessel. Therefore, if a biomaterial is placed at the wall, the protein adsorption rate should be governed by diffusion alone. However, a number of experiments with blood proteins have found that there was a high initial adsorption rate correlating to diffusion-controlled mechanisms, but after some time, a plateau value was reached (Fig. 8.14). It is now

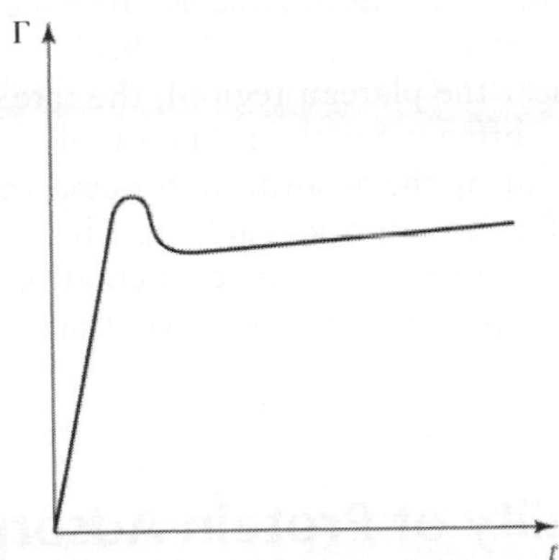

Figure 8.14
Diagram showing the total amount of adsorbed blood proteins (Γ) onto a surface as a function of time (t). There is a high initial adsorption rate correlating to diffusion-controlled mechanisms, and after some time, a plateau value is reached. The "overshoot", or "hump" in the adsorption curve has been explained in a variety of ways, including that during the rearrangement on the surface that occurs as more protein is absorbed, proteins that are less strongly bound may desorb. (Adapted with permission from [1].)

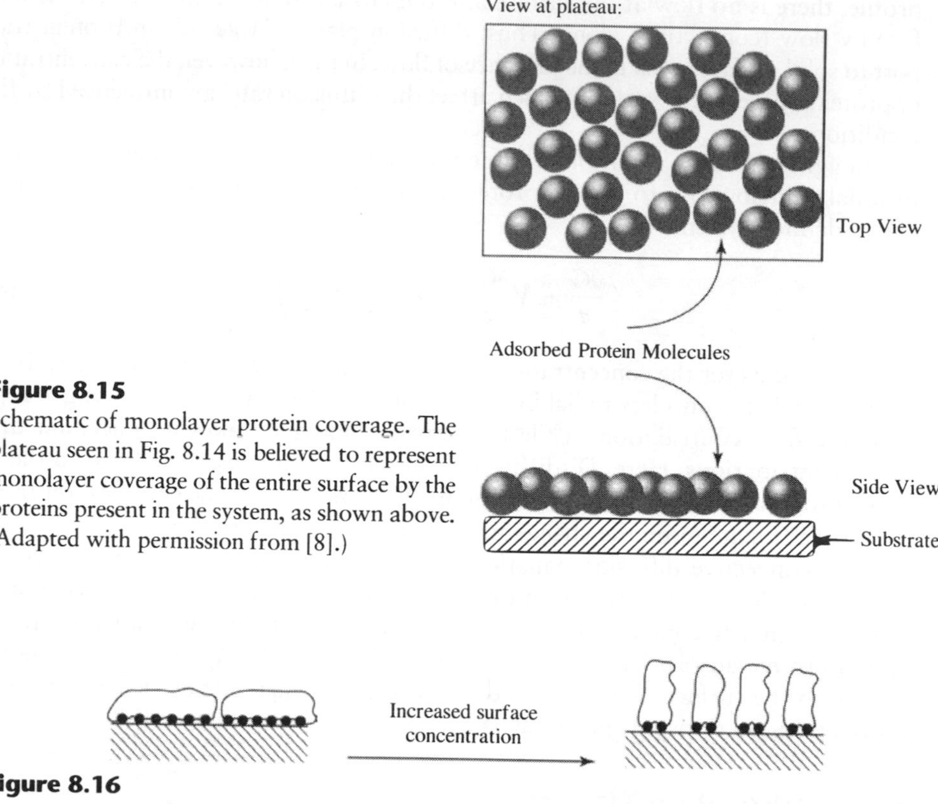

Figure 8.15
Schematic of monolayer protein coverage. The plateau seen in Fig. 8.14 is believed to represent monolayer coverage of the entire surface by the proteins present in the system, as shown above. (Adapted with permission from [8].)

Figure 8.16
Rearrangement of proteins on a surface. The rate of adsorption slows in the vicinity of the plateau region. Presumably, it is more difficult for protein molecules to find a free space on the surface at this point. Rearrangement of proteins (specifically change in their orientation) on the surface occurs to improve packing, thereby increasing the concentration of the protein on the surface. (Adapted with permission from [1].)

believed that this plateau represents monolayer coverage of the entire surface by the proteins present in the system, as shown in Fig. 8.15.

At longer times (near the plateau region), the rate of adsorption slows since, presumably, it is more difficult for the protein molecules to find a free space on the surface. At points during the adsorption process, there may be rearrangement of proteins on the surface to improve packing. This concept is illustrated in Fig. 8.16. In this figure, the molecules change orientation in response to increasing surface concentration of protein, as would occur at later times in the adsorption process.

8.4 Reversibility of Protein Adsorption

8.4.1 Reversible and Irreversible Binding

Whether the protein arrives early or near the plateau value in the adsorption process, there is always a short period of **reversible** binding before it attaches permanently to the surface. It is thought that the protein first makes a few contacts (a "handhold") for initial attachment. As its residence time on the biomaterial increases, the protein changes conformation to promote interactions with the surface. This

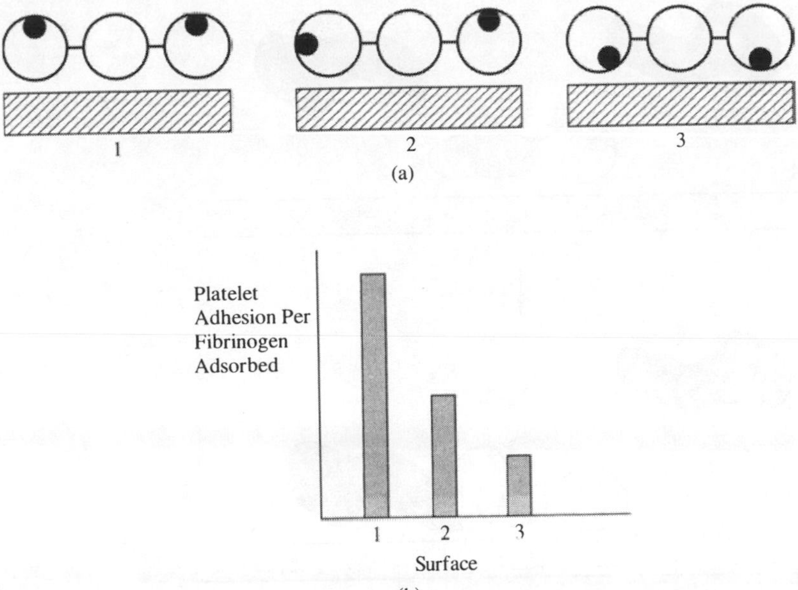

Figure 8.17
Impact of protein adsorption on biological activity. (a) In this example, the darkened regions within the circles indicate biologically active regions of fibrinogen that promote platelet binding. (b) The final conformation of a protein on the surface, and hence where the active regions are located, has a strong impact on its activity. For example, in group 1 there are two biologically active surfaces opposite of the biomaterial surface, hence more activity is observed, whereas when the active regions are oriented toward the biomaterial surface (like in group 3) less activity is observed. (Adapted with permission from [8].)

may be a reaction to characteristics of the surface itself, or to neighboring proteins in the adsorbate (**lateral interactions**). This usually involves some degree of protein unfolding and spreading on the material.

After these conformational changes, eventually protein adsorption becomes **irreversible** (permanent). However, the time required for this to occur depends on the exact protein/surface combination. After this point, protein **desorption** is unlikely because all contacts between the surface and protein would have to be broken simultaneously (see following section).

The final conformation of the protein on the surface has a strong impact on its activity, and, thus, usefulness after adsorption. For example, a series of studies indicates that the ability of fibrinogen (a protein found in the blood) to bind platelets (cell fragments important in blood clotting, see Chapter 13) is affected by the characteristics of the surface to which it is adsorbed [8]. As depicted in Fig. 8.17, this can be due to alterations in the conformation of the adsorbed protein, which on some materials may be such that the binding sites are oriented downward toward the surface and therefore cannot be recognized by the platelets.

8.4.2 Desorption and Exchange

While desorption is unlikely, exchange of adsorbed protein molecules does occur in systems like blood that contain multiple protein types. It is believed that this happens because of the dynamic nature of protein attachment to surfaces. It is possible that while a protein breaks contact for an instant due to fluctuations in bonds that govern its attachment to the surface, another protein could form an interaction in

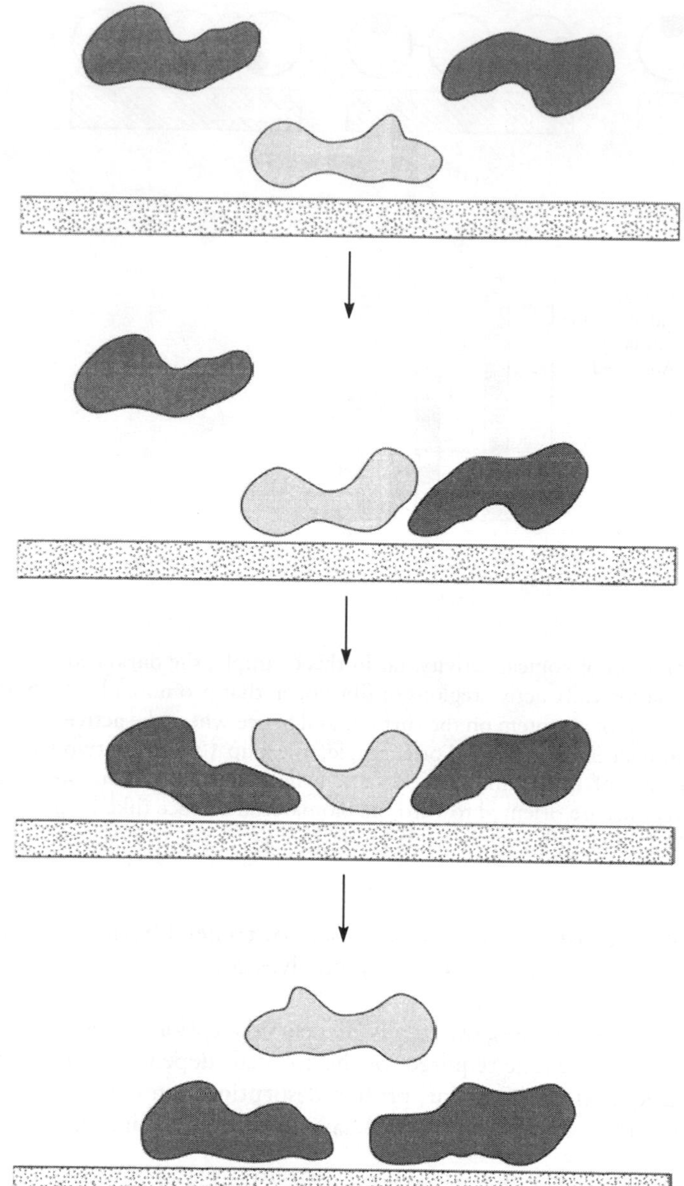

Figure 8.18
A schematic of proteins exchanged on a material surface. The initial protein (light gray) is wedged out of the way by the newer proteins (dark gray), which have a greater affinity for the material. (Adapted with permission from [2] and [4].)

the vacated space. If the second protein can place enough "feet" on the surface in this manner, it will displace the first protein (Fig. 8.18).

Due to this phenomenon, the final protein composition on a surface not only depends on the concentration of protein in the solution, but also its surface affinity. As discussed earlier in this chapter and summarized in Table 8.1, surface affinity can be influenced by the size, charge, hydrophobicity, structural stability, and unfolding rate of the protein. Since the diffusion rate is dependent on concentration, it follows that proteins with higher concentration will arrive and adsorb first, but they will eventually be replaced by those with greater surface affinity. This exchange is known as the **Vroman effect**. A summary of the Vroman effect with selected plasma proteins on glass and metal oxide surfaces is found in Fig. 8.19.

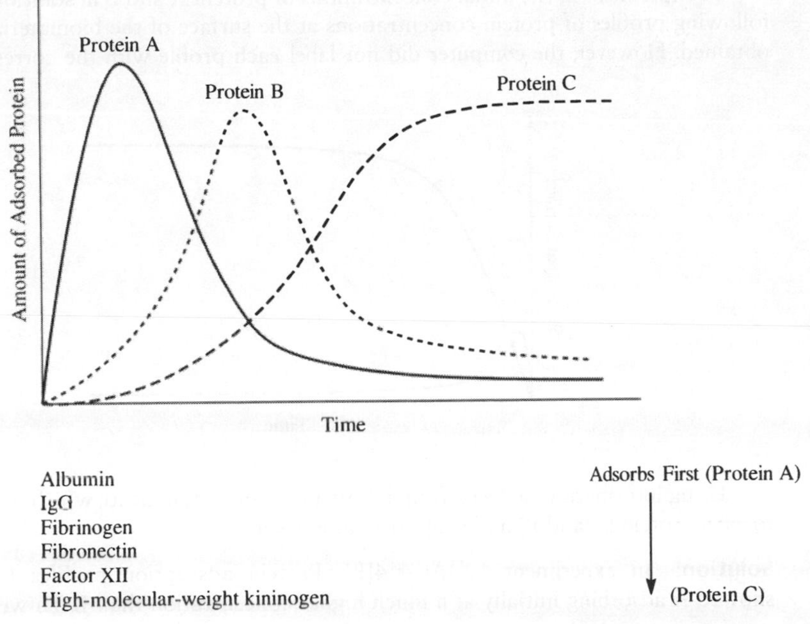

Figure 8.19
A diagram of the Vroman effect. Proteins with higher concentration (such as albumin in the case of blood) will rapidly attach, and then be replaced over time by proteins with greater surface affinity. (Adapted with permission from [2].)

EXAMPLE PROBLEM 8.4

An experimental biomaterial is placed into an aqueous solution containing protein A (10 kDa) at an initial solution concentration of [A] and protein B (100 Da) at an initial solution concentration of [B]. It can be assumed for this exercise that the protein adsorption rate is governed by diffusion alone. Consider the results of the following experiments:

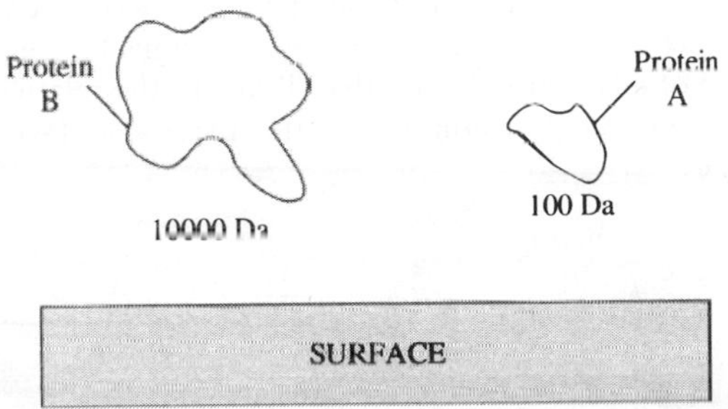

In experiment 1, the initial concentration of protein A in solution was four times the initial concentration of protein B in solution. The following profiles of protein concentration at the surface of the biomaterial with time were obtained.

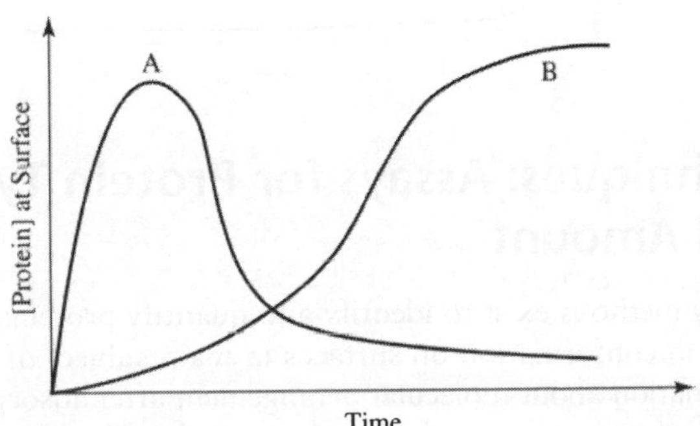

In experiment 2, the initial concentrations of protein A and B in solution were equal. The following profiles of protein concentrations at the surface of the biomaterial with time were obtained. However, the computer did not label each profile with the corresponding protein.

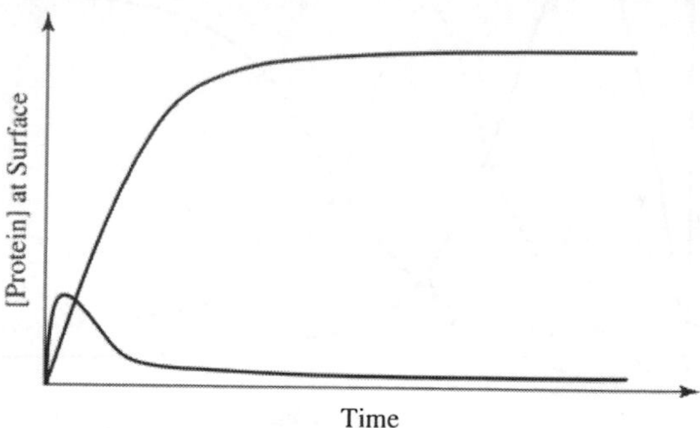

Using information deduced from the first experiment, indicate which profile corresponds to each protein (A and B) and support your answer.

Solution: In experiment 1, [A] = 4[B]. Protein adsorption profiles for experiment 1 showed A adsorbing initially at a much higher concentration than B. However, with time, B was present at high concentrations at the material surface and A was scarcely present. Considering that the initial concentration of A was high relative to B, the high initial adsorption of A relative to B can be explained in terms of the availability of many more molecules of A than B to interact with the surface. However, as time progressed, protein B adsorbed to the surface at a much higher concentration than A, despite the lower initial solution concentration. Thus, B exhibited a higher affinity for the material surface and displaced the lower affinity A molecules from the surface with time. This is an example of the Vroman Effect. In experiment 2, [A] = [B]. Considering that protein B demonstrated a higher affinity for the material surface than A in experiment 1, one would expect that it would be present on the material surface at higher concentrations than A with time. However, A might be expected to show an initial rate of adsorption higher than B due to the relatively smaller molecular size, which could facilitate initial diffusion of A to the material surface. Thus, the profiles should be labeled as follows: ■

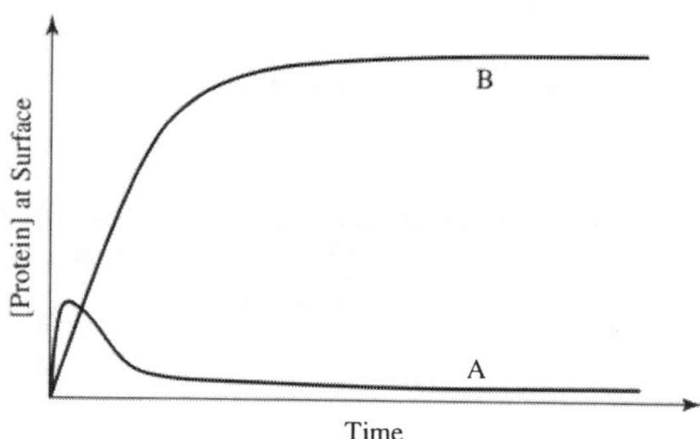

8.5 Techniques: Assays for Protein Type and Amount

Although many methods exist to identify and quantify proteins in solution, determination of protein conformation on surfaces (a main subject of this chapter) is more difficult. Information about molecular arrangement after adsorption can be obtained using a number of the surface analysis techniques described in Chapter 7. ATR-FTIR and other, more advanced surface methods have been employed to probe protein coatings on materials.

Therefore, rather than surface analysis, the focus of this section is on established techniques to identify specific proteins and determine their amount in a given sample. Although these methods are most commonly used to assess a liquid sample containing proteins, some, especially those using antibodies (see below) may be modified for applications involving surface-adsorbed proteins. Alternatively, these techniques can provide information about the protein constitution of the liquid phase over the surface before and after adsorption and, thus, give an indication of the composition of the adsorbate.

This section first discusses affinity chromatography, which achieves quantification and protein purification through the use of the thermodynamic parameters discussed earlier in this chapter. The remainder of the section describes general characterization techniques to determine protein type and quantity, including colorimetric and fluorescent assays, enzyme-linked immunosorbent assays (ELISAs), and Western blotting. It should be noted that a combination of methods are often required to identify/quantify the amount of a particular protein in a sample. For example, a sample that has been fractionated via affinity chromatography (see below) can then be subjected to an ELISA to confirm that a certain protein is found in that portion of the sample.

8.5.1 High-Performance Liquid Chromatography (HPLC): Affinity Chromatography

As shown in Fig. 2.55, there are many different types of liquid chromatography. Size exclusion chromatography (SEC) was described in Chapter 2. We will focus in this section on one type of **affinity chromatography** known as adsorption chromatography. **Ion exchange chromatography** is another important kind of affinity chromatography that separates compounds based on charge, but discussion of this technique is beyond the scope of this book.

8.5.1.1 Basic Principles **Adsorption chromatography** employs the concept of separation by preferential adsorption of the analyte (often proteins) based on hydrophobic and polar interactions. Like SEC, the system contains both a mobile and a stationary phase. The mobile phase is a liquid solvent into which the dissolved sample is injected. The stationary phase is composed of small (diameter 3–10 μm) porous silica or polymer beads. However, unlike SEC, in affinity chromatography, there is no physical entrapment of the analyte in the porous beads. For adsorption chromatography, the beads are coated with either a very hydrophobic (non-polar) or very hydrophilic (polar) polymer that is covalently bonded to their surface. The analyte molecules then adsorb to the beads in differing degrees, depending on their own hydrophobicity.

Retention time is highly affected by the chemical composition of the analyte. The first species to exit the stationary phase is the molecule with the least affinity for the column, and that with the most affinity is eluted last (Fig. 8.20). In between, molecules are retained for varying amounts of time depending on the extent of their interaction with the beads. However, what constitutes "least" and "most" affinity depends on the configuration of the HPLC system.

Normal-phase chromatography employs a polar stationary phase, and a non-polar mobile phase, such as hexane. In contrast, **reversed-phase chromatography** generally uses a non-polar stationary phase and a polar (often aqueous) mobile phase. Therefore, in normal-phase chromatography, more hydrophilic molecules are eluted later since they have more affinity for the stationary than the mobile

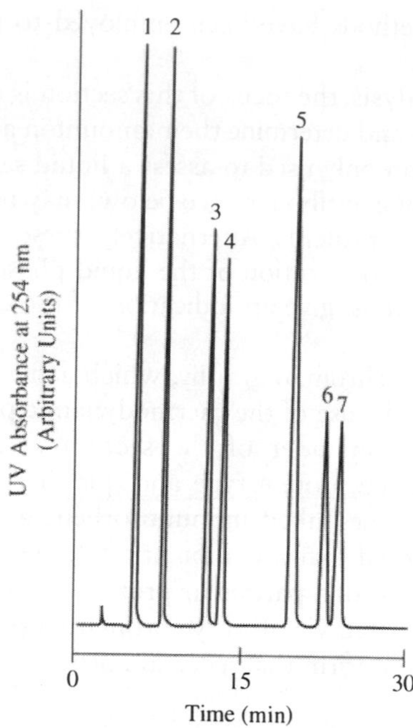

1. Methylparaben (R: —CH_3)
2. Ethylparaben (R: —CH_2CH_3)
3. Isopropylparabene (R: —$CH(CH_3)_2$)
4. n-Propylparabene (R: —$CH_2CH_2CH_3$)
5. sec.-Butylparabene (R: —$CHCH3C_2H_5$)
6. Isobutylparabene (R: —$CH_2CH(CH_3)_2$)
7. n-Butylparaben (R: —$CH_2CH_2CH_2CH_3$)

HO O O R

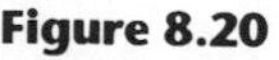

Figure 8.20
HPLC trace of a mixture of parabens (p-hydroxybenzoic acid esters—parabens are widely used antimicrobial agents) on a reversed phase column using a water-methanol (50:50) mixture as the mobile phase. Overall, parabens with increasing hydrophobicity (longer hydrocarbon chains in R group) demonstrate greater retention time due to increased interactions between the molecule and the column. (Adapted with permission from [9].)

phase. However, in reversed-phase chromatography, more hydrophilic species are eluted first, as they have more affinity for the mobile than for the stationary phase (Fig. 8.21).

8.5.1.2 Instrumentation As depicted in Fig. 8.22, the instrumentation required for affinity chromatography is identical to that used for SEC, and includes five basic components: a pump, an injector, a column to separate samples based on hydrophobicity, a detector, and a processor/computer to translate signals from the detector into the appropriate plot. As for SEC, there are a wide variety of detectors used in affinity chromatography, including those based on UV, refractive index or fluorescence.

8.5.1.3 Information Provided Affinity chromatography is often used to determine the amount of a certain separated species present in the original sample. This is accomplished by first integrating the area under the peak for that species. In a similar manner, a standard curve can be generated by integrating the area under the peaks representing increasing amounts of the substance of interest (Fig. 8.23). By comparing the area from the unknown to that recorded on the standard curve, the amount of the unknown species can be quantified. Unlike SEC, where time to elution is used to assign molecular weight, in affinity chromatography, the area under the peak is of most importance for quantification.

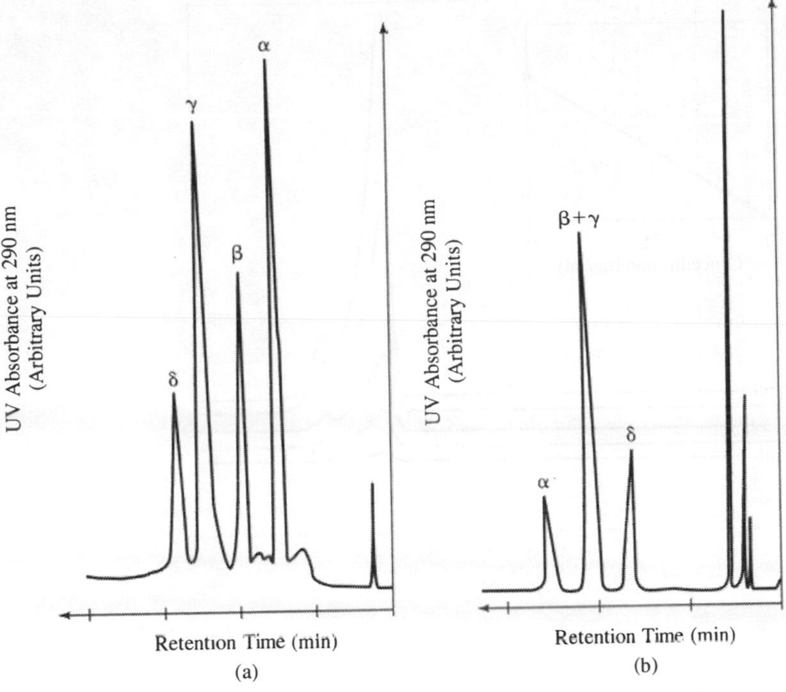

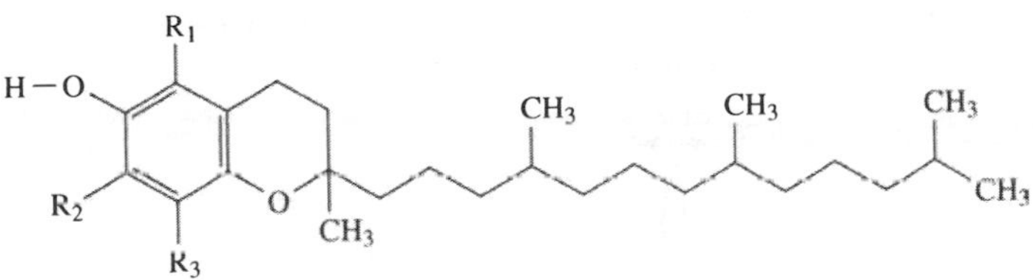

Compound	R_1	R_2	R_3	
α-Tocopherol	—CH_3	—CH_3	—CH_3	
β-Tocopherol	—CH_3	—H	CH_3	
γ-Tocopherol	—H	—CH_3	—CH_3	
δ-Tocopherol	—H	—H	—CH_3	← **Most hydrophilic**

Figure 8.21
(a) Normal-phase chromatogram [mobile phase: hexane–amyl alcohol (99.5:0.5)] of a mixture of α-, β-, γ-, and δ-Tocopherol (four isoforms of vitamin E). In this case, the most hydrophilic substance (δ-Tocopherol) exits the column last because it has a relatively low affinity for the hydrophobic mobile phase. (b) Reversed-phase chromatogram [mobile phase: methanol-water (9:1)] of a mixture of α-, β-, γ-, and δ-Tocopherol. Here the most hydrophilic substance (δ-Tocopherol) exits the column first because it has a relatively high affinity for the hydrophilic mobile phase. (Adapted with permission from [10].)

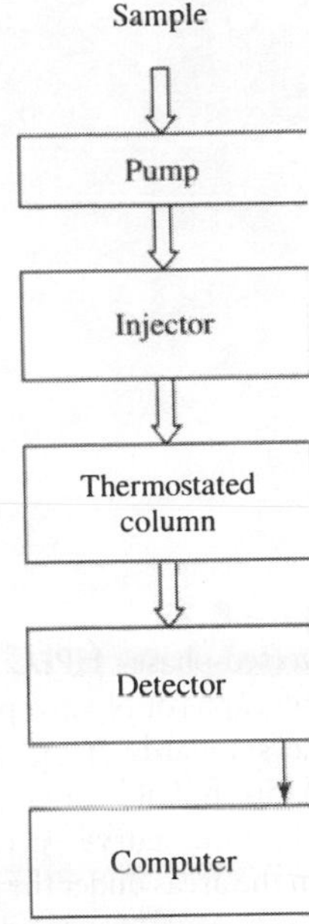

Figure 8.22
Block diagram of affinity chromatography instrumentation. Five basic components are included: a pump, an injector, a column to separate samples based on hydrophobicity, a detector, and a processor/computer to translate signals from the detector into the appropriate plot.

However, elution time is a key element in **fractionation**, another application of affinity chromatography. Such procedures are commonly used for purification of proteins (Fig. 8.24). For example, if the elution time of a pure protein is determined, fractions of the mobile phase can be collected around this time. Because this chromatographic method is non-destructive, these fractions can be reconstituted and used for further studies as a source of uncontaminated sample material.

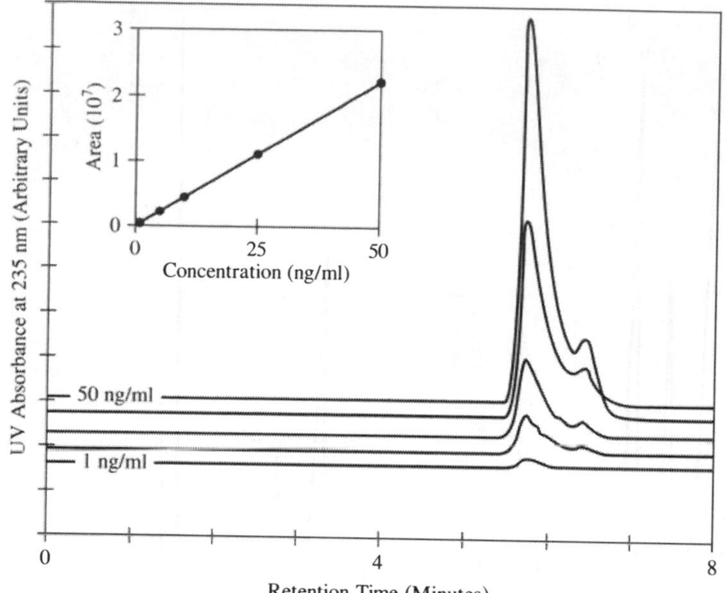

Figure 8.23
Reversed-phase HPLC chromatographs of N-vinyl pyrrolidone standards (1, 5, 10, 25, and 50 ng/ml). Inset graph: Calibration curve generated from the areas under the peaks.

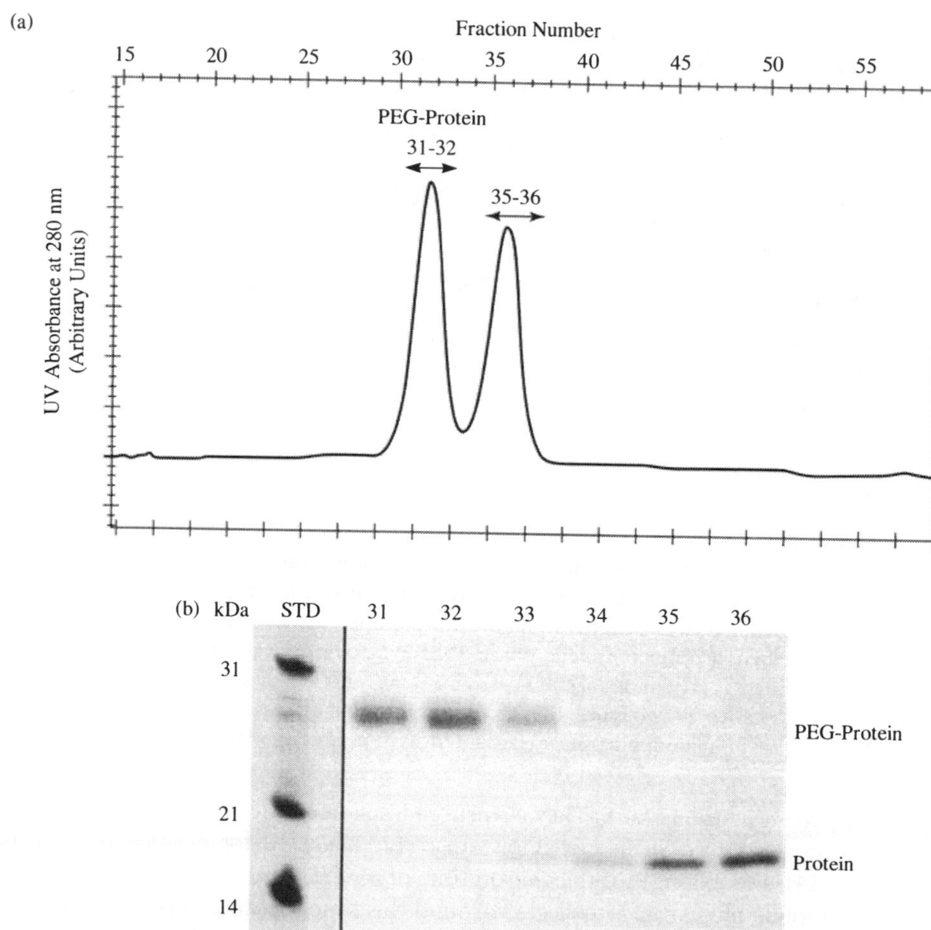

Figure 8.24
Fractionation of a poly(ethylene glycol) (PEG)-protein conjugate by ion exchange chromatography. (a) Elution profile for the PEG/protein reaction mixture applied to a chromatography column. (b) SDS-PAGE analysis of fractions 31–36 recovered from the column. Fractions 31 and 32 contain predominantly the PEG-protein conjugate. Fractions 34–36 contain the unreacted protein. Molecular weight markers are shown in the lane labeled STD. (Adapted with permission from [11].)

EXAMPLE PROBLEM 8.5

Five standard samples of known concentrations of protein X were run through a reversed-phase HPLC system. The data that follow were obtained. After running the standards, three samples (A, B and C) of protein X of unknown concentration were run through the system. Calculate the concentrations of each of the unknown protein solutions, given that the area under the absorbance curve of sample A was 0.87×10^7, of sample B was 1.32×10^7, and of sample C was 0.21×10^7. What would you predict the area under the curve to be for a sample of protein X of concentration 29.0 ng/ml? A sample of a second protein (protein Y) was run on the sample column under the same conditions and eluted approximately 2 minutes after protein X. Based on this observation, which protein has the largest molecular weight? Which protein has greater hydrophilic character?

[X] (ng/ml)	Area Under the Absorbance Curve (Arbitrary Units)
1.0	0.05×10^7
5.0	0.25×10^7
10.0	0.50×10^7
25.0	1.25×10^7
50.0	2.50×10^7

Solution: Given the information for the standards, a standard curve can be generated from a linear regression of the data, with the concentration being the variable "*x*" and the area under the absorbance curve being the variable "*y*" in the linear equation $y = mx + b$, where "*m*" is the slope and "*b*" is the y-intercept.

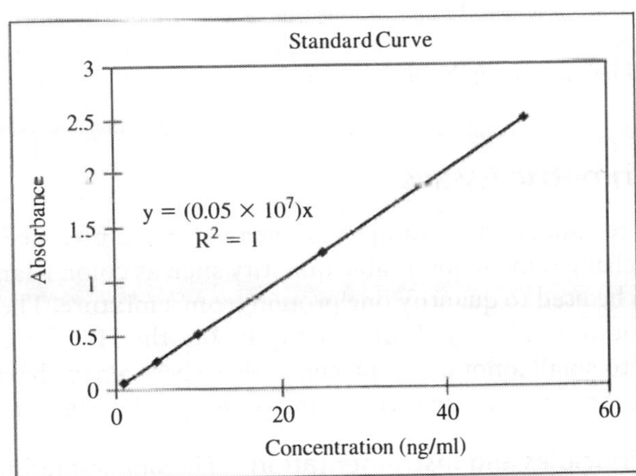

In this case, the slope is 0.05×10^7 ml/ng and the y-intercept is 0, with a correlation coefficient of 1. The equation can be verified for each data point as illustrated below for the first data point:

$$y = mx + b$$

$$0.05 \times 10^7 = m \cdot (1.0 \text{ ng/ml}) + b$$

$$0.05 \times 10^7 = 0.05 \times 10^7 \text{ ml/ng} \cdot (1.0 \text{ ng/ml}) + 0$$

$$0.05 \times 10^7 = 0.05 \times 10^7 \ldots \text{ as was to be shown.}$$

Thus, the linear equation for the calibration curve is as follows:

$$(\text{Area Under the Absorbance Curve}) = (0.05 \times 10^7 \text{ ml/ng})^*[X]$$

$$[X] = (\text{Area Under the Absorbance Curve})/(0.05 \times 10^7 \text{ ml/ng})$$

The unknown concentration of each sample can be calculated by substituting into this equation the corresponding area under the absorbance curve.

For sample A,

$$[X] = 0.87 \times 10^7/(0.05 \times 10^7 \text{ ml/ng}) = \underline{17.4 \text{ ng/ml}}$$

For sample B,

$$[X] = 1.32 \times 10^7/(0.05 \times 10^7 \text{ ml/ng}) = \underline{26.4 \text{ ng/ml}}$$

For sample C,

$$[X] = 0.21 \times 10^7/(0.05 \times 10^7 \text{ ml/ng}) = \underline{4.2 \text{ ng/ml}}$$

The area under the absorbance curve for a 29.0 ng/ml sample of protein X would be predicted to be

$$\text{Area Under the Absorbance Curve} = (0.05 \times 10^7 \text{ ml/ng}) \cdot 29.0 \text{ ng/ml}$$

$$\text{Area Under the Absorbance Curve} = \underline{1.45 \times 10^7 \text{ arbitrary units}}$$

The elution times of various proteins do not give any indication of the molecular weight of the proteins in HPLC, as it is an affinity-based assay and not a size-exclusion assay. Thus, no determination can be made with respect to the relative sizes of proteins X and Y based upon the HPLC information given. However, there is sufficient information to comment on the relative hydrophilicity of the proteins. Since this is reversed-phase HPLC, it can be assumed that a nonpolar stationary phase and polar mobile phase were used. Therefore, hydrophilic species are eluted first, as they have greater affinity for the mobile phase than the stationary phase. As protein X eluted before protein Y, protein X is more hydrophilic than protein Y based upon the given results. ■

8.5.2 Colorimetric Assays

The following techniques are examples of assays for the presence of a certain protein, based on changes in an observable quantity such as color. Many of these are robust enough to be used to quantify one protein from a mixture. These assays provide similar information to affinity chromatography, but the HPLC technique is usually more sensitive to small amounts of protein. Also, these assays have not been developed for all types of proteins, so certain samples may still be best detected via HPLC.

8.5.2.1 Basic Principles and Instrumentation The simplest test for the presence of a given protein involves direct reaction of the component with a marker chemical to cause a specific color change. The molecule causing this specific color (**chromophore**) will absorb UV-VIS radiation in a manner similar to that described in Chapter 2. Therefore, a UV-VIS spectrophotometer (or, often, an automated plate reader with an attached spectrophotometer) can be used to read the absorbance of the sample at a known wavelength. Beer-Lambert's law is then employed to determine the concentration of the protein in the sample as compared to a standard curve (see Chapter 2).

Colorimetric assays have been designed for proteins that are either enzymes or non-enzymes, although the mechanism of color formation varies slightly. Since the job of an **enzyme** is to cleave substrate materials (see Chapter 9 for more information), this can be exploited to form the basis of the colorimetric assay. If a substrate can be added, that, when cleaved, alters color dramatically (or changes from colorless to colored), the color change can easily be quantified. Since the amount of substrate cleaved is directly proportional to the amount of enzyme present, there is usually a linear correlation between the degree of color change and the amount of enzyme of interest.

Detection of non-enzymatic components may involve a reaction that attaches a chromophore directly to the protein of interest. Alternatively, a portion of the protein to be quantified may react to change the conformation or other chemical characteristics of a dye, thus producing a color change.

8.5.3 Fluorescent Assays

8.5.3.1 Basic Principles Fluorescent assays for proteins are similar in concept to colorimetric assays, but there are key differences in instrumentation. In this case, the reaction causes the attachment of a fluorescing molecule (**fluorophore**) to the protein of interest. Visible light fluorescence (like X-ray fluorescence discussed in Chapter 7), involves excitation of the fluorophore molecule through absorption of a specific amount of energy (visible light of a given wavelength). On a molecular level, for visible light fluorescence, the excitation often involves the transition of electrons from the π bonding to anti-bonding orbital. The excited molecule undergoes collisions and interactions with surrounding molecules, which causes **radiationless decay** (loss of energy) until the lowest excited energy state is reached. The molecule then returns to the ground state (see Chapter 2), and, in so doing, emits energy of the same order of magnitude as that absorbed (in this case, a slightly different wavelength of visible light due to the loss of energy via radiationless decay).

8.5.3.2 Instrumentation The instrumentation for a fluorometer is similar to that for the UV-VIS spectrophotometer described in Chapter 2. Like a spectrophotometer, a fluorometer includes four main components: a source of visible light, a filter to select the appropriate wavelength, a detector, and a processor/computer to translate signals from the detector into the appropriate values. However, as seen in Fig. 8.25, the light source sample and detector are not collinear, in order to minimize the effect of emission beam scattering. Also in contrast to UV-VIS spectrophotometers, the instrumentation is configured to analyze light intensity from the sample near a certain wavelength (the expected emission wavelength) only, instead of providing values for the entire spectrum. Because fluorescent phenomena are

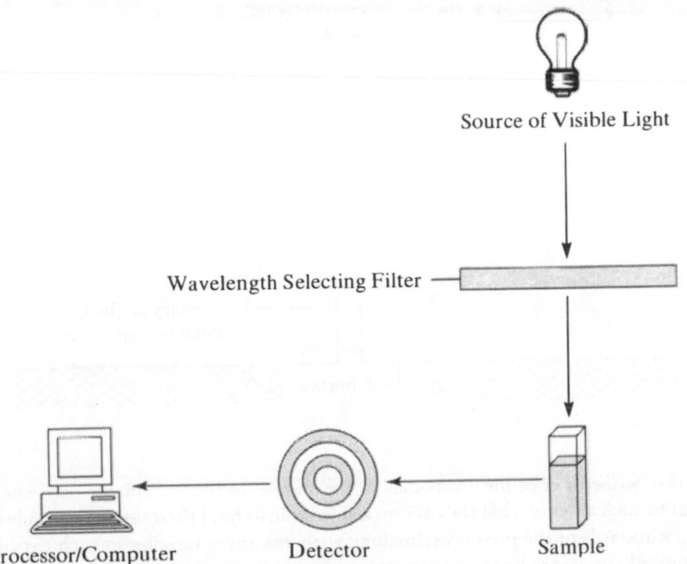

Figure 8.25
Schematic of a fluorometer. A fluorometer includes four main components: a source of visible light, a filter to select the appropriate wavelength, a detector, and a processor/computer to translate signals from the detector into the appropriate values. However, in contrast to UV-VIS spectrophotometers, the instrumentation is configured to analyze light intensity from the sample near a certain wavelength (the expected emission wavelength) only, instead of providing values for the entire spectrum.

short-lived, the fluorometer must be able to provide the excitation wavelength and detect at the emission wavelength simultaneously.

8.5.3.3 Information Provided A derivative of Beer-Lambert's law can be used with fluorescence intensity values, thus allowing the quantification of fluorescently labeled protein molecules, given appropriate standards. Advantages of fluorescent assays include that fluorescent phenomena are detectable at one to three orders of magnitude lower concentration than that observable with traditional colorimetric (absorbance) techniques. Additionally, certain amino acids, such as tryptophan or tyrosine, are intrinsic fluorophores. Therefore, if the protein of interest contains enough of these amino acids, an additional reaction to label the protein is unnecessary.

8.5.4 Enzyme-linked Immunosorbent Assay (ELISA)

8.5.4.1 Basic Principles and Procedures For very specific identification of a protein, the enzyme-detection approach described above can be combined with the use of antibodies in an **enzyme-linked immunosorbent assay** (**ELISA**). The most common type of ELISA is the **sandwich ELISA**. Antibodies, discussed further in Chapter 12, have a unique structure designed to recognize specific portions of proteins and bind tightly to them. Therefore, in the sandwich ELISA, well plates are first coated with an antibody[1] (called the **primary antibody**) designed to attach to the protein of interest. The following steps are then performed (Fig. 8.26):

1. The sample (containing the possible protein of interest) is added.
2. A second antibody (the **secondary antibody**) that is conjugated to an enzyme is added. The secondary antibody will bind to another specific site on the protein of interest. (The enzymes most commonly used for these assays include alkaline phosphatase, horseradish peroxidase and *p*-nitrophenol phosphatase.)

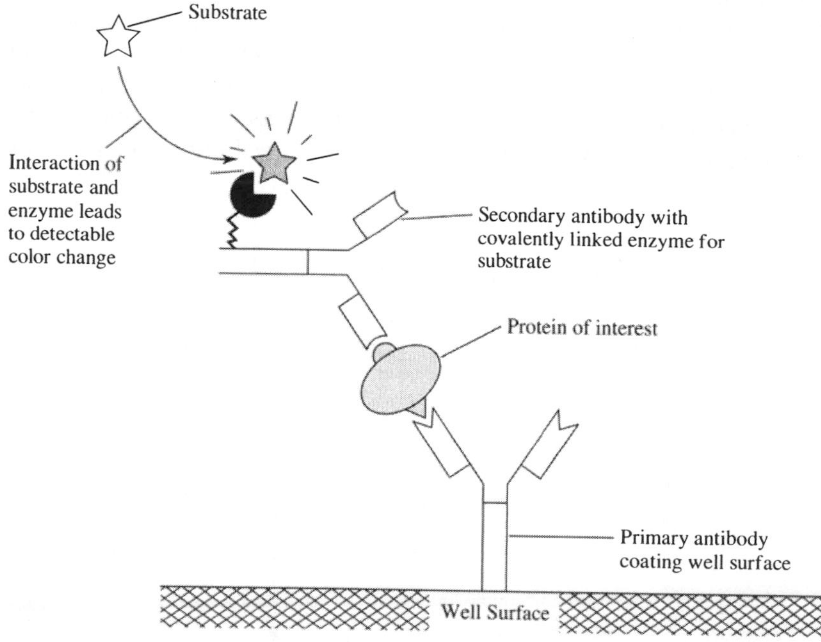

Figure 8.26
Process used in a sandwich ELISA. First, the primary antibody is attached to a well, after which the sample is added. The proteins of interest will then attach to the primary antibody. A secondary antibody is then added, which will attach to the protein of interest. A substrate is added. The well is rinsed after each step, and color change produced by the secondary antibody is measured on a spectrophotometer. This measurement corresponds to the amount of protein of interest in the initial solution.

[1]This method assumes that adsorption of the antibodies to the surface of the well plates does not cause structural rearrangement to such a degree that they are no longer able to bind their target molecules. This is confirmed by running standards of the pure protein along with unknown samples in each experiment to ascertain that the standard curves are linear with respect to protein concentration.

3. The substrate for the enzyme is added and the color change is quantified on a plate reader/spectrophotometer.

Similar to colorimetric assays, the color change is proportional to the amount of protein present. Quantification occurs as the color change for the sample is compared to that which occurs in the presence of different concentrations of the pure protein of interest (standards) after the standards are subjected to the same procedure as described above. It is also common to fluorescently label or radio-label the secondary antibody in this procedure, rather than conjugating it to an enzyme. In these cases, the amount of the protein of interest is quantified by fluorometric-based methods as described previously or by using a radiation detector (such as a gamma counter).

A modification of this technique, in which soluble antibodies are added to a protein adsorbed on a biomaterial surface, can be used to probe the conformation of the adsorbed protein. If the antibodies do not bind to the same degree as they would if the protein were in solution, this is an indication that the protein has unfolded or the regions recognized by the antibody are masked by the surface.

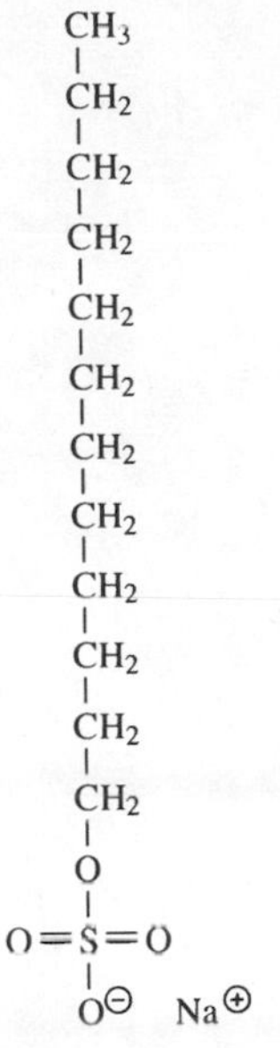

CH_3–CH_2–CH_2–CH_2–CH_2–CH_2–CH_2–CH_2–CH_2–CH_2–CH_2–CH_2–O–$S(=O)_2$–$O^{\ominus}$ $Na^{\oplus}$

Figure 8.27
Structure of sodium dodecyl sulfate (SDS).

8.5.5 Western Blotting

8.5.5.1 Basic Principles and Procedures Antibodies can also be used to identify a certain protein after separation of the many proteins contained in a sample through the use of gel electrophoresis. This procedure is called **Western blotting.** In this case, the sample is first treated with sodium dodecyl sulfate (SDS) (Fig. 8.27), an **amphiphilic** molecule (one that has both hydrophilic and hydrophobic regions). SDS binds to the hydrophobic regions of proteins and causes them to unfold. The SDS-treated sample is then loaded on a poly(acrylamide) gel and exposed to an electric field. SDS is highly negatively charged and effectively masks any charge on the protein, so in the presence of an electric field, the SDS protein will migrate toward the positive pole. Larger molecules will experience more drag while moving through the pores of

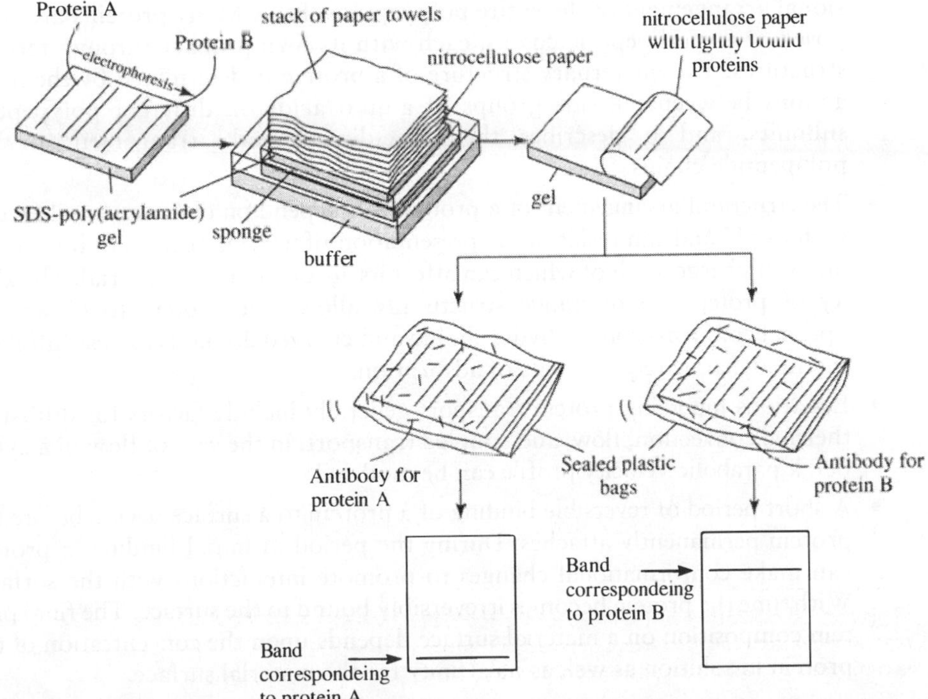

Figure 8.28
Process used in a Western blot assay. The sample is run on a poly(acrylamide) gel, and then transferred to a nitrocellulose sheet. This sheet is then reacted with antibodies (in this case antibodies for proteins A and B) to determine what proteins were present in the initial sample.

the gel, and thus will migrate more slowly. The result is discrete bands in the gel, representing proteins with different molecular weights. This procedure, called **SDS-poly(acrylamide)-gel electrophoresis (SDS-PAGE)**, is a means to separate proteins based solely on molecular weight, and is often used to purify a protein of interest.

To confirm that a certain band contains the target protein, a Western blot can then be performed (Fig. 8.28). This involves the following steps:

1. The bands are transferred to nitrocellulose paper by pressing the gel firmly against the paper. Since nitrocellulose binds proteins nonspecifically, the bands are transferred and appear in the same order as on the original gel.
2. A primary antibody in solution is added on top of the blotted paper.
3. A labeled secondary antibody is added that binds the primary antibody.
4. If the secondary antibody is enzyme-conjugated, the substrate is then added.

Color change, fluorescence, or radioactivity is recorded via camera or other means.

Summary

- Protein adsorption involves a system composed of the protein, solvent, and surface. In order to assess the likelihood of a specific adsorption event, the thermodynamics of the event are evaluated in terms of the total change in Gibbs free energy (G) from before to after the event. An adsorption event is deemed energetically favorable if it lowers ΔG.
- The factors of the entire protein adsorption system that have the greatest impact on adsorption are dehydration of the surface and protein, redistribution of charged groups, and structural rearrangement of the protein.
- The primary structures of proteins are dictated by the linear order of their constituent amino acids. The secondary structure can result in the formation of α-helices and β-pleated sheets. The tertiary structure depends upon how the secondary structural elements are folded, and it entails the three-dimensional arrangement of the entire polypeptide chain. Many proteins are composed of several peptide chains, each with its own primary through tertiary structures. The quaternary structure of a protein is determined by the interactions between the side groups of amino acids on different polypeptide subunits, and it describes the three-dimensional arrangement of the polypeptide chains.
- The structural arrangement of a protein can depend on environmental factors such as pH and can result in the presentation of varying regions of hydrophobicity or charge, each of which can affect its adsorption to a material. The ability of proteins to rearrange structurally allows the protein to obtain the optimal conformation for hydrophobic and charged domains to best fulfill the thermodynamic requirements of adsorption.
- Equations modeling protein transport generally include factors for diffusion, thermal convection, flow, and coupled transport. In the case of flow in a cylinder, a parabolic velocity profile can be modeled.
- A short period of reversible binding of a protein to a surface occurs before the protein permanently attaches. During the period of initial binding, a protein can make conformational changes to promote interactions with the surface. With time the protein becomes irreversibly bound to the surface. The final protein composition on a material surface depends upon the concentration of the protein in solution as well as its affinity for the material surface.

- Affinity chromatography techniques such as adsorption chromatography and ion exchange chromatography allow for protein quantification and purification/fractionation through the application of thermodynamic principles.
- Colorimetric and fluorescent assays can be used to determine and quantify the presence of a certain protein based upon observable changes in the color or fluorescence of the assay solution, respectively. ELISA techniques provide for very specific identification of a protein through the interaction and subsequent detection (colorimetric, fluorescent, or radiographic) of antibodies specific for the protein of interest.
- Western blotting provides a means for separation of proteins through electrophoresis and identification of the protein of interest through use of a detectible antibody specific for the protein of interest.

Problems

8.1 Consider a material for a vascular graft application with proteins adsorbed to its surface and a second material with proteins covalently attached to its surface. For which material would you expect the protein layer to be more stable under flow conditions similar to those found in a blood vessel? Why?

8.2 You are performing an *in vitro* experiment in which you will expose a material you are considering for a medical device to synovial fluid, which contains the proteins albumin, transferrin, and IgM at concentrations of 5, 0.5, and 0.05 mg/ml, respectively. Each of these components has a particular affinity for your material, with IgM being the highest and albumin being the lowest.

(a) Describe the kinetics of protein adsorption to your material and how the surface concentration of each protein will change with time.

(b) Subsequently in the experiment, more albumin is added to the synovial fluid. What effect will this have on the proteins adsorbed to the surface?

(c) The graph below shows the amount of IgM adsorbed to the material surface as a function of time. What will happen on the material surface with the addition of more IgM?

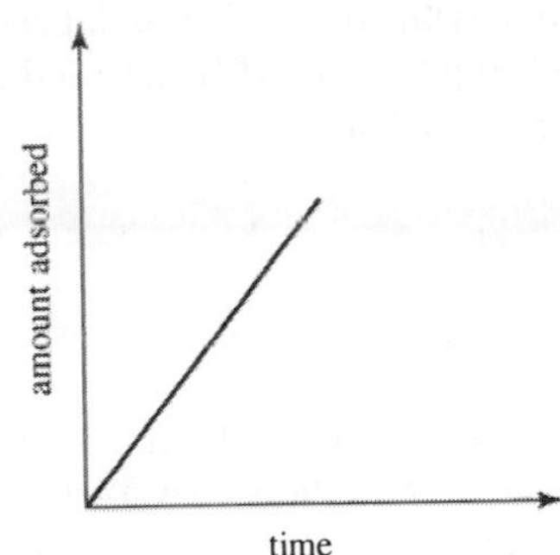

8.3 What determiners of protein structure have the largest impact on protein adsorption to a material? Why?

8.4 You are performing an *in vitro* test to determine protein adsorption to a material. Your testing solution has a pH of 7.2. Partway through your test an assistant accidentally adds some HCl to the solution, resulting in a pH change to 6.7. Will this affect the experiment? Why or why not? (Explain in terms of the response of proteins to changes in pH.)

8.5 You are performing an *in vitro* test in which you are testing the adsorption of three proteins (X, Y, and Z) to a material. After you have exposed the proteins to the material surface, how do you determine which proteins adsorbed? What assay(s) would be suited to analyze the solution and the material surface?

8.6 (a) Describe the similarities and differences between two types of HPLC: size-exclusion chromatography and adsorption chromatography.

(b) Assume the graph below was produced using reversed-phase adsorption chromatography. One of the curves represents a polysaccharide (sugar), while the other represents the same polysaccharide covalently linked to poly(styrene) for a drug delivery application. Which curve is associated with each and why? Explain in terms of molecular interactions with the stationary phase of the column.

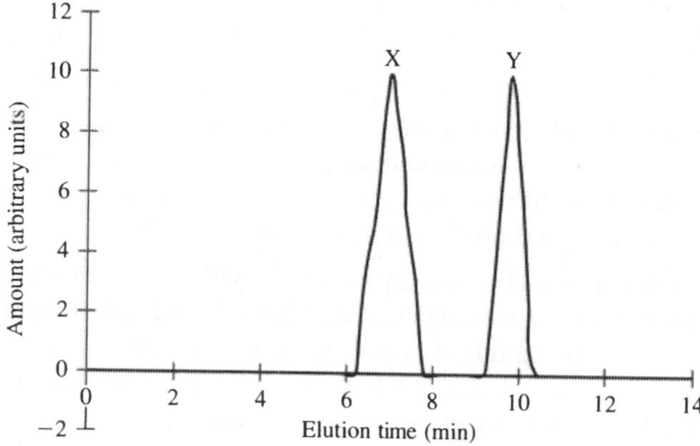

(c) Now assume that the graph above was produced using gel permeation chromatography (a type of size exclusion chromatography) for the same molecules as described above. Which curve is associated with each and why? Explain in terms of molecular interactions with the stationary phase of the column.

8.7 You are interested in surface modification of a material with both a protein and a peptide for a tissue engineering application. However, the affinity of one biomolecule for the material surface is much greater than the other. What surface modification technique(s) could be applied to allow the presence of both biomolecules on the material surface?

References

1. Andrade, J.D. and V. Hlady. "Protein Adsorption and Materials Biocompatibility: A Tutorial Review and Suggested Hypotheses." In *Biopolymers/Non-Exclusion HPLC*, K. Dusek, C.G. Overberger, and G. Heublein, Eds. New York: Springer-Verlag, pp. 1–63, 1986.
2. Dee, K.C., D.A. Puleo, and R. Bizios. *An Introduction to Tissue-Biomaterial Interactions*. Hoboken: Wiley-Liss, 2002.
3. Norde, W. and J. Lyklema. "Why Proteins Prefer Interfaces." *Journal of Biomaterials Science Polymer Edition*, vol. 2, pp. 183–202, 1991.
4. Andrade, J.D. *Surface and Interfacial Aspects of Biomedical Polymers: Volume 2: Protein Adsorption*. New York: Plenum Press, 1985.
5. Schulz, G.E. and R.H. Schirmer. *Principles of Protein Structure*. New York: Springer-Verlag, 1985.
6. Wierenga, R.K. "The TIM-Barrel Fold: A Versatile Framework for Efficient Enzymes." *FEBS Letters*, vol. 492, pp. 193–198, 2001.
7. Bird, R.B., W.E. Stewart, and E.N. Lightfoot. *Transport Phenomena*, 2nd ed. New York: John Wiley and Sons, 2002.
8. Horbett, T.A. "Principles Underlying the Role of Adsorbed Plasma Proteins in Blood Interactions with Foreign Materials." *Cardiovascular Pathology*, vol. 2, pp. 137S–148S, 1993.
9. Maeda, Y., M. Yamamoto, K. Owada, S. Sato, T. Masui, H. Nakazawa, and M. Fujita. "High-Performance Liquid Chromatographic Determination of Six P-Hydroxybenzoic Acid Esters in Cosmetics Using Sep-Pak Florisil

Cartridges for Sample Pre-Treatment." *Journal of Chromatography*, vol. 410, pp. 413–418, 1987.
10. Pyka, A. and J. Sliwiok. "Chromatographic Separation of Tocopherols." *Journal of Chromatography: A*, vol. 935, pp. 71–76, 2001.
11. Rosendahl, M.S., D.H. Doherty, D.J. Smith, S.J. Carlson, E.A. Chlipala, and G.N. Cox. "A Long-Acting, Highly Potent Interferon Alpha-2 Conjugate Created Using Site-Specific PEGylation." *Bioconjugate Chemistry*, vol. 16, pp. 200–207, 2005.

Additional Reading

Alberts, B., A. Johnson, J. Lewis, M. Raff, K. Roberts, and P. Walter. *Molecular Biology of the Cell*, 4th ed. New York: Garland Publishing, 2002.

Atkins, P. and J. de Paula. *Physical Chemistry*, 8th ed. New York: WH Freeman and Co., 2006.

Horbett, T.A. "Principles Underlying the Role of Adsorbed Plasma Proteins in Blood Interactions with Foreign Materials." *Cardiovascular Pathology*, vol. 2, pp. 137S–148S, 1993.

Hubbell, J.A. "Matrix Effects." In *Principles of Tissue Engineering*, R.P. Lanza, R. Langer, and J. Vacanti, Eds., 2nd ed. Austin: Academic Press, pp. 237–250, 2000.

Kuby, J. *Immunology*, 3rd ed. New York: W.H. Freeman, 1997.

Rouessac, F. and A. Rouessac. *Chemical Analysis: Modern Instrumental Methods and Techniques*. New York: John Wiley and Sons, 2000.

Skoog, D.A. and J.J. Leary. *Principles of Instrumental Analysis*, 4th ed. Orlando: Saunders College Publishing, 1992.

Voet, D. and J.G. Voet. *Biochemistry*, 3rd ed. New York: John Wiley and Sons, 2004.

CHAPTER 9 Cell Interactions with Biomaterials

Main Objective

To understand the components and important functions of eukaryotic cells, as well as methods to quantify how cells interact with the biomaterial environment.

Specific Objectives

1. To understand the basic components of a eukaryotic cell.
2. To understand the types of receptor–ligand interactions.
3. To compare and contrast properties of the major components of the extracellular matrix.
4. To understand how receptor signaling can result in changes in gene expression, which in turn can alter important cellular functions.
5. To distinguish among four major cellular functions.
6. To understand and use DLVO theory to model nonspecific interactions between cells and surfaces.
7. To understand and use basic equations describing receptor–ligand interactions to model specific interactions involved in cell adhesion.
8. To understand important parameters in models of cell migration.
9. To identify components that may affect cytotoxicity of a biomaterial.
10. To understand the theory behind and possible limitations to the cytotoxicity and cellular function assays presented.

9.1 Introduction: Cell-Surface Interactions and Cellular Functions

As discussed at length in the previous two chapters, biomaterial surface properties affect protein attachment and, in turn, the composition of the adsorbed layer dictates cell recruitment and attachment. Therefore, surface characteristics play a large role in the overall biological response to a material. In this chapter, we will explore cellular responses to surfaces and/or attached proteins. It is important to keep in mind that, while protein–surface interactions are often nonspecific, protein–cell interactions are, in many instances, specific, and usually occur via receptor-ligand interactions (see following section).

Regardless of the type of interaction, it is imperative to the success of the implant that the chosen biomaterial (and adsorbed proteins) support all the required functions of the attached (or neighboring) cells. Among these functions are the following:

1. Viability (all cell types, often associated with adhesion/spreading on substrate)
2. Communication (all cell types)
3. Protein synthesis (all cell types)
4. Proliferation (some cell types)
5. Migration (some cell types)
6. Activation/differentiation (some cell types)
7. Programmed cell death (some cell types)

However, before we discuss in more detail how cell–substrate interactions can influence each of the above functions, we will first review the basic components of a cell and how these allow for communication with the extracellular environment.

9.2 Cellular Structure

There exists a wide variety of cell types in human tissues, each type having different functions. Some cells' main action is secretion of soluble factors, others are electrically active, and still others act to destroy invading pathogens. Both **differentiated (committed)** and **non-differentiated (progenitor)** cells can be found in the body. Differentiated cells are those that have attained tissue-specific functions, while progenitor cells remain uncommitted and can **differentiate** (undergo a controlled series of changes, usually involving alterations in gene expression and protein synthesis) into a variety of cell types. Further discussion of the process of differentiation is found in Section 9.4.3.

All of these cells, however, have certain functions, and thus certain structural parameters, in common. The basic cellular components found in mammalian cells are described in this section and summarized in Fig. 9.1. A key aspect to maintaining cell viability is that each of the main cellular tasks is compartmentalized in a different **organelle**, which is usually bounded by a selectively permeable membrane. In many cases, several organelles work together to perform one of the functions found on the above list (e.g. the nucleus, the endoplasmic reticulum/Golgi apparatus, and cellular vesicles all play a role in protein synthesis).

9.2.1 Cell Membrane

The cell is divided from its external environment by the **cell membrane**, a bilayered structure (Fig. 9.1) composed primarily of phospholipids. **Phospholipids** are molecules possessing a polar (hydrophilic) head group and a nonpolar (hydrophobic) tail composed of fatty acids. Figure 9.2 depicts both the chemical structure and the three-dimensional conformation of one of the phospholipids commonly found in the cell membrane. Because of the differences in polarity between the regions of the molecule, when exposed to an aqueous environment, the most thermodynamically stable structure for phospholipids is a bilayer wherein the hydrophobic tails are effectively "hidden" from the water and the polar head groups interact with the environment. (This is based on the same principles as self-assembly techniques described for surface modification in Chapter 7.)

As shown in Fig. 9.1, the cell membrane also contains a number of proteins. Some of these have both hydrophilic and hydrophobic domains and thus can span the entire membrane (called **transmembrane proteins**), while others are

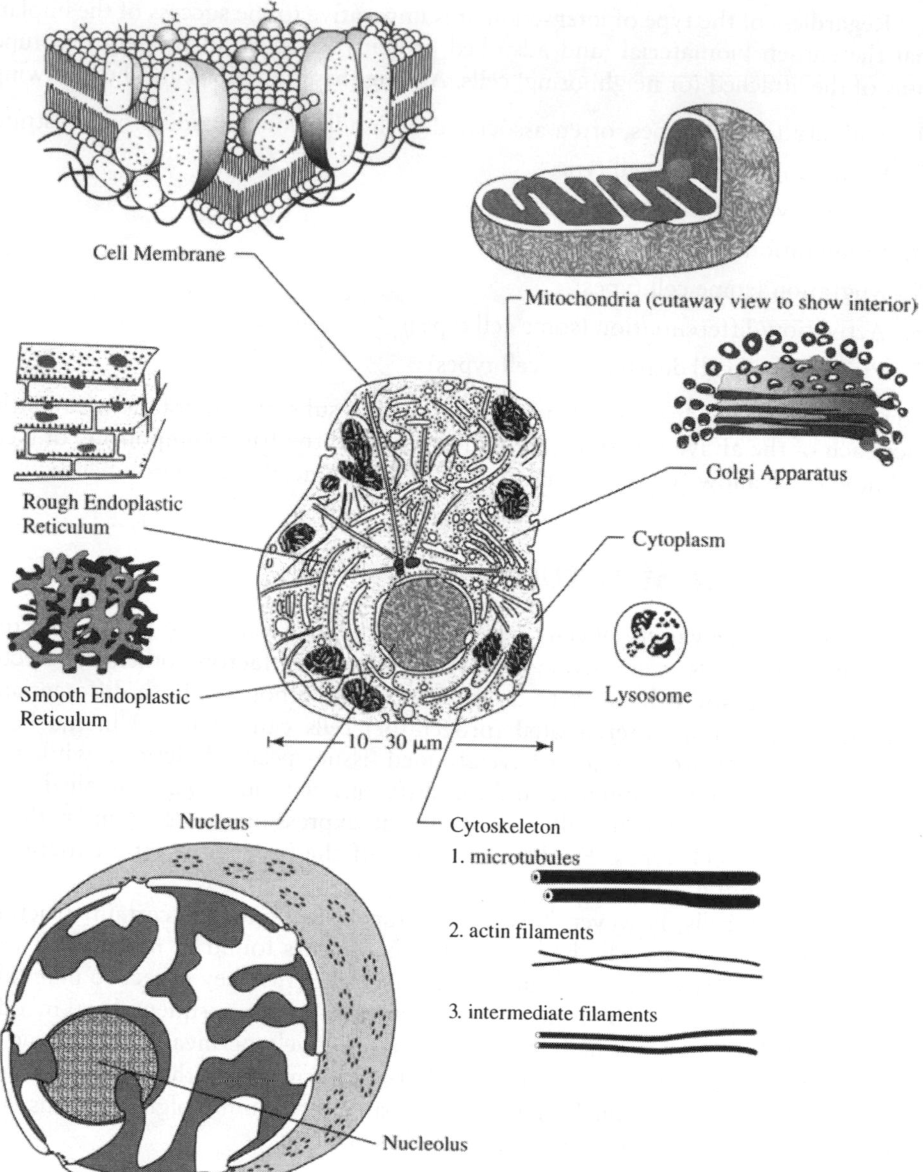

Figure 9.1
A mammalian cell showing the main cellular components: the plasma cell membrane, mitochondria, Golgi apparatus, cytoplasm, lysosome, cytoskeleton, nucleus, smooth endoplasmic reticulum, and rough endoplasmic reticulum. The nucleus contains the nucleolus, an area where ribosomes are assembled. (Adapted with permission from [1] and [2].)

anchored in the cell membrane, but project primarily either into the extracellular or intracellular space. Many transmembrane proteins act as channels or pumps for specific molecules to maintain a well-defined chemistry within the cell. Transmembrane **channel proteins** do not bind to the transported molecules, but form small pores in the phospholipid bilayer to allow (usually) inorganic ions such as Na^+, K^+, Ca^{2+} or Cl^- to pass down their concentration gradients into or out of the cell. In contrast, transmembrane **carrier proteins** such as ion pumps physically bind to the molecule to be transported and often require an expenditure of energy to cause transport opposite the concentration gradient. A common example of this is the Na^+/K^+ pump that is required to maintain osmotic pressure and regulate cell volume.

Proteins projecting into the extracellular space are often receptors for specific extracellular molecules, and will be discussed later in this section (9.2.7). In addition, there are a number of carbohydrate-derived molecules covalently attached to

1-Stearoyl-2-oleoyl-3-phosphatidylcholine

(a)

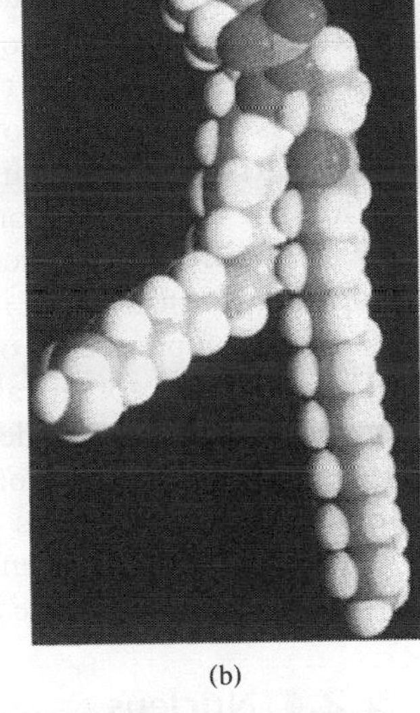

(b)

Figure 9.2
(a) The chemical structure and (b) the three dimensional conformation of one of the phospholipids commonly found in the cell membrane. (Image in (b) courtesy of Richard Pastor, NIH, Bethesda, MD.)

the cell surface to form the cell **glycocalyx.** The importance of this coating to the prevention of unwanted blood clotting is addressed in Chapter 12. The positions of the molecules within the membrane are not fixed, but, rather, are quite fluid, and the locations of specific molecules on the cell surface can easily be rearranged in response to external stimuli.

Maintenance of the integrity of the cell membrane is extremely important because it divides the aqueous environment outside the cell (extracellular space) from that within the cell (the **cytoplasm**). As mentioned above, the cytoplasm has a unique chemical composition, which can be very different from that found outside the cell and which is crucial to cell survival. Additionally, the cell membrane is the point of contact between the extracellular and intracellular environments and therefore represents the main mechanism by which a cell communicates with other cells and its surroundings.

9.2.2 Cytoskeleton

A brief overview of cytoskeletal elements is given in this section, but the reader may consult resources at the end of the chapter for more extensive information. There are three general types of cytoskeletal elements: 6–8-nm-diameter actin **microfibrils,** 10-nm-diameter **intermediate filaments,** and 25-nm-diameter **microtubules** (Fig. 9.1). They are all protein-based structures that can be lengthened or shortened in response to cellular needs. Like the skeleton of the body, they impart shape to the cell and play a large role in cell motility. For example, they allow the extension of finger-like portions of the cell membrane called **pseudopodia** in response to external stimuli or as the first step in cell locomotion (see later sections of this chapter).

In addition to their contribution to cell structure, microtubules play a significant role in separation of duplicated DNA before cell division (see section 9.4.2 for more on cell proliferation). Intermediate filaments also attach to a number of receptor proteins that project into the extracellular space and are therefore an important means for the cell to "translate" external signals (see section below on membrane receptors).

9.2.3 Mitochondria

Several **mitochondria**, which produce energy for cellular functions via a process called oxidative phosphorylation, are usually found in each cell. They have a unique structure that involves two phospholipid membranes (Fig. 9.1). The **inner membrane** is highly folded to increase its surface area, and surrounds the **matrix space**. The matrix contains a mixture of enzymes to break down molecules such as glucose, while the final generation of energy through redox reactions culminating in oxidative phosphorylation occurs at the inner membrane. The **outer membrane** serves to separate the matrix and inner membrane from the rest of the cytoplasm.

The end product of oxidative phosphorylation is **adenosine triphosphate (ATP)**. This molecule is often called the "energy currency" of the cell since it can be transported to the area needed and then hydrolyzed to **adenosine diphosphate (ADP)**. This reaction is very exothermic, and the energy produced can be used to drive required cellular processes (such as pumping ions against a concentration gradient to maintain the proper chemistry in the cytoplasm). The ADP is then recycled back to the mitochondria, where it once again undergoes phosphorylation to ATP.

9.2.4 Nucleus

9.2.4.1 Structure and Function of the Nucleus The **nucleus** can be considered the control center for the cell and contains genetic information in the form of **DNA (deoxyribonucleic acid)** that is condensed into **chromatin**. The nucleus is separated from the rest of the cell by the **nuclear envelope**, which consists of two phospholipid membranes (Fig. 9.1). The outer membrane is contiguous with the endoplasmic reticulum (see below) and is connected with the inner membrane at specific locations called **nuclear pores**. The pores are composed of proteins that form gates to allow only specific molecules in and out of the nucleus.

As shown in Fig. 9.1, the nucleus also contains an area called the **nucleolus**, where ribosomes are assembled. Ribosomes are important to the process of protein assembly in the endoplasmic reticulum and are discussed further later in this chapter.

9.2.4.2 Structure of DNA Due to its particular structure, DNA carries thousands of information-containing elements called **genes**. In essence, DNA forms a template for all proteins synthesized by the cell. When a gene is **expressed**, the cell is actively producing the protein encoded by the gene. DNA remains in its condensed (or **supercoiled**) form in the nucleus, except in the areas where genes are being expressed to produce proteins. Additionally, before a cell divides, the DNA opens up to a less tightly coiled form so that it can be replicated.

As mentioned in Chapter 8, genes contain **codons** that code for specific amino acids and thus determine the primary structure of a protein (see Section 9.4.4 for a more detailed description of how protein synthesis occurs). This is possible due to the unique structure of the DNA double helix. DNA is a polymer of **nucleic acid** subunits. As shown in Fig. 9.3, each nucleic acid is composed of a phosphate group, a sugar and a base. In DNA, the bases can be either double-ring structures (the **purines**) or single-ring structures (the **pyrimidines**). As depicted in Fig. 9.4, the two

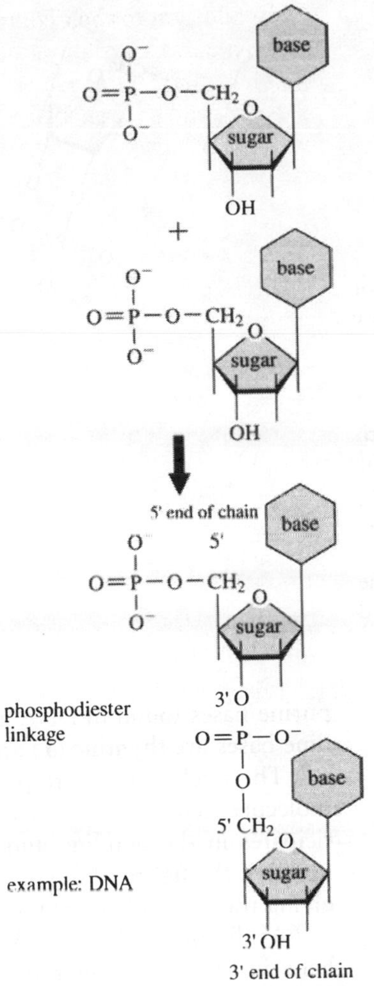

Figure 9.3
A nucleic acid is composed of a phosphate group, a sugar and a base. Nucleic acids can be combined to create structures like DNA. (Adapted with permission from [1].)

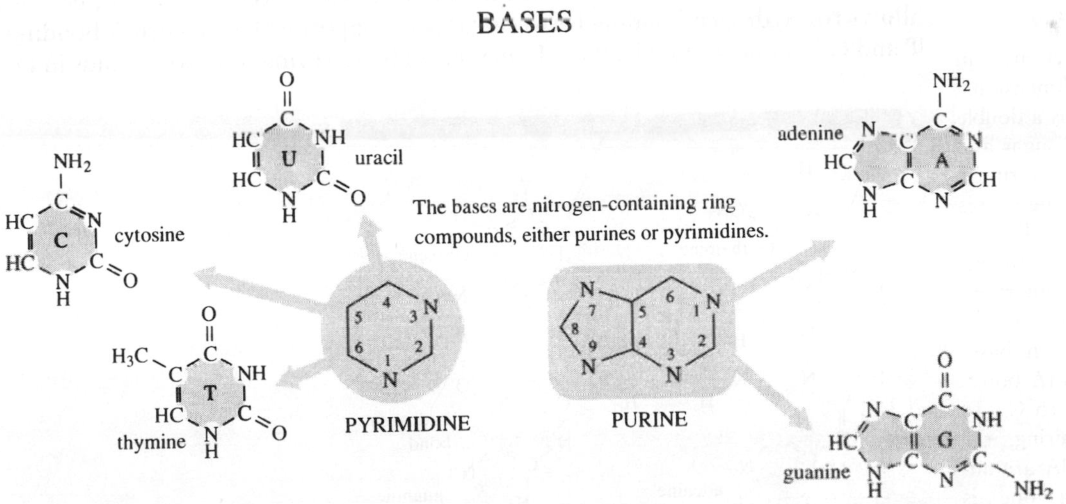

Figure 9.4
Schematic of the bases of DNA/RNA. These bases can be either single-ring structures (pyrimidines) or double-ring structures (purines). The two pyrimidine bases in DNA are thymine (T) and cytosine (C), while the two purine bases are adenine (A) and guanine (G). Uracil (U) replaces thymine in RNA. (Adapted with permission from [1].)

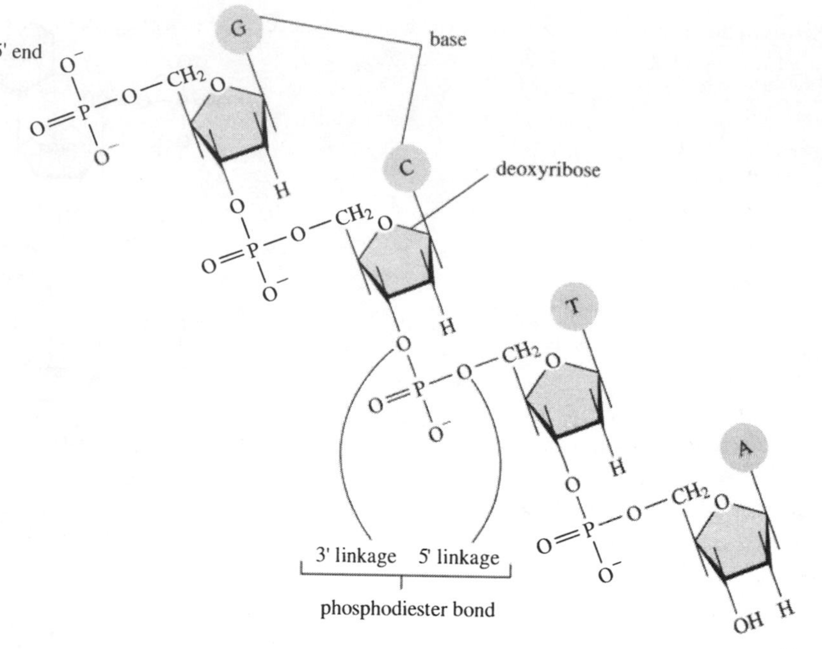

Figure 9.5
Sugar backbone of DNA. For DNA, the nucleic acids are polymerized using a phosphodiester linkage to form the molecule. The 3′ and 5′ designate the carbon on each sugar that participates in the bonding and indicates the orientation of the chain. The type of sugar is the deoxyribose sugar, thus giving the molecule its name. (Adapted with permission from [1].)

purine bases found in DNA are **adenine (A)** and **guanine (G)**, while the two pyrimidine bases are **thymine (T)** and **cytosine (C)**.

The nucleic acids are polymerized using a phosphodiester linkage to form the molecule seen in Fig. 9.5. The 3′ and 5′ designate the carbon on each sugar that participates in the bonding and are used to indicate the orientation of the chain. As noted in the figure, the type of sugar present in DNA is the *deoxyribose sugar*, thus giving the molecule its name.

As discovered in the 1950's, the three-dimensional structure of DNA is a double helix in which the sugar and phosphate groups form a backbone, while the bases from each chain are directed toward the interior. This is very important, because it allows for hydrogen bonding between bases on opposite chains, with A bonding to T and G bonding to C (Fig. 9.6). To maximize base pairing, the two strands in DNA

Figure 9.6
Base–base interactions in DNA. The three-dimensional structure of DNA is a double helix in which the sugar and phosphate groups form a backbone, while the bases from each chain are directed toward the interior. This orientation is very important, because it allows for hydrogen bonding between bases on opposite chains (A bonds to T and G bonds to C). To maximize base pairing, the two strands in DNA are antiparallel, so that one is aligned in the 3′ to 5′ direction, while its complementary strand is aligned in the 5′ to 3′ direction. (Adapted with permission from [1].)

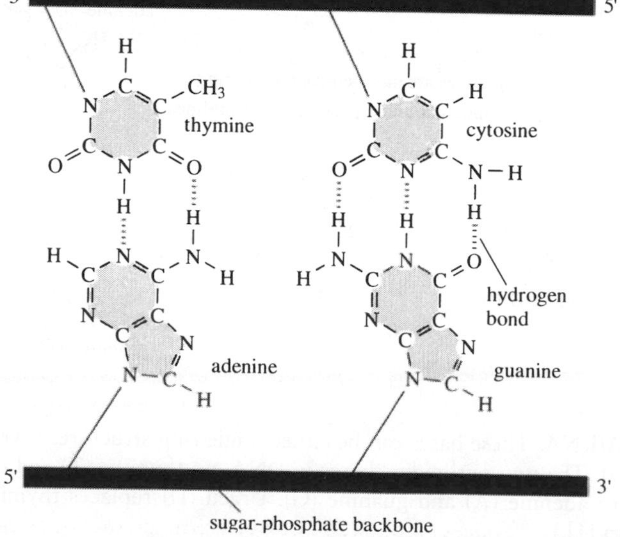

are antiparallel, so that one is aligned in the 3′ to 5′ direction, while its complementary strand is aligned in the 5′ to 3′ direction (Fig. 9.6).

A three-dimensional illustration of the structure of DNA is found in Fig. 9.7. The right-handed double helix has approximately 10 base pairs per turn and is held together predominately by hydrophobic interactions. Besides imparting additional structural stability through hydrogen bonds, the bases are the key to the genetic information found within DNA. A set of three bases comprises a codon for a specific amino acid and thus can be directly related to protein structure if the proper transcription and translation machinery is in place (see Section 9.4.4).

9.2.4.3 Structure of RNA In addition to DNA, some types of **ribonucleic acid (RNA)** are found in the nucleus. Although both molecules are polymers of nucleic acids and thus share many structural characteristics, there are several points in which RNA differs from DNA. From a chemical standpoint, the sugar in the backbone of RNA contains an additional oxygen (the ribose sugar, see Fig. 9.8), and the pyrimidine base thymine found in DNA has been replaced by **uracil (U)** in RNA (Fig. 9.4). However, probably the most striking difference between DNA and RNA is that, as depicted in Fig. 9.9, RNA is single stranded and therefore does not form a regular helical structure.

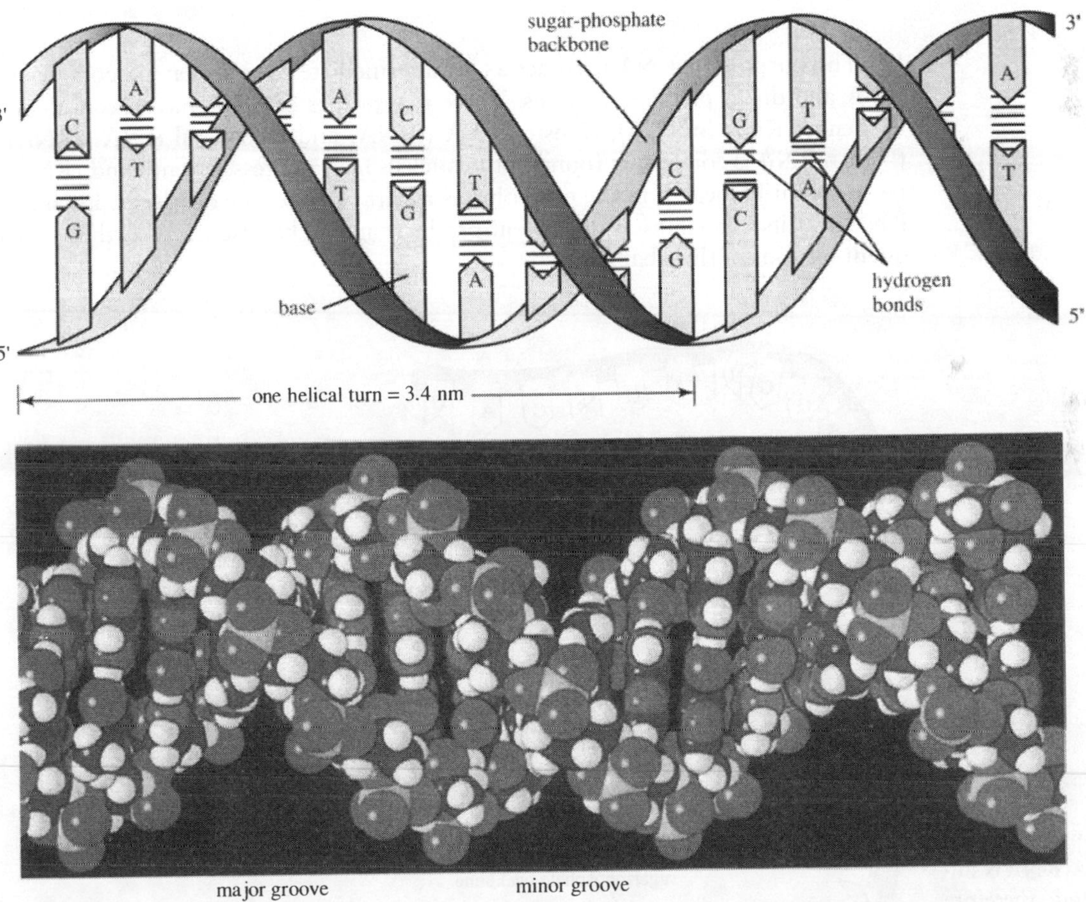

Figure 9.7
The chemical structure and three-dimensional conformation of DNA. (Adapted with permission from [1].)

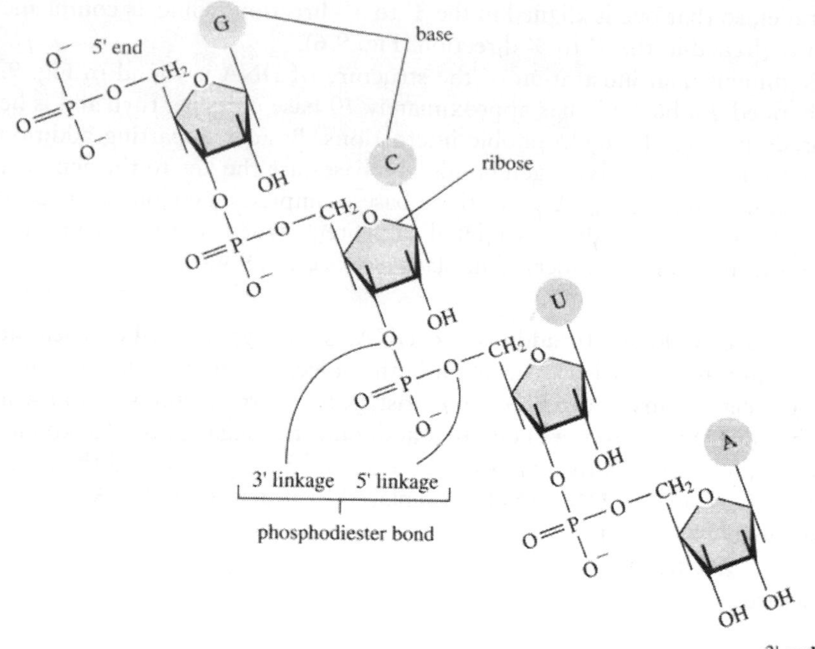

Figure 9.8
Sugar backbone of RNA. For RNA, the nucleic acids are polymerized using a phosphodiester linkage to form the molecule, just like in DNA. However, the type of sugar present in the backbone of RNA is ribose. (Adapted with permission from [1].)

The purpose of RNA is to act as an intermediate for the genetic code found in DNA and direct protein synthesis. Three main types of RNA have been identified: **messenger RNA (mRNA)**, **transfer RNA (tRNA)** and **ribosomal RNA (rRNA)**. Of these, mRNA is commonly found in the nucleus near expressed genes and rRNA may be temporarily located in the nucleolus as a part of ribosome synthesis. Each type of RNA and its contribution to protein production will be discussed further in subsequent sections of this chapter.

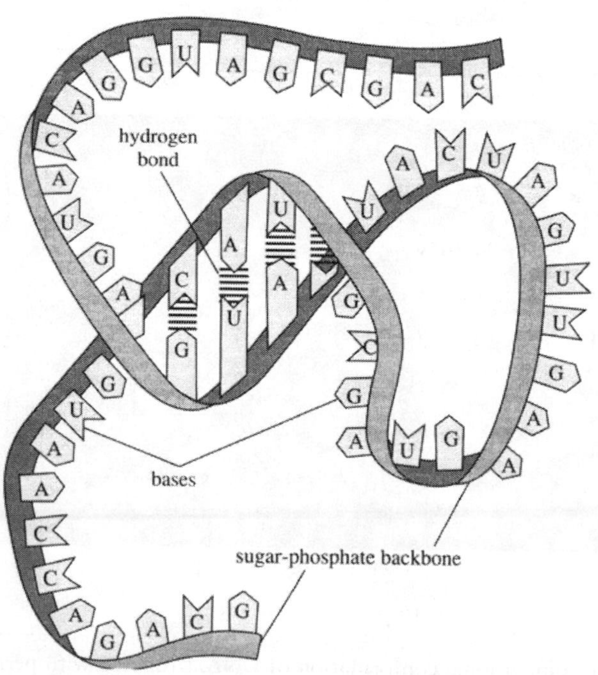

Figure 9.9
Structure of RNA. RNA is single stranded and therefore does not form a regular helical structure. (Adapted with permission from [1].)

9.2.5 Endoplasmic Reticulum

As mentioned above, the outer membrane of the nuclear envelope is connected to the **endoplasmic reticulum (ER)** of the cell (Fig. 9.10). These long, flattened sheets made of phospholipid membranes are where protein synthesis occurs. The ER is generally divided into two separate but connected domains: the **rough ER**, which contains a large number of ribosomes on its external surface, and the **smooth ER**, which is more tubular in structure and includes no ribosomes.

Ribosomes are composed of two subunits containing rRNA and associated proteins, each of which is assembled in the nucleolus. In their final form, they are globular structures that catalyze the reaction in which mRNA, possessing the information derived from DNA, is used as a template to synthesize a particular protein (see Section 9.4.4 for more details).

After the protein is formed, it is released into the interior (**lumen**) of the rough ER where it is directed to the smooth ER and packaged into small phospholipid vesicles (see below) for transport to the **Golgi apparatus** (Fig. 9.10). In the Golgi apparatus, the different proteins are further modified, sorted and packaged for transport to their final destinations. In this manner, proteins can either be targeted to a certain organelle within the cell, or can be tagged for release into the extracellular space.

9.2.6 Vesicles

Vesicles containing proteins encased in a phospholipid bilayer are found throughout the cytoplasm, trafficking proteins from the ER to the Golgi, or from the Golgi to a target destination. If the proteins are to be secreted, the vesicles will join the cell membrane and release their contents in a process known as **exocytosis**. Vesicles are also important to the opposite process, **endocytosis**, where particles from the extracellular environment are taken in via infolding of the cell membrane. During endocytosis, specialized vesicles with digestive enzymes (**lysosomes**, see Fig. 9.1) may join with the newly formed endocytotic vesicle. Lysosomes are designed to help break down the ingested particles and are particularly important to the actions of granulocytes and neutrophils in the acute inflammatory response (see Chapter 10).

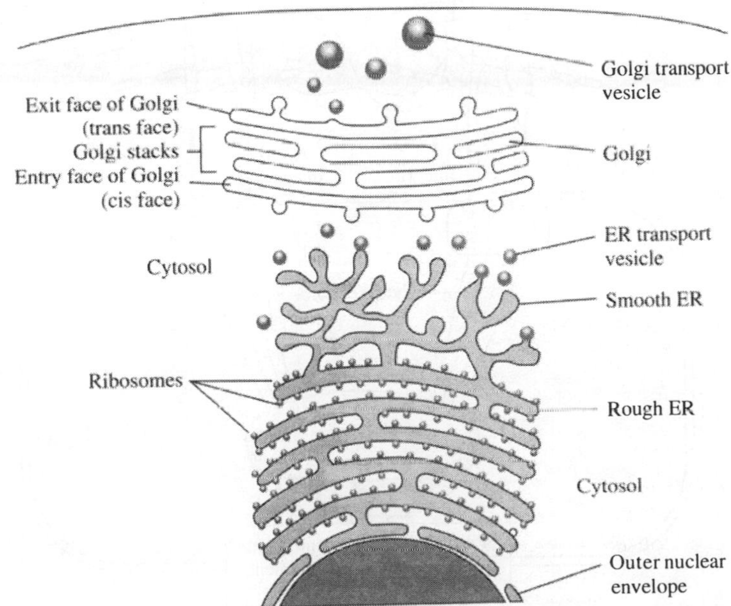

Figure 9.10 Schematic of the endoplasmic reticulum (ER), which is responsible for protein synthesis. The rough ER, which contains a large number of ribosomes, is attached to the nuclear envelope. The rough ER transforms into the smooth ER away from the nucleus. Pieces of the ER will then split off and transfer to the Golgi apparatus, where the proteins created in the ER are further modified and transported to their final destinations. (Adapted with permission from [2].)

9.2.7 Membrane Receptors and Cell Contacts

Interactions between a cell and other cells or its extracellular environment can result in alterations in functions such as cell spreading, migration, communication, differentiation and/or activation (Fig. 9.11). This is often referred to as "*outside-in*" signaling. Conversely, for a variety of reasons, the cell may secrete different molecules or rearrange its contacts and thus change its extracellular environment ("*inside-out*" signaling). In either case, these cell–cell and cell–**extracellular matrix (ECM)** interactions are enabled by protein-based receptors on the cell membrane. In this section we describe several categories of cell contacts as well as the receptors that facilitate them.

9.2.7.1 Types of Cell Contacts As shown in Fig. 9.12, cells can form various contacts with other cells. These include tight junctions, gap junctions, and desmosomes. **Tight junctions** form when adjacent cell membranes adhere to each other, preventing even small molecules from passing between the cells. **Gap junctions** are small, hydrophilic channels created by a plaque-like structure that connects two different cell membranes. **Desmosomes** are mechanical attachments of two cells, either in broad bands (**belt desmosomes**) or in specific spots (**spot desmosomes**). They are caused by the association of cadherin receptors on each cell.

Similarly, cells can be attached in various ways to the ECM. The most common contacts are **hemidesmosomes** and **focal adhesions**. Both hemidesmosomes and focal adhesions have structures similar to the desmosome, but, here, the receptor mediating the adhesion is of the integrin class (see below). These interactions are indicative of strong adhesion to the ECM.

9.2.7.2 Types of Membrane Receptors and Ligands The varied cellular interactions described above are facilitated by different cell membrane receptors, each of which is specific for a small range of target molecules (**ligands**). Some of the most common receptor molecules are grouped into the following categories:

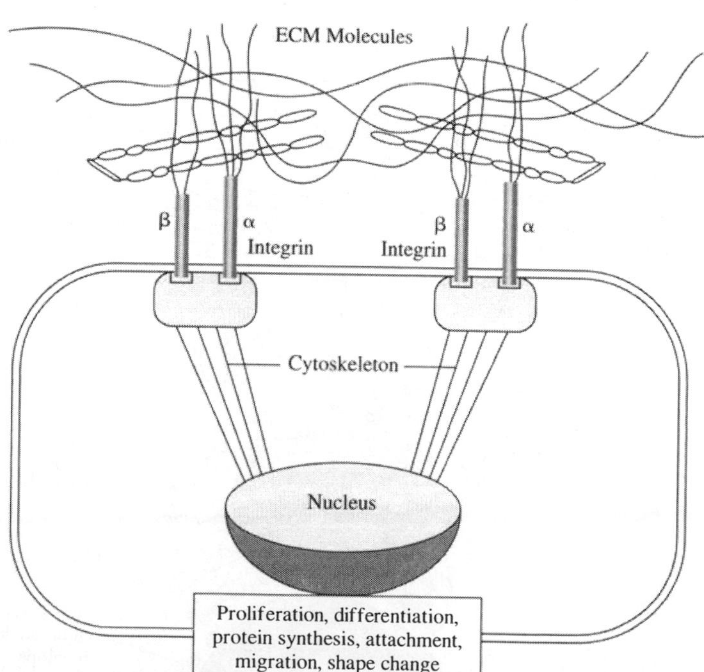

Figure 9.11
Cell interactions with the external environment can result in an alteration of cellular function ("outside-in" signaling). Conversely, because of changes in cellular functions such as differentiation and migration, the cell may change its extracellular environment ("inside-out" signaling). All of these interactions are enabled by protein-based receptors on the cell membrane, such as the integrins. (Adapted with permission from [3].)

1. Cadherins
2. Selectins
3. Mucins
4. Integrins
5. Other cell adhesion molecules (CAMs)

As mentioned above, the transmembrane **cadherins** are responsible for cell–cell contacts in the form of desmosomes (Fig. 9.13). They undergo calcium-dependent **homophilic** binding (a cadherin molecule on one cell binds to a cadherin molecule on a second cell), while their cytoplasmic regions attach to intermediate filaments, thus linking the extracellular and intracellular environments.

Like cadherins, the **selectins** are involved in cell–cell binding, but selectins take part in **heterophilic** binding. Instead of binding to other selectins, these receptors are specific for certain carbohydrate groups present on target cell membranes. An illustration of selectin structure is found in Fig. 9.14.

Mucins are protein-based molecules that contain covalently bound carbohydrate moieties and, thus, present ligands for binding to selectins. As such, they are also involved in heterophilic cell–cell interactions. Mucin–selectin interactions (depicted in Fig. 9.14) play a large role in the early stages of white blood cell migration to sites of injury (see Chapter 10).

Integrins are transmembrane proteins involved in both cell–cell and cell–matrix contacts. These receptors are linked intracellularly to the intermediate filaments, thereby

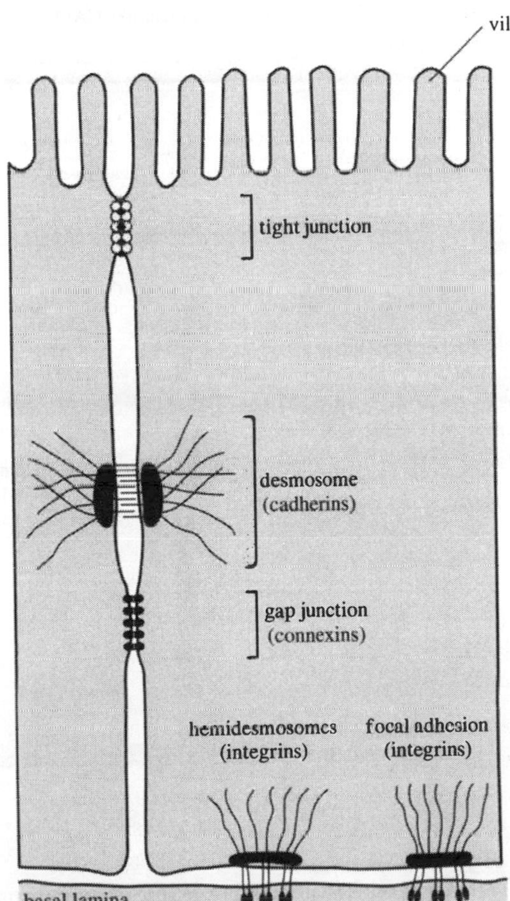

Figure 9.12
Schematic showing the different types of cell contacts in epithelial cells. Tight junctions, desmosomes and gap junctions form as a part of cell–cell contacts, whereas hemidesmosomes and focal adhesions occur during cell-ECM contacts. (Adapted with permission from [1].)

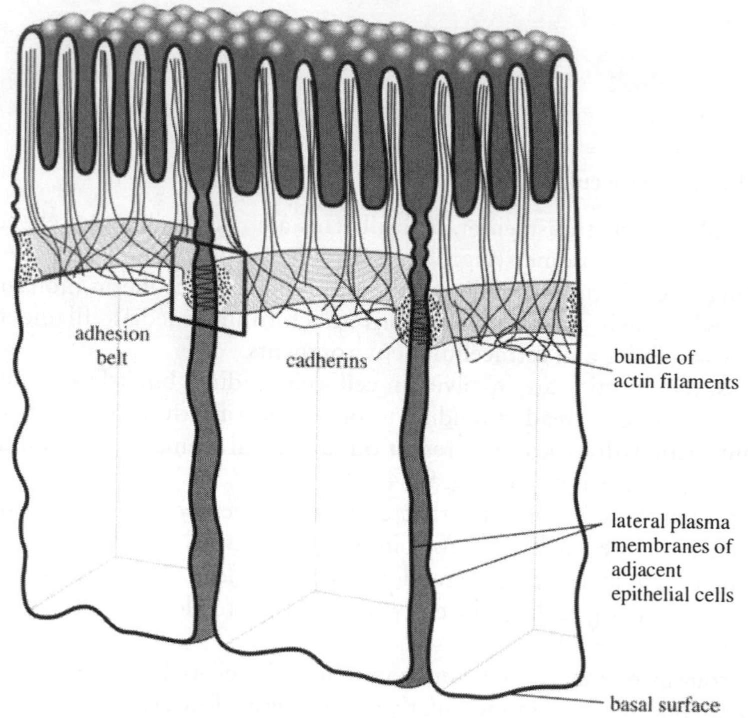

Figure 9.13
Location of cadherins in epithelial cells. Transmembrane cadherins are responsible for cell-cell contacts in the form of desmosomes. They undergo calcium-dependent homophilic binding (cadherin molecules on the two cells bind to each other), while their cytoplasmic regions attach to intermediate filaments, thus linking the extracellular and intracellular environments. (Adapted with permission from [1].)

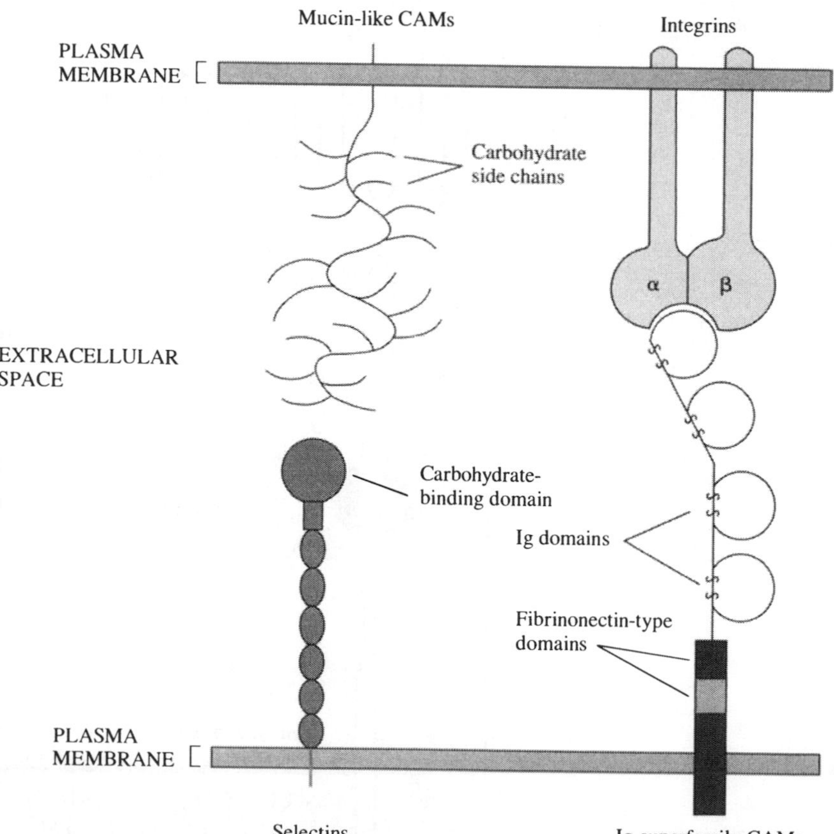

Figure 9.14
Various types of cell membrane receptors: mucins, integrins, selectins, and Ig-cell adhesion molecules (Ig-CAMs). (Adapted with permission from [4].)

directly coupling extracellular binding events to cellular structure. As shown in Fig. 9.14, these proteins are **heterodimers**, possessing two distinct subunits (α and β). There are variations in the composition of both the α and β chains, and, therefore, different subunit combinations result in adhesion to different ligands. For example, some integrin receptors bind ECM proteins like collagen and thus form an important mediator of focal adhesions, as described previously. Other combinations of subunits lead to specificity for the cell adhesion molecules described in the following paragraph.

Other **cell adhesion molecules (CAMs)** comprise a large group of membrane proteins that mediate cell–cell interactions via both hetero- and homophilic binding. Many of these are considered part of the immunoglobulin (Ig) superfamily, based on the structure of the molecule. As indicated in Fig. 9.14, CAMs interact with integrin receptors on neighboring cells. Like the mucin-selectin interactions, CAM–integrin binding is important in cell migration that occurs early in the inflammatory response (see Chapter 10).

While the receptors described above consist mainly of protein with a small amount of attached carbohydrate (sugar), other receptors contain only a small protein core and extensive amounts of attached carbohydrates. These molecules are called **proteoglycans** and their structure is described further in the following section. Proteoglycan receptors are important to a wide range of cell functions. An important one in cardiovascular tissues is the thrombomodulin receptor, which is expressed on cells that line blood vessels and aids in blood clotting (see Chapter 13).

9.3 Extracellular Environment

Contacts between a cell and the surrounding ECM are dynamic and crucial to cell survival. Alterations to the ECM, such as may occur during biomaterial implantation, can result in changes to the shape and/or function of neighboring cells. In addition, as key cell-matrix interactions are further understood, it may be possible to select important aspects of the ECM to include in new biomaterials in order to better direct the tissue response to the implant. This section describes in more detail the most common components of the ECM.

The ECM can be conceptualized as a fiber-reinforced matrix, with fiber-forming elements (collagen and elastin) surrounded by various space-filling molecules (glycoproteins and proteoglycans). This matrix also contains both free and sequestered soluble mediators, such as growth factors. We begin our discussion with the contributions of the fibrous proteins to the structure of the ECM.

9.3.1 Collagen

Collagen is the most abundant protein in mammals and is primarily responsible for tissue tensile strength. As shown in Fig. 9.15, collagen is formed from a triple helix of polypeptide chains called ***α* chains.** Combinations of different α chains form the nearly 20 different collagen types now identified. The most common are the fibrillar collagens (Types I, II, and III), and, of these, Type I is the most abundant. Other collagens, such as Types IX and XII, are nonfibrillar but play an important role in the assembly of the fibers formed from Types I-III.

Examining Fig. 9.15 in more detail, it can be seen that each α chain is composed of alternating amino acids in a gly-X-Y pattern. Because glycine is the smallest amino acid, its position at every third residue allows for tight packing of the three chains in a helical conformation. Although X and Y can be any amino acids, they are often proline and hydroxyproline, respectively. As discussed in Chapter 8, the unique ring structure of proline causes kinks in the polypeptide chain, which, in this instance, is used to stabilize the helical structure.

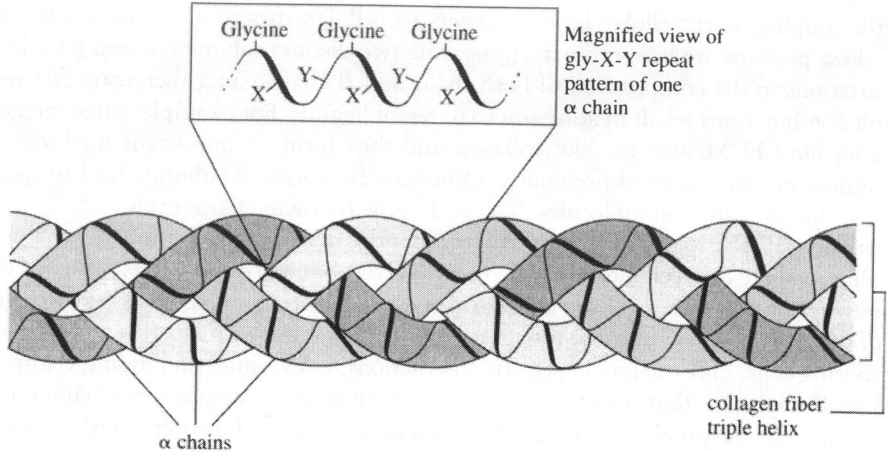

Figure 9.15
Schematic representation of three collagen α chains combining to form a collagen fiber triple helix. Each α chain has a unique shade in this figure to facilitate visualization. It can be seen in the magnified view that each α chain is composed of alternating amino acids in a gly-X-Y pattern.

Because the final collagen fibers are usually too large to be completely assembled within the cell, **procollagen** molecules are secreted into the extracellular space, where they undergo self-assembly into mature fibers. As illustrated in Fig. 9.16, upon exiting the cell, small peptide sequences of the procollagen molecule are cleaved to allow for more efficient packing of the collagen molecules into **fibrils** (diameter 10–300 nm). Individual fibrils then further assemble into larger **fibers** (final diameter 0.5–3 μm). Fibrils and fibers are stabilized by the formation of lysine-lysine covalent crosslinks via the actions of the protein **lysyl oxidase.** Further information about the formation of collagen molecules can be found in Section 9.4.4.

Collagen molecules, particularly the fibrillar collagens, possess many of the same physical properties as other polymeric materials (discussed in Chapters 3–4). For example, if the crosslinking of collagen is prevented, the tensile strength of the material is significantly reduced because the fibers are allowed to slide past one another, much like the blocks of a semicrystalline polymer undergoing tensile testing (see Fig 4.17). Therefore, methods are currently being explored to increase the crosslinking of collagen to improve mechanical properties and handling characteristics for such applications as tissue engineering scaffolds and wound dressings.

9.3.2 Elastin

As mentioned in Chapter 4, **elastin** forms fibers that allow large elastic deformation at low stresses and that are responsible for the resiliency and extensibility of the ECM (Fig. 9.17). Elastin consists of a large number of hydrophobic amino acids (~85%), particularly valine (~15%). **Elastic fibers** consist of elastin as well as auxiliary (nonelastin) proteins, including lysyl oxidase, which creates a complex three-dimensional network by crosslinking lysine residues both within and between chains. Like with other rubbery materials, these covalent crosslinks are key to the elasticity of the fibers. As discussed in Chapter 4, thermodynamic considerations drive the return of elastin to its unstretched state and result in the unique mechanical properties of this ECM element.

9.3.3 Proteoglycans

Other (amorphous) components of the ECM include proteoglycans and glycoproteins. These molecules are important to the matrix structure due to their extensive

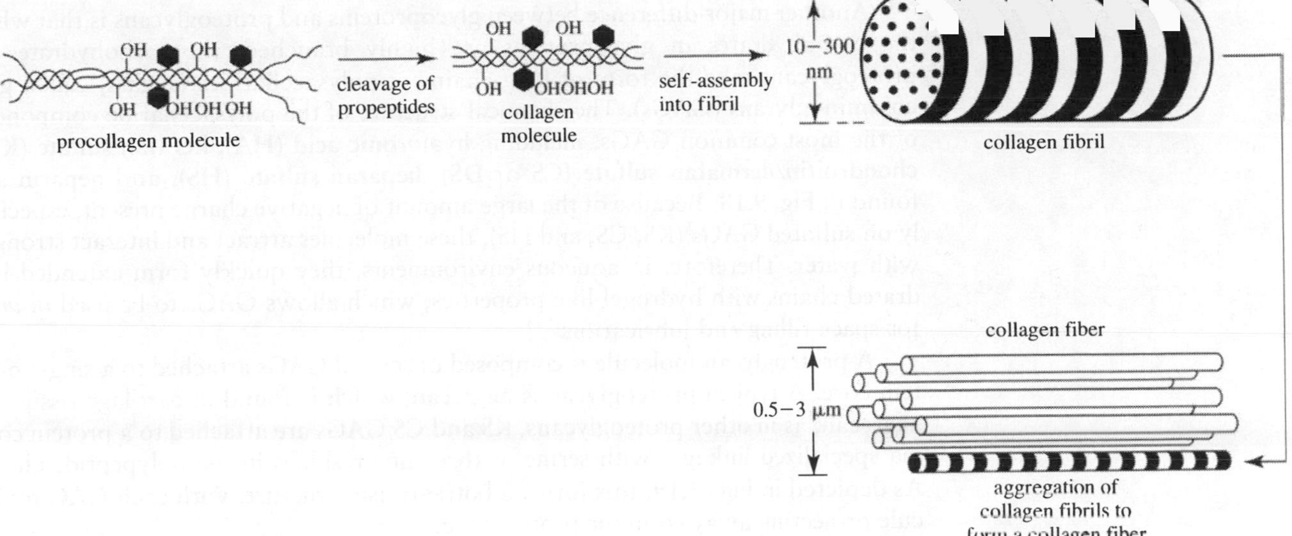

Figure 9.16
Assembly of collagen fibers. Because the final collagen fibers are usually too large to be completely assembled within the cell, the process occurs in stages both in the intracellular and extracellular environment. Procollagen molecules, which are created in the intracellular space, are secreted into the extracellular space, where they undergo self-assembly into mature fibers. Upon exiting the cell, small peptide sequences of the procollagen molecule are cleaved to allow for more efficient packing of the collagen molecules into fibrils (diameter 10–300 nm). Individual fibrils then further assemble into larger fibers (final diameter 0.5–3 μm). (Adapted with permission from [1].)

interactions with water and other ECM elements. Although their names are similar, and both contain protein and carbohydrate constituents, **proteoglycans** can be considered mainly carbohydrate (glycan) with small amounts of attached protein, while **glycoproteins** are polypeptides having attached carbohydrate chains. (Glycoproteins are discussed further in the next section.)

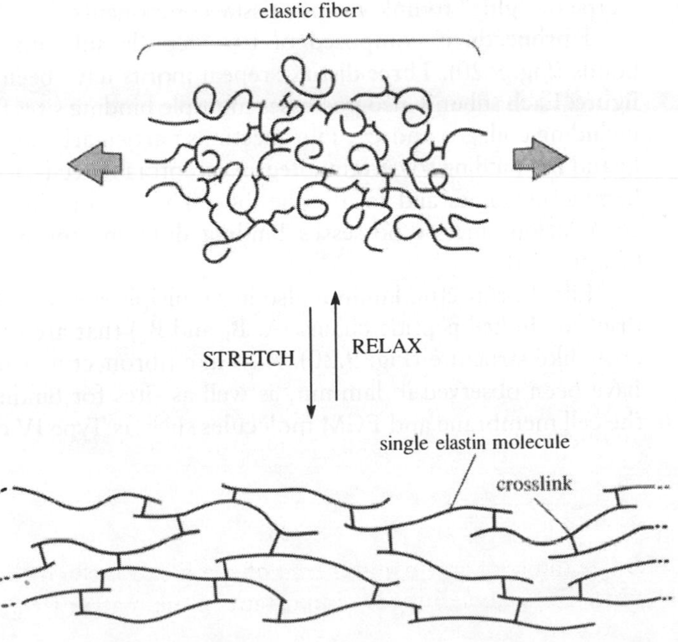

Figure 9.17
Diagram of elastin showing the relaxed and stressed states. Tensile forces cause the individual elastin molecules to unfold and align in the direction of loading. The network is held together by the crosslinks between the elastin molecules. (Adapted with permission from [1].)

Another major difference between glycoproteins and proteoglycans is that while the carbohydrates in glycoproteins are highly branched, the carbohydrates in proteoglycans take the form of long chains of polysaccharides (sugars) called **glycosaminoglycans (GAGs)**. The chemical structure of the polysaccharide component of the most common GAGs, including **hyaluronic acid (HA)**, **keratan sulfate (KS)**, **chondroitin/dermatan sulfate** (CS or DS), **heparan sulfate** (HS), and heparin are found in Fig. 9.18. Because of the large amount of negative charge present, especially on sulfated GAGs (KS, CS, and HS), these molecules attract and interact strongly with water. Therefore, in aqueous environments, they quickly form extended hydrated chains with hydrogel-like properties, which allows GAGs to be used *in vivo* for space filling and lubrication.

A proteoglycan molecule is composed of several GAGs attached to a single protein core. A typical proteoglycan is **aggrecan**, which is found in cartilage tissue. In aggrecan, as in other proteoglycans, KS and CS GAGs are attached to a protein core via specialized linkages with serine or threonine residues in the polypeptide chain. As depicted in Fig. 9.19, this forms a bottle-brush structure, with each GAG molecule projecting away from the protein core.

Like KS and CS, proteoglycans containing heparan sulfate GAGs are also found in the ECM, where they are often used to interact with and retain soluble bioactive molecules (see Section 9.3.5). In addition, heparan sulfate is found on the surface of many mammalian cells. Heparan sulfate and its cousin heparin, which has a similar chemical structure (see Fig 9.18), are best known for their anticoagulant properties (see Chapter 13). Thus, as discussed in Chapter 7, heparin-based surface coatings have been widely explored to improve blood compatibility of cardiovascular devices.

9.3.4 Glycoproteins

Although a variety of glycoproteins are found in the ECM, this section will focus on two representative molecules, fibronectin and laminin. Both of these, like many other glycoproteins, contain several repeating motifs as well as binding domains for cells or a number of ECM constituents. Glycoproteins are therefore often considered a type of "glue" to link various tissue components.

Fibronectin is composed of two peptide subunits held together by disulfide bonds (Fig. 9.20). Three distinct repeat motifs have been identified, as shown in the figure. Each subunit also possesses multiple binding sites for various ECM molecules, including collagen and CS. Fibronectin is particularly important because it contains a ligand for binding to certain integrin receptors on cells, thus facilitating formation of hemidesmosomes and focal adhesions. This glycoprotein also plays a role in blood coagulation since it possesses binding domains for both fibrin and heparin (see Chapter 13).

Like fibronectin, **laminin** also has multiple subunits. In this case, there are three disulfide-linked peptide chains (A, B_1 and B_2) that are arranged in a loosely woven, cross-like structure (Fig. 9.20). Also like fibronectin, a number of repeating motifs have been observed in laminin, as well as sites for binding to integrin receptors on the cell membrane and ECM molecules such as Type IV collagen.

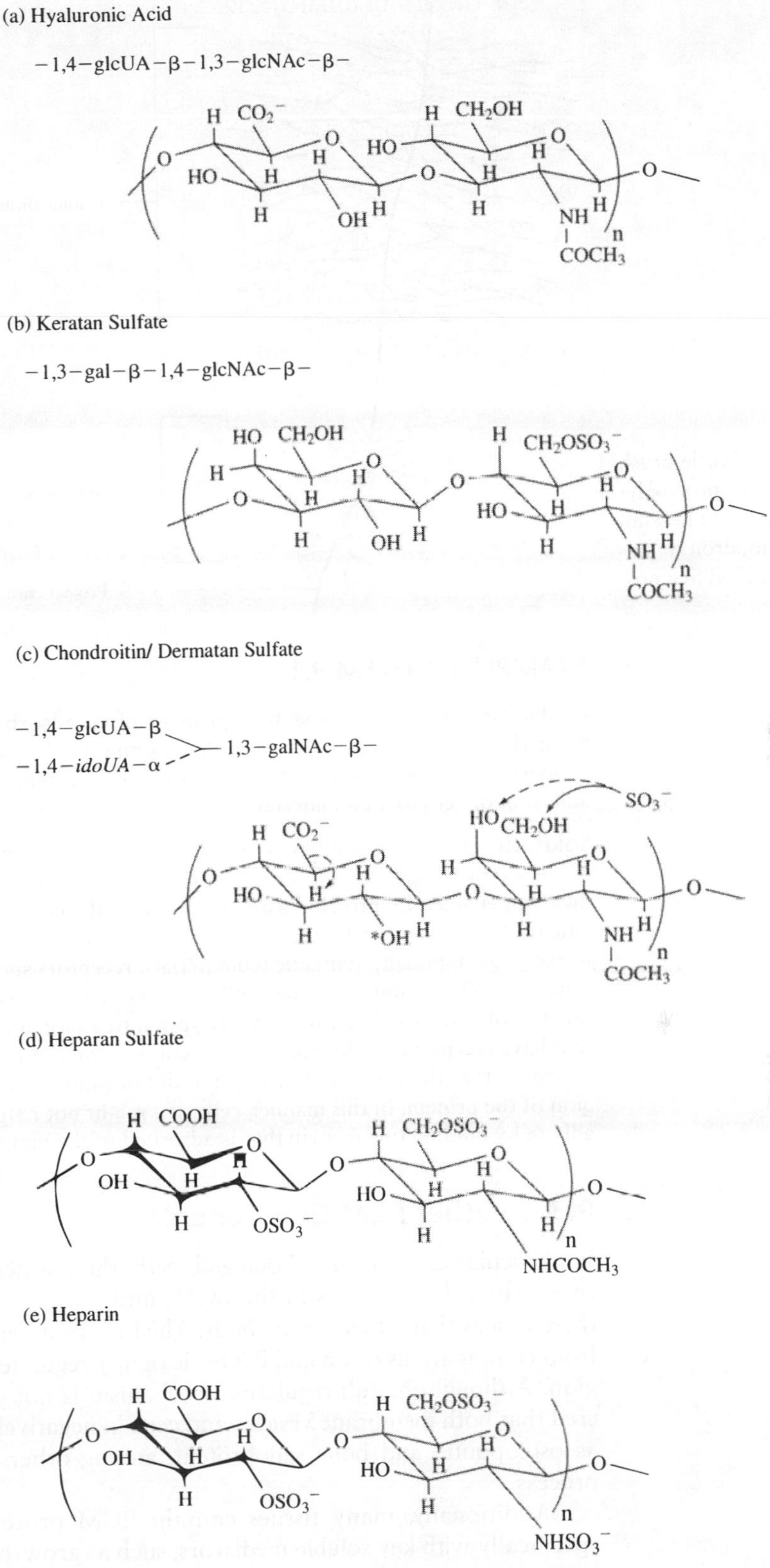

(a) Hyaluronic Acid

−1,4−glcUA−β−1,3−glcNAc−β−

(b) Keratan Sulfate

−1,3−gal−β−1,4−glcNAc−β−

(c) Chondroitin/ Dermatan Sulfate

−1,4−glcUA−β
−1,4−*idoUA*−α
1,3−galNAc−β−

(d) Heparan Sulfate

(e) Heparin

Figure 9.18
The chemical structure of (a) hyaluronic acid, (b) keratan sulfate, (c) chondroitin/dermatan sulfate, (d) heparan sulfate, and (e) heparin. For (a)-(c), "glcUA" denotes D-glucuronic acid, "glcNAc" denotes N-acetyl glucosamine, "gal" denotes D-galactose, and "idoUA" denotes L-iduronic acid. The dashed lines and asterisk in (c) denote the positions of the indicated elements for −1,4-*idoUA*-α −1,3-galNAc-β-. (Adapted with permission from [5] and [6].)

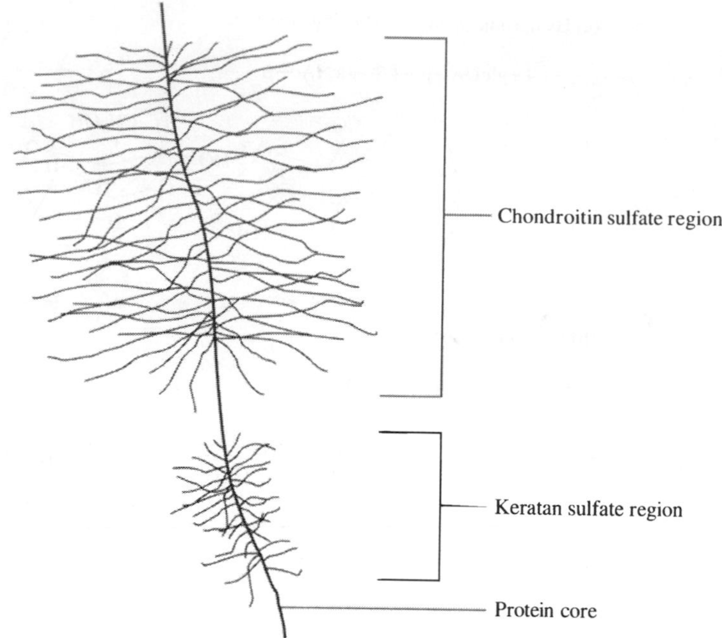

Figure 9.19
Example of the bottle-brush structure of a large proteoglycan including areas of keratan sulfate and chondroitin sulfate that are attached to a protein core.

EXAMPLE PROBLEM 9.1

As discussed in previous chapters, proteins often adsorb to biomaterial surfaces when implanted *in vivo* or exposed to serum-containing media *in vitro*. Many biomaterials do not support cell adhesion prior to the adsorption of a protein layer. How might proteins facilitate adhesion of cells to a biomaterial?

Solution: In the natural physiological environment, cells attach to other cells and elements of the extracellular environment. Many of these cell–cell and cell–extracellular matrix contacts are enabled by protein-based receptors on the cell membrane. These receptors are specific for binding with a limited range of target molecules. As many biomaterials are not native to the body, especially synthetic biomaterials, receptors specific for binding to these biomaterials generally do not occur naturally. However, receptors are naturally present for a large number of proteins. Thus, protein adsorption to a biomaterial can facilitate adhesion of cells that have receptors specific for the adherent proteins, and/or regions of the adherent proteins, assuming that the process of adsorption did not distort or sterically occlude the binding region of the protein. In this manner, cells that might not naturally adhere to a biomaterial may adhere by binding to a protein that is adsorbed to the material. ■

9.3.5 Other ECM Components

In particular cases, such as bone and teeth, there is deposition of *mineral crystals* between the collagen fibers in the ECM, imparting a significantly higher modulus to these tissues than others in the body. The localized deposition of these crystals, made from combinations of Ca and P ions, is tightly regulated by the cells inhabiting the region. Although the full regulation mechanism is not yet known, it has been discovered that both membrane vesicles and certain negatively charged ECM proteins, such as osteopontin and bone sialoprotein, among others, play important roles in this process.

Additionally, many tissues contain ECM proteins with motifs that interact specifically with key soluble mediators, such as growth factors. The result of these interactions is to *sequester* the soluble factor and store it until it is needed to stimulate a specific cellular function through binding to the proper cell membrane receptor.

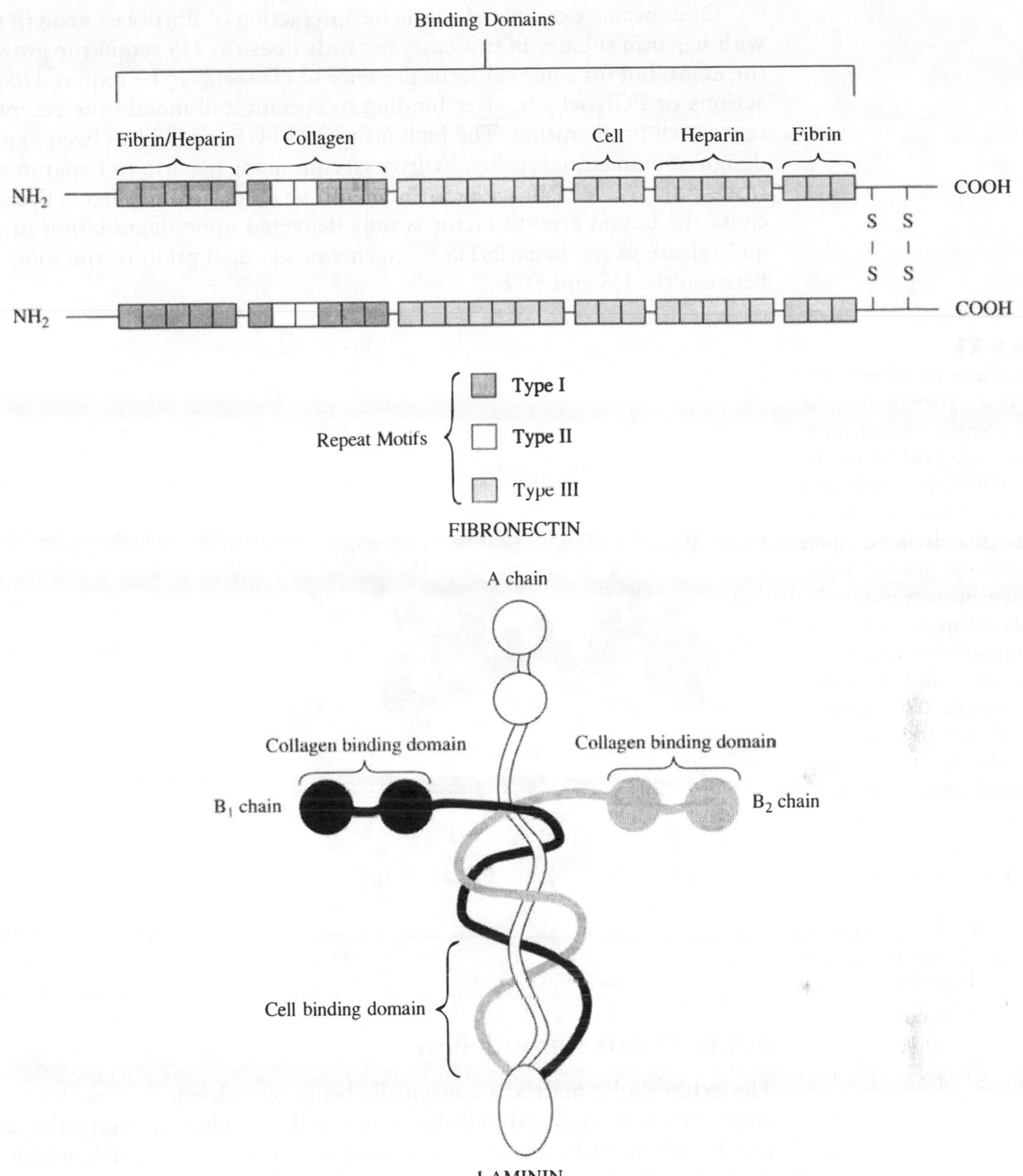

Figure 9.20
Structure of fibronectin and laminin. Fibronectin is composed of two peptide subunits held together by disulfide bonds. Three distinct repeat motifs (indicated by Type I, Type II, and Type III in the figure) have been identified in fibronectin. Laminin also has multiple subunits: three disulfide-linked peptide chains (A, B_1 and B_2) are arranged in a loosely woven, cross-like structure. Although not depicted here, within the laminin subunits repeat motifs can be observed, as in fibronectin.

Release of these soluble factors often occurs during matrix remodeling, when the cells digest part of the protein binding the bioactive molecule (see below) or as a part of matrix injury. In this way, cells can be directed to alter their functions in response to localized changes in their environment.

One specific example of this is the interaction of fibroblast growth factor (FGF) with heparan sulfate. In this case, not only does the HS retain the growth factor in the ECM, but for some cells, the presence of HS seems to be required to promote the actions of FGF, which, after binding to specific cell membrane receptors, usually causes cell proliferation. The high affinity of FGF for HS has been exploited in the design of biomaterials (often hydrogels) containing heparin or heparan sulfate. After loading these materials with FGF, they can be used as controlled delivery devices because the bound growth factor is only delivered upon degradation of the material and release of the heparin/HS fragments or via disruption of the ionic interactions between the HS and FGF.

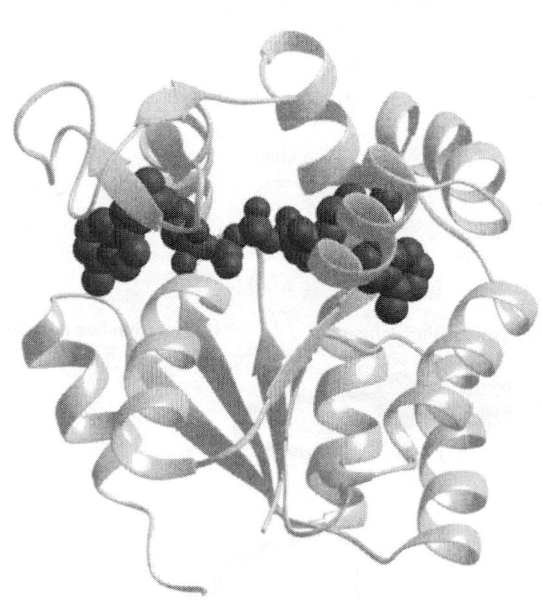

Figure 9.21
The structure of an enzyme, in this case Q1999R *Bacillus subtilis* adenylate kinase (grey ribbons). The folding of the polypeptide chains results in a small pocket into which the molecule that is acted upon by the enzyme (the substrate, in this case bis-(adenosine)-5'-pentaphosphate, shown in the dark grey spheres) can insert. This pocket, called the active site, is specific for a certain portion of the substrate. After the appropriate reaction has been catalyzed, the substrate is released and the enzyme can bind to additional molecules to begin the process again. (Image courtesy of R. Couñago, J.S. Olson, Y. Shamoo, and J. Soman, Rice University.)

9.3.6 Matrix Remodeling

The extracellular matrix is continually being **remodeled.** During this process, older components are digested and the amino acids recycled back into the cells for later use. Simultaneously, the cells synthesize new matrix molecules, which are further modified after being deposited extracellularly. The molecules responsible for most of these actions are a subset of proteins called **enzymes**, which catalyze specific reactions, either within the cell, or in the ECM. As mentioned above, the enzyme lysyl oxidase catalyzes crosslinking of collagen and elastin. Like other catalysts, enzymes act to promote certain reactions by lowering the required activation energy. In particular, these molecules function by bringing the reactants physically closer, and potentially weakening existing interactions, thus facilitating the formation of new bonds, or the breakage of bonds at specific points.

Enzymes are globular proteins with complex tertiary and quaternary structures. As shown in Fig. 9.21, folding of the polypeptide chains results in a small pocket into which the molecule that is acted upon by the enzyme (the **substrate**) can insert. This cleft is called the **active site**, and is specific for a certain portion of the substrate. After the appropriate reaction has been catalyzed, the substrate or pieces of cleaved substrate are released and the enzyme can bind to additional molecules to begin the process again.

Matrix degradation in humans is primarily the result of the enzyme family called the **matrix metalloproteinases (MMPs)**. These molecules catalyze the cleavage of collagens and proteoglycans, among others. In healthy tissue, matrix remodeling is strictly regulated so that matrix degradation does not occur at a higher rate than the synthesis of new ECM molecules. One of the means to do this is through alterations in the localized concentrations of inhibitors of the MMPs, called **tissue inhibitors of metalloproteinases (TIMPs)**. Therefore, the relative concentrations of MMPs and TIMPs in a particular region will determine to what extent the ECM is degraded in that area.

9.3.7 ECM Molecules as Biomaterials

As mentioned in Chapter 1, many ECM molecules have been employed as biomaterials, particularly collagen and certain types of proteoglycans. These molecules, either with or without further chemical modification, have been used in a wide variety of tissues. It is also possible to utilize the entire intact ECM, rather than just one specific ECM molecule, to replace damaged tissue. Although unwanted immune responses are a potential problem with ECM-derived materials, decellularization and fixation procedures have been developed to reduce the risk of material "rejection." Examples of this type of biomaterial currently used in clinical procedures include decellularized bone grafts and decellularized heart valve replacements (see Chapter 14 for more about the problem of pathologic calcification of naturally derived tissue replacements).

EXAMPLE PROBLEM 9.2

A researcher developed a synthetic hydrogel material for cartilage tissue engineering applications, but discovered that the material takes 200 years to degrade under physiological conditions *in vitro*. The researcher then developed a method to add a chemically reactive group to each end of gelatin (a type of denatured collagen), such that it can serve as a crosslinker in the hydrogel. The researcher subsequently showed that the gelatin crosslinker could be incorporated into the hydrogels at high weight percentages.

(a) A study was conducted to characterize the degradation of the hydrogel material *in vivo*. In one group (Group A) hydrogels containing the gelatin crosslinker were implanted for twelve weeks. Control hydrogels containing a nongelatin, nondegradable crosslinker were implanted for twelve weeks in Group B. The hydrogels from one group degraded completely over the course of the study, whereas the samples from the other group did not degrade at all. From which group do you suppose the samples degraded? Why?

(b) It was found that the concentration of tissue inhibitors of metalloproteinases (TIMPs) at the implantation site for one subject in Group A was an order of magnitude higher than that of the other subjects. Also, it was found that the degradation profile of the sample in this subject was different from the other samples in Group A. Did the sample in this subject degrade more rapidly or more slowly than the others from this group? Support your answer.

Solution

(a) The samples from Group A likely degraded as they contained gelatin crosslinkers at high weight percentages. Thus, the majority of the hydrogel for samples in Group A was gelatin by weight. Recalling that gelatin is processed collagen and that collagen can be enzymatically degraded through the action of matrix metalloproteinases (specifically, collagenases), it follows that the gelatin crosslinkers can be degraded by the collagenases normally present in the physiological environment *in vivo*. Thus, the hydrogel likely degraded through the enzymatic cleavage of the gelatin crosslinkers, which were not present in samples from Group B.

(b) TIMPs inhibit the action of matrix metalloproteinases and are a natural regulator of remodeling of the extracellular matrix. It follows that the hydrogel sample from the subject in which high levels of TIMPs were detected degraded more slowly than the samples from the other subjects in Group A, as the enzymatic degradation of the gelatin crosslinkers in the hydrogel was impeded by the higher concentration of TIMPs. ■

9.4 Cell–Environment Interactions that Affect Cellular Functions

A cell's microenvironment, including localized cell–cell and cell–ECM contacts, is extremely important because these interactions can result in alterations of cellular functions via complex intracellular pathways. Examining a more detailed picture of cell-environment interactions (Fig. 9.11), the binding of ECM molecules to integrin receptors to form focal adhesions causes changes in the cytoskeleton that ultimately affect gene expression in the nucleus. Similarly, cells also possess receptors for soluble mediators, such as growth factors, that can act through a cascade of intracellular factors (**secondary messengers**) to alter gene expression. The effects of soluble factors are particularly important in the immune and inflammatory responses to biomaterials, as described in Chapters 10–12.

Alterations in gene expression can affect the four major cellular functions—cell viability, proliferation, differentiation, and protein synthesis—as well as other functions like communication. The pathways involved in these cellular functions that may be regulated by cell-environment interactions are described in this section, while cell migration is addressed in the following section. Specific examples of how these processes may be altered by changes in the extracellular environment due to biomaterials implantation are found in subsequent chapters.

9.4.1 Cell Survival

In extreme cases, changes in the extracellular environment can result in cell death, either through the more traditional necrosis, or via a type of programmed cell death termed **apoptosis**. This can occur due to general changes in the chemistry of the surroundings (e.g. decrease in pH), or due to the presence of a specific factor that binds to the cell membrane to expressly direct cell death (more common for apoptosis).

Necrosis is a series of changes in cell structure, including increased permeability of the membrane and a leakage of important intracellular enzymes, eventually resulting in cell lysis (disintegration). Microscopically, this type of cell death is characterized by cell swelling and a disintegration of organelles. The area is cleared when expired cells are phagocytosed (consumed) by inflammatory cells (see Chapter 10).

In contrast, apoptosis involves a series of more controlled changes that can also be observed microscopically. Important characteristics include cell shrinkage, the formation of cytoplasmic buds and finally, fragmentation into **apoptotic bodies** comprised of vesicles containing small groups of organelles. These vesicles are then phagocytosed by neighboring cells, and, unlike necrosis, no inflammatory response is initiated. This type of cell death is particularly important in embryogenesis and development, as well as in the deletion of autoreactive immune cells, discussed further in Chapter 12.

9.4.2 Cell Proliferation

Although the events governing the cell cycle are not completely understood, the presence of the proper extracellular environment (e.g. enough "space") is an important factor in determining whether a cell will divide at a given time. Cells can be classified as labile, permanent, or stable, depending on their propensity for proliferation. **Labile**

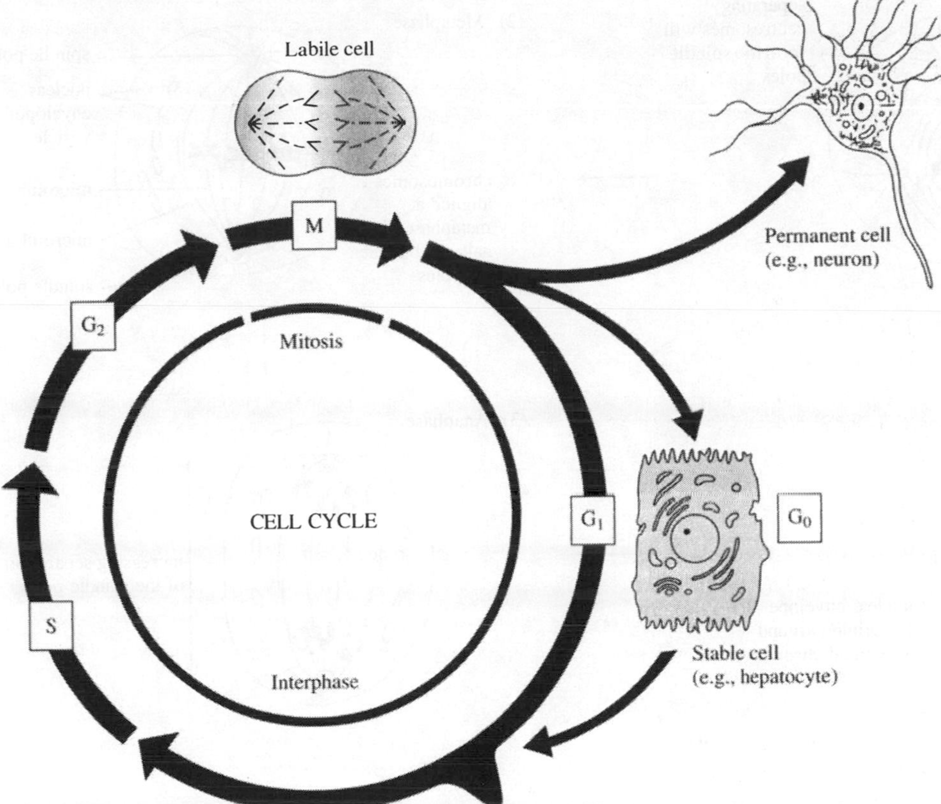

Figure 9.22 Diagram of the typical cell cycle. The cell cycle is divided into mitosis (M phase), when the cell divides, and interphase (phases G_1, S and G_2), in which cellular DNA and organelles are replicated in preparation for mitosis. The G_1 phase is a time of general cell growth and fabrication of additional organelles. During the S phase, the nuclear DNA is replicated. In the G_2 phase the proteins and structures enabling cell division are assembled. Instead of G_1, stable cells may enter a G_0 phase and be considered quiescent (resting). During this period, these cells do not increase in size or replicate their organelles, but, rather, perform a specific function within a tissue. (Adapted with permission from [7].)

cells replicate continuously, while **permanent** cell types are terminally differentiated (see next section) and have lost the ability to divide. **Stable** cells fall somewhere between these two extremes. After one division, they take on a specific function, but they can be induced by cues, such as the loss of nearby cells, to reenter the cell cycle and proliferate.

9.4.2.1 Cell Cycle: Interphase Each of these cell types and their relation to the cell cycle is depicted in Fig. 9.22. The cell cycle is divided into **mitosis (M phase)**, when the cell divides, and **interphase** (phases G_1, S and G_2), in which cellular DNA and organelles are replicated in preparation for mitosis. The **G_1 phase** is considered a time of general cell growth and fabrication of additional organelles, including an increase in the size of the cell membrane. During the **S phase**, the nuclear DNA is replicated. This is followed by the **G_2 phase**, in which proteins and structures enabling cell division are assembled.

Instead of G_1, stable cells may enter a **G_0 phase** and be considered **quiescent** (resting). During this period, these cells do not increase in size or replicate their organelles, but, rather, perform a specific function within a tissue. As discussed above, particular stimuli may encourage them to return to the cycle at G_1 and continue replication.

9.4.2.2 Cell Cycle: Mitosis After the G_2 phase is completed, the cell is ready to begin mitosis (M phase). Mitosis is subdivided into several characteristic periods, illustrated in Fig. 9.23(a):

1. Prophase
2. Metaphase
3. Anaphase
4. Telophase

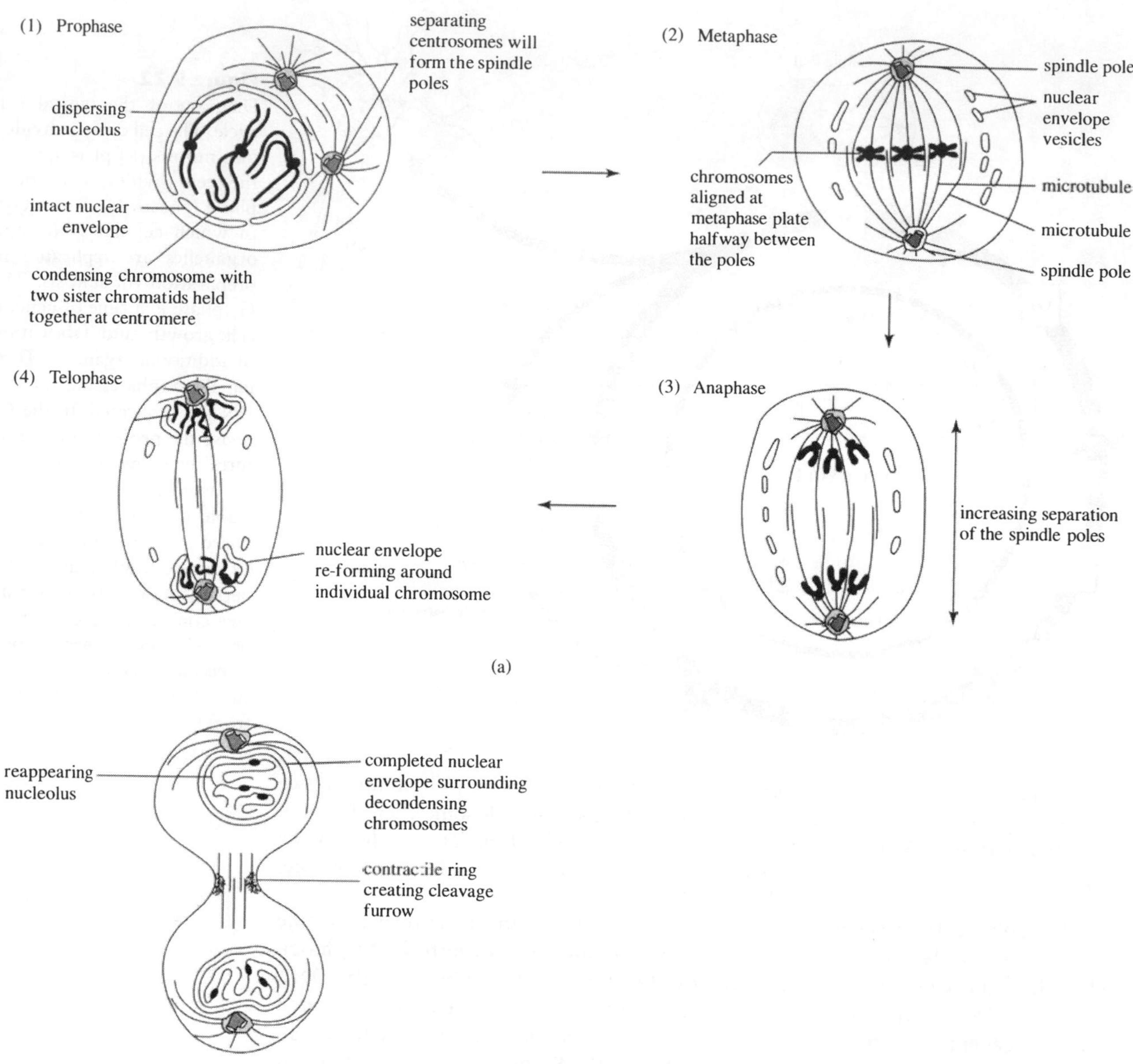

Figure 9.23
(a) Mitosis is subdivided into four main characteristic periods: prophase, metaphase, anaphase, and telophase. Prophase is marked by the dissipation of the nucleolus and formation of the mitotic spindles. During metaphase, the chromosomes are aligned between the two mitotic spindles. Anaphase is the period when the chromosomes are pulled apart by the spindle microtubules and arrange themselves at the spindle poles. Telophase is the period of time when the nuclear envelope begins to reform and the cell starts to undergo cytokinesis. (b) Cytokinesis, the division of the cytoplasm, occurs after mitosis and consists of the development of a cleavage furrow and eventual separation into the two daughter cells. (Adapted with permission from [1].)

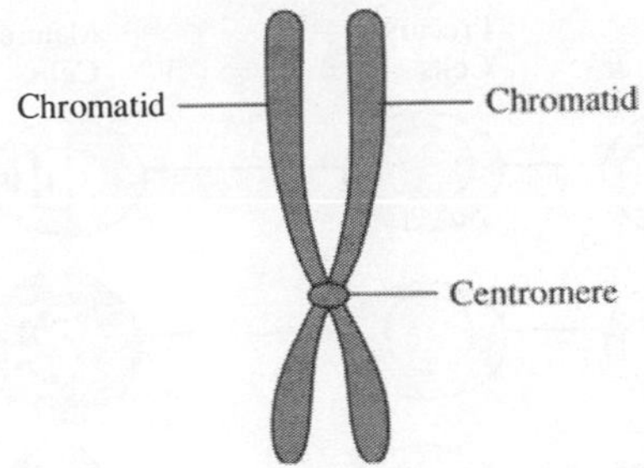

Figure 9.24
Schematic of a chromosome, which consists of two chromatids and a centromere. (Adapted with permission from [8].)

The transition from G_2 to **prophase** is marked by the dissipation of the nucleolus and condensation of chromatin in the nucleus into **chromosomes** (Fig. 9.24). After replication in the S phase, each chromosome contains two identical sister **chromatids**. After mitosis, one chromatid of each chromosome will be found in the nucleus of one of the daughter cells. The separation of two pairs of centrosomes with their attached microtubules is also observed outside the nuclear envelope. These will form the **mitotic spindle**, necessary for equally dividing the chromosomes in later phases of mitosis.

As the cell moves into the next stage of mitosis, **metaphase**, the nuclear envelope disintegrates and the spindle microtubules can now attach directly to the chromosomes. This portion of mitosis is sometimes called **prometaphase**. After attachment to the mitotic spindle, the chromosomes are tugged back and forth in the cell until they align near the equator of the cell [Fig. 9.23(a)]. This alignment marks the end of metaphase.

Anaphase begins abruptly when the sister chromatids are pulled apart by the spindle microtubules and visibly separate [Fig. 9.23(a)]. Each chromatid (now called a chromosome) then travels toward the closest spindle pole (centrosome). Simultaneously, the cell begins to elongate, producing more distance between poles.

In the last stage of mitosis, **telophase**, the divided chromosomes have reached their respective poles and the spindle microtubules begin to disassemble [Fig. 9.23(a)]. The nuclear envelope reforms and the nucleolus reappears. **Cytokinesis**, or division of the cytoplasm, usually begins in anaphase and ends after telophase [Fig. 9.23(b)]. This process is characterized by a slow infolding of the plasma membrane around the center of the cell (the cleavage furrow) and results in two separate daughter cells with cytoplasmic constituents identical to that of the parent cell.

9.4.3 Cell Differentiation

As mentioned earlier in the chapter, in many tissues, there exists a type of **progenitor** or **stem cell**. Stem cells possess the capability to self-renew as well as to form more than one cell type. Stem cells can produce **differentiated** or **committed** cells, which usually perform a particular function within a tissue. They may be labile, stable, or permanent, but can only reproduce their own cell type. Alternatively, stem cells may divide to create additional **pluripotent** cells that can produce several cell types, or **totipotent** cells that can produce all cell types.

A major difference between **embryonic stem cells** and **adult stem cells** is that embryonic stem cells, found in embryos, have not yet been committed to a certain type of tissue. Thus, depending on the age of the embryo, they can be thought of as more or less totipotent. In contrast, adult stem cells are isolated from the adult and are tissue specific, suggesting they are more pluripotent. Two common examples of adult stem cells are found in the bone marrow: **hematopoietic stem cells** form both red and white blood cells (Fig. 9.25), while **mesenchymal stem cells** can differentiate into cells from various connective tissues (such as bone, cartilage and tendon/ligament) (Fig. 9.26).

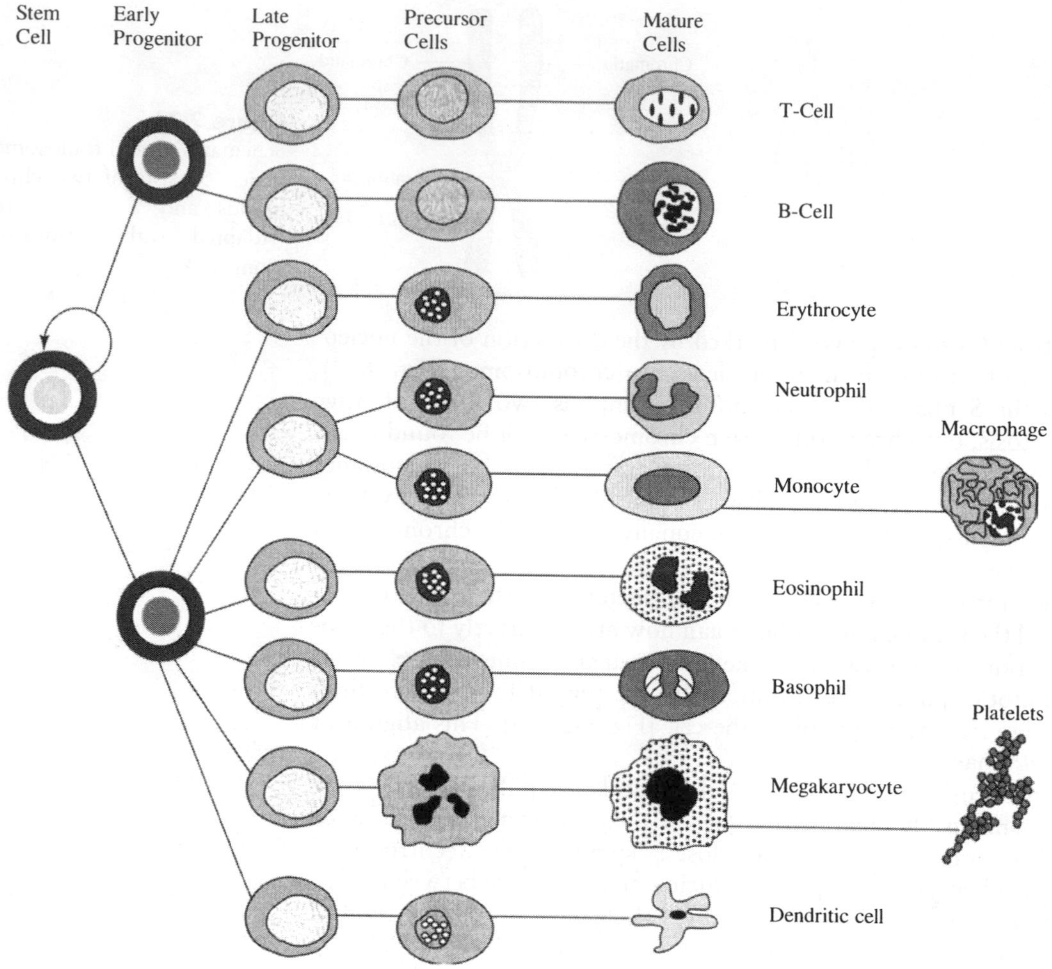

Figure 9.25
Production of blood cells from a hematopoietic stem cell. The stem cell can either replicate itself (curved arrow), or differentiate into various cell types. (Adapted with permission from [9].)

When stem cells (either pluripotent or totipotent) are required to differentiate (such as to regenerate tissue that has been lost due to injury), they undergo a controlled set of changes, usually involving alterations in gene expression and levels of protein synthesis, which result in transformation of their **phenotype.** A cell's phenotype refers to its observable characteristics, including its **morphology**, or cell shape, as well as quantifiable parameters, such as production of a specific protein.

It has been found that these differentiation stages can be initiated and controlled by soluble and insoluble elements from the extracellular environment, including both chemical and mechanical factors, through binding to transmembrane receptors on the cell surface. Understanding these stimuli and incorporating them into the design of novel biomaterials is a focus of much current research, especially in the field of tissue engineering.

9.4.4 Protein Synthesis

In addition to affecting cellular differentiation, receptor-ligand binding can cause changes in the function of committed cells, which, like differentiation, is usually associated with alterations in the amount or type of protein synthesized.

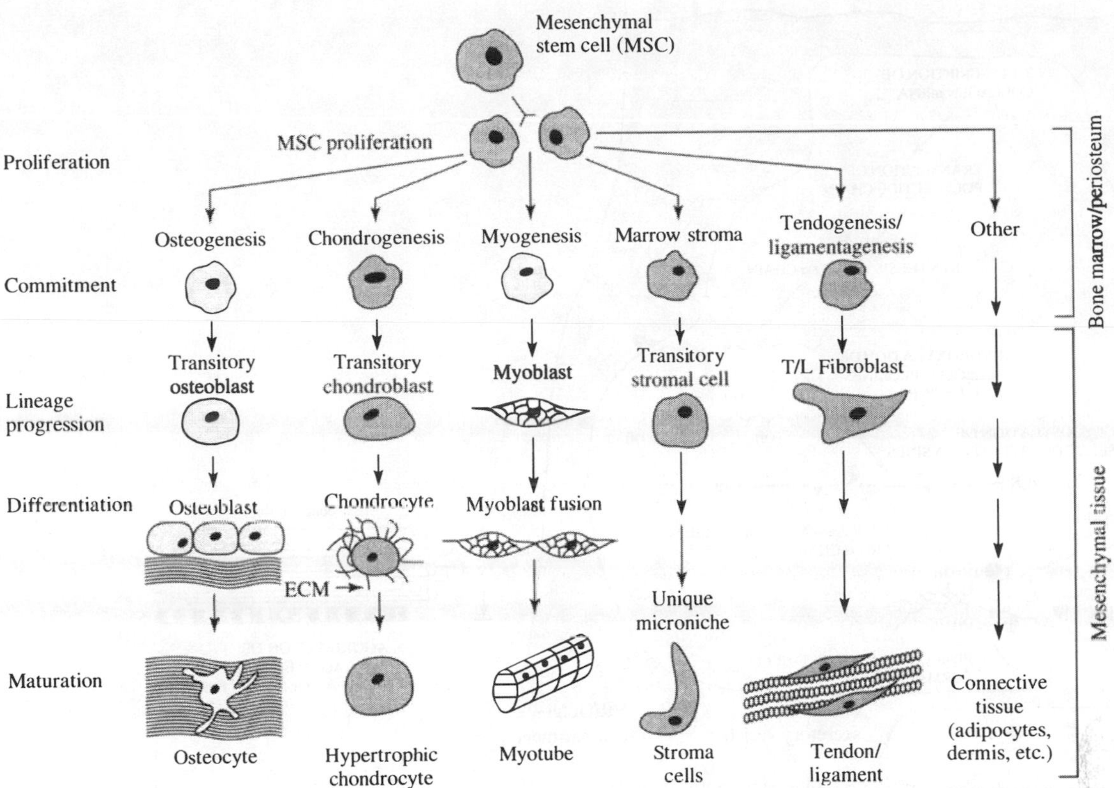

Figure 9.26
Mesenchymal stem cells (MSCs) have the potential to differentiate through a number of different pathways (as shown) to form mesenchymal tissues such as bone, cartilage, muscle, tendon, ligament, and adipose tissue. The MSCs can proliferate to produce additional MSCs, or they can commit to a specific lineage for tissue-specific differentiation. The commitment and progression of an MSC to and through a specific lineage involves the action of bioactive molecules, such as growth factors and cytokines. In the process of differentiation and maturation the cell increases its production of tissue-specific molecules. Terminally differentiated cells, such as osteocytes, may alter their levels of synthesis of matrix molecules to play an increased role in tissue maintenance or homeostasis. (Adapted with permission from [10].)

For example, protein production is important in cellular functions such as communication and activation, as well as in the creation and remodeling of the ECM surrounding the cell.

The general steps that are required to create and secrete a protein starting from its genetic code are described in this section. As an example, we will focus on the production of an important extracellular matrix protein, collagen (see Section 9.3.1). An overview of this process is given in Figs. 9.27 and 9.28.

9.4.4.1 Collagen Synthesis: Transcription Collagen synthesis begins when the portion of chromatin coding for collagen becomes less compact, allowing enzymes that "unzip" the double helix to separate the DNA strands. These enzymes, called **RNA polymerases,** then synthesize linear mRNA strands that are complementary to the collagen gene on the DNA using the base-pairing technique described previously (Fig. 9.29). This process is **transcription.** (A similar process occurs during replication of the chromatin before cell division, but in this case the new molecules generated are complementary DNA strands and the enzymes that form them are **DNA polymerases.**)

The linear, single-stranded mRNA molecules can be 1,000 to 10,000 bases long and contain the complement to the DNA code. For example, if a base sequence in DNA was CCAGGA, the corresponding mRNA bases would be GGUCCU. Since three bases form the codon for a specific amino acid, in this example, this section

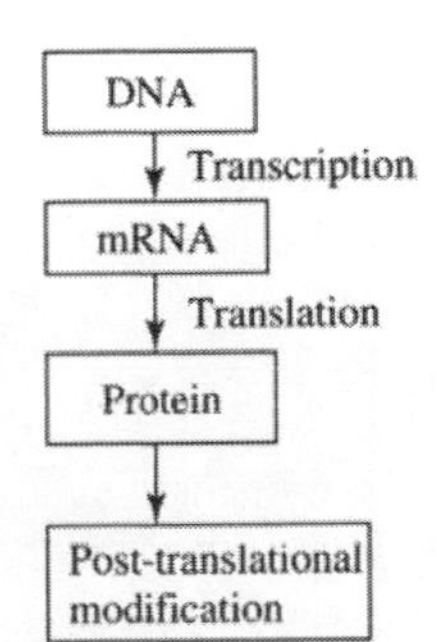

Figure 9.27
Block diagram of the steps for the creation and modification of proteins.

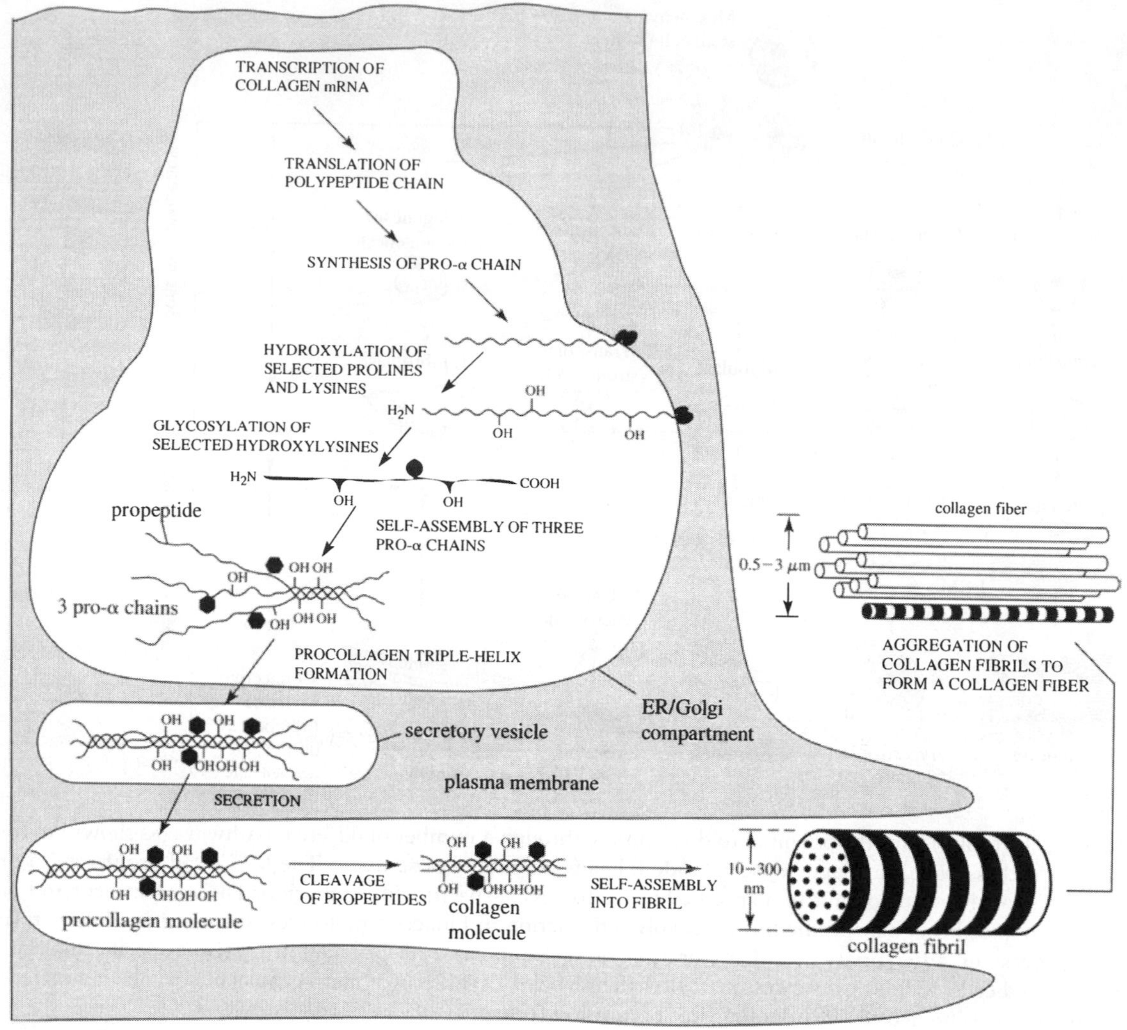

Figure 9.28
Summary of the steps of collagen synthesis. Transcription, translation, synthesis to create the α-chain, and the joining of three of these chains to create the collagen triple helix occur within the cell. The procollagen molecule is then secreted and assembled into fibrils and finally fibers. (Adapted with permission from [1].)

of mRNA (and thus DNA) would code for glycine (GGU codon on mRNA) and proline (CCU codon on mRNA). The entire list of mRNA codons is found in Fig. 9.30. After fabrication, the mRNA strand moves out of the nucleus through nuclear pores and into the ER.

9.4.4.2 Collagen Synthesis: Translation and Post-Translational Modification

Once in the ER, another type of RNA, tRNA, is required in addition to the mRNA. tRNA is also single-stranded, but it is folded into a complex "hairpin" structure that is stabilized by base pairings within the molecule (Fig. 9.31). tRNAs act as adaptor molecules and possess binding sites for a specific amino acid on one end and the mRNA molecule on the other. The binding site for the mRNA is a series of three bases known as the **anticodon.** The anticodon is complementary to the mRNA code for that particular amino acid. In the above example, a tRNA containing glycine and the anticodon CCA could bind to the first part of the mRNA molecule, followed by a second

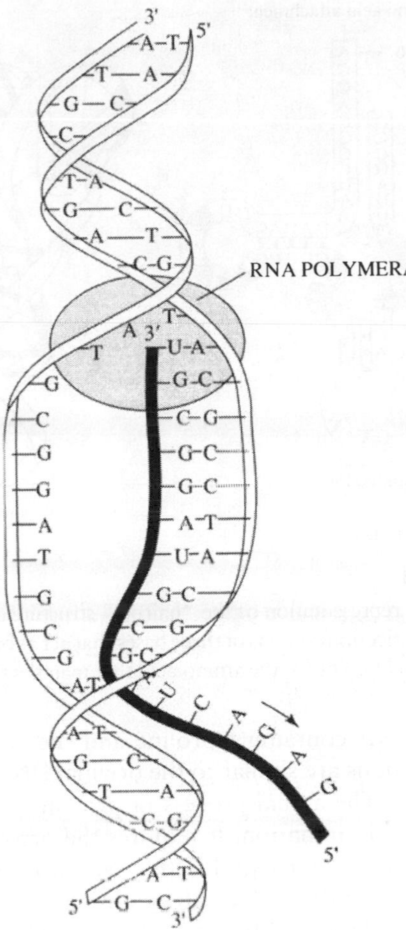

Figure 9.29
Schematic showing the transcription process on a separated DNA stand. RNA polymerase (shaded region) is responsible for "unzipping" the strand and synthesizing the linear mRNA strand. (Adapted with permission from [8].)

1st position (5' end) ↓	2nd position U	2nd position C	2nd position A	2nd position G	3rd position (3' end) ↓
U	Phe	Ser	Tyr	Cys	U
	Phe	Ser	Tyr	Cys	C
	Leu	Ser	STOP	STOP	A
	Leu	Ser	STOP	Trp	G
C	Leu	Pro	His	Arg	U
	Leu	Pro	His	Arg	C
	Leu	Pro	Gln	Arg	A
	Leu	Pro	Gln	Arg	G
A	Ile	Thr	Asn	Ser	U
	Ile	Thr	Asn	Ser	C
	Ile	Thr	Lys	Arg	A
	Met	Thr	Lys	Arg	G
G	Val	Ala	Asp	Gly	U
	Val	Ala	Asp	Gly	C
	Val	Ala	Glu	Gly	A
	Val	Ala	Glu	Gly	G

Figure 9.30
List of mRNA codons. (Adapted with permission from [1].)

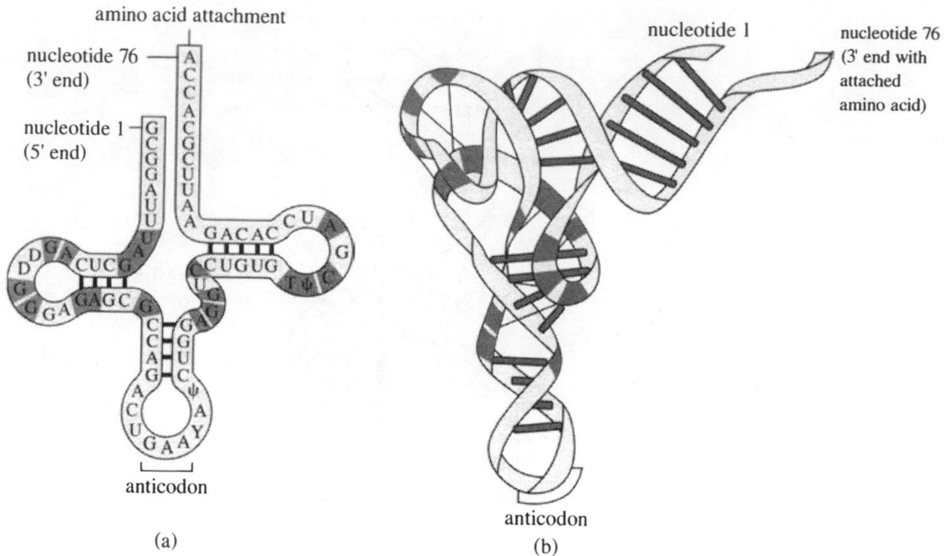

Figure 9.31
(a) Schematic representation of the "hairpin" structure of tRNA. (b) Actual three-dimensional conformation of tRNA. The anticodon consists of three bases that act as binding sites for the mRNA, while the opposite end serves as an attachment point for the amino acid that matches the anticodon. (Adapted with permission from [1].)

tRNA containing proline and the anticodon GGA (Fig. 9.32). Note that the anticodons are similar to the original DNA sequence, except for the use of U instead of T.

The actual process of protein assembly has three stages: initiation, elongation, and termination. It requires the presence of ribosomes located on the external surface of the rough ER (Fig. 9.33). In the **initiation** stage, the smaller ribosomal subunit binds to a specific codon (a **start codon**) on the mRNA and this promotes the attachment of the second, larger ribosomal subunit. As shown in Fig. 9.34(a), there are two distinct domains on the ribosome: the **P site** binds the growing peptide, while the **A site** contains the next amino acid to be added to the chain.

During the **elongation** phase, two tRNA molecules, one in the P site and one in the A site on the ribosome, are bound to the mRNA [Fig. 9.34(b)]. The ribosome catalyzes the formation of a peptide bond between the amino acids and the tRNA in

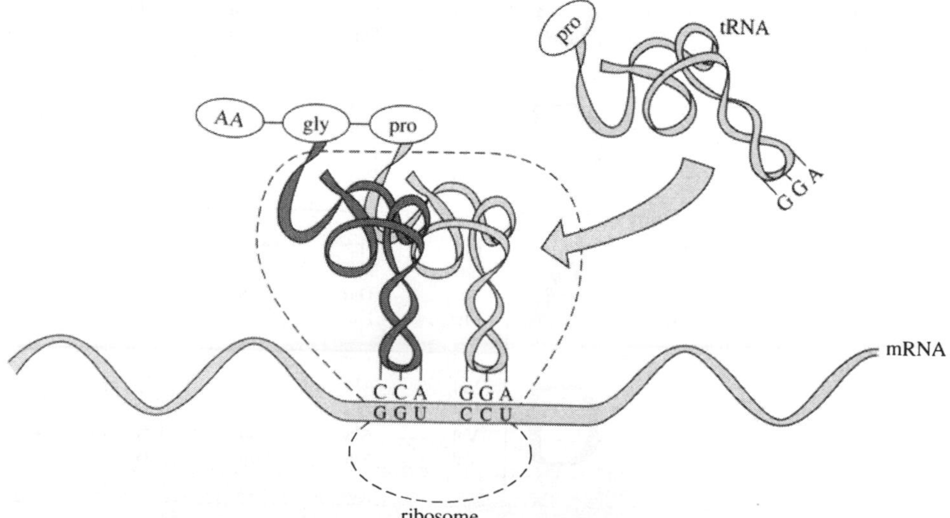

Figure 9.32
Addition of proline to a growing peptide chain. The tRNA carrying the proline and exhibiting an appropriate anticodon (GGA) is able to bind to the codon (CCU) of the mRNA. The proline is then attached to the glycine residue via a peptide bond.

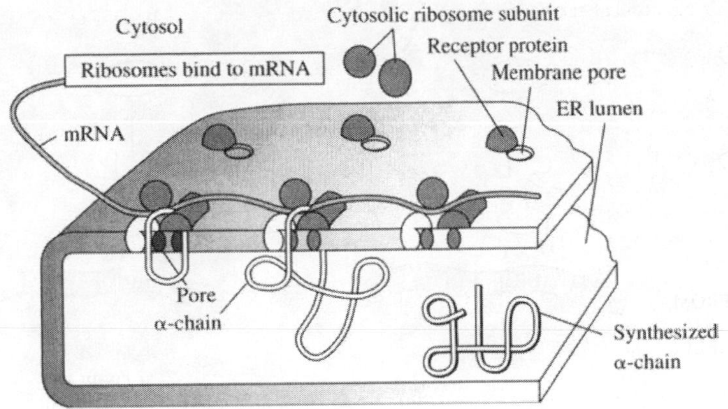

Figure 9.33 Diagram of collagen pro α-chain synthesis. The ribosomes bind to the mRNA, and the pro α-chain is formed and then released into the ER lumen after translation. (Adapted with permission from [2].)

the P site is released. The tRNA previously in the A site moves to the P site and a third tRNA molecule attaches in the newly open A site. A peptide bond again forms and the process is repeated.

When the ribosome reaches particular codons on the mRNA (**termination codons**) that are recognized by release factors, protein synthesis is **terminated.** The polypeptide chain is cleaved from the last tRNA and the tRNA is released [Fig. 9.34(c)]. The release factor then initiates the dissociation of the ribosomal subunits. The entire process of converting the codons from the mRNA to a polypeptide chain is called **translation.**

After translation is completed, the protein, now a fully formed collagen pro-α chain, moves into the ER lumen (Fig. 9.33). Further **post-translational processing** in the ER and Golgi, illustrated in Fig. 9.28, results in the association of three pro-α chains to form a procollagen molecule. As discussed in Section 9.3.1, additional reactions occur after procollagen secretion into the ECM to further stabilize the triple-helical structure, and eventually, fibril and fiber assembly.

EXAMPLE PROBLEM 9.3

Some approaches for tissue regeneration involve the application of a biomaterial to deliver bioactive factors to promote a specific biological response. For instance, some strategies involve the delivery of the protein Bone Morphogenetic Protein-2 (BMP-2) to promote local bone formation. Several researchers, however, are developing methods to deliver DNA specifically engineered to contain the gene encoding BMP-2 in addition to sequences that promote expression of the gene. One approach to deliver the DNA to the cell is to complex it with a polycationic polymer, such as poly(ethylenimine). Another approach is to encapsulate the DNA within phospholipid microspheres.

(a) In terms of structural stability and duration of bioactive effect, what are the potential advantages of delivering DNA that encodes a therapeutic protein, rather than delivering the protein directly?
(b) Discuss the mechanism of complexation of DNA with a polycationic polymer. If the complex carries a net positive charge, how might this facilitate cellular entry of the DNA?
(c) Discuss a possible mechanism of cellular entry of lipid-encapsulated DNA.
(d) Is cellular entry of the DNA alone sufficient for protein expression, or must the DNA enter a specific part of the cell for expression? If it must reach a specific part of the cell, name that part.

Solution

(a) Proteins generally require maintenance of a complex three-dimensional structure to retain biological activity. As discussed in previous chapters, this overall structure includes the primary, secondary, tertiary, and quarternary structure of the protein. The structure of the protein is highly susceptible to environmental factors, such as the pH

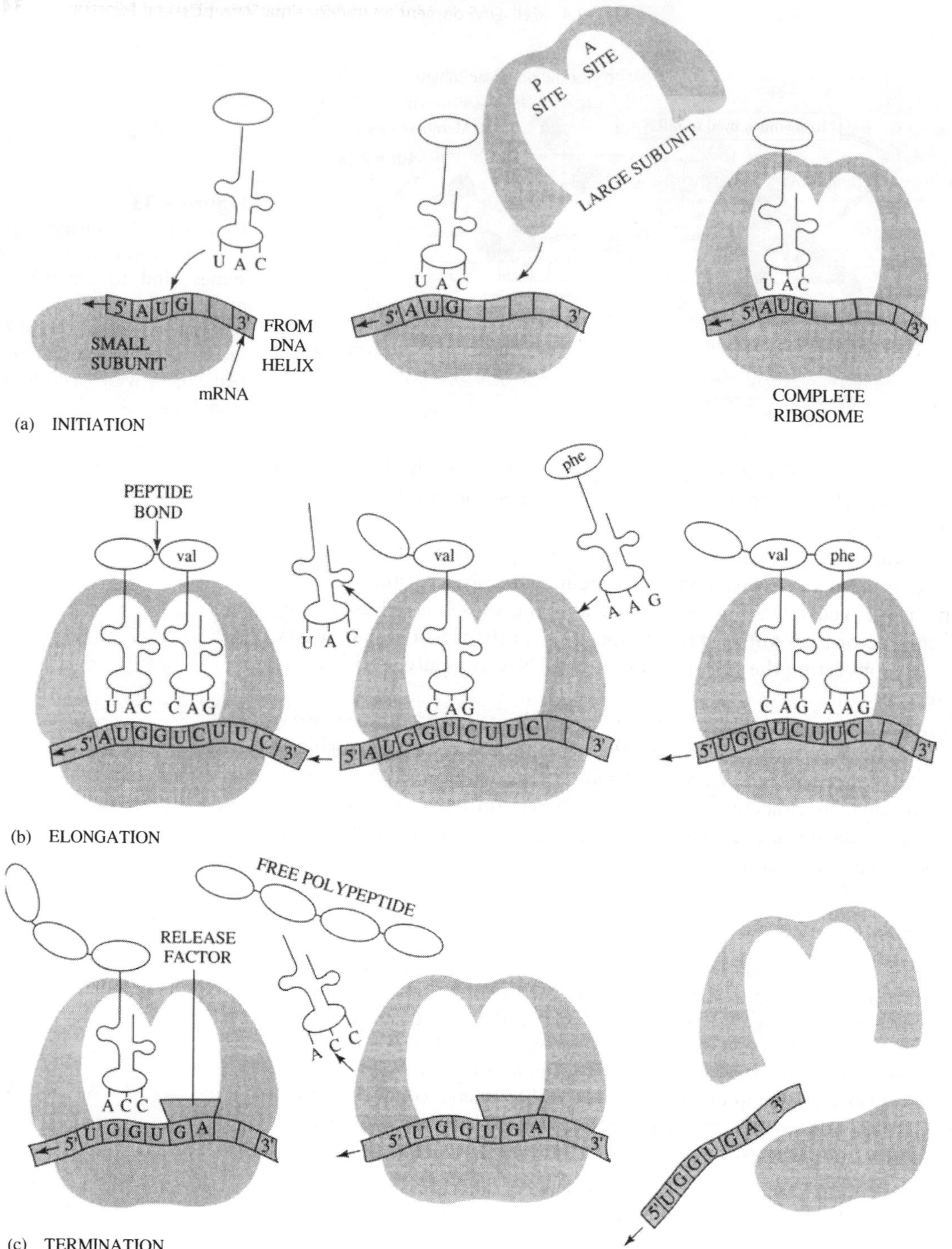

Figure 9.34

Diagram of the translation process. There are three main stages: initiation, elongation, and termination. (a) In the initiation stage, the smaller ribosomal subunit binds to a specific codon (a start codon) on the mRNA and this promotes the attachment of the second, larger ribosomal subunit. (b) During the elongation phase, two tRNA molecules, one in the P site (which binds the growing peptide) and one in the A site (which contains the next amino acid to be added to the chain), are bound to the mRNA. The ribosome catalyzes the formation of a peptide bond between the amino acids and the tRNA in the P site is released. The tRNA previously in the A site moves to the P site and a third tRNA molecule attaches in the newly open A site. This process then repeats. (c) When the ribosome reaches particular codons on the mRNA (termination codons) that are recognized by release factors, protein synthesis is terminated. The polypeptide chain is cleaved from the last tRNA and the tRNA is released. The release factor then initiates the dissociation of the ribosomal subunits. (Adapted with permission from [8].)

of the solution and the presence of enzymes. In the extracellular environment, proteins can be degraded by the action of enzymes and the effects of pH, such as the acidic pH of the wound-healing environment. DNA is generally more stable than proteins, and it depends, primarily, on its sequence of bases, for maintenance of function. The double-stranded structure of DNA is driven by the hydrophobic effect to have the negatively charged phosphate backbone exposed to the (aqueous) solution, while the ring structures of the nucleotides form stabilizing hydrogen bonds in the interior of the double helix. Thus, DNA is generally more structurally stable than proteins in the aqueous physiological environment, and consequently, it is generally better able to maintain bioactivity than proteins. In terms of duration of bioactive effect, proteins are only effective as long as they are present in a bioactive form. As therapeutic proteins are degraded and cleared from the target site, additional proteins must be delivered to maintain the desired biological effect with time. DNA, however, can be expressed to form the protein of interest. As it is essentially a blueprint for protein production, many copies of a protein can be produced from one gene. The protein expression can potentially continue in a cell as long as the cell and the DNA are viable. Thus, plasmid DNA presents the potential for a sustained bioavailability of the desired therapeutic protein when compared to delivery of the protein itself.

(b) DNA is a polyanionic macromolecule due to the negative charges of the phosphate groups along the backbone of the DNA. As a result, polycationic polymers can form electrostatic complexes with plasmid DNA in proper conditions through charge-charge interaction of the negative DNA and the positive polymer. If the complex carries a net positive charge, the positive charge can potentially interact with the negatively charged cell membrane through electrostatic attraction. This electrostatic interaction of the complex with the cell membrane may facilitate cellular entry of the DNA, as DNA alone would likely be repelled by the cell membrane (negative charges repelling each other).

(c) The cell membrane is composed of a dynamic and fluid phospholipid bilayer. If DNA is encapsulated in microspheres composed of comparable phospholipids, the phospholipids of the microsphere could potentially approach and fuse with the cell membrane, thereby transferring the DNA cargo into the interior of the cell.

(d) Cellular entry of DNA alone is not sufficient for gene expression. The DNA must enter the nucleus to be expressed. DNA in the nucleus of a cell can be transcribed to messenger RNA (mRNA). Translation of the mRNA to the encoded protein subsequently occurs outside the nucleus with the assistance of ribosomal RNA (rRNA) and transfer RNA (tRNA). ■

9.5 Models of Adhesion, Spreading and Migration

Besides affecting cell viability, proliferation, differentiation, and protein synthesis, cell-ECM interactions have a large impact on the degree of cell adhesion and migration across/through a substrate. These aspects of cell function must be considered in biomaterial design in order to assure implant integration and prevent unwanted scarring around the device.

The steps involved in cellular adhesion and migration have been extensively studied for a variety of cell types. These experiments have given us a better understanding of the role of membrane receptors and the cytoskeleton in these processes, and have allowed for the development of a number of increasingly complex mathematical models for adhesion, spreading, and migration. Key aspects of simple models for these processes are reviewed here.

9.5.1 Basic Adhesion Models: DLVO Theory

A basic model for cell adhesion to a surface is centered on **DLVO theory**, based on work from Derjaguin, Landau, Verway, and Overbeek. First developed to explain coagulation of charged colloidal particles, this theory is based on thermodynamic arguments, like those explained in Chapter 8 for protein adsorption. This is a highly simplified model for contact between a cell and a surface, since it does not take into account any specific receptor-ligand interactions between molecules on the cell membrane and those on the substrate. Therefore, it may be used only as a first approximation to understand how cells react to a biomaterial. Similarly, it may also be employed to model bacterial adhesion to biomedical implants (see Chapter 14).

Figure 9.35 depicts the free energy of interaction, $G(z)$, between a particle and the surface as determined by DLVO theory as a function of separation distance (z). Similar to force-distance curves for atomic bonding (Chapter 1), this curve is the result of several competing forces, two of which are shown as dashed lines in the graph. As a particle approaches a surface, there is a drop in potential energy (called the **secondary minimum**) which represents a balance between long-range electrostatic interactions (repulsive) and long-range van der Waals interactions (attractive). As discussed previously, overall electrostatic interactions are influenced by the charge of the surface, charge of the cell, and composition of the surrounding media, while van der Waals forces are caused by dipolar interactions between the cell and the substrate. Hydrophobic (dehydration) effects are not considered in DLVO theory since they exist over much shorter ranges than electrostatic and van der Waals forces and thus do not significantly contribute to the energy of interaction between the particle and the surface.

The particle (cell) may remain loosely attached to the surface as a result of this secondary minimum; however, it will never become firmly adherent unless it can overcome the potential energy barrier (shown in Fig. 9.35) and move into the **primary minimum** (not shown in Fig. 9.35). The primary minimum is caused by the balance of short-range electrostatic and van der Waals forces at the point of contact. The energy needed to overcome the barrier is provided by random motion of the particle and is dependent on the temperature of the system (Brownian motion).

9.5.2 DLVO Theory Limitations and Further Models

While the DLVO theory provides an estimate of cell-surface binding, it does not take into account several important factors, including steric repulsion. Much like proteins, cells will not be able to attach to surfaces with bulky, hydrophilic groups that

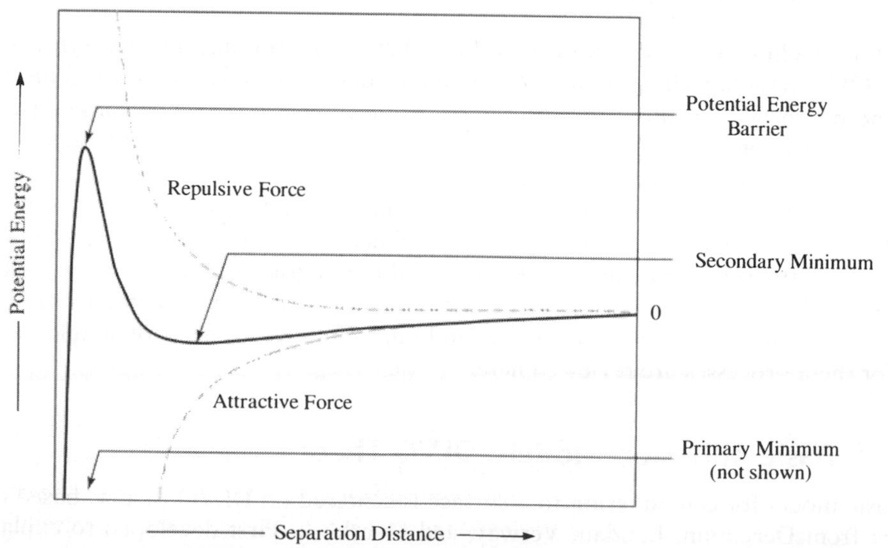

Figure 9.35
Particle adhesion modeled with DLVO theory. The graph depicts the free energy of interaction as a function of separation distance. As a particle approaches a surface, there is a drop in potential energy, which represents a balance between long-range electrostatic interactions (repulsive) and long-range van der Waals interactions (attractive). The particle (cell) may remain loosely attached to the surface as a result of this secondary minimum; however, it will never become firmly adherent unless it can overcome the potential energy barrier (shown in the figure by the peak) and move into the primary minimum (not shown).

extend into the environment and are in constant motion near the surface. In addition, the role of surface topography is not addressed in this model. Also similar to protein adsorption, rough surfaces may physically trap cells in grooves on the surface. It is important to note, however, that cells are several orders of magnitude larger than proteins, so what is "rough" from the perspective of proteins may appear smooth on the length scale that would be sensed by the cell.

Also, as discussed above, DLVO theory does not consider specific ligand-receptor interactions, which are extremely important in cell adhesion. Thus, additional models have been developed to address this topic, many of which include terms involving the kinetics of receptor–ligand binding. Although the details of these models are beyond the scope of this book, equations have been formulated to provide information about the number of ligand–receptor complexes formed over time in a variety of situations if the total number of receptor molecules and original ligand amounts are known. For example, the receptor–ligand binding can be modeled as a reversible chemical reaction:

$$R + L \underset{k_r}{\overset{k_f}{\rightleftarrows}} C$$

In this reaction, R is the free receptor, L is the free ligand, C is the receptor–ligand complex, and k_f and k_r are the reaction rates of complex formation and dissociation, respectively. k_f and k_r can be related to the thermodynamic principles of binding discussed above and in Chapter 1. Therefore, it is possible to model the change in receptor–ligand complex concentration over time as

$$\frac{dC}{dt} = k_f RL - k_r C \tag{9.1}$$

where R, L, and C represent the concentrations of the free receptor, free ligand, and receptor–ligand complex, respectively. However, it is possible to combine these models with the DLVO theory to make a more accurate prediction of cell–substrate adhesion, taking into account both specific and nonspecific interactions.

9.5.3 Models of Cell Spreading and Migration

9.5.3.1 Cell Spreading After attachment, cells may extend finger-like pseudopodia along the substrate surface. At this point, integrin receptors in the cell membrane may interact with ligands on the material surface to firmly anchor the cell in place. This process is known as **cell spreading** and occurs to a greater or lesser degree with all cell types. Since this is a complex phenomenon involving internal cytoskeletal rearrangement as well as production and/or adsorption of adhesive proteins on the substrate, simple models of cell spreading have not yet been developed.

However, there is experimental evidence that, at least for certain cell types, there is a correlation between degree of spreading and the free energy of the surface. The existence of such a correlation is logical since surface free energy affects protein adsorption (see Chapter 8) and it is the interaction between the protein coating and membrane receptors that results in cell spreading.

9.5.3.2 Cell Migration Cell migration begins with similar events as those involved in cell spreading. As depicted in Fig. 9.36, extension of the cell membrane in long pseudopodia is directed by polymerization of actin microfibrils near the leading edge of the cell. This is followed by attachment of membrane integrin receptors to the substrate. After the pseudopodia are firmly adhered, there is generation of a contractile force and a concomitant release of rear receptors, leading to forward cellular

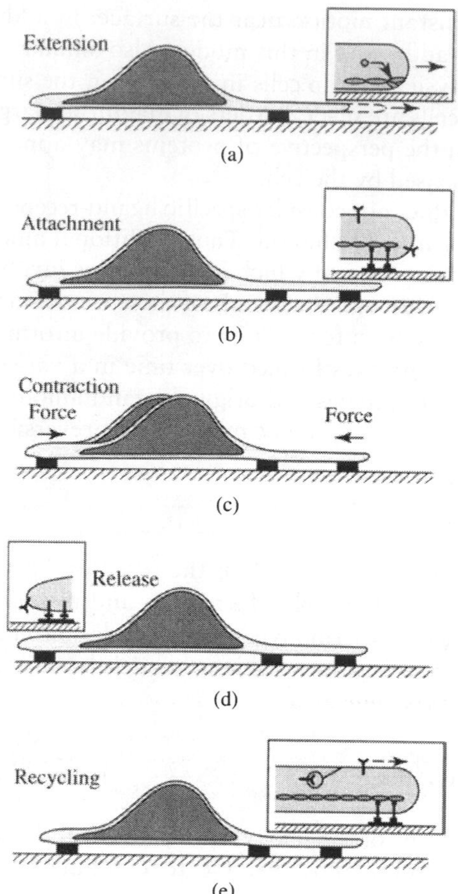

Figure 9.36
Diagram of cell migration. (a) First, extension of the cell membrane in long pseudopodia is directed by polymerization of actin microfibrils near the leading edge of the cell. (b) The membrane then attaches to the substrate via integrin receptors. (c, d) After the pseudopodia are firmly adhered, there is generation of a contractile force and a concomitant release of rear receptors, leading to forward cellular motion. (e) Finally, the integrin receptors are recycled to the leading edge so that they may be used again as the process continues. (Adapted with permission from [11].)

motion. Finally, the integrin receptors are recycled to the leading edge so that they may be used again as the process continues.

Because this is an extremely complicated process, models of cell migration that describe events at various levels of detail have been developed, and parameters calculated in one model can be used to determine constants in larger-scale models. The diagram in Fig. 9.37 demonstrates that information about detailed intracellular events may eventually be used to predict the movement of entire cell populations.

At the top of the hierarchy, mathematical models have been designed to provide information about the migration of a population of cells. As introduced in Chapter 2 for diffusion of atoms in a metallic biomaterial, the number of cells migrating across a particular location can also be modeled using a flux equation. In the simplest case, cell migration is the result of a combination of random cell motility and directed movement in response to soluble chemical signals (**chemotaxis**). Therefore, the flux of cells M (cells/distance/time) for a two-dimensional system can be represented as

$$M = random\ motility + chemotaxis \tag{9.2}$$

or

$$M = -\sigma \frac{dN}{dx} + \chi N \frac{dC}{dx} \tag{9.3}$$

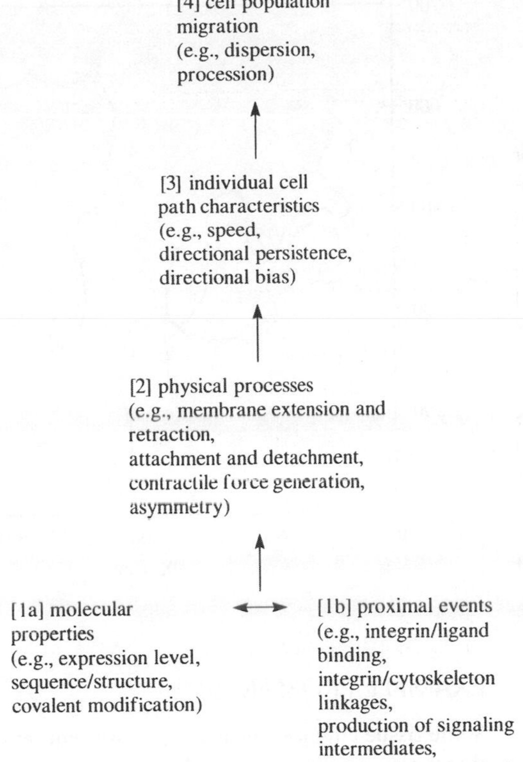

Figure 9.37
A diagram demonstrating the relationship between different levels of modeling of cellular movement. Information about detailed intracellular events may eventually be used to predict the movement of entire cell populations. (Adapted with permission from [12].)

where σ is the random motility coefficient, N is the cell number, χ is the chemotactic coefficient, C is the concentration of the chemical signal, and x is the distance coordinate.

The random motility term, as the name suggests, models the random nature of nondirected cell movement. If no chemical factor is present to induce cell movement in a particular direction, the second term is 0 and it is assumed that the cells move in a random-walk pattern. If a soluble agent is present, migration depends on the concentration of the substance at the location of interest, which is included in the second term.

On a more detailed level, the migration of individual cells can be modeled. The paths of individual cells are tracked and plotted in Fig. 9.38. From these plots, two main parameters, **translocation speed** (s) and **persistence time** (p) are determined. Translocation speed is the speed of cell movement over any straight-line portion of the graph, between changes in direction. Persistence time is the length of time that the cell moves along the substrate without a drastic change in direction. At times much longer than p, these parameters can be related to the random motility coefficient in the population model (assuming a two-dimensional system) by the formula

$$\sigma = \frac{1}{2}s^2p \tag{9.4}$$

Models of increasingly detailed intracellular events, such as actin polymerization and integrin binding, are also possible, but their descriptions are beyond the scope of this text. Experimental means of tracking movements of both individual cells and cell populations are discussed in the following section.

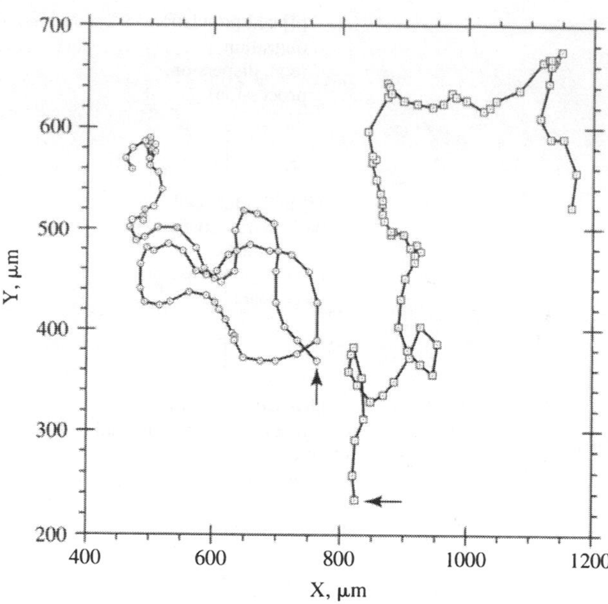

Figure 9.38
Typical trajectories for bovine pulmonary artery endothelial cells migrating in a uniform environment. Symbols represent the location of the centroid of each cell at 30 minute intervals. The arrows indicate the starting point for each trajectory. Two main parameters can be determined from these plots: translocation speed and persistence time. (Image courtesy of Y. Lee and K. Zygourakis, Rice University.)

EXAMPLE PROBLEM 9.4

Some tissue engineering strategies use synthetic polymer hydrogel scaffolds to promote and direct tissue regeneration. However, many hydrogel materials, such as those based upon poly(ethylene glycol) (PEG), do not readily support cell adhesion unless modified to do so. One method of modification of hydrogels is the covalent attachment of a specific peptide sequence or sequences promoting cell attachment. The peptide sequence RGD (arginine-glycine-aspartic acid) is a motif found in a number of extracellular matrix proteins. Recognition of the RGD sequence by integrins can lead to cell binding. Consider a tissue engineering hydrogel scaffold composed from a poly(ethylene glycol)-*co*-poly(α-hydroxy acid) diacrylate macromer [13]. The acrylate moieties allow for the covalent crosslinking of the macromers upon proper initiation to form a hydrogel, while the ester groups allow for hydrolytic degradation of the resulting hydrogels. Assume that the hydrogels have been modified through the covalent inclusion of macromer chains of poly(ethylene glycol) acrylate modified with a terminal RGD sequence.

(a) Given that poly(ethylene glycol)-*co*-poly(α-hydroxy acid) diacrylate hydrogels are biodegradable, should the peptide modification be limited to the surface of the material or should it occur throughout the bulk of the material to promote long-term cell adhesion? Justify your answer.

(b) The peptide sequence will be chemically coupled to a reactive acrylate group that will allow for covalent incorporation of the peptide moiety into the hydrogel network. You are given the choice between having (a) a PEG spacer (molecular weight of 3,400 Da) between the acrylate group and the peptide or (b) no spacer between the acrylate group and the peptide. Which method will yield the highest cell attachment per given number of peptides? Why? Assume that the PEG-*co*-poly(α-hydroxy acid) diacrylate used to fabricate the hydrogels has a molecular weight of 8,000 Da.

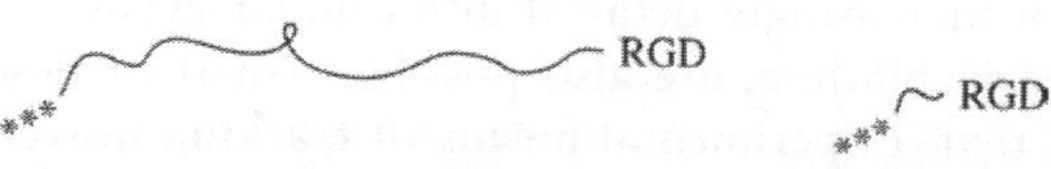

(c) Assume now that a sheet of the peptide modified PEG-*co*-poly(α-hydroxy acid) diacrylate hydrogel will be tested for cell adhesion to the surface of the material in a tissue culture experiment. Three groups are examined. The surface concentration of the RGD peptide is 0.001 pmole/cm^2 in Group A, 0.1 pmole/cm^2 in Group B, and 1 pmole/cm^2 in Group C. Which group will likely result in the highest cell adhesion? Which group will likely result in the highest degree of cell spreading on the material? How is cell migration affected by the concentration of the ligand (in this case, the peptide) on the material surface?

Solution

(a) Given that the hydrogel is intended for tissue engineering applications in which long-term cell adhesion to the material is desirable, the peptide modification should be present in the bulk of the material, rather than limited to the surface of the material. If the modification is limited to the surface of the material, the cell adhesive properties of the material will be greatly diminished when the modified surface is lost to degradation. However, if the bulk of the material is modified with the peptide sequence, the peptide will be present in the material throughout the course of degradation of the material, be it through surface erosion or a bulk degradation mechanism. Thus, cell adhesion will be promoted throughout the course of material degradation through bulk incorporation of the peptide sequence.

(b) Use of the peptide moiety with the PEG spacer will likely result in greater cell attachment per given number of peptides. The hydrogel surface will present free ends and exposed sections of the constituent PEG-*co*-poly(α-hydroxy acid) diacrylate polymer chains. These free ends and sections of the polymer chains will have some mobility. In the case of a peptide moiety with no spacer, the peptide sequence will likely be sterically blocked from exposure to cells due to the presence of the PEG-*co*-poly(α-hydroxy acid) diacrylate chain segments and ends at the hydrogel surface. However, a PEG spacer will likely allow for the peptide sequence to be tethered from the bulk of the material. The 3,400-Da molecular weight of the spacer is nearly half that of the PEG-*co*-poly(α-hydroxy acid) diacrylate chains and will likely be sufficient to allow for presentation of the peptide sequence with minimal steric hindrance from the free chain ends at the surface. Thus, it will promote cell adhesion.

(c) The group with the highest surface concentration of the peptide (Group C) will generally result in the highest degree of cell adhesion and the highest degree of cell spreading. As the number of ligands on the material surface increases, the number of ligands available for cell attachment generally increases, so the degree of cell adhesion increases. As adherent cells become capable of making increasing numbers of contacts, the degree of cell spreading increases. Cells require interactions with the ligands on the surface for adhesion. Increasing concentrations of ligands on the surface will allow for increasing cell motility up to a point, beyond which the motility decreases with increasing surface concentrations of ligands. This is due to the fact that, at higher concentrations of ligands on the surface, the cells will be highly spread upon the surface and will have many points of contact that must be broken to allow for motility. ■

9.6 Techniques: Assays to Determine Effects of Cell-Material Interactions

In this chapter, we have examined the basic constituents of the cell and the ECM and discussed how their interactions affect various cell functions. In this section, assays to determine to what extent certain functions have been altered are described. These include measurements of **cytotoxicity** (cell death), cell adhesion and spreading, cell migration, and changes in gene expression (DNA/RNA assays). As mentioned previously, the production of proteins is also important to cellular differentiation and function, and can be quantified using the same methods described in Chapter 8 (colorimetric or fluorescent assays, ELISAs, or Western blotting).

The location of various proteins in the ECM may be detected through immunostaining, which is described later in this section.

9.6.1 Cytotoxicity Assays

At the most basic level, cell–environment interactions affect the viability of the cell. Therefore, cytotoxicity is a large concern in developing new substrata for cells, and *in vitro* assays for cytotoxicity are often a required first step in biocompatibility testing for novel biomaterials. A number of regulatory boards, including the ASTM, (mentioned in Chapter 4 for mechanical testing protocols) and the International Organization of Standardization (ISO) have developed standard procedures for cytotoxicity experiments and analysis of the resulting data.

As shown in Table 9.1, a number of accepted cytotoxicity assays have been developed, including direct contact, agar diffusion, and elution tests. One of the reasons that alternative testing procedures exist is that there are several characteristics of a biomaterial that can affect its overall cytotoxicity. Often, the aspects of the material that determine its cytotoxicity are different from those that determine its interactions with the cell surface. Therefore, a particular material may promote cell adhesion and spreading, while at the same time be deleterious to viability over days or weeks. Anything present in a biomaterial (on the surface or in the bulk) that interferes with cellular metabolism or protein synthesis machinery is considered cytotoxic. This includes the material itself, any additives or processing agents used in fabrication, and potential degradation products.

It is important to note that both the type and differentiation state of the surrounding cells, as well as the final use of the product, must be taken into account when selecting which combinations of cytotoxicity tests are most appropriate. An example of this is found with zinc eugenol cements in dentistry, which produce cell death in elution assays, but are commonly used in current dental procedures where the material is separated from surrounding cells by a thick layer of calcified tissue called dentin.

9.6.1.1 Direct Contact Assay The conceptually simplest cytotoxicity test is the **direct contact assay**. Here, the test material is fabricated to specific dimensions and placed on top of a layer of cells cultured in a cell culture plate. After 24 hours in a culture incubator, the cells in the area around the sample are examined microscopically to evaluate the extent of swelling and lysis. Those cells that are no longer living will often lift up from the surface and float in the media, resulting in a cell-less ring around the material. In some protocols, the size of this ring (including both dead and damaged cells) is measured. Because this assay is primarily qualitative, the inclusion of positive (non-cytotoxic) and negative (completely cytotoxic) controls is crucial so that the relative degree of cytotoxicity for the sample material can be estimated.

TABLE 9.1

Cytotoxicity Assays Used on Materials

Description	Material Form	ASTM Standard Number
Direct contact	Bulk or extract	F-813
Agar diffusion	Bulk or extract	F-895
Elution	Extract	F-619

(Adapted with permission from [14].)

Although not required by ASTM standards in this and other assays, additional tests may be performed on the cells after exposure to the biomaterial to provide more information about the cytotoxic properties of the sample. For example, qualitative assessment of the fraction of dead cells in a sample is also possible via the use of dyes that are not able to permeate the cell membrane of living cells. The stained cells are those that have died and are no longer able to maintain the integrity of their cell membranes.

A more quantitative approach is obtained by measuring the amount of an intracellular enzyme, such as **lactate dehydrogenase (LDH)**, in the media. This enzyme, important in cellular metabolism, can only be detected in the supernatant after the cell has lysed and released its intracellular contents. A standard curve is then used to convert LDH amounts to number of lysed cells.

Alternatively, viability can be quantified by using dyes that change color only in the presence of viable cells. The color change can then be read at a specified wavelength on a microplate reader equipped with a spectrophotometer, similar to the method that was described for protein assays in Chapter 8. The amount of viable cells is then represented as a fraction based on the ratio of color generation in the sample wells to the color found in wells with no treatment (positive control). The most common compound used for such measurements is (3-(4,5-dimethylthiazolyl-2)-2,5-diphenyltetrazolium bromide) (MTT), which produces a purple color in the presence of living cells.

9.6.1.2 Agar Diffusion Assay The **agar diffusion assay** is similar to the direct contact assay, except in this case, the cells are allowed to adhere to culture dishes and are then covered with agar before exposure to the sample material. Agar is a natural polymer derived from red algae and will not harm the cells below it. However, it does provide a physical barrier to keep the sample from crushing or disturbing the cell layer, as may occur in direct contact testing.

The agar is combined with cell culture media to insure the survival of the cells. However, soluble products from the sample may diffuse into the agar and result in cell death in localized regions under the material. The cells are then divided into zones, depending on their distance from the sample, and viability is examined 1–3 days after exposure (Fig. 9.39). The greater the number of affected zones and/or the farther away from the specimen effects are observed, the greater the cytotoxicity of the sample. As in the direct contact assay, cellular dyes indicating viability may be included in the media to provide a better estimate of the number of dead cells in each zone. Positive and negative controls are often included to aid in comparison of results.

9.6.1.3 Elution Assay **Elution** or **extract assays** are performed to determine the cytotoxicity of leachable molecules found in biomaterials, such as nonreacted monomers or degradation products. The most common version of this procedure is completed by eluting any soluble molecules in aqueous media, since this is closest to the biological environment.

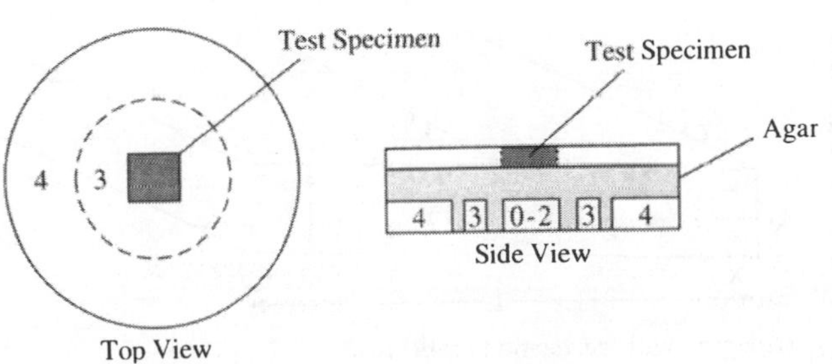

Figure 9.39
Schematic of the agar diffusion assay, used to determine cytotoxicity of a material sample. Cells adhered to a well plate are covered with agar. The test specimen is then placed on top of the agar and the cells are kept in culture for 1–3 days. The cells are then divided into zones, depending on their distance from the sample, and viability is examined. The greater the number of affected zones and/or the farther away from the specimen the effects are observed, the greater the cytotoxicity of the sample. (Adapted with permission from [14].)

In these assays, cells are plated and allowed to adhere to cell culture wells for 24 hours. Simultaneously, extract media is prepared by placing a known amount of material in a given amount of fresh cell culture media and allowing any soluble products to diffuse into the media for 24 hours at 37°C. After this period, the extract media is added to the wells containing cells and viability is monitored over 1–3 days using the techniques described previously.

9.6.2 Adhesion/Spreading Assays

Cell adhesion to various surfaces is often quantified by allowing cells to attach to the sample material for a set amount of time and then rinsing away nonadhered cells in a controlled manner. The amount of cell adhesion is then measured by recording either the number of cells that remain on the surface, or the number of cells washed away. For the latter case,

$$\begin{pmatrix} \textit{Number of} \\ \textit{cells on surface} \end{pmatrix} = \begin{pmatrix} \textit{Total number} \\ \textit{of seeded cells} \end{pmatrix} - \begin{pmatrix} \textit{Number of cells in} \\ \textit{washing media} \end{pmatrix}$$

In either instance, the number of cells can be determined by staining the cells with a dye such as MTT, radioactively labeling them, or lysing them and assaying for intracellular enzymes like LDH.

Examination of cell spreading is more qualitative and usually involves staining the cells and looking at representative fields via light microscopy. In some cases, analysis software can be used with images obtained by the microscope to determine the surface area of cells under different conditions, thus providing a more quantitative assessment of spreading.

A major disadvantage to these adhesion assays is that it is difficult to reproduce the force exerted in the washing step, which can cause high experimental error between samples. To overcome this limitation, a number of means to provide controlled flow during the washing step have been developed. One of these is to place the specimen in a parallel plate flow chamber (Fig. 9.40). For such a system, the shear stress (τ) at the wall (where the sample is inserted) is proportional to the volumetric flow

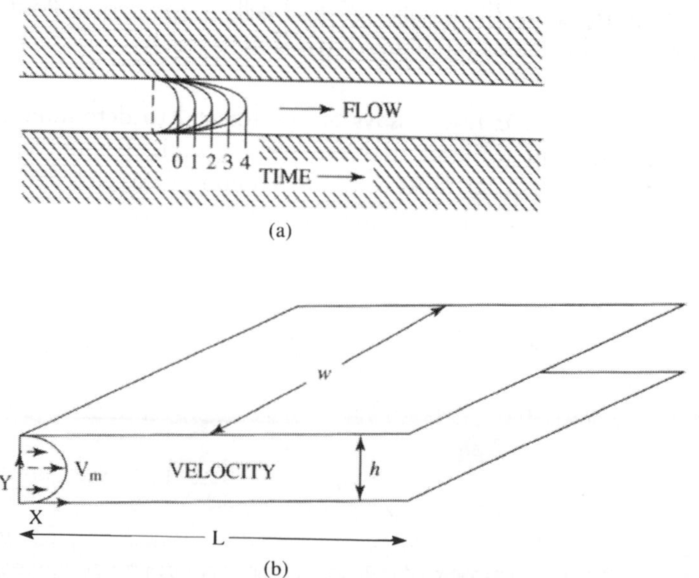

Figure 9.40
Schematic of a parallel plate flow chamber, which can be used to control shearing forces imparted on cells during adhesion/spreading assays. The parameter h indicates the distance between the plates, w indicates the width of the plates in the test setup and V_m denotes the velocity of the flow of the solution. As shown in (a), V_m changes with time upon initiation of fluid flow until a parabolic steady-state V_m profile is reached. (Adapted with permission from [15].)

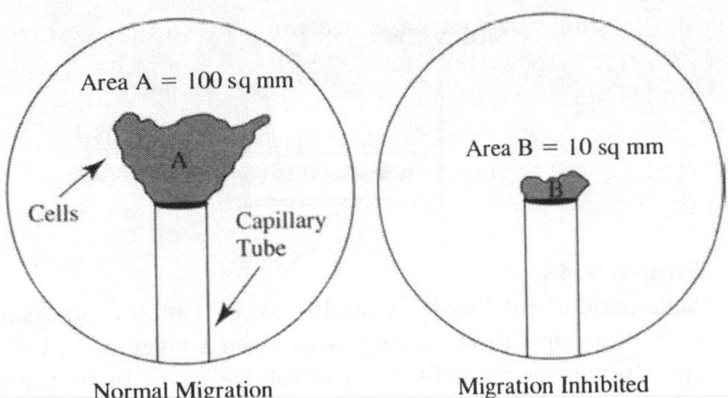

Figure 9.41
Schematic of the capillary tube test, a type of migration assay. In this instance cells are originally contained in the capillary tube, which is then placed on a cell culture surface. The migration of the cells is then monitored microscopically over 2–4 days. (Adapted with permission from [16].)

rate (Q) as well as the viscosity (μ) of the solution (h and w are dimensional parameters defined in Fig. 9.40):

$$\tau = \mu \frac{6Q}{h^2 w} \tag{9.5}$$

Therefore, the force imparted on the specimen can be controlled by altering either of these parameters in the washing step. Other methods of producing controlled shear during sample rinsing include the use of radial flow chambers or centrifugation techniques.

9.6.3 Migration Assays

Several procedures for assessing cell migration have been developed and may be used in combination with the mathematical models described above to characterize cell movement on various surfaces. In particular, a number of means to examine the migration of cell populations can be used, including those that record the average distance migrated and others that record the number of cells that have moved away from the point of origin. Examples of assays that measure distance of migration include the **capillary tube** test. The capillary tube method was one of the first developed and involves confinement of cell populations in a small tube (a capillary tube). The opening of the tube is then placed against a surface (often a cell culture well), allowing the cells to migrate out of the tube in a fan-like shape (Fig. 9.41). After 2–4 days, the area of the fan shape is measured to provide a quantitative assessment of distance migrated.

In a modification of this technique, the cells may be confined within a physical barrier (such as a ring), and then the barrier lifted (Fig. 9.42). The increase in the radius of the cell population over several days can be monitored and measured using a light microscope and appropriate image analysis software. The main drawback to these and other population migration assays is that it is difficult to distinguish what portion of the increase in area is attributable to migration, and what portion is caused by cell proliferation. This is a particular problem if the experiment is performed over several days, when cell proliferation may have a significant effect.

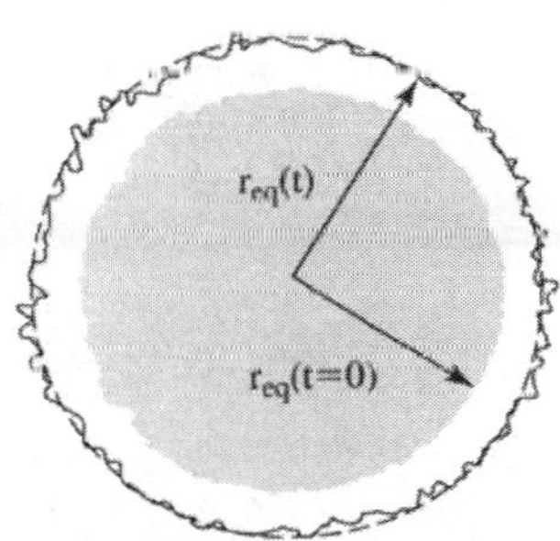

Figure 9.42
Schematic of an alternative migration assay. The cells are seeded in the bottom of a cell culture dish surrounded by a ring of known diameter (grey area in diagram). The ring is removed, and the radius of the cell colony r_{eq} is monitored over time to determine the extent of migration. (Adapted with permission from [17].)

The number of cells in a population migrating away from a given area can be quantified using the **Boyden chamber assay**. This assay is most often employed to determine the effects of soluble factors on migration, rather than examining the impact of the substrate. In the Boyden chamber (or transwell chamber) test, a porous filter separates the cells from the soluble agent to be tested. As seen in Fig. 9.43, the cells are originally seeded in the top layer, and the test substance placed in

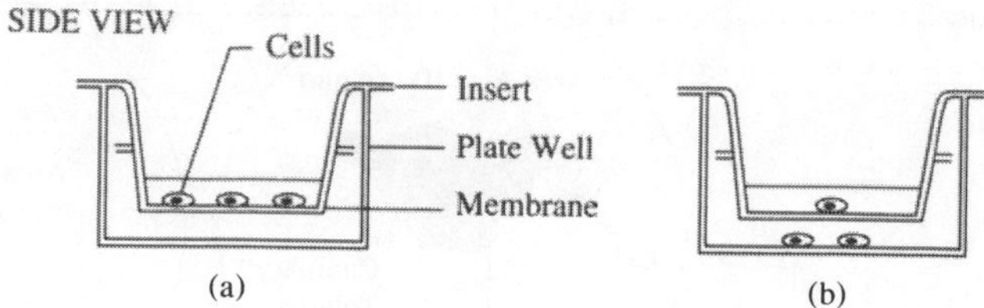

Figure 9.43
Schematic of the Boyden chamber assay, a migration assay that can quantify the number of cells in a population moving away from a given area. In the Boyden chamber test, a porous filter separates the cells and the soluble agent to be tested. The pores are large enough to allow cells to migrate through (~3–8 μm), but small enough to prevent cells from dropping through due to gravity (<12–20 μm). (a) The cells are originally seeded in the top layer, and the test substance is placed in the bottom chamber. This setup allows the soluble agent to diffuse through the filter (membrane) and interact with the cells. (b) After a specified period of time, the number of cells that have migrated through the membrane and that are found in the bottom chamber are quantified via light microscopy. (Adapted with permission from [11].)

the bottom chamber, where it can diffuse through the filter and interact with the cells. After a specified period of time, the number of cells that have migrated through the filter and are found in the bottom chamber are quantified via light microscopy. Further refinements of this technique (Zigmond chamber, Dunn chamber) allow for more direct microscopic visualization of the cells as they migrate through the barrier in response to the attractive agent.

Test methods examining movement of individual cells usually involve an apparatus that allows the incubation of the cells with the test surface on top of a microscope stage. Images of cell locations at given time intervals up to several hours are then captured and processed to determine the precise location of the cell centers at each time point, thus forming a "cell track" over the culture period. Using mathematical models like those described above and comparing cell positions between time points, parameters such as cell speed (s) and persistence time (p) can be calculated.

9.6.4 DNA and RNA Assays

DNA and RNA assays can be used to determine if there is direct damage to a cell's DNA caused by a biomaterial (this is a test for mutagenicity, discussed further in Chapter 14), but, they are most often employed to see how the biomaterial environment affects gene expression, and thus cellular function. Dramatic changes in gene expression may not be desired, because this may result in altered protein production, which could cause problems in the surrounding tissue. However, in diseased tissues, alteration of gene expression to increase production of a certain protein may be desired. (This forms the basis of gene therapy techniques, which are beyond the scope of this text.) Both down- and up-regulation of specific genes can be detected using the following techniques.

9.6.4.1 Polymerase Chain Reaction (PCR) and Reverse-Transcription Polymerase Chain Reaction (RT-PCR) Before the presence of a certain gene can be confirmed or quantified, it is first necessary to expand the amount of DNA or RNA for that gene to detectable levels. For DNA, this procedure uses the **polymerase chain reaction (PCR)** and for RNA, the **reverse-transcription polymerase chain reaction (RT-PCR)**. For these techniques to be useful, the DNA base sequences on each end of the gene of interest must be known, so that a set of DNA-binding **primers**

(short oligonucleotide sequences) can be synthesized. For PCR, the following steps are then performed (Fig. 9.44):

1. The double-stranded genomic DNA (dsDNA) is denatured via heat treatment to produce two single strands of DNA (ssDNA).
2. The ssDNA is cooled with an excess of primers to promote primer-DNA **hybridization** (binding).
3. A heat-stable DNA polymerase (Taq polymerase) and the four deoxyribonucleotide triphosphates (bases) are added.
4. The DNA polymerase then replicates each strand, starting at the primers.
5. The newly formed dsDNA is then heated to separate the strands and the reaction continues.

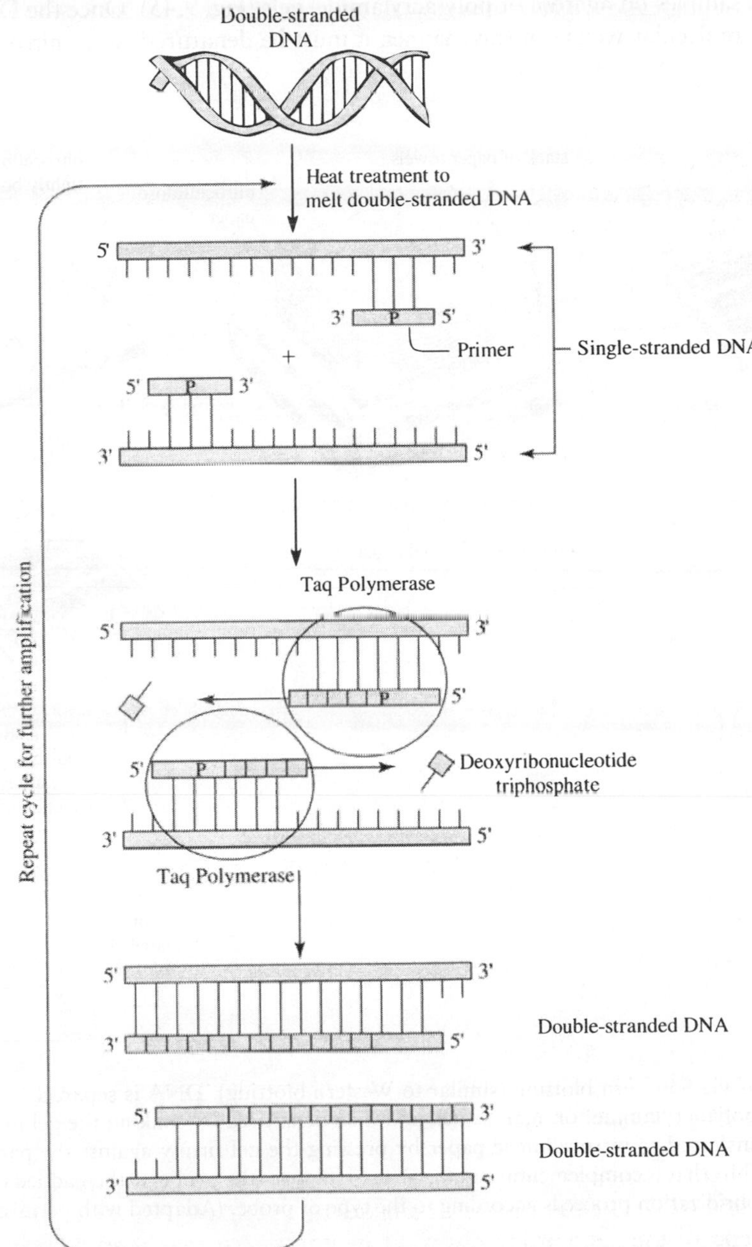

Figure 9.44
Diagram of the steps for PCR processing. First, the double-stranded genomic DNA is denatured via heat treatment to produce two single strands of DNA. A heat-stable DNA polymerase (Taq polymerase) and the four deoxyribonucleotide triphosphates (bases or dNTPs) are subsequently added and the DNA polymerase replicates each strand, starting at the primers. The newly formed dsDNA is then heated to separate the strands and the reaction continues for a second cycle. This procedure can be repeated for many cycles, resulting in a large number of copies of the gene of interest in a relatively short time.

This procedure can be repeated for many cycles to produce a large number of copies of the gene of interest in a relatively short time.

RT-PCR follows the same steps as described above, with one additional step at the beginning of the procedure. In this case, the starting material is mRNA, so it must first be transcribed into DNA before PCR can proceed. This is done with an enzyme, reverse transcriptase, derived from viruses. Here, the enzyme generates ssDNA complementary to the mRNA present in the sample. This ssDNA is then placed into the PCR reaction starting at step 2, where the specific gene of interest can be expanded.

9.6.4.2 Southern and Northern Blotting The DNA amplified with PCR can now be analyzed via **Southern blotting**, a procedure similar to Western blotting (see Chapter 8). However, since DNA is already negatively charged, no SDS is added before running samples on agarose or poly(acrylamide) gels (Fig. 9.45). Once the DNA is separated by molecular weight in this manner, it must be denatured, since nitrocellulose only binds

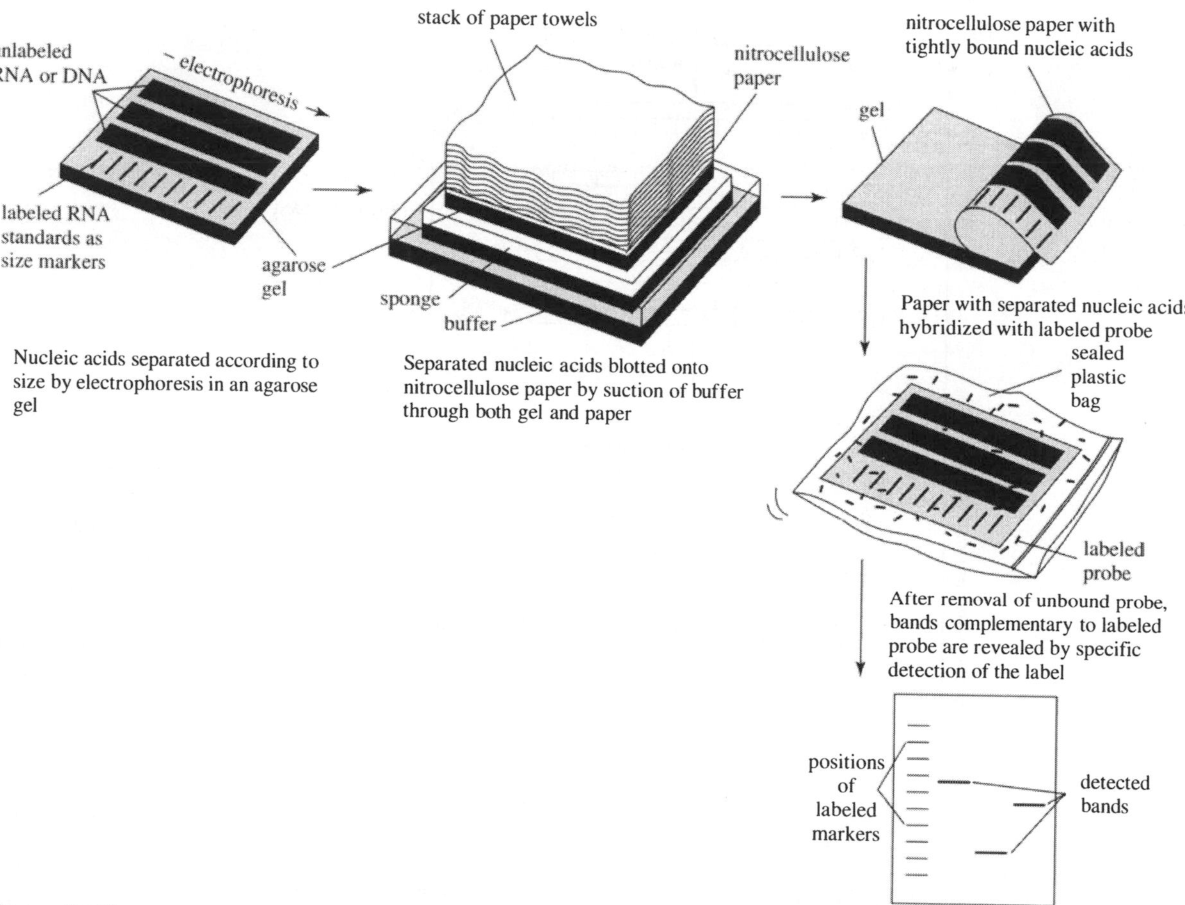

Figure 9.45

Diagram of DNA analysis via Southern blotting (similar to Western blotting). DNA is separated by molecular weight via electrophoresis on a poly(acrylamide) or agarose gel, and then denatured by soaking the gel in NaOH. The resulting ssDNA bands are transferred to nitrocellulose paper by pressing the gel firmly against the paper. A solution containing labeled DNA or RNA that is complementary to the gene of interest (the probe) is then added on top of the blotted paper, and detection of hybridization proceeds according to the type of probe. (Adapted with permission from [1].)

ssDNA. This is accomplished by soaking the gel in NaOH. The sample then undergoes the following steps:

1. The resulting ssDNA bands are transferred to nitrocellulose paper by pressing the gel firmly against the paper.
2. A solution containing labeled DNA or RNA that is complementary to the gene of interest (the **probe**) is added on top of the blotted paper.
3. Detection of hybridization then proceeds according to the type of probe (usually either labeled with a fluorescent molecule or radioisotope).

If desired, mRNA may be analyzed similarly through **Northern blotting.** The procedure is identical to that for Southern blotting, but no denaturation step is required after gel electrophoresis, since mRNA is single stranded. Again, either complementary DNA or RNA probes may be used to verify the presence of a certain RNA sequence.

Although it may be possible, through the use of image-analysis software or radioisotopes, to determine the relative intensity of DNA or RNA bands and thus provide an idea of alterations in gene expression, quantification via Southern/Northern blotting is difficult. To obtain more quantitative estimates of mRNA content in a sample, researchers now often use **real-time RT-PCR,** which operates using similar principles to RT-PCR, but tracks the fold expansion of the DNA after each polymerization cycle using a fluorescent probe.

9.6.5 Protein Production Assays: Immunostaining

There are a number of means to quantify protein synthesis, including those described in Chapter 8, such as colorimetric and fluorescent assays. These methods, based on changes in color or fluorescence of a marker molecule once it has bound to the protein of interest, have been developed to detect both enzymes and non-enzymatic molecules. In addition, they may be readily used for ECM components with

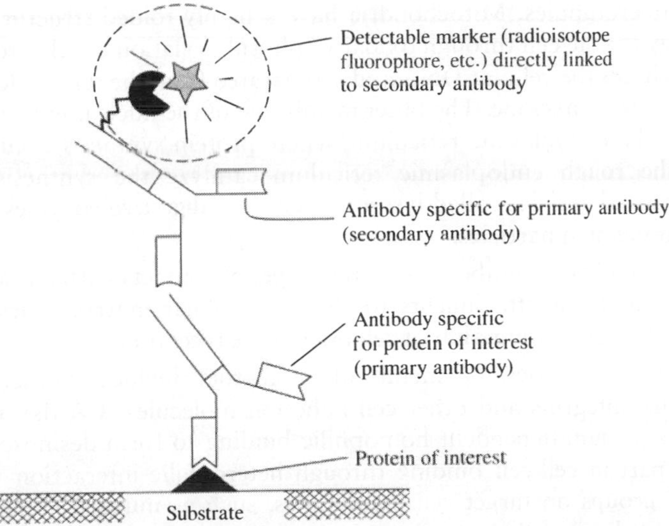

Figure 9.46
Diagram of the technique used in immunohistochemistry. First, a primary antibody is added to the sample section, which then binds to the protein of interest. A labeled secondary antibody is then added that can bind to a portion of the primary antibody. The secondary antibody can be monitored via a variety of means.

low amino acid contents, such as proteoglycans. Additional techniques described in the previous chapter that are common for protein detection are antibody-based methods like ELISAs and Western blotting.

In a method similar to that described for ELISAs and Western blots, antibodies can be used to identify the location of proteins in tissues, particularly in thin sections taken and visualized via light microscopy. This technique is called **immunohistochemistry**, and the sections are said to be **immunostained**. The process is depicted in Fig. 9.46:

1. A primary antibody is added to the section, which then binds to the protein of interest.
2. A labeled secondary antibody is then added that can bind to a portion of the primary antibody. The secondary antibody can be linked to an enzyme, or can be tagged directly with a **chromophore** (colored molecule).
3. The enzyme's substrate is added, if necessary, and then the section is imaged under visible light to detect areas of the sample where the protein is present (should demonstrate a characteristic color).

This is the **indirect method** of immunostaining. It is the most commonly used, since there is the possibility of signal amplification, depending on the design of the primary and secondary antibodies. *Amplification* occurs if many tagged secondary molecules bind to the primary antibody, thus giving a strong localized color, even in the presence of only a small amount of protein. Similar techniques can be used to fluorescently label proteins in a section and visualize them with a fluorescent microscope.

Summary

- Eukaryotic cells contain a number of specialized components. The cell membrane is a bilayered phospholipid barrier that divides the cytoplasm of the cell from the extracellular environment. The cytoskeleton generally consists of dynamic protein-based structures, including microfibrils, intermediate filaments, and microtubules. Mitochondria have a highly folded structure and produce energy for the cell through oxidative phosphorylation of ADP to ATP. The nucleus holds the cellular DNA and is separated from the remainder of the cell by the nuclear envelope. The outer membrane of the nuclear envelope is connected to the endoplasmic reticulum, where protein synthesis occurs. Ribosomes on the rough endoplasmic reticulum catalyze the synthesis of proteins. Specialized vesicles called lysosomes contain digestive enzymes used to break down ingested particles.
- Cells can form a number of different types of contacts with one another as well as a variety of attachments to the extracellular matrix. These connections occur through interaction of cell membrane receptors.
- General categories of membrane receptors include cadherins, selectins, mucins, integrins and other cell adhesion molecules (CAMs). Cadherins undergo calcium-dependent homophilic binding to form desmosomes. Selectins take part in cell-cell binding through heterophilic interaction with carbohydrate groups on target cell membranes, such as mucins. Different combinations of the two distinct subunits of membrane-spanning integrins can lead to interactions to form either cell-cell or cell-matrix contacts. CAMs mediate cell-cell interactions through both heterophilic and homophilic binding.
- Glycoproteins are mainly proteins with small amounts of attached carbohydrates, whereas proteoglycans are largely carbohydrates with small protein

components. The carbohydrates attached to the polypeptide in a proteoglycan are called glycosaminoglycans and can include hyaluronic acid, keratin sulfate, and chondroitin/dermatan sulfate.

- The binding of extracellular matrix molecules to integrins, which are linked intracellularly to intermediate filaments, can cause changes in the cytoskeleton that can affect gene expression in the cell. Also, soluble mediators can interact with receptors on the cell membrane and lead to alterations in gene expression through secondary messenger cascades.
- Four major cellular functions are viability, proliferation, differentiation, and protein synthesis.
- Cell death can occur by one of two general mechanisms: necrosis, which involves swelling and lysis of the cell and clearance of the debris by inflammatory cells; and apoptosis (programmed cell death), in which the cell fragments in a controlled manner to form apoptotic bodies that are phagocytosed by surrounding cells without inducing an inflammatory response.
- Cellular proliferation proceeds through a number of steps, which include mitosis (M phase) and interphase (phases G_1, S and G_2). Cells that are not proliferating are in phase G_0.
- Differentiated or committed cells can only reproduce their own cell type, whereas pluripotent cells can produce several cell types and totipotent cells can produce all cell types.
- Protein synthesis involves RNA polymerase transiently separating the strands of DNA in the region encoding the protein of interest and subsequent transcription to form the respective mRNA. The mRNA moves to the ER, and specific tRNA molecules and ribosomes interact with it to translate the protein of interest. Post-translational processing then occurs in the ER and the Golgi apparatus.
- DLVO theory entails a basic model for cell adhesion to a surface through nonspecific hydrostatic and van der Waals interactions. Models have also been developed to describe specific receptor–ligand interactions based upon thermodynamic principles and concentrations of ligands and receptors. It is possible to combine these models with DLVO theory to result in a more accurate model of cell–substrate adhesion, which considers both specific and nonspecific interactions.
- Migration of a population of cells on a surface can be random or in response to specific stimuli, such as soluble chemical signals (chemotaxis). Cell population motility can be modeled in terms of the flux of cells across a particular location on a surface, with separate terms included for random motility and chemotaxis.
- The migration of individual cells can be modeled with the inclusion of the translocation speed (speed of cell movement between changes in direction) and persistence time (length of time that the cell moves along the substrate without changing direction).
- Biomaterial cytotoxicity is a complex topic that involves consideration of the cytotoxicity of the material, its leachable products, and its degradation products.
- A variety of cytotoxicity assays exist, including direct contact assays, agar diffusion assays, and elution assays, and involve the quantification of either the number of dead cells, the number of living cells, or both.

- Cell adhesion assays entail counting the number of adherent cells on a material with respect to the number of seeded cells, either visually through microscopic examination, or through the use of wash and cytometry techniques. Cell spreading assays involve staining and, with the aid of a microscope, counting the cells that have spread on a material.
- Migration assays can include characterization of the migration of cell populations with techniques such as the Boyden chamber assay, or the movement of individual cells through the use of complex imaging systems capable of tracking individual cells over time in culture.
- The integrity of nucleic acids can be assessed through PCR (for DNA), RT-PCR (for RNA), Southern blotting (for DNA) and Northern blotting (for RNA).
- The quantification of protein production can be accomplished through colorimetric and fluorescent methods. Immunostaining provides a method for qualitatively visualizing protein expression.

Problems

9.1 (a) What are the various types of cell membrane receptors and ligands? What type of contacts does each form (cell-cell or cell-ECM)?

(b) How do these different receptors and ligands interact with a biomaterial?

9.2 Some ECM components, such as collagen, can be larger than cells, yet cells are responsible for their formation. How does this occur? Draw a diagram and describe the synthesis of collagen, including all key steps from transcription to formation of fibers in the extracellular matrix. Provide the location at which each of these steps takes place.

9.3 Most tissues in the body are relatively soft compared with bone. What is responsible for the high modulus of bone? How could you apply this knowledge when designing a synthetic scaffold material to replace bone via a tissue engineering approach?

9.4 How would you test the cytotoxicity of the following materials *in vitro*?

(a) metal for a hip implant

(b) degradable scaffold for use in tissue engineering

9.5 You have a material that you are testing as a potential tissue engineering scaffold. You have previously attempted to characterize cell attachment to the material using an MTT assay, however the material is interfering with the assay. Name an alternative method to determine the number of cells attached to the material.

9.6 You decide to use a tissue engineering approach where a scaffold with no cells is implanted, and the surrounding cells will infiltrate the implant and start the regeneration process. To aid in cell infiltration, a chemical agent will be loaded into the scaffold and released upon implantation to attract neighboring cells. How would you determine whether this chemical agent has the desired effect in an *in vitro* test?

9.7 You are evaluating a synthetic scaffold for repair of cartilage defects. Following the implantation of the material and the formation of new tissue within the defect, which techniques would you use to determine the protein content of the newly formed tissue?

9.8 The data below show the effect of the composition of a new block copolymer XY upon the water contact angle and percent cell attachment from a cell adhesion assay in the presence of the protein fibronectin.

Copolymer Composition (% X)	Water contact angle (°)	% Cell Attachment
5	120	55
10	95	70
25	80	90
50	65	65
75	40	45
100	15	20

(a) What is the relative hydrophobicity of the X and Y blocks in the copolymer? Justify your answer based on the data presented above.

(b) Explain the dependence of cell attachment on copolymer composition. In particular, provide a justification for the amount of cell attachment observed at 5% X, 25% X, and 100% X.

9.9 The pictures shown below are from an experiment in which osteoblasts (bone forming cells) were cultured on a poly(ethylene glycol)-based hydrogel material with different concentrations of a covalently linked RGD peptide sequence (designated as Acr-PEG-RGD) for 2 or 24 hours. This peptide sequence is known to bind to integrin receptors to promote cell attachment and spreading. (Figure reprinted with permission from [18].)

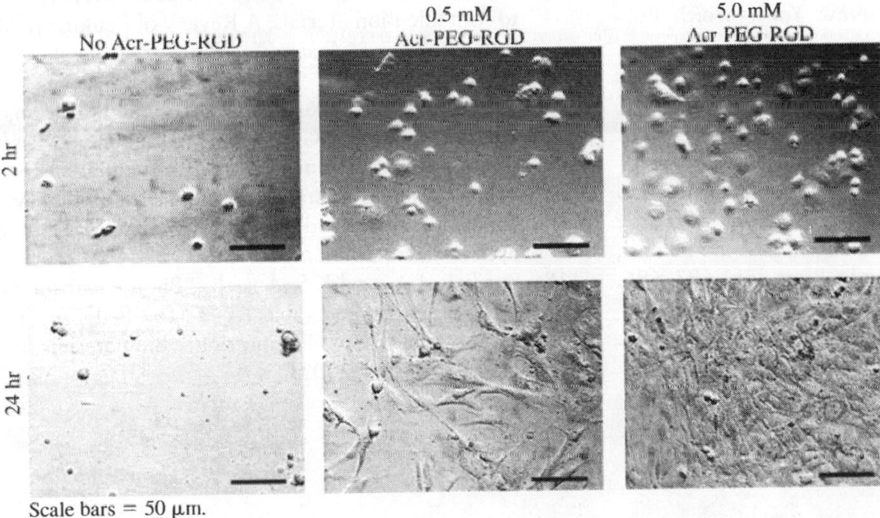

Scale bars = 50 μm.

(a) Describe two ways in which the RGD peptide could be linked to the surface of the material.
(b) The above experiment was performed in the presence of a mixture of blood serum proteins in the cell culture medium. If twice as much of the same protein mixture were added to the culture medium, would cell attachment and spreading be affected for the no-RGD or the 5 mM RGD samples? Explain your reasoning in both cases.
(c) Explain why it appears that there is a larger number of cells in the 24-hour image than in the 2-hour image for the 5-mM RGD sample.

References

1. Alberts, B., D. Bray, J. Lewis, M. Raff, K. Roberts, and J. Watson. *Molecular Biology of the Cell*, 3rd ed. New York: Garland Publishing, 1994.
2. Bergman, R.A., Afifi, A.K., and P.M. Heidger. *Histology*. Philadelphia: W.B. Saunders Company, 1996.
3. Cotran, R.S., Kumar, V., Collins, T., and S.L. Robbins. *Robbins Pathologic Basis of Disease*, 2nd ed. Philadephia: W.B. Saunders Company, 1999.
4. Kuby, J. *Immunology*, 3rd ed. New York: W.H. Freeman, 1997.
5. Hay, E.D. *Cell Biology of Extracellular Matrix*, 2nd ed. New York: Plenum Press, 1991.
6. Bhat, S.V. *Biomaterials*, 2nd ed. Harrow: Alpha Science International Ltd., 2005.
7. Martinez-Hernandez, A. "Repair, Regeneration, and Fibrosis." In *Pathology*, E. Rubin and J.L. Farber, Eds., 2nd ed. Philadelphia: J.B. Lippincott, 1994.
8. Curtis, H. *Biology*, 4th ed. New York: Worth Publishers, 1983.
9. Koller, M.R., and B.O. Palsson. "Tissue Engineering: Reconstituting Human Hematopoiesis *Ex Vivo*." *Biotechnology and Bioengineering*, vol. 42, pp. 909–930, 1993.
10. Bruder, S.P. and A.I. Caplan. "Bone Regeneration through Cellular Engineering." In *Principles of Tissue Engineering*, R.P. Lanza, R. Langer, and J. Vacanti, Eds., 2nd ed. Austin: Academic Press, pp. 683–696, 2000.
11. Palsson, B.O. and S.N. Bhatia. *Tissue Engineering*. Upper Saddle River: Pearson Prentice Hall, 2004.
12. Maheshwari, G. and D.A. Lauffenburger. "Deconstructing (and Reconstructing) Cell Migration." *Microscopy Research and Technique*, vol. 43, pp. 358–368, 1998.
13. Sawhney, A.S., P.P. Chandrashekkar, and J.A. Hubbell. "Bioeradible Hydrogels Based on Photopolymerized Poly(ethylene glycol)-co-poly(α hydroxy acid) Diacrylate Macromers", Macro-molecules, vol.26, pp. 581–587, 1993.
14. Shalaby, S.W. and K.J.L. Burg. *Absorbable and Biodegradable Polymers*. Boca Raton: CRC Press, 2004.
15. Andrade, J.D. and V. Hlady. "Protein Adsorption and Materials Biocompatibility: A Tutorial Review and Suggested Hypotheses." In *Biopolymers/Non-Exclusion HPLC*, K. Dusek, C.G. Overberger, and G. Heublein, Eds. New York: Springer-Verlag, pp. 1–63, 1986.
16. Hallab, N., J.J. Jacobs, and J. Black. "Hypersensitivity to Metallic Biomaterials: A Review of Leukocyte Migration Inhibition Assays," *Biomaterials*, vol. 21, pp. 1301–1314, 2000.
17. Shin, H., K. Zygourakis, M.C. Farach-Carson, M.J. Yaszemski, and A.G. Mikos. "Attachment, Proliferation, and Migration of Marrow Stromal Osteoblasts Cultured on Biomimetic Hydrogels Modified with an Osteopontin-Derived Peptide," *Biomaterials*, vol. 25, pp. 895–906, 2004.
18. Burdick, J.A. and K.S. Anseth. "Photoencapsulation of Osteoblasts in Injectable RGD-Modified PEG Hydrogels for Bone Tissue Engineering." Biomaterials, vol. 23, pp. 4315–4323, 2002.

Additional Reading

Asthagiri, A.R. and D.A. Lauffenburger. "Bioengineering Models of Cell Signaling," *Annual Review of Biomedical Engineering*, vol. 2, pp. 31–53, 2000.

Bruck, S.D. *Properties of Biomaterials in the Physiological Environment*. Boca Raton: CRC Press, 1980.

Cai, S., Y. Liu, X. Zheng Shu, and G.D. Prestwich. "Injectable Glycosaminoglycan Hydrogels for Controlled Release of Human Basic Fibroblast Growth Factor," *Biomaterials*, vol. 26, pp. 6054–6067, 2005.

Chan, B.P. and K.F. So. "Photochemical Crosslinking Improves the Physicochemical Properties of Collagen Scaffolds," *Journal of Biomedical Materials Research Part A*, vol. 75, pp. 689–701, 2005.

Charulatha, V. and A. Rajaram. "Influence of Different Crosslinking Treatments on the Physical Properties of Collagen Membranes," *Biomaterials*, vol. 24, pp. 759–767, 2003.

Couñago, R. Chen, S., and Y. Shamoo. "*In Vivo* Molecular Evolution Reveals Biophysical Origins of Organismal Fitness." *Molecular Cell*, vol. 22, pp. 441–449, 2006.

Dee, K.C., D.A. Puleo, and R. Bizios. *An Introduction to Tissue-Biomaterial Interactions*. Hoboken: Wiley-Liss, 2002.

Dickinson, R.B., A.G. Ruta, and S.E. Truesdail. "Physiochemical Basis of Bacterial Adhesion to Biomaterial Surfaces." In *Antimicrobial/Anti-Infective Materials: Principles, Applications, and Devices*, S.P. Sawan and G. Manivannan, Eds. Lancaster: Technomic Publishing, pp. 67–93, 2000.

Edelman, E.R., E. Mathiowitz, R. Langer, and M. Klagsbrun. "Controlled and Modulated Release of Basic Fibroblast Growth Factor," *Biomaterials*, vol. 12, pp. 619–626, 1991.

Fujisawa, R. and Y. Kuboki. "Preferential Adsorption of Dentin and Bone Acidic Proteins on the (100) Face of Hydroxyapatite Crystals," *Biochimica et Biophysica Acta*, vol. 1075, pp. 56–60, 1991.

Guyton, A.C. and J.E. Hall. *Textbook of Medical Physiology*, 11th ed. Philadelphia: W.B. Saunders, 2006.

Hartgerink, J.D., E. Beniash, and S.I. Stupp. "Self-Assembly and Mineralization of Peptide-Amphiphile Nanofibers," *Science*, vol. 294, pp. 1684–1688, 2001.

Horbett, T.A. "Principles Underlying the Role of Adsorbed Plasma Proteins in Blood Interactions with Foreign Materials," *Cardiovascular Pathology*, vol. 2, pp. 137S–148S, 1993.

Horbett, T.A. "The Role of Adsorbed Proteins in Tissue Response to Biomaterials." In *Biomaterials Science: An Introduction to Materials in Medicine*, B.D. Ratner, A.S. Hoffman, F.J. Schoen, and J.E. Lemons, Eds., 2nd ed. San Diego: Elsevier Academic Press, pp. 237–246, 2004.

Huang, F.M., K.W. Tai, M.Y. Chou, and Y.C. Chang. "Cytotoxicity of Resin-, Zinc Oxide-Eugenol-, and Calcium Hydroxide-Based Root Canal Sealers on Human Periodontal Ligament Cells and Permanent V79 Cells," *International Endodontic Journal*, vol. 35, pp. 153–158, 2002.

Hubbell, J.A. "Matrix Effects." In *Principles of Tissue Engineering*, R.P. Lanza, R. Langer, and J. Vacanti, Eds., 2nd ed. Austin: Academic Press, pp. 237–250, 2000.

Hunter, G.K. and H.A. Goldberg. "Modulation of Crystal Formation by Bone Phosphoproteins: Role of Glutamic Acid-Rich Sequences in the Nucleation of Hydroxyapatite by Bone Sialoprotein," *The Biochemical Journal*, vol. 302 (Pt 1), pp. 175–179, 1994.

Lin, X. "Functions of Heparan Sulfate Proteoglycans in Cell Signaling During Development," *Development*, vol. 131, pp. 6009–6021, 2004.

Martins-Green, M. "Dynamics of Cell-ECM Interactions." In *Principles of Tissue Engineering*, R.P. Lanza, R. Langer, and J. Vacanti, Eds., 2nd ed. Austin: Academic Press, pp. 33–55, 2000.

Mitchell, R.N. and F.J. Schoen. "Cells and Cell Injury." In *Biomaterials Science: An Introduction to Materials in Medicine*, B.D. Ratner, A.S. Hoffman, F.J. Schoen, and J.E. Lemons, Eds., 2nd ed., San Diego: Elsevier Academic Press, pp. 246–260, 2004.

Salih, E., S. Ashkar, L.C. Gerstenfeld, and M.J. Glimcher. "Identification of the Phosphorylated Sites of Metabolically 32P-Labeled Osteopontin from Cultured Chicken Osteoblasts," *Journal of Biological Chemistry*, vol. 272, pp. 13966–13973, 1997.

Saltzman, W.M. "Cell Interactions with Polymers." In *Principles of Tissue Engineering*, R.P. Lanza, R. Langer, and J. Vacanti, Eds., 2nd ed. Austin: Academic Press, pp. 221–235, 2000.

Schakenraad, J.M. "Cells: Their Surfaces and Interactions with Materials." In *Biomaterials Science: An Introduction to Materials in Medicine*, B.D. Ratner, A.S. Hoffman, F.J. Schoen, and J.E. Lemons, Eds., 1st ed. San Diego: Elsevier Academic Press, pp. 141–147, 1996.

Schoen, F.J. and R.N. Mitchell. "Tissues, the Extracellular Matrix, and Cell-Biomaterial Interactions." In *Biomaterials Science: An Introduction to Materials in Medicine*, B.D. Ratner, A.S. Hoffman, F.J. Schoen, and J.E. Lemons, Eds., 2nd ed. San Diego: Elsevier Academic Press, pp. 260–281, 2004.

Scott-Burden, T. "Extracellular Matrix: The cellular Environment," *News in Physiological Sciences*, vol. 9, pp. 110–115, 1994.

Voet, D. and J.G. Voet. *Biochemistry*, 3rd ed. New York: John Wiley and Sons, 2004.

Watts, A. and R.C. Paterson. "Pulpal Response to a Zinc Oxide-Eugenol Cement," *International Endodontic Journal*, vol. 20, pp. 82–86, 1987.

Zygourakis, K. "Quantification and Regulation of Cell Migration," *Tissue Engineering*, vol. 2, pp. 1–16, 1996.

Biomaterial Implantation and Acute Inflammation

CHAPTER 10

Main Objective

To become familiar with the cells involved in the various stages of the acute inflammatory response and to understand the interplay of inflammation with the acquired immune response.

Specific Objectives

1. To distinguish between innate and acquired immunity.
2. To compare and contrast the formation and actions of the four types of leukocytes.
3. To understand the physiological response of acute inflammation.
4. To learn the clinical signs of inflammation and their physiologic causes.
5. To understand the steps and signals involved in migration of neutrophils and their action in neutralizing foreign invaders.
6. To understand the role of macrophages in destroying foreign particles and interaction with the acquired immune system.
7. To understand the concepts behind and possible limitations to the *in vitro* techniques presented.

10.1 Introduction: Overview of Innate and Acquired Immunity

In the next few chapters, we will examine the specific protein and cellular interactions with biomaterials involved in various common responses, such as inflammation, immunity, and blood clotting. An example of the biological response to a material implanted for several weeks is found in Fig. 10.1. Implantation of a biomaterial is regarded as an assault on the body's status quo, or **homeostasis**. The body has developed several defense mechanisms against invasion in an attempt to return to homeostasis. Although originally intended to protect against assault from pathogens, many of the same cells and signaling molecules also respond to biomaterials.

One is born with **innate (nonspecific) immunity** and this is the first line of defense. If the invading organism is not cleared by the innate immune response, then

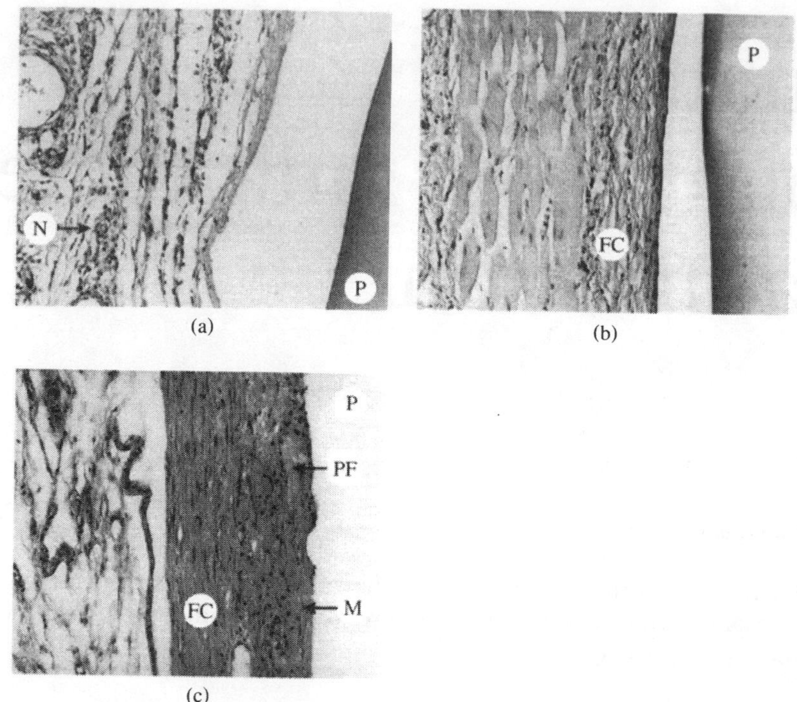

Figure 10.1
Sequence of images of *in vivo* response to a biodegradable, polymeric biomaterial (poly(propylene fumarate-co-ethylene glycol)) implanted subcutaneously in a rat for up to 12 weeks: (a) four days post-implantation, (b) three weeks post-implantation, (c) 12 weeks post-implantation. Hemotoxylin and eosin stain. The letter P indicates polymer or space left by polymer, N represents neutrophils, FC denotes fibrous capsule, M designates macrophages, and PF signifies polymer fragments embedded in the fibrous capsule. A typical wound-healing response is shown in this example. Within the first few days, infiltration of neutrophils into the implantation area is seen (acute inflammation), followed by the slower development of a fibrous capsule surrounding the implant (fibrous encapsulation/healing). Because this material is biodegradable, evidence of polymer fragmentation is also present at the later time points. (Reprinted with permission from [1].)

the body engages the **acquired (specific) immune response,**[1] which involves the activation of a type of white blood cell called the lymphocyte. In contrast to innate immunity, which resides in an individual at birth, the acquired immune response is activated when children are given vaccinations for specific diseases or develop immunity following exposure to particular pathogens.

If the organism persists after exposure to both the innate and acquired immune response, **infection** may develop. However, it is important to recognize that aspects of the innate response, such as inflammation, can occur without the presence of infection, as is often the case with biomaterial implantation. The two types of immune responses are highly intertwined, often sharing signaling molecules, as discussed later in the chapter. Both responses also depend, in large part, on the activity of various white blood cells (**leukocytes**).

[1]Innate and acquired immunity are terms developed by immunologists to describe these two different responses to foreign organisms. In a clinical setting, inflammation is often used as a synonym for innate immunity, and the "immune response" to a pathogen refers to the acquired immune response only.

10.1.1 Characteristics of Leukocytes

10.1.1.1 Leukocyte Types There are four main types of leukocytes usually encountered in blood, each performing a unique function:

1. **Granulocytes.** These cells, so named because of their granular appearance under light microscopy, can be subdivided into neutrophils, eosinophils and basophils. Their nuclei have multiple lobes (making them appear to have several nuclei) and their main function is to phagocytose foreign invaders and aid in the inflammatory response.
2. **Monocytes.** Unlike the granulocytes, these cells do not have nuclei divided into lobes. They have a large phagocytic capability and play a central role in the inflammatory response.
3. **Lymphocytes/plasma cells.** These cells, including T and B cells, function as a part of the acquired immune response, and will be discussed further in Chapter 12. Lymphocytes can be divided into memory cells, which are responsible for a more rapid response if one is exposed to the same pathogen for a second time, and effector cells, which produce antibodies or take other actions to remove foreign invaders.
4. **Megakaryocytes.** This cell type is found only in the bone marrow, where it fragments to produce **platelets.** These nonnucleated fragments circulate in the blood and aid in blood clotting (discussed in Chapter 13).

10.1.1.2 Leukocyte Formation The genesis of leukocytes begins with the pluripotent hematopoetic stem cell, which forms two different types of early precursor cells: one that eventually differentiates into red blood cells (erythrocytes), granulocytes, monocytes, and megakaryocytes, and one that differentiates into lymphocytes (Fig. 9.25). Granulocytes, monocytes and megakaryocytes are formed in the bone marrow. Lymphocytes are created in the bone marrow and mature in the lymphoid tissue (lymph glands, spleen, thymus, and tonsils). Granulocytes are usually stored in the bone marrow there until needed by the body. Lymphocytes are often stored in lymphoid tissue, but a fraction of them circulate in the blood at all times.

10.1.1.3 Life Span of Leukocytes Generally, leukocytes are only present in the blood to be transported to a tissue where they are needed. Granulocytes, for example, usually spend 4–8 hours in the blood and 4–5 days in the target tissue, unless they expire while combating an invading organism. Monocytes are present for 10–20 hours in the blood, and then migrate into the tissues, where they become **tissue macrophages.** Macrophages are larger than monocytes, possess more killing potential, and can live months to years. These cells provide a continual, resident defense against infection.

Lymphocytes enter the circulation with drainage of lymph fluid, stay in the blood for only a few hours, and then reenter the lymphoid tissue. Here, the cells can remain for some time or can almost immediately return to the bloodstream through the lymph drainage. This cycle is repeated again and again, so there is continual circulation of lymphocytes throughout the body. The life span of a single lymphocyte is weeks to years, depending on the body's need.

10.1.2 Sources of Innate Immunity

While the details of acquired immunity are discussed further in Chapter 12, the remainder of this chapter will focus on innate immunity. There are four main components of the defense provided by innate immunity:

1. Anatomic barriers (skin and mucous membranes)
2. Physiologic barriers (temperature of body, low pH in stomach)

3. Phagocytic cells (granulocytes)
4. Inflammation

It is important to note that a typical innate immune response will use a combination of these defenses to reduce the number of invading organisms, such as with the recruitment of phagocytic cells (number 3 on the list above) during the inflammatory process (number 4).

10.2 Clinical Signs of Inflammation and their Causes

Clinically, inflammation is characterized by certain symptoms, called the four **cardinal signs.** These signs have Latin names, indicating that they have been observed for centuries as a part of the inflammatory process. Inflamed tissue often exhibits

1. Rubor (redness)
2. Tumor (swelling)
3. Calore (tissue heating)
4. Dolore (pain)

As medical knowledge has progressed, the causes of these particular symptoms have been determined. They are a result of physiological changes that help to define **acute inflammation.** Acute inflammation, a part of innate immunity, is an immediate response to tissue injury. The associated physiological changes occur in the first hours to days after the assault, so acute can be distinguished from **chronic inflammation,** in which changes persist over weeks to months. Both acute and chronic inflammation can be observed in the response to the implanted material in Fig. 10.1. Chronic inflammation will be discussed further in Chapter 11.

Acute inflammation is controlled via substances released from the complement system and T-type lymphocytes, both discussed further in Chapter 12, or via byproducts of the blood-clotting cascade (see Chapter 13). These soluble substances are listed in Table 10.1 and cause a variety of responses.

After injury, blood vessels in nearby regions will **vasodilate,** or expand. This is one of the reasons for both the development of redness and tissue heating during inflammation. There is also an increase in the permeability of nearby capillaries,

TABLE 10.1

Mediators of Inflammatory Effects

Inflammatory Effect	Mediators
Vasodilation of local blood vessels	Kinins, fibrinopeptides, histamine, prostaglandins
Increased permeability of capillaries	Bradykinin, fibrinopeptides, prostaglandins
Clotting in the interstitial spaces	Fibrinogen and other plasma proteins
Migration of neutrophils into tissue	IL-8, platelet activating factor (PAF), complement split products C3a, C5a, C5b67, fibrinopeptides, prostaglandins, leukotrienes
Migration of macrophages into tissue	Macrophage inflammatory protein (MIP): 1a and 1b

leading to leakage of fluid into the surrounding (**interstitial**) space. Certain blood proteins, such as fibrinogen, that have found their way to this interstitial space then encourage clotting to wall off the injured area and form an anatomical barrier to invading organisms. Other soluble factors act to attract large numbers of granulocytes and monocytes into the tissue to begin to phagocytose debris and foreign organisms. Individual tissue cells can also swell at this time. This combination of events is a main cause of the observed tumor, or tissue swelling, during inflammation. The pain associated with the inflammatory response is a by-product of the release of certain substances called **kinins** from the blood clotting cascade (see Chapter 13).

10.3 Role of Tissue Macrophages and Neutrophils

A key portion of the defense mechanism presented by the inflammatory response is the influx of phagocytic cells to combat foreign invaders. The body's first line of cellular defense is the actions of the tissue macrophages residing in the area. This response occurs within an hour after injury. Also during this time, there is an invasion of granulocytes, especially neutrophils, from the bloodstream in response to soluble factors in the inflamed tissue. The movement of the neutrophils out of the blood vessels and into the tissue is called **extravasation**.

10.3.1 Migration of Neutrophils

To extravasate, neutrophils must first bind to vascular endothelium, then penetrate the endothelial layer lining the blood vessel, and finally, migrate to the area of inflammation. This involves four major steps: **rolling, activation, arrest and adhesion**, and **migration** (Fig. 10.2). Rolling occurs because, as the neutrophils are carried along by the blood, they can bind briefly to the vascular endothelium through low-affinity selectin–carbohydrate interactions. As discussed in Chapter 9, selectins are receptors found on endothelial cells that have a carbohydrate-like portion to interact with proteoglycans (mucins) on the surface of the neutrophils. Selectins are upregulated on inflamed endothelium, facilitating the binding of neutrophils. However, since these are not strong interactions, the cells are tethered briefly to the endothelium, and then the flowing blood dislodges them. This is repeated over and over, giving the appearance that the cells are rolling along the surface of the blood vessel.

As the neutrophils are rolling, they can be activated by **chemoattractants**, substances that cause the migration of neutrophils toward the damaged tissue. Movement of cells in response to chemical stimuli is called **chemotaxis**, and extravasation is the first part of this process for neutrophils. The two most prominent activating chemoattractants for neutrophils are interleukin-8 (IL-8) and macrophage inflammatory protein-1b (MIP-1b). IL-8 and MIP-1b can bind to specific receptors on the neutrophil's surface and activate intracellular pathways that induce a conformational change in integrin molecules in the cell membrane. The integrins now have a higher affinity for the immunoglobulin superfamily of cell adhesion molecules (CAM) found on the surface of the endothelium.

The strong interaction between integrin receptors on the neutrophil and CAMs presented by endothelial cells leads to the cessation of cellular rolling and a firm adhesion to the endothelium (arrest and adhesion). The final stage of extravasation occurs as the neutrophil undergoes **transendothelial migration** into the inflamed tissue. The cell accomplishes this through **diapedesis,** or by squeezing parts of the cell at a time though small spaces between endothelial cells (Fig. 10.2). Although the

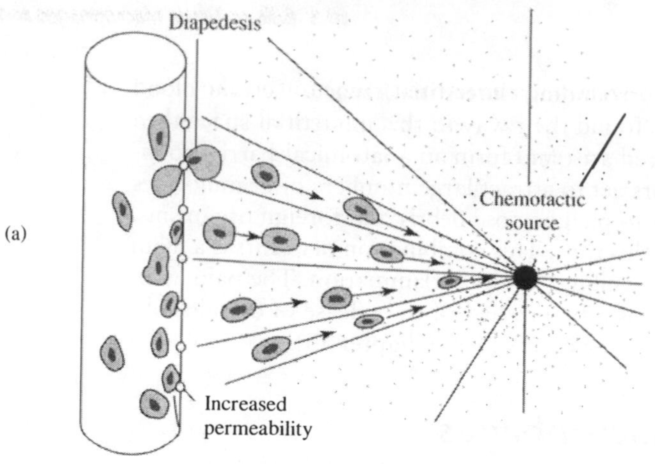

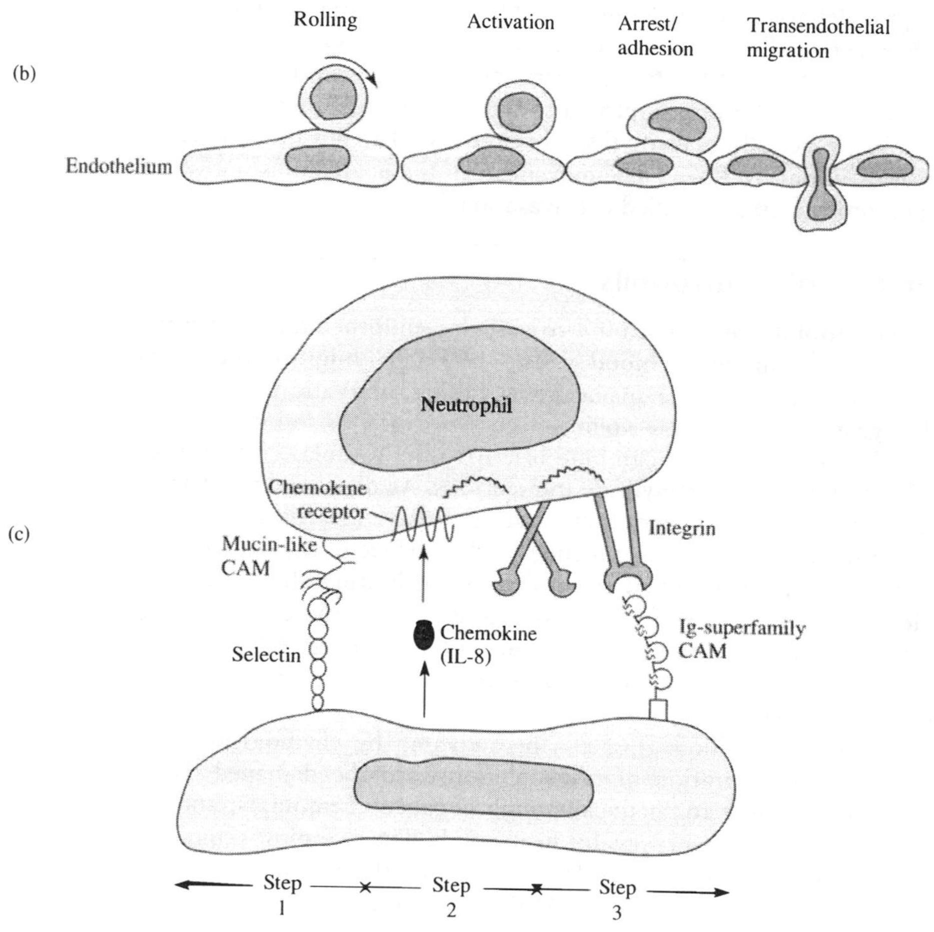

Figure 10.2
Extravasation of neutrophils. (a) To extravasate, neutrophils must bind to vascular endothelium, penetrate the endothelial layer lining the blood vessel, and migrate to the area of inflammation. (b) This involves four major steps: rolling, activation, arrest/adhesion, and migration. (c) Rolling occurs because, as the neutrophils are carried along by the blood, they can bind briefly to the vascular endothelium through low-affinity selectin–carbohydrate interactions (step 1 in diagram). Neutrophils can then be activated by chemoattractants. Chemoattractants (such as IL-8 and MIP-1b) bind to specific receptors on the neutrophil's surface and activate intercellular pathways that induce a conformational change in integrin molecules in the cell membrane (step 2). The integrins now have a higher affinity for the immunoglobulin superfamily of cell adhesion molecules (CAMs) found on the surface of the endothelium, which results in the cessation of rolling and a firm adhesion to the endothelium (arrest and adhesion, step 3). (Adapted with permission from [2] and [3].)

precise stimulus for transendothelial migration is unknown, once in the target tissue, neutrophils express high levels of receptors for further chemoattractants, allowing them to home to the area where they are needed.

10.3.2 Actions of Neutrophils

Once at the site of injury, neutrophils can perform several functions to deter invasion of foreign organisms and aid in the wound-healing response. These functions include killing mechanisms based on phagocytosis, a respiratory burst, or secretion of signaling molecules.

10.3.2.1 Phagocytosis The main task of neutrophils is to phagocytose foreign agents. In addition to the normal steps of phagocytosis, as outlined in Chapter 9, neutrophils contain granules containing bactericidal agents and enzymes that join with the phagosome (a large vesicle through which large particles are injested) to digest foreign matter. Activated neutrophils also express a greater number of receptors for antibody- and complement-coated foreign particles to help in their removal from the area. These coatings, to be discussed further in later chapters, are used specifically to speed the elimination of foreign substances. In this case, the activating chemical that upregulates the receptors for the coatings is a by-product of the complement cascade (see Chapter 12).

10.3.2.2 Respiratory Burst Activated neutrophils also exhibit a respiratory burst, in which glucose metabolism increases up to tenfold and oxygen consumption increases two- to threefold. This leads to the formation of reactive oxygen and nitrogen species (radicals and strong oxidizers) in intracellular granules. These can be released as another means to kill foreign organisms, and are also the compounds that promote corrosion and oxidative degradation of biomaterials in the body (see Chapter 5). However, such reactive species may also cause unwanted tissue damage, so it is important to contain the inflammatory response to localized areas. Means of inflammation control are discussed later in this chapter.

10.3.2.3 Secretion of Chemical Mediators In addition to their role in eliminating foreign invaders, neutrophils secrete a number of factors, called **cytokines**, that have specific effects on several cell types. The actions of selected cytokines are listed in Table 10.2, while a summary of cytokines and their target cells is found in Table 10.3.

TABLE 10.2
Actions of Cytokines

Interleukin-1 (IL-1)	Promotes granulocyte migration, increases production of IL-8, activates lymphocytes, promotes release of tissue factor
Interleukin-6 (IL-6)	Activates lymphocytes
Interleukin-8 (IL-8)	Attracts neutrophils, promotes neutrophil integrin/CAM interaction
Macrophage inflammatory protein 1a (MIP-1a)	Attracts monocytes
Macrophage inflammatory protein 1b (MIP-1b)	Same effect as IL-8 on neutrophils, attracts monocytes
Transforming growth factor-β (TGF-β)	Limits inflammatory response
Tumor necrosis factor-α (TNF-α)	Promotes granulocyte migration, increases production of IL-8, promotes release of tissue factor

TABLE 10.3

Cytokines Involved in Inflammation/Immunity

Cytokines produced by inflammatory cells to act on inflammatory cells	IL-1, IL-8, MIP-1a, MIP-1b, TGF-β, TNF-α
Cytokines produced by inflammatory cells to act on lymphocytes	IL-1, IL-6, TNF-α

Activated neutrophils in tissues release mediators like MIP-1a and MIP-1b to recruit monocytes to the area, and also IL-8 to attract more neutrophils. Many of these factors are also chemotactic for lymphocytes, which provides a point of communication, or crossover, between the innate and acquired immune response.

EXAMPLE PROBLEM 10.1

A company developed a new synthetic material for use in small diameter vascular graft applications. Initial studies conducted *in vitro* to examine the potential inflammatory response to the material involved the culture of cells isolated from whole blood in the presence of the material for 48 hours. The media was analyzed with the use of an ELISA following the culture period. It was found that the expression levels of IL-8 and MIP-1b were approximately four times the normal physiological levels. A control material cultured in the same manner in the presence of the cells did not present an increase in IL-8 and MIP-1b expression. Based on these results, will the material be expected to induce a stronger inflammatory response than the control material when implanted as a vascular graft *in vivo*? Why or why not? Does the material seem well suited for use in long-term vascular graft applications from an inflammation standpoint?

Solution: An inflammatory response is to be expected with any surgical implantation of a material, as tissue disruption is a necessary part of the implantation procedure. However, some factors can instigate a more severe inflammatory response than would normally occur. In this case, it is stated that the experimental material invokes heightened expression of IL-8 and MIP-1b, relative to a control material. Recalling that IL-8 and MIP-1b are strong chemoattractants for neutrophils, it follows that heightened expression of IL-8 and MIP-1b in the presence of the material will likely result in increased neutrophil activation and adhesion close to the implant. The neutrophils can then migrate through the epithelium and release cytokines to recruit additional inflammatory cells to the site. Thus, the experimental material results in a heightened IL-8 and MIP-1b expression that will likely produce a greater inflammatory response *in vivo* than the control material, due to the recruitment, activation, and adhesion of neutrophils. The problem does not give adequate information to comment on the expected time frame of the inflammatory response. However, a large initial inflammatory response could decrease the long-term viability of the implant, as it may be exposed to low pH, oxidizing species, and radical species that could potentially damage and/or alter the material. ■

10.4 Role of Other Leukocytes

10.4.1 Monocytes/Macrophages

Partially due to the signals released by the neutrophils, about five to six hours after the inflammatory response begins, monocytes arrive at the injury site. They then start to enlarge to form tissue macrophages. Macrophage maturation can take up to eight hours and involves swelling of the cell and formation of a large quantity of lysosomes. Over days to weeks, the macrophage will become the dominant cell type. The functions of the macrophage are similar to that of the neutrophil, although macrophages have greater and more sustainable killing capacities.

10.4.2 Actions of Macrophages

Like neutrophils, macrophages act to phagocytose foreign agents, as well as secrete chemical mediators to coordinate the responses from a number of body systems. However, the macrophage is also essential in the interaction of the innate and acquired immune response through its role as an antigen-presenting cell, as discussed below.

10.4.2.1 Phagocytosis and Biomaterials Although phagocytosis proceeds in the same way as for neutrophils, an individual macrophage can engulf many more bacteria or particles than a neutrophil. However, because macrophages remain at the site of injury longer, a number of events can occur that interfere with their phagocytic processes, especially if the injury is associated with implantation of a biomaterial. For example, if phagocytosed biomaterial particles resist degradation, they can remain sequestered in the macrophage until it dies and lyses, when they are re-released into the environment. If the number of these indigestible particles is small, this process may be repeated over a long period of time, with several cycles of macrophages recruited to the area in an attempt to eliminate the particles.

However, if there is a large number of indigestible particles, a clinical condition can develop due to the many macrophages continually dying and being replaced in a localized region. **Silicosis** is an example of such a condition caused by inhaled silica particles that remain in the lung tissue. As the macrophages lyse after being unable to digest the silica, not only are the particles returned to the tissue, but other cellular contents, such as cytokines, are also released. One of the actions of these cytokines is to stimulate fibroblasts to form fibrous tissue in the afflicted areas. These fibrotic regions in the lungs reduce the surface area available for oxygen transfer, thus severely impairing oxygen intake by the patient.

In contrast, if the size of the nondegradable material is much larger than that of the cell, another event, **frustrated phagocytosis**, may be observed. This can occur either with neutrophils or macrophages, and involves the release of lysosomal enzymes and other products into the environment around the foreign material, as the particle is too large to be taken into the cell and degraded intracellularly. This usually occurs if the particle is greater than 5 μm along its largest dimension. The amount of enzymes released during this process has been linked to the size of the particle, suggesting that larger implants may induce a greater response.

10.4.2.2 Secretion of Chemical Mediators Activated macrophages secrete many chemical mediators, but to provide examples of how these cells affect the responses of other systems, we will focus on three main cytokines: interleukin-1 (IL-1), interleukin-6 (IL-6), and tumor necrosis factor-α (TNF-α). Some or all of these factors have the following effects, in three general areas:

1. Effects on the inflammatory response (IL-1 and TNF-α)
2. Effects on the acquired immune response (IL-1 and IL-6)
3. Systemic effects (all)

Examining these responses in more detail, in inflammation, both IL-1 and TNF-α act to promote cell migration by increasing the expression of adhesion molecules on the vascular endothelium. They are also implicated in increasing the expression of CAMs that bind integrins on the granulocyte surface, and increasing production of IL-8, the cytokine that promotes neutrophil integrin–CAM interactions. In addition, TNF-α can directly activate both neutrophils and macrophages.

Secretion of these cytokines also provides communication with the acquired immune response (Chapter 12) in that all of the above-mentioned substances have been found to activate and/or promote migration of lymphocytes. Systemic effects are also possible. These cytokines induce production of acute-phase proteins by the liver, which results in a rise in body temperature (fever) to reduce the viability of an invading pathogen. IL-1 and TNF-α also promote synthesis and release of tissue factor from endothelial cells and macrophages, which causes activation of the blood-clotting cascade (Chapter 13).

10.4.2.3 Role as Antigen-Presenting Cells A key function of the macrophage is its role as an **antigen-presenting cell (APC)**, which provides a direct connection between the innate and acquired immune responses. Activated macrophages exhibit increased expression of a certain receptor (major histocompatibility complex class II) that allows the presentation of foreign proteins (antigens) to lymphocytes. The interaction of certain lymphocytes with a macrophage having the protein attached to this receptor triggers the activation of the acquired immune response (discussed further in Chapter 12).

EXAMPLE PROBLEM 10.2

Several patients who had undergone spinal fusion surgeries in the past three months were complaining to their orthopedic surgeon of excessive swelling and heat in the area of the surgery. After review of the patient charts, it was discovered that titanium pedicle screws and rods were implanted in each case. The surgeon hypothesized that motion between the screws and the rods could have led to the formation of debris particles [4] immediately surrounding the implants. Upon further investigation, it was found that the amount of debris particles was proportional to the degree of motion between the pedicle screws and the rods. Also, the presence of macrophages was noted to be directly proportional to the amount of debris particles present. How would the expected tissue response to the wear debris particles from the implants differ from the expected response to the bulk implants?

Solution: An inflammatory response ensues upon the tissue injury induced by any surgical implantation of a biomaterial. In the ideal case, the inflammatory response is resolved in a number of days. However, many biomaterials are recognized as foreign objects and result in a prolonged inflammatory response, as phagocytic cells such as macrophages attempt to remove the material. Materials much larger than macrophages in size, such as a pedicle screw, are too large to be phagocytosed. As a result, macrophages surround the material and release lysosomal enzymes into the extracellular environment in an attempt to degrade the material in a process called frustrated phagocytosis. On the other hand, micrometer scale wear debris particles from the implants are capable of being endocytosed by the macrophages. As titanium is not biodegradable, the particles will remain in the macrophages in this case until cell death and lysis, at which time the particles will be reintroduced into the environment, where they can be endocytosed by other macrophages. Additionally, the creation of wear debris increases the total amount of surface area of the implant material being presented, thereby increasing the degree of biological response. ■

10.4.3 Other Granulocytes

Although the cellular events of inflammation are associated primarily with the actions of neutrophils and macrophages, other granulocytes are also involved to a lesser degree. Eosinophils respond to chemoattractants in a similar manner as neutrophils/macrophages, but their phagocytic capacities are relatively small. They are important, however, in that they can attach to and destroy parasites. In addition, they may detoxify some of the inflammation-inducing agents, thus preventing the spread of inflammation outside a localized area.

Basophils are found in the blood, and are similar in function to mast cells found in various tissues. These cells can be activated to release heparin, histamine, bradykinin and serotonin, which are soluble mediators of inflammation (some of the actions of these substances can be found in Table 10.1). Basophils and mast cells also play a large role in the allergic reaction, discussed further in Chapter 12.

10.5 Termination of Acute Inflammation

The acute inflammatory response is well designed to help in recovering homeostasis and preventing the invasion of foreign organisms after injury. However, several of the physiological changes associated with this response would prove detrimental to the function of the tissue if they were widespread or continued for a long period of time. Therefore, several means to reduce or end acute inflammation are found in all tissues.

Throughout the inflammatory process, the interaction of a variety of chemical mediators provides a system of checks and balances to ensure that the effects are localized. One example of this is the production of IL-1 receptor agonist (IL-1ra) by the same cells that produce IL-1 (macrophages, among others). This molecule has a similar chemical structure to IL-1 and thus binds to the same receptors on target cells, but, unlike IL-1, does not stimulate them. In this way, target cells' activation can be inhibited by binding IL-1ra (Fig. 10.3). Therefore, the relative amount of IL-1 and IL-1ra produced by macrophages aids in determining how severe the inflammatory response becomes.

An alternative means of controlling the extent of inflammation is production of a substance that limits the inflammatory response. In some cases, transforming growth factor-β (TGF-β), produced by both macrophages and lymphocytes, has been known to have this effect by inhibiting activation of certain cell types involved in the inflammatory response. Finally, it is important to note that the chemical mediators involved in inflammation are quickly inactivated or destroyed in solution, meaning they must act within a small radius from where they were produced. This further promotes a localized response to injury.

As the stimulus for acute inflammation is removed, the response may terminate in several ways. Acute inflammation may progress to chronic inflammation, which, as discussed in Chapter 11, is characterized by the presence of lymphocytes

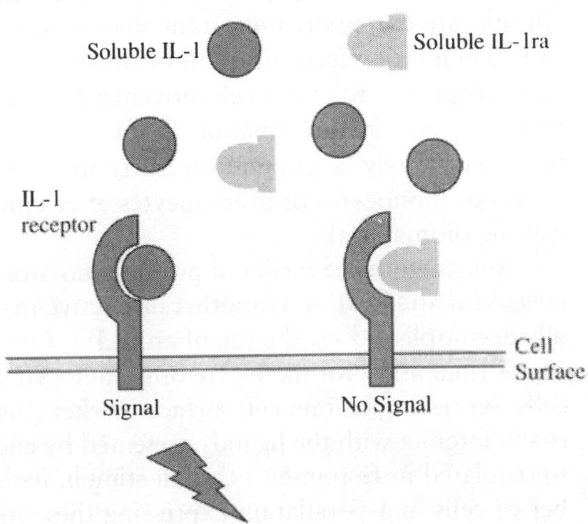

Figure 10.3
Schematic showing a cell's response to IL-1 receptor agonist (IL-1ra) and IL-1. IL-1ra has a similar chemical structure to IL-1 and thus binds to the same receptors on target cells. However, unlike IL-1, IL-1ra does not stimulate the cells. In this way, binding IL-1ra can inhibit a target cell's activation. The severity of the inflammatory response is determined by the relative amounts of IL-1 and IL-1ra.

and other mononuclear cells. Alternatively, it may be more successfully resolved by the formation of granulation tissue and a foreign body reaction. This reaction, described in detail in the next chapter, is considered to be a normal wound-healing response in the presence of a nondegradable biomaterial.

10.6 Techniques: *In Vitro* Assays for Inflammatory Response

Many of the *in vitro* assays performed to gain information about how or to what extent biomaterials provoke an inflammatory response fall into the categories described in Chapter 9. In most cases, cells are isolated from human blood and cultured in the presence of the sample material for hours to days before testing for cellular activation. It is expected that with a greater level of activation, the biomaterial will be more pro-inflammatory *in vivo*. These experiments can be performed on a variety of cells involved in the inflammatory response, including endothelial cells and several types of leukocytes.

10.6.1 Leukocyte Assays

In vitro techniques involving leukocytes (most commonly neutrophils or macrophages) generally examine one or more of the following as indicators of cell activation:

1. Cell adhesion and spreading
2. Cell death
3. Cell migration
4. Cytokine release
5. Cell surface marker expression

Cell adhesion can be quantified in a number of ways, as discussed in the previous chapter. These means include radioactively or fluorescently labeling the cells or lysing the cells and then measuring the release of a particular intracellular molecule (such as LDH). Also as mentioned in Chapter 9, judging the extent of cell spreading is more qualitative and involves staining and then imaging the adherent cells with a light microscope.

Assays for migration of inflammatory cells, both in response to degradation products from biomaterials and along biomaterial surfaces in response to other stimuli, are extremely important since movement to areas of need is a key function of this cell type. Versions of all of the migration assays described in Chapter 9 have been employed to study cell movement. Direct observation of individual cells over time may provide information about the effect of material properties on cell motility. Alternatively, a population assay may be used to examine the migration of a group of monocytes or granulocytes after culture with and without exposure to the sample biomaterial.

Release into the media of pro-inflammatory cytokines, including several of the interleukins and TNF-α, is another distinctive marker of cell activation. Detection is usually accomplished via the use of an ELISA (see Chapter 8) for the cytokine of interest.

A final assay for monocyte or granulocyte activation requires the identification of cells expressing certain cell surface markers, usually specific receptors that will eventually interact with the ligands presented by endothelial cells. Since these receptors are upregulated in response to certain stimuli, including those discussed above, the number of cells in a population expressing these markers after exposure to a biomaterial provides a means of quantifying the ability of the material to induce activation. Cell counting is accomplished using a **fluorescence-activated cell sorter (FACS)** or **flow cytometry** techniques.

FACS machines and flow cytometry operate on similar principles and are based on immunostaining techniques (see Chapter 9). After a fluorescently tagged antibody to the receptor of interest has been incubated with the inflammatory cells, the entire population is then placed in the FACS (Fig. 10.4). The cells are passed one at a time from a vibrating nozzle past a laser that is set to emit a wavelength of light that will excite the fluorophore. The intensity of the fluorescence for each leukocyte (number of antibody molecules attached to the cell) is monitored and sent as output to a computer, enabling quantification of relative amounts of fluorescing (activated) and nonfluorescing (nonactivated) cells.

Physical separation of the activated and nonactivated cells is also possible via FACS. The laser excitation causes a cell to possess a negative charge in proportion to the intensity of the fluorescence. Cells can therefore be deflected from electrically charged plates. Depending on the configuration of these plates, cells

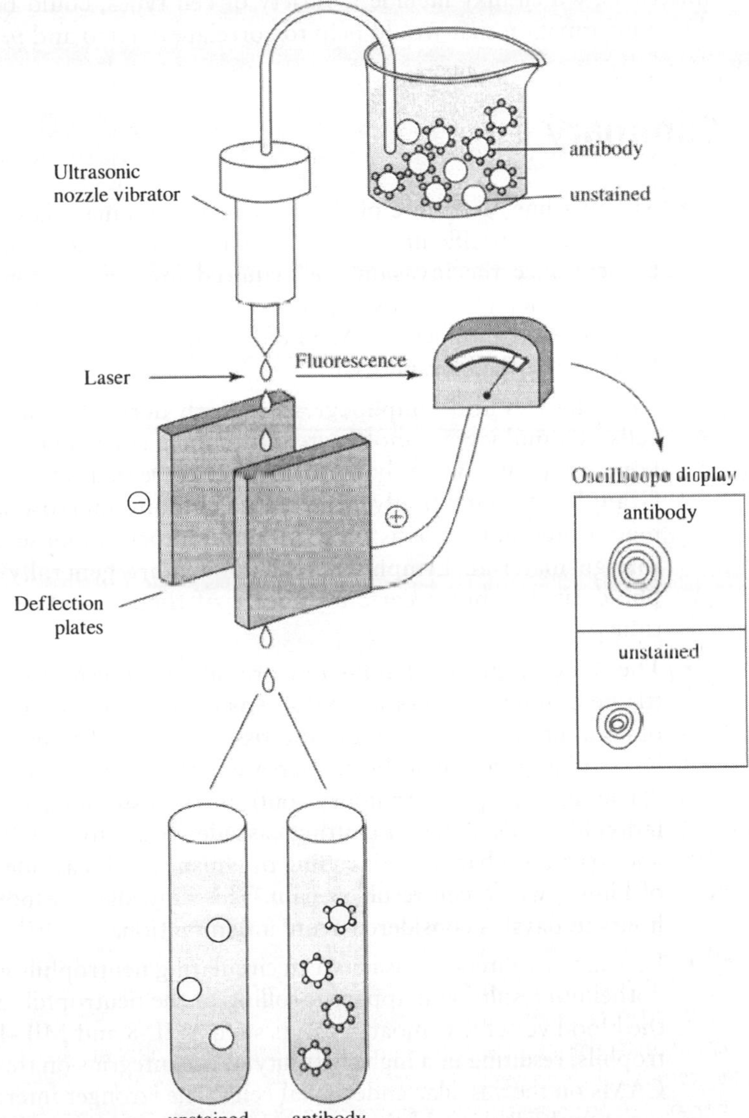

Figure 10.4
Cell characterization via fluorescence-activated cell sorting (FACS). First, fluorescently tagged cells are placed in the FACS. The cells are passed one at a time from a vibrating nozzle past a laser that is set to emit a wavelength of light that will excite the fluorophore. The intensity of the fluorescence for each cell (number of antibody molecules attached to the cell) is monitored and sent as output to a computer, enabling quantification of relative amounts of fluorescing (expressing receptor) and nonfluorescing cells (not expressing receptor). Physical separation of the two cell populations is also possible. The laser excitation causes a cell to possess a negative charge in proportion to the intensity of the fluorescence. Cells can therefore be deflected from electrically charged plates. Depending on the configuration of these plates, cells can be separated into two or more groups displaying varying degrees of fluorescence. (Adapted with permission from [3].)

can be separated into two or more groups displaying varying degrees of fluorescence (Fig. 10.4).

10.6.2 Other Assays

A further *in vitro* assay for the inflammatory potential of biomaterials tests the response of endothelial cells. The upregulation of cell surface receptors (e.g. selectins) or ligands (e.g. CAMs) on endothelial cells promotes the migration of neutrophils and macrophages and thus is a key step in the inflammatory response. Therefore, after exposure to a biomaterial, the presence of these cell surface markers is examined using similar methods (FACS or flow cytometry) as described for leukocytes.

A recent development in *in vitro* assays utilizes model systems derived from tissue-engineered constructs to examine the inflammatory response. For example, a tissue-engineered skin replacement can be cocultured with a potential skin-contacting biomaterial and the release of inflammatory cytokines by the cells in the construct may be monitored via ELISA or other means [5]. These three-dimensional constructs, which may include a variety of cell types, could be a future means to obtain information that would help to correlate *in vitro* and *in vivo* responses.

Summary

- The first line of defense of the body to foreign materials and organisms is innate or non-specific immunity. If the innate immune response is not sufficient to neutralize the invasion, an acquired immune response can be invoked. Innate immunity depends in part on the actions of white blood cells like granulocytes and monocytes. Acquired immunity involves the action of white blood cells called lymphocytes.
- Granulocytes and lymphocytes are both derived from hematopoetic stem cells. Granulocytes, monocytes, and megakaryocytes are formed in the bone marrow, while lymphocytes are created in the lymphoid tissue. Granulocytes commonly remain in the bone marrow until needed. Their main function is to assist in the inflammatory response and to phagocytose foreign material. Lymphocytes, however, are generally stored in the lymphoid tissues, but a certain number of them circulate in the blood at all times.
- The clinical signs of inflammation are rubor (redness), tumor (swelling), calore (tissue heating), and dolore (pain). Vasodilation of blood vessels in the vicinity of an injury results in redness and tissue heating. The leaking of fluid into the interstitial space caused by an increase in the permeability of surrounding capillaries in response to an injury contributes to swelling, as does the swelling of individual cells. A blood clotting cascade ensues to segregate the injured area and to create a barrier to invading organisms. This cascade involves the release of kinins, which can result in pain. This immediate response (in the range of hours to days) is considered acute inflammation.
- Low affinity interactions between circulating neutrophils and the vascular endothelium result in an apparent rolling of the neutrophils along the surface of the blood vessel. Chemoattractants such as IL-8 and MIP-1b can activate neutrophils, resulting in a higher affinity of the integrins on the neutrophils for the CAMs on the vascular endothelial cells. The stronger interactions result in the arrest and adhesion of the neutrophils to the vascular endothelial cells. Once

adhered, the neutrophils undergo transendothelial migration by a process of diapedesis to enter the extravascular space, where they encounter further chemoattractants to direct them to the site of injury.

- Neutrophils can deter invasion of foreign organisms through phagocytosis, a respiratory burst, or secretion of chemical mediators. Phagocytosis involves the engulfment and ingestion of the insulting material by the cell, where it can be digested by enzymes and bactericidal agents. Activated neutrophils can form granules containing highly reactive nitrogen and oxygen species as a result of the respiratory burst, which can be released to kill foreign organisms. Additionally, activated neutrophils secrete a number of cytokines to recruit monocytes and other neutrophils to the area of insult.
- Macrophages phagocytose materials as neutrophils do; however, macrophages can engulf many more bacteria or particles than a neutrophil. Macrophages and neutrophils both can be involved in frustrated phagocytosis in response to a nondegradable material much larger than the cell. Activated macrophages secrete cytokines that can have systemic effects as well as effects on the inflammatory and/or acquired immune responses. A key function of the activated macrophage is its role as an antigen-presenting cell, which provides a direct connection between the innate and acquired immune responses.
- A variety of *in vitro* techniques can be employed to gain information regarding the inflammatory response that a biomaterial may invoke. *In vitro* techniques involving leukocytes generally examine cell adhesion and spreading, cell death, cell migration, cytokine release, and/or cell surface markers as indicators of cell activation. Fluorescence-activated cell sorting and flow cytometry techniques provide a means for quantifying the number of cells (leukocytes or endothelial cells) expressing certain surface markers. Additional *in vitro* assays for inflammatory potential include the use of model systems derived from tissue engineering constructs.

Problems

10.1 Describe the differences between innate and acquired immunity.

10.2 Of the different components of innate immunity, which is the least likely to have an effect on the response to an implanted biomaterial?

10.3 In experiments to evaluate the tissue response to a biomaterial, a control group is often included involving the complete surgical procedure but without implanting the biomaterial. What is the rationale for the inclusion of this control group, and what is the expected tissue response?

10.4 What are some of the phagocytic complications that can occur after material implantation?

10.5 You are examining three materials—poly(tetrafluoroethylene), poly(ethylene terephthalate), and poly(propylene)—for potential use as a vascular graft. How would you determine which of the three materials induces the least activation of granulocytes?

10.6 Describe the major steps of neutrophil extravasation and list the important biomolecules involved in each step. Patient X has a rare disease that prevents the expression of selectins on endothelial cells. Patient Y has a related disease that prevents expression of Ig-superfamily CAMs on endothelial cells. What would be expected in each patient in terms of neutrophil extravasation and why?

References

1. Suggs, L.J., R.S. Krishnan, C.A. Garcia, S.J. Peter, J.M. Anderson, and A.G. Mikos. "*In Vitro* and *In Vivo* Degradation of Poly(Propylene Fumarate-Co-Ethylene Glycol) Hydrogels," *Journal of Biomedical Materials Research*, vol. 42, pp. 312–320, 1998.
2. Guyton, A.C. and J.E. Hall. *Textbook of Medical Physiology*, 9th ed. Philadelphia: W.B. Saunders, 1996.
3. Kuby, J. *Immunology*, 3rd ed. New York: W.H. Freeman, 1997.
4. Wang, J.C., W.D. Yu, H.S. Sandhu, F. Betts, S. Bhuta, and R.B. Delamarter. "Metal Debris from Titanium Spinal Implants," *Spine*, vol. 24, pp. 899–903, 1999.
5. Trasciatti, S., A. Podesta, S. Bonaretti, V. Mazzoncini, and S. Rosini. "*In Vitro* Effects of Different Formulations of Bovine Collagen on Cultured Human Skin," *Biomaterials*, vol. 19, pp. 897–903, 1998.

Additional Reading

Alberts, B., A. Johnson, J. Lewis, M. Raff, K. Roberts, and P. Walter. *Molecular Biology of the Cell*, 4th ed. New York: Garland Publishing, 2002.

Anderson, J.M. "Mechanisms of Inflammation and Infection with Implanted Devices," *Cardiovascular Pathology*, vol. 2, pp. 33S–41S, 1993.

Black, J. *Biological Performance of Materials: Fundamentals of Biocompatibility*, 4th ed. New York: CRC Press, 2005.

Colman, R.W., J. Hirsh, V.J. Marder, A.W. Clowes, and J.N. George. *Hemostasis and Thrombosis: Basic Principles and Clinical Practice*. Philadelphia: Lippincott, Williams, and Wilkins, 2001.

Dee, K.C., D.A. Puleo, and R. Bizios. *An Introduction to Tissue-Biomaterial Interactions*. Hoboken: Wiley-Liss, 2002.

Granchi, D., E. Cenni, E. Verri, G. Ciapetti, S. Gamberini, A. Gori, and A. Pizzoferrato. "Flow-Cytometric Analysis of Leukocyte Activation Induced by Polyethylene-Terephthalate with and without Pyrolytic Carbon Coating," *Journal of Biomedical Materials Research*, vol. 39, pp. 549–553, 1998.

Gretzer, C., K. Gisselfalt, E. Liljensten, L. Ryden, and P. Thomsen. "Adhesion, Apoptosis and Cytokine Release of Human Mononuclear Cells Cultured on Degradable Poly(Urethane Urea), Polystyrene and Titanium in Vitro," *Biomaterials*, vol. 24, pp. 2843–2852, 2003.

Hallab, N., J.J. Jacobs, and J. Black. "Hypersensitivity to Metallic Biomaterials: A Review of Leukocyte Migration Inhibition Assays," *Biomaterials*, vol. 21, pp. 1301–1314, 2000.

Jenney, C.R., K.M. DeFife, E. Colton, and J.M. Anderson. "Human Monocyte/Macrophage Adhesion, Macrophage Motility, and Il-4-Induced Foreign Body Giant Cell Formation on Silane-Modified Surfaces In Vitro. Student Research Award in the Master's Degree Candidate Category, 24th Annual Meeting of the Society for Biomaterials, San Diego, CA, April 22–26, 1998," *Journal of Biomedical Materials Research*, vol. 41, pp. 171–184, 1998.

Mitchell, R.N. "Innate and Adaptive Immunity: The Immune Respinse to Foreign Materials." In *Biomaterials Science: An Introduction to Materials in Medicine*, B.D. Ratner, A.S. Hoffman, F.J. Schoen, and J.E. Lemons, Eds., 2nd ed. San Diego: Elsevier Academic Press, pp. 304–318, 2004.

Palsson, B.O. and S.N. Bhatia. *Tissue Engineering*. Upper Saddle River: Pearson Prentice Hall, 2004.

Pu, F.R., R.L. Williams, T.K. Markkula, and J.A. Hunt. "Expression of Leukocyte-Endothelial Cell Adhesion Molecules on Monocyte Adhesion to Human Endothelial Cells on Plasma Treated PET and PTFE In Vitro," *Biomaterials*, vol. 23, pp. 4705–4718, 2002.

Shen, M. and T.A. Horbett. "The Effects of Surface Chemistry and Adsorbed Proteins on Monocyte/Macrophage Adhesion to Chemically Modified Polystyrene Surfaces," *Journal of Biomedical Materials Research*, vol. 57, pp. 336–345, 2001.

Silver, F.H. and D.L. Christiansen. *Biomaterials Science and Biocompatibility*. New York: Springer, 1999.

Trindade, M.C., M. Lind, D. Sun, D.J. Schurman, S.B. Goodman, and R.L. Smith. "*In Vitro* Reaction to Orthopaedic Biomaterials by Macrophages and Lymphocytes Isolated from Patients Undergoing Revision Surgery," *Biomaterials*, vol. 22, pp. 253–259, 2001.

Wound Healing and the Presence of Biomaterials

CHAPTER 11

Main Objective

To understand the stages and types of resolution after biomaterial implantation and how this differs from wound healing without the presence of an implant.

Specific Objectives

1. To identify the characteristics of granulation tissue.
2. To understand how implant properties affect the foreign body response.
3. To compare and contrast fibrous encapsulation and chronic inflammation.
4. To distinguish among four different types of resolution and characterize them as successful or unsuccessful outcomes.
5. To compare and contrast wound repair and regeneration.
6. To compare and contrast the stages of normal wound healing with the stages after biomaterial implantation.
7. To understand the concerns and possible limitations associated with the choice of animal models for assessment of inflammatory response and biocompatibility.

11.1 Introduction: Formation of Granulation Tissue

In this chapter, we will continue to examine the body's response to an implanted biomaterial with a focus on events that occur starting approximately 24 hours after implantation. (Acute response to implantation was discussed in Chapter 10.) As early as one day postimplantation (or injury), macrophages and other cells involved in the inflammatory process provide chemoattractive signals to promote migration of fibroblasts and vascular endothelial cells into the area (Fig. 11.1). Within three to five days, microscopic observation of the beginning of granulation tissue formation is possible.

Granulation tissue is characterized histologically by a pebbly, granular appearance (thus its name) (Fig. 11.2). This is caused by the creation of many vascular buds sprouting from existing blood vessels. This process is called **neovascularization** or **angiogenesis.** At its peak, granulation tissue has more capillaries per volume than any other tissue type.

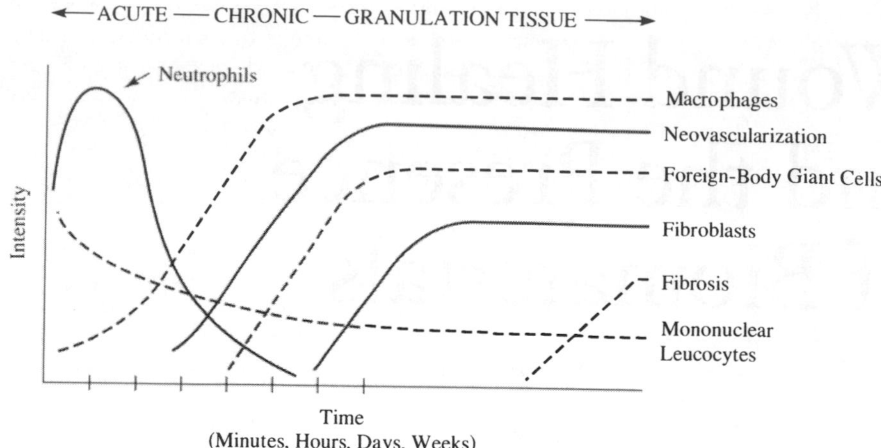

Figure 11.1
Wound-healing response of the body after injury or biomaterial implantation. (Adapted with permission from [1].)

This stage of wound healing is also characterized by the proliferation of **fibroblasts.** Fibroblasts, mentioned briefly in the previous chapter, are a committed cell type found in many tissues. One of their main functions is to synthesize and maintain connective tissues by producing an extracellular matrix rich in collagen and proteoglycans. In granulation tissue, some of these fibroblasts may take on features of smooth muscle cells and are termed **myofibroblasts.** Myofibroblasts are responsible for wound contraction, which results in faster healing due to a decrease in the overall defect size.

EXAMPLE PROBLEM 11.1

Blood vessels can be formed *de novo* during development in a process termed **vasculogenesis.** In this process vascular progenitor cells migrate and differentiate to form blood vessels in response to cues presented through the extracellular matrix and cytokines. How does angiogenesis differ from vasculogenesis? Why might the likelihood of vasculogenesis occurring decrease with age? Why is a blood supply important for developing and regenerating tissue?

Solution: Angiogenesis involves the creation of new blood vessels through a process of budding or sprouting from existing blood vessels. Thus, angiogenesis is not a *de novo* process. Vasculogenesis, however, does not involve sprouting or budding of new blood vessels

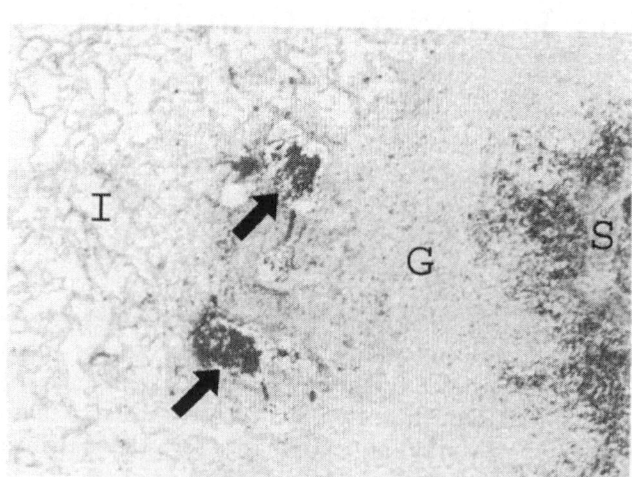

Figure 11.2
Granulation tissue formation at the tissue/material interface. Large surface wounds in the spleen were treated with a porous sodium amylose succinate material in a canine model. A well-developed zone of granulation tissue (G) separates the spleen (S) and the polymer (I). Blood-vessel-like areas are at the leading edge of the granulation tissue (arrows). The sample is stained with hematoxylin and eosin, which highlights the nuclei of the cells (black dots). Original magnification 60X. (Reprinted with permission from [2].)

from existing ones. Rather, it entails the creation of new vessels from vascular progenitor cells guided by cellular and extracellular matrix signals. The number of stem or progenitor cells present in the body decreases with age. Thus, the number of vascular progenitor cells available to participate in vasculogenesis decreases with age. It follows that the likelihood of vasculogenesis occurring would decrease with age. The embryonic environment, on the other hand, is rich in stem cells and facilitates vasculogenesis. Blood vessels are necessary in developing and/or regenerating tissue to provide cells with nutrients and to remove cellular waste products. ■

11.2 Foreign Body Reaction

Granulation tissue may form part of the **foreign body reaction**. This reaction involves **foreign body giant cells** (FBGCs) and the elements of granulation tissue discussed previously. Foreign body giant cells are multinucleated cells formed by the fusion of monocytes/macrophages in an attempt to phagocytose the biomaterial, which is much larger than a single cell.

The relative composition of the foreign body reaction is dependent on several factors associated with the implant. One of these is the surface properties of the material. This includes the topography (roughness) and surface chemistry of the implant. For example, for smooth implants, such as silicone breast prostheses, layers of macrophages one to two cells in thickness can be observed. However, for rough implants, such as the outer surfaces of degrading biomaterials, a mixture of macrophages and FBGCs are seen (Fig. 11.3, Fig. 11.4).

The shape of the implanted material (in particular, its surface area to volume ratio) can also have an effect on the foreign body reaction. Implants with a high surface area to volume ratio (e.g., fabrics or porous materials) have higher ratios of macrophages and FBGCs at the tissue-material interface, while implants with a lower surface area to volume ratio show more fibrous (granulation) tissue production. FBGCs and/or macrophages may remain surrounding a biomaterial for the lifetime of the implant, but it is not clear if these cells are actively secreting

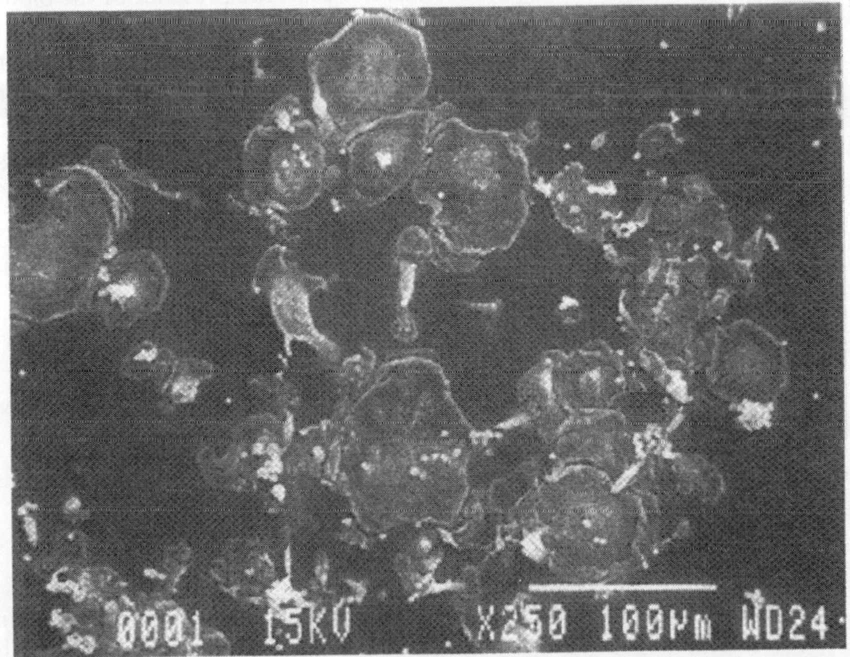

Figure 11.3
Scanning electron micrograph demonstrating a foreign body reaction to poly(propylene fumarate-co-ethylene glycol) implanted subcutaneously in a rat model. Both macrophages (smaller cells) and foreign body giant cells (larger cells) can be seen in the image. (Reprinted with permission from [3].)

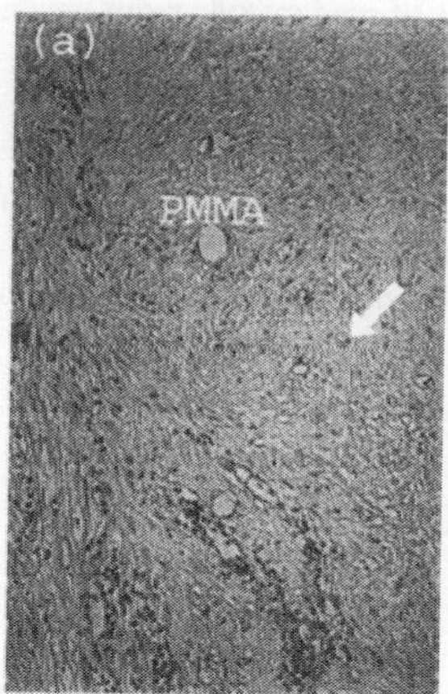

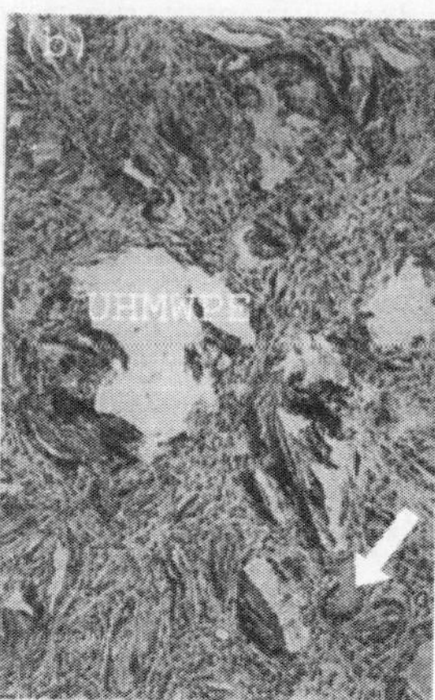

Figure 11.4
Histological sections from a rabbit wound chamber. (a) Foreign-body reaction to particulate PMMA (round voids) with numerous macrophages (small arrow) identified in the tissue. (b) Foreign-body reaction to large particles of UHMWPE (irregular voids) with macrophages and foreign-body giant cells (large arrow). Basic Oil Red O Stain, original magnification 60X. (Reprinted with permission from [4].)

bioactive factors, such as degradative enzymes or chemotactic agents, during this entire period.

11.3 Fibrous Encapsulation

The final stage of healing for implants made from nondegradable materials is fibrous encapsulation (Fig. 11.1). This involves granulation tissue maturation, which is marked by the presence of larger blood vessels and alignment of collagen fibers in response to local mechanical forces. In this case, the presence of the biomaterial prevents both the collapse of the capsule surrounding the implant and the subsequent formation of a scar, as would occur in normal wound healing (see later in this chapter for an in-depth discussion of scar formation). Fibrous encapsulation is considered an acceptable result after implantation of many biomaterials.

The degree of long-term (four weeks postimplantation and later) capsule formation depends on several factors:

1. Degree of original injury during implantation
2. Amount of subsequent cell death
3. Location of implant site
4. Degradation time of implant (if degradable)

More specifically, the thickness of the capsule may be affected by the following factors:

1. Amount and composition of small particulates produced
2. Mechanical factors at implant site
3. Shape of implant
4. Electrical currents (if produced)

The size of the fibrous capsule increases in proportion to the rate of shedding of small particulates, which can be caused by corrosion, degradation, and wear. The chemical composition of these fragments, particularly their cytotoxicity, is also a large factor in capsule formation. In addition, the capsule becomes thicker in response to mechanical factors like motion between the implant and the surrounding tissue.

Thicker capsules have been observed over edges and distinct changes in surface features of the material and, thus, are affected by the shape of the implant. Finally, in implants producing electrical currents, such as stimulating electrodes, capsule thickness corresponds to current density. In this case, functioning electrodes can mediate changes in local pH and O_2 concentrations and encourage corrosion, so capsule formation may be caused by these indirect effects as well as the presence of the electric current.

EXAMPLE PROBLEM 11.2

A pharmaceutical laboratory developed a nondegradable synthetic polymer implant for controlled drug delivery. The researchers envision subcutaneous implantation of the delivery device, with the release of the drug being controlled by diffusion. They determined the release kinetics of the drug from the carrier in studies conducted *in vitro*, but have found that the release kinetics differ when the device is implanted *in vivo*. Specifically, the drug is found to release more slowly *in vivo*. What are some possible factors that could contribute to the differences in the observed release kinetics? Would a cube-shaped form of the implant or a spherical form of the implant of the same volume likely result in a thicker fibrous capsule formation? Why?

Solution: The complex environment encountered *in vivo* is difficult to replicate in experiments conducted *in vitro*. Consequently, it is common for experimental results obtained from *in vitro* studies to differ from studies conducted *in vivo*. The final stage of the tissue response to the implantation of the nondegradable synthetic polymer drug delivery device will be fibrous encapsulation of the device. The fibrous capsule could potentially serve as a barrier to the diffusion of the drug out of the device, thereby slowing the release. Fibrous encapsulation would be very difficult to replicate *in vitro;* thus, the observed release *in vitro* likely did not entail a diffusional barrier presented by a tissue element. Additionally, the presence and concentrations of enzymes could differ between the cases studied *in vitro* and *in vivo*, and could affect the release kinetics. A cube-shaped implant would probably result in a thicker fibrous capsule formation than a spherical implant of the same volume, as the distinct edges and corners of the cubic implant could promote a greater fibrous tissue formation response to isolate the implant. Additionally, the surface area presented by a cube is greater than the surface area presented by a sphere of the same volume; thus, the presentation of more surface area of a foreign material with sharp corners could elicit a more pronounced fibrous encapsulation and possibly an increased presence of macrophages and foreign body giant cells. ■

11.4 Chronic Inflammation

Chronic inflammation is less uniform histologically than acute inflammation (Fig. 11.5). It is characterized by the presence of mononuclear cells, including lymphocytes and plasma cells, which may also indicate that the material has triggered an acquired immune response (discussed further in the following chapter). Although it is common to see a short-lived chronic inflammatory response between the end of acute inflammation and the full development of granulation tissue (Fig 11.1), persistence of chronic inflammation beyond this point is considered pathologic.

In some cases, chronic inflammation can include the presence of **granulomas.** Granulomas consist of a layer of FBGCs surrounding a nonphagocytosable particle. The FBGCs are themselves contained within a ring of large modified macrophages called **epitheloid cells.** This cell mass is then surrounded by a layer of lymphocytes.

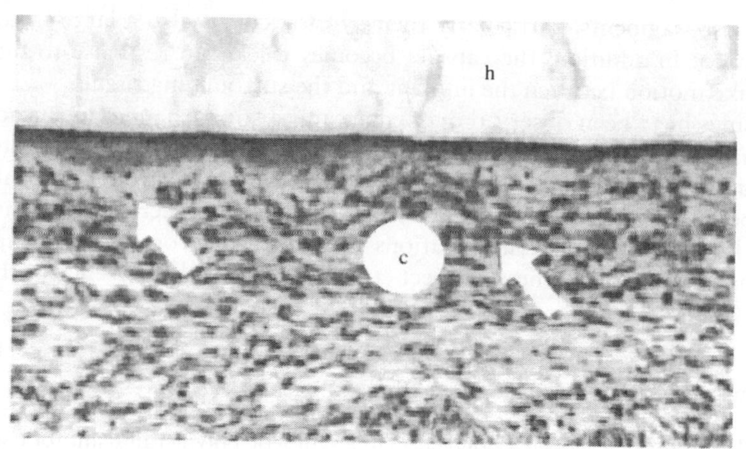

Figure 11.5
Chronic inflammation of a natural polymer (dextran) hydrogel (h) in a subcutaneous rat model. Macrophages (arrow on right), lymphocytes (arrow on left) and elongated fibroblasts are identified in the surrounding tissue. C represents the area in which the fibrous capsule is beginning to form. Toluidine blue stain. Original magnification 100X. (Reprinted with permission from [5].)

Chronic inflammation can be a result of the chemical or physical properties of the biomaterial, or can be caused by motion at the implant site.

11.5 Four Types of Resolution

As mentioned in the previous chapter, the overall goal of the inflammation and wound healing response is to restore the body's status quo after injury. Therefore, the formation of a new equilibrium state can be considered a **resolution** of this response. There are four main types of possible resolutions, some of which were discussed previously:

1. Extrusion
2. Resorption
3. Integration
4. Encapsulation

In extrusion, if the implant is in contact with epithelial tissue (the top layer of the skin), a pouch contiguous with this tissue can be formed and the material can be forced out of the body. This is how a splinter "works itself out."

If an implant is biodegradable (resorbable), it is possible that no fibrous capsule will form, depending on the rate of degradation. Alternatively, if a capsule does form, after implant resorption, the capsule can either collapse and remain this way or can be replaced with appropriate tissue.

Integration occurs in limited cases, such as the implantation of pure titanium in bone. This resolution type is characterized by a close approximation of host tissue to the implant, with no intervening fibrous capsule.

Encapsulation is the traditional response to nonresorbable materials, as described previously. Chronic inflammation/granuloma generation is not included in this category, since in this case there is not a return to the status quo (no resolution has occurred).

Each of the resolution types described above can be considered a failure or a success, depending on the reason for biomaterial implantation. For example, resorption and integration are the two most ideal resolutions for tissue engineering applications, whereas encapsulation, normally considered an acceptable outcome for biomaterial implantation, would represent failure of the tissue-engineered product. This is due to the nature of tissue engineering, a field in which the overriding goal is to create a fully functional tissue, rather than to replace damaged tissue with synthetic materials.

11.6 Repair vs. Regeneration: Wound Healing in Skin

As mentioned above, tissue engineering uses biomaterials to create functional tissue. Two processes can form functional tissue: **repair** and **regeneration.** Either can have a successful result, depending on the goal of the tissue engineering treatment. In tissue repair, the defect is replaced by scar tissue, which may have a different structure, biochemical composition, and/or mechanical properties from native tissue. In tissue regeneration, the defect is replaced by tissue identical to that which was there before the wound occurred. In this case, the normal tissue structure, composition, and properties are completely restored. In this section, we will use wound healing in the skin as an example to illustrate differences in repair vs. regeneration and to highlight how normal wound healing differs from healing near a non-degradable biomaterial.

11.6.1 Skin Repair

Skin is composed of two regions, the internal **dermal layer,** and the outer **epidermal layer,** as shown in Fig. 11.6. If injury involves only the epidermal layer, defect regeneration is possible (see below). However, many cuts and burns extend into the dermal layer, where the primary means of wound healing is repair.

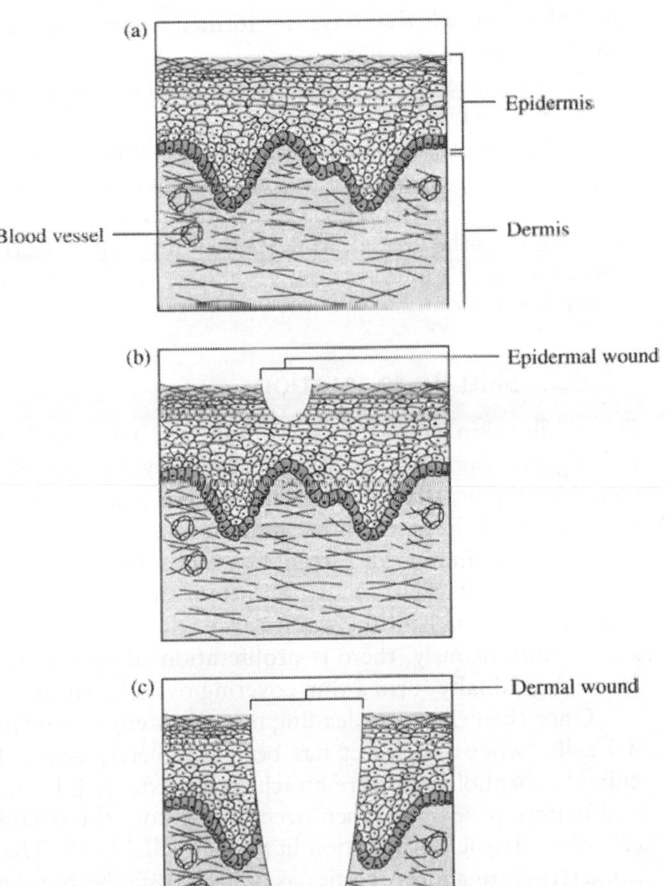

Figure 11.6
(a) Schematic of skin representing the internal dermal layer and the outer epidermal layer. If injury involves only the epidermal layer, as shown in (b) defect regeneration is possible. However, if cuts or burns extend into the dermal layer, as shown in (c) the primary means of wound healing is repair.

After injury, the first response is blood clotting and the formation of a fibrin network to prevent fluid loss (see Chapter 13 for a more in-depth discussion). This is followed by acute inflammation, including the same sequence of localized response and cellular migration as described previously for biomaterial implantation (Chapter 10). This stage is characterized by removal of tissue debris and deposition of hyaluronic acid, a glycosaminoglycan, in the extracellular matrix.

The inflammatory response triggers an influx of fibroblasts, which proliferate and deposit extracellular matrix, and mark the beginning of granulation tissue formation. As described previously, a large number of new blood vessels are also formed during this time. A particular characteristic of the tissue at this stage is that the collagen fibers (type III) deposited in the extracellular matrix are thin and randomly oriented. As new extracellular matrix is deposited, the fibrin clot is dissolved via release of specific enzymes and phagocytosis from the remaining macrophages.

The final stage of skin wound repair is *remodeling*, or scar formation. Starting approximately one week after injury, there is turnover of collagen molecules in the extracellular matrix, characterized by degradation of collagen type III via enzymes and/or phagocytosis and its eventual replacement by collagen type I. The new collagen bundles are larger and oriented along the principal lines of stress in the tissue. Similarly, there is an increase in the ratio of glycosaminoglycans such as chondroitin and dermatan sulfate to hyaluronic acid.

Collagen accumulation in scar tissue can continue for two to three months after injury. Additionally, the mechanical properties of the neotissue continue to increase over several months due to further crosslinking of the collagen fibers. During this time, blood vessels that have not formed connections are resorbed, and the scar becomes pale and avascular.

This represents the completion of skin repair: A functional tissue replacement has been generated, that, in many cases, may be entirely adequate. It should be noted that this stage cannot be fully completed in the presence of a nondegradable material since the capsule around the material remains and is never remodeled into scar tissue. As the defect in the dermis is being filled, the wound may concurrently be reepithelialized, as described in the next section. This does not represent regeneration of the defect, however, due to the presence of the scar tissue in the dermal layer.

11.6.2 Skin Regeneration

For smaller skin wounds that are contained in the epidermal layer (termed erosions), full regeneration of the defect is possible via **reepithelialization.** As in the case of complete repair, this process cannot take place with the continued presence of a nondegradable implant in the epidermis.

As shown in Fig. 11.7, reepithelialization begins as the cells at the edge of defect change shape (flatten) to cover more of the wound. Dissolution of attachments to extracellular matrix at the wound edge allows migration of these cells into the defect site. Simultaneously, there is proliferation of epithelial cells behind the advancing front to gradually form a thin covering over the entire wound site.

Once the cells at the leading migratory edge come in contact with other epithelial cells (when the defect has been completely covered), they recover their more cuboid morphology and re-attach to the extracellular matrix. Further proliferation and matrix production then occurs to restore the original thickness of tissue. This completes tissue regeneration in the epithelial layer. The resulting neotissue has the same structure and properties as did the tissue before the injury.

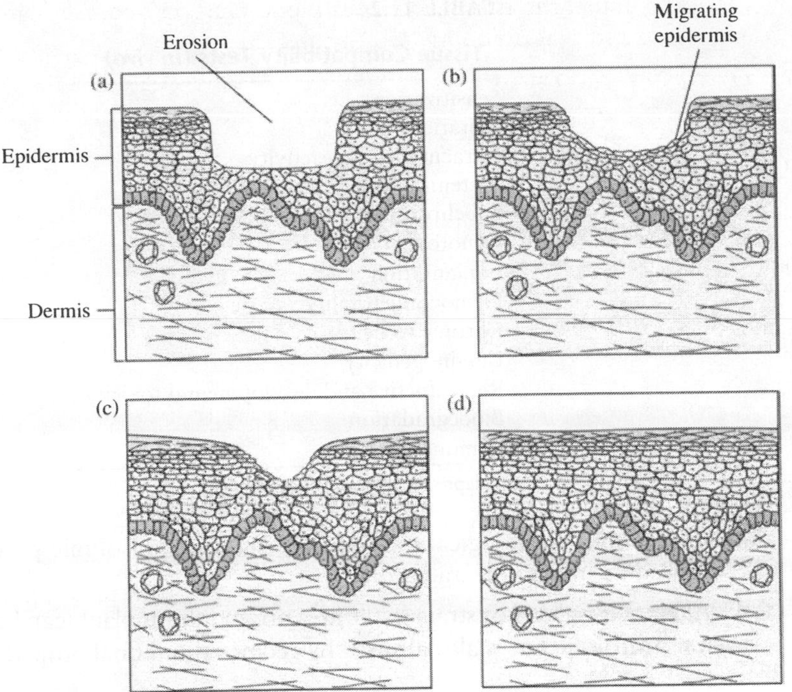

Figure 11.7 Regeneration of skin wounds contained in the epidermal layer. (a) Reepithelialization begins as the cells at the edge of the defect change shape (flatten) to cover more of the wound. (b) These cells then migrate into the defect site. (c) Once the cells at the leading migratory edge come in contact with other epithelial cells (when the defect has been completely covered), they recover their more cuboid morphology and reattach to the extracellular matrix. (d) Further proliferation and matrix production then occurs to restore the original thickness of the tissue. (Adapted with permission from [6].)

11.7 Techniques: *In Vivo* Assays for Inflammatory Response

While *in vitro* evaluation of the inflammatory response (see previous chapter) can be useful as an indicator of material biocompatibility, it cannot replace *in vivo* testing due to the complex interplay of cell types and signaling molecules that comprise the inflammatory response. Table 11.1 lists factors related to a biomedical implant that may affect the *in vivo* response. The items on this list may cause a specific biological response through a variety of means:

1. Interactions of biological molecules (such as proteins and ions) or cells with the implant (this includes both the topography and chemistry of the material).
2. Interactions of biological molecules or cells with soluble agents leached from the implant (leaching may occur due to the original chemical properties, additives, or degradation of the material).

TABLE 11.1

Relevant Factors of *in vivo* Tissue Compatibility Evaluation
The material(s) of manufacture
Intended additives, process contaminants, and residues
Leachable substances
Degradation products
Other components and their interactions in the final product
The properties and characteristics of the final product

(Adapted with permission from [7].)

TABLE 11.2

Tissue Compatibility Tests (*in vivo*)
Sensitization
Irritation
Intracutaneous reactivity
Systemic toxicity (acute toxicity)
Subchronic toxicity (subacute toxicity)
Genotoxicity
Implantation
Hemocompatibility
Chronic toxicity
Carcinogenicity
Reproductive and developmental toxicity
Biodegradation
Immune responses

(Adapted with permission from [7].)

3. Interactions of biological molecules or cells with insoluble particulates (usually caused by implant degradation).
4. Alterations in load or strain in the area around the implant (can be caused by material properties, but is also affected by geometry and final properties of the device).

Given the complexity of these interactions and the importance of biocompatibility testing, a number of regulatory agencies (U.S. Food and Drug Administration, ASTM, ISO) have proposed guidelines and procedures for *in vivo* biocompatibility assessment [8–11]. According to these standards, **biocompatibility** can be considered "the ability of a medical device to perform with an appropriate host response in a specific application" and thus, **biocompatibility assessment** is "a measurement of the magnitude and duration of the adverse alterations in homeostatic mechanisms that determine the host response."

A wide variety of tests fall under this broad definition of biocompatibility assessment, which includes examination of carcinogenicity, hemocompatibility, immune response, and the inflammatory response (see Table 11.2). Many of these studies will be discussed in later chapters. In this section, we will focus on *in vivo* examinations most directly assessing the inflammatory response. As per the ISO standards, this involves tests for localized reactivity and toxicity, as well as systemic toxicity (acute, subacute, and chronic). Additionally, it is recommended that these effects be determined both after injection of extracts of the biomaterial and after implantation.

The subsequent discussion follows after Spector and Lalor [12] and is intended to point out some of the major concerns in devising *in vivo* studies for biomedical devices, particularly those involving implantation of a biomaterial into a specific tissue. Although these parameters should be considered for relatively "inert" implants as well as tissue engineered products, it should be noted that biocompatibility testing of devices including active molecules, such as cells and growth factors, further complicates the screening procedure, so additional *in vitro* and *in vivo* tests may be required for tissue engineered products. Of course, as with all animal studies, *in vivo* biocompatibility examinations must follow proper animal care guidelines for concerns such as sterility and mitigation of pain both during and after surgery.

11.7.1 Considerations in Development of Animal Models

11.7.1.1 Choice of Animal To study the inflammatory response *in vivo*, the animal species should be selected based on a similarity in physiology and healing response to

TABLE 11.3

Medical Devices and the Corresponding Animal Models Used for *in vivo* Testing

Device Classification	Animal
Cardiovascular	
Heart valves	Sheep
Vascular grafts	Dog, pig
Stents	Pig, dog
Ventricular assist devices	Calf
Artificial hearts	Calf
Ex vivo shunts	Baboon, dog
Orthopedic/bone	
Bone regeneration/substitutes	Rabbit, dog, pig, mouse, rat
Total joints—hips, knees	Dog, goat, nonhuman primate
Vertebral implants	Sheep, goat, baboon
Craniofacial implants	Rabbit, pig, dog, nonhuman primate
Cartilage	Rabbit, dog
Tendon and ligament substitutes	Dog, sheep
Neurological	
Peripheral nerve regeneration	Rat, cat, nonhuman primate
Electrical stimulation	Rat, cat, nonhuman primate
Ophthalmological	
Contact lens	Rabbit
Intraocular lens	Rabbit, monkey

(Adapted with permission from [7].)

that which would occur in humans for a given application. Of course, there is often no animal that will completely match the course of healing in humans, so it may be impossible to entirely predict human responses to a biomaterial based on animal experiments. For the development of new materials, investigators usually start with a small animal model (rat, rabbit) and then move to a larger model (goat, dog, sheep, cow) if results from the first study show an acceptable amount of localized inflammation. Table 11.3 shows common animal models for testing various medical devices.

11.7.1.2 Choice of Implant Site For the majority of studies, the implant site should be as close as possible to that which will be used in the final application. Sometimes a more accessible site, such as a subcutaneous pouch, is used for a first screening of the inflammatory response to a new material. In any case, the implant site should be assessed for several parameters that may affect the amount of inflammation perceived. For example, if there is a reduction in the number of macrophages and other inflammatory cells observed at a site that is not well vascularized, this may represent a lack of access to these cells, rather than anti-inflammatory properties of the material. Other important factors are the surrounding cells' ability to proliferate and migrate, and the effect of alterations in mechanical factors on the behavior of the surrounding cells.

11.7.1.3 Length of Study As per ISO standards, several types of toxicity should be addressed if appropriate for the final application of the material. **Acute toxicity** refers to negative effects appearing up to 24 hours after administration, while **subacute toxicity** involves effects occurring 14–28 days after administration. **Subchronic toxicity** refers to responses occurring usually within the first 90 days (or less than 10% of the lifetime of the animal), while **chronic toxicity** involves effects appearing after this time. These studies can be performed using extracts of the biomaterial, or direct implantation at an appropriate location, depending on the final device design.

In addition to toxicity tests, implantation followed by histological analysis (see below) can provide important information about the localized inflammatory response to the biomaterial. For these implantation tests, the response measured is actually a combination of responses to surgery, inflammation, and finally tissue remodeling around the implant (resolution), so assessment at multiple time points is preferred.

11.7.1.4 Biomaterial Considerations: Dose and Administration Because the form of an implant affects the biological response, it is important to test not only new materials, but materials in the same shape as will be used in the final device. In essence, the shape of the material affects its "dose" as seen by the body. It should be noted that biocompatibility testing may be carried out for two primary reasons: either to screen novel materials to gain insight into the degree and type of inflammatory response (in which case the shape of the material is of little concern) or to assess the inflammatory response to the material in a form very similar to that which will be implanted (in which case shape is more important).

For experiments that involve direct implantation of a material into a specific location, the following factors in addition to overall shape can affect the dose of the material received by the animal:

1. Implant weight and/or bulk size
2. Implant surface area
3. Implant topography
4. Number of implants per animal

As explained previously, biomaterial samples can be administered to an animal via direct implantation. Alternatively, extracts of the material may be injected into the animal to assess the response to soluble products. In this case, the extraction media as well as the site of injection may affect the inflammatory response.

A method falling between these two means of administration is the cage implant model. Here, the biomaterial is placed in a stainless steel cage, which is then implanted (Fig. 11.8). This enables investigators to examine the inflammatory response without providing direct contact between the material and the surrounding tissue. The method is particularly suited to assessing the reaction to the soluble (extractable) fraction of the biomaterial. A possible drawback is that the addition of the cage material may alter the inflammatory response in the localized area around the cage.

11.7.1.5 Inclusion of Proper Controls In many cases, the addition of appropriate controls can provide useful information about the relative response to the test sample. Depending on the application and comparison desired, controls may include intact contralateral tissue (from the opposite limb) or an unfilled surgical implant site. At other times, material and device controls (comparison of the new implant with a standard material or a previous version of the device) may be recommended.

11.7.2 Methods of Assessment

The method of assessment for biological response to biomaterials should be selected to provide the most pertinent information possible and should be included as a part

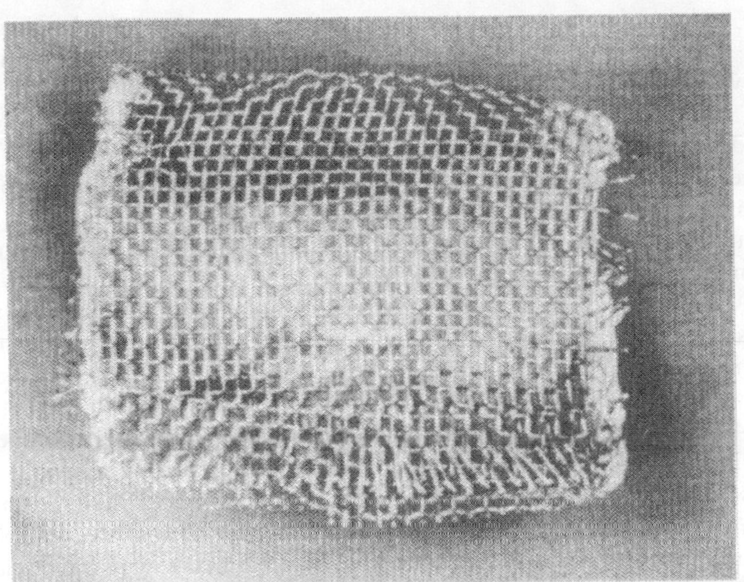

Figure 11.8
Image of a stainless steel cage implant model. The cage implant system was developed by James M. Anderson and his associates at Case Western Reserve University [13] and involves the placement of an experimental biomaterial in a stainless steel cage, which is then implanted. This system allows investigators to examine the inflammatory response without direct contact between the implanted experimental biomaterial and the surrounding tissue. (Reprinted with permission from [14].)

of the design of the experiment. For biocompatibility studies involving direct implantation of a material, there are a number of assessment methods, described below. The use of several methods concurrently is encouraged in order to obtain a full picture of the degree and nature of the inflammatory response to the implant.

11.7.2.1 Histology/Immunohistochemistry After explantation, the tissue containing the implant can be sectioned and stained, either with conventional dyes or antibodies, as described in Chapter 9. This technique is very common and allows for visualization of the tissue reaction at various stages through the identification of specific cell types and/or extracellular matrix molecules. However, due to variation between samples or suboptimal staining protocols, quantification of the amount or intensity of stain can be difficult using this technique. This has improved in recent years with the addition of computer-aided analysis of stained sections.

11.7.2.2 Electron Microscopy Both transmission electron microscopy (TEM) and scanning electron microscopy (SEM) can be employed to examine tissue response to an implant. The principles behind the operation of this equipment are discussed in Chapter 7 and the same procedures are used for samples containing explanted materials. TEM allows the interface of the implant to be examined at the ultrastructural level. If used in conjunction with X-ray analysis (see Chapter 7), this method may also be used to determine what types of materials have leached from the sample and where they are located. At later time points, TEM can be employed to assess integration with the surrounding tissue. However, a major drawback to using this technique is the difficulty in obtaining the ultrathin sections required. Additionally, since samples must be imaged under vacuum, special care must be used to fix and dehydrate the specimens prior to sectioning to maintain tissue morphology.

SEM, which does not require sectioning of the sample, may be an alternative to provide topographical images of the implant–tissue interface. As with TEM, soluble products that have leached away from the implant can be located via X-ray analysis associated with SEM. Also like TEM, because most SEM imaging is done *in vacuo*, proper fixation and dehydration protocols are very important to preserve the integrity of the sample. Recent development of environmental SEMs that allow imaging in the presence of water are a means to overcome this limitation.

11.7.2.3 Biochemical Assays Biochemical assays can also help assess inflammation after biomaterial implantation. As described in Chapter 9, a number of techniques are used, including colorimetric assays for production of bioactive molecules, or immuno-based assays for identification of a specific protein. For example, using biochemical assays, it may be possible to assess amounts of inflammatory mediators in the tissue surrounding the implant. Major advantages of this method are that it is quantitative and a large number of samples can be examined at one time with the use of an automated plate reader.

11.7.2.4 Mechanical Testing Mechanical testing of explanted specimens including the implant and surrounding tissue is often performed on a testing frame like that described in Chapter 4. Tensile, bending, or "push out" tests are particularly common. This method is useful to assess the longer-term response to implants, such as the time course of remodeling around the device, or how well the implant is integrated with the neighboring tissue. While this technique is quantitative, the results depend heavily on whether the samples are tested fresh, frozen, or after fixation. Thus, consistent sample handling is extremely important to allow for comparison of data between time points or between studies.

EXAMPLE PROBLEM 11.3

A study was conducted to evaluate the inflammatory response to a novel degradable implant material. The material has been designed to degrade by a bulk process after six weeks. One group of mice (Group A) received implantation of discs of the material under the skin on their backs (dorsal subcutaneous implantation). Another group (Group B) of the study received dorsal subcutaneous injection of a volume of degradation products of the material equal to the volume of the disk implanted in Group A. In both cases, the tissue response to the material was evaluated after 24 hours of implantation via histology, immunohistochemistry, and biochemical assays. A profound inflammatory response was observed in Group B, while a minor inflammatory response was observed in Group A. Assuming that no difference exists in the inflammatory response due to surgical implantation versus injection in this case, what conclusions can be drawn regarding the compatibility of the material?

Solution: The minor inflammatory response observed in Group A indicates that the whole discs do not induce a significant inflammatory response after 24 hours. As the material was designed to degrade over the course of six weeks via a bulk degradation process, little to no degradation products would be expected to be present in or around the material after 24 hours of implantation. However, in the case of Group B, in which degradation products of the material were injected, a large inflammatory response was observed after 24 hours. This indicates that the degradation products of the implant material induce an inflammatory response. Thus, the implant material will likely induce a more pronounced inflammatory response as it degrades. However, it is difficult to project how severe the inflammatory response to the material would be after six weeks of implantation of the whole discs versus that observed in Group B, as not all degradation products will be presented at once when the actual material degrades *in vivo*.

■

Summary

- Granulation tissue generally develops several days after an injury. It is characterized histologically by a pebbly, granular appearance due to the sprouting of many vascular buds from existing blood vessels in a process called angiogenesis.
- The foreign body reaction to an implant involves the action of elements of granulation tissue and foreign body giant cells (multinucleated cells formed by the fusion of macrophages).
- Fibrous encapsulation is the final stage of healing in response to nondegradable implants. It involves the maturation of granulation tissue and formation of a fibrous capsule surrounding the implant. The degree of capsule formation can be influenced by the degree of original injury during implantation, the amount of subsequent cell death, the type of material implanted, and the location of the implant.
- Chronic inflammation has a less uniform histological appearance than acute inflammation/fibrous encapsulation, and it is characterized by the presence of lymphocytes, plasma cells, and, in some cases, granulomas.
- There are four primary types of resolution to the inflammatory and wound healing response following injury and/or implantation: extrusion, resorption, integration, and encapsulation. Extrusion involves the foreign material being forced out of the body. Resorbable implants disappear with time and may or may not involve the formation of a fibrous capsule. Integration involves the close approximation of the native tissue to the implant, with no intervening fibrous capsule. Encapsulation entails the fibrous encapsulation of the material, but does not include chronic inflammation. The intended application of the material determines if the generated response is a success or failure.
- Wound repair can be achieved through either tissue repair or tissue regeneration. In tissue repair, the defect is replaced by scar tissue, which may have different structure, biochemical composition, and/or mechanical properties from the native tissue. In tissue regeneration, the defect is replaced by tissue identical to that which was there prior to the wound. Normal repair or regeneration of wounds cannot be fully completed in the presence of a nondegradable implant material, as the capsule around the material remains and is not remodeled.
- Due to the complex interplay of cells and signaling molecules involved, the inflammatory response and biocompatibility associated with a biomaterial is often assessed through *in vivo* studies using appropriate animal models. Examination of the inflammatory response is only one of a number of tests required for determination of biocompatibility.
- Design of *in vivo* experiments should consider the type of animal, location of implant site, length of study, dose and administration of the biomaterial, inclusion of proper controls, and methods of assessment.
- The material can be assessed following explantation by a variety of means, including histology, immunohistochemistry, electron microscopy (TEM and/or SEM), biochemical assays, and mechanical testing.

Problems

11.1 List the stages of wound healing after biomaterial implantation.

11.2 List the differences in the tissue response at the wound site following implantation of a nondegradable biomaterial as compared to a simple lesion.

11.3 You have been instructed to design the outer case for an implantable cardioverter–defibrillator, a device that attempts to halt the progression of ventricular fibrillation. What material structure and surface properties can influence the level of the foreign body giant cell response, and what is the effect of each?

11.4 What type of resolution response occurs with each of the following?

(a) Splinter
(b) Degradable tissue engineering scaffold
(c) Titanium bone screw
(d) Degradable meniscal arrow (used to repair meniscal tears)
(e) Breast implant
(f) Artificial heart valve leaflet
(g) Catheter
(h) Surface scar tissue (scab)
(i) Coral implant for bone repair

11.5 Is tissue regeneration necessary to repair a defect?

11.6 The company you work for has developed a modified poly(urethane) material for a potential vascular graft application. You have been instructed to examine the body's inflammatory response to the material and determine whether an implant can be created such that the inflammatory response would not hinder the implant's function. What experiment would you conduct to characterize the inflammatory response to the material and to evaluate its suitability for this application?

11.7 A new polymeric material was being considered for use as part of a drug delivery system. In order to evaluate the tissue response to the implantation of the material, nonporous compositions in the form of a disc were implanted subcutaneously in an animal model for 4 weeks. Describe the host response to the implantation of the material as a function of time as well as any potential adverse effects.

11.8 Your company has just developed an electrode to be implanted in the brain to measure electrical activity in terms of electrical current. After implantation in a rat brain *in vivo*, you record the following results as indicated by the solid line (A) below.

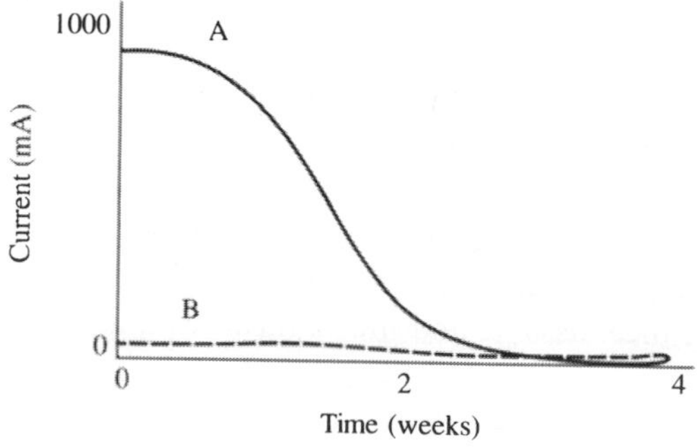

(a) Formulate a mechanism to explain these observations.
(b) After implanting an electrode with its surface modified by covalent attachment of poly(ethylene glycol) in the rat brain, you obtain the data shown by the dashed line above (line B). Why does the surface modification of the electrode alter the results? Would you recommend marketing the surface modified electrode?

References

1. Anderson, J.M. "Mechanisms of Inflammation and Infection with Implanted Devices," *Cardiovascular Pathology*, vol. 2, pp. 33S–41S, 1993.
2. Jeffery, D.L., D.P. Dressler, J.M. Anderson, and M.J. Gallagher. "Hemostatic and Healing Studies of Sodium Amylose Succinate (Ip760)," *Journal of Biomedical Materials Research*, vol. 16, pp. 51–61, 1982.
3. Suggs, L.J., M.S. Shive, C.A. Garcia, J.M. Anderson, and A.G. Mikos. "*In Vitro* Cytotoxicity and *In Vivo* Biocompatibility of Poly(Propylene Fumarate-Co-Ethylene Glycol) Hydrogels," *Journal of Biomedical Materials Research*, vol. 46, pp. 22–32, 1999.
4. Schmalzried, T.P., M. Jasty, A. Rosenberg, and W.H. Harris. "Histologic Identification of Polyethylene Wear Debris Using Oil Red O Stain," *Journal of Applied Biomaterials*, vol. 4, pp. 119–125, 1993.
5. Cadee, J.A., M.J. van Luyn, L.A. Brouwer, J.A. Plantinga, P.B. van Wachem, C.J. de Groot, W. den Otter, and W.E. Hennink. "*In Vivo* Biocompatibility of Dextran-Based Hydrogels," *Journal of Biomedical Materials Research*, vol. 50, pp. 397–404, 2000.
6. Martinez-Hernandez, A. "Repair, Regeneration, and Fibrosis," in *Pathology*, E. Rubin and J.L. Farber, Eds., 2nd ed. Philadelphia: J.B. Lippincott, 1994.
7. Anderson, J.M. and F.J. Schoen. "*In Vivo* Assessment of Tissue Compatibility." In *Biomaterials Science: An Introduction to Materials in Medicine*, B.D. Ratner, A.S. Hoffman, F.J. Schoen, and J.E. Lemons, Eds., 2nd ed. San Diego: Elsevier Academic Press, pp. 360–367, 2004.
8. ASTM F763-99, *Standard Practice for Short-Term Screening of Implant Materials*, ASTM International.
9. ASTM F1904-98e1, *Standard Practice for Testing the Biological Responses to Particles* In Vivo, ASTM International.
10. ASTM F1983-99, *Standard Practice for Assessment of Compatibility of Absorbable/Resorbable Biomaterials for Implant Applications*, ASTM International.
11. ASTM F981-04, *Standard Practice for Assessment of Compatibility of Biomaterials for Surgical Implants with Respect to Effect of Materials on Muscle and Bone*, ASTM International.
12. Spector, M. and P.A. Lalor. "*In Vivo* Assessment of Tissue Compatibility." In *Biomaterials Science: An Introduction to Materials in Medicine*, B.D. Ratner, A.S. Hoffman, F.J. Schoen, and J.E. Lemons, Eds., 1st ed. San Diego: Elsevier Academic Press, pp. 220–228, 1996.
13. Marchant, R., A. Hiltner, C. Hamlin, A. Rabinovitch, R. Slobodkin, and J.M. Anderson. "*In Vivo* Biocompatibility Studies. I. The Cage Implant System and a Biodegradable Hydrogel," *Journal of Biomedical Materials Research*, vol. 17, pp. 301–325, 1983.
14. Peppas, N.A., and R. Langer. "New Challenges in Biomaterials," *Science*, vol. 263, pp. 1715–1720, 1994.

Additional Reading

Bhat, S.V. *Biomaterials.* Boston: Kluwer Academic Publishers, 2002.

Black, J. *Biological Performance of Materials: Fundamentals of Biocompatibility*, 4th ed. New York: CRC Press, 2005.

Clark, R.A.F. and A.J. Singer. "Wound Repair: Basic Biology to Tissue Engineering." In *Principles of Tissue Engineering*, R.P. Lanza, R. Langer, and J. Vacanti, Eds., 2nd ed. Austin: Academic Press, pp. 857–878, 2000.

Dee, K.C., D.A. Puleo, and R. Bizios. *An Introduction to Tissue-Biomaterial Interactions.* Hoboken: Wiley-Liss, 2002.

Jenney, C.R. and J.M. Anderson. "Alkylsilane-Modified Surfaces: Inhibition of Human Macrophage Adhesion and Foreign Body Giant Cell Formation." *Journal of Biomedical Materials Research*, vol. 46, pp. 11–21, 1999.

Kuby, J. *Immunology*, 3rd ed. New York: W.H. Freeman, 1997.

Matthews, B.D., G. Mostafa, A.M. Carbonell, C.S. Joels, K.W. Kercher, C. Austin, H.J. Norton, and B.T. Heniford. "Evaluation of Adhesion Formation and Host Tissue Response to Intra-Abdominal Polytetrafluoroethylene Mesh and Composite Prosthetic Mesh," *The Journal of Surgical Research*, vol. 123, pp. 227–234, 2005.

Silver, F.H. *Biomaterials, Medical Devices, and Tissue Engineering: An Integrated Approach*. New York: Chapman and Hall, 1994.

Silver, F.H. and D.L. Christiansen. *Biomaterials Science and Biocompatibility*. New York: Springer, 1999.

Yannas, I.V. "Synthesis of Tissues and Organs," *Chembiochem*, vol. 5, pp. 26–39, 2004.

Immune Response to Biomaterials

CHAPTER 12

Main Objective

To understand the steps involved in and the results of stimulation of the acquired immune response and the complement cascade after biomaterial implantation.

Specific Objectives

1. To distinguish between humoral and cellular immunity.
2. To understand the process of antigen presentation in the immune response, including the roles of antigens, haptens and adjuvants.
3. To understand the steps of lymphocyte maturation and of expansion of clonal populations.
4. To understand the characteristics and functions of antibodies.
5. To compare and contrast actions of stimulated B and T cells.
6. To distinguish between the roles of different types of T cells.
7. To understand the steps involved in the complement cascade and potential interactions with the inflammatory and acquired immune responses.
8. To understand the effects of activation of the complement system and its regulation.
9. To distinguish among the four types of allergic responses and understand which are of major concern for biomaterials development.
10. To understand the concepts behind and possible limitations to the *in vitro* and *in vivo* techniques presented.

12.1 Introduction: Overview of Acquired Immunity

The previous few chapters have described the innate (nonspecific) response to an implanted material. However, it is also possible that the body could respond to specific portions of the biomaterial (or proteins adsorbed on the biomaterial). This is the **acquired immune response**, and is mediated by lymphocytes circulating constantly in the blood and tissues.

In terms of the acquired immune response, of most concern to the biomaterialist is the issue of immunotoxicity. **Immunotoxicity** is a broad term that refers to adverse effects on the function of the immune system or other body systems as a result of alterations in immune system function [1]. For example, both allergies (immune system dysfunction) and autoimmune diseases (destruction of other tissues due to the immune system attacking "self" cells) have developed after biomaterial implantations. The acquired immune response to tissue-engineered products, which contain a mixture of materials and possibly foreign cells or proteins, is especially complex and should be a design criterion for these devices. In order to mitigate potentially immunotoxic responses to such products, we must first understand the basics of the structure of the acquired immune response, the focus of the first part of this chapter. Material hypersensitivity (allergy) is discussed later in the chapter.

The acquired immune response is adaptive and has four characteristics [2]:

1. Specificity
2. Diversity
3. Self/nonself recognition
4. Immunologic memory

There are two types of acquired immunity, humoral and cellular. **Humoral immunity** is based on the actions of antibodies against foreign substances. It plays a large role in the response to foreign agents such as bacteria. In contrast, **cellular immunity** utilizes specialized lymphocytes (T cells) and its primary function is in the detection of altered self cells (such as from viral infections or cancer).

The specificity of acquired immunity comes from the fact that lymphocytes (B and T cells) involved in an immune reaction are activated in response to antigens. An **antigen** is a substance (usually foreign and having a molecular weight greater than 8,000 Da) that binds specifically to an **antibody** (an **immunoglobulin** glycoprotein) or **T cell receptor (TCR)** to initiate the acquired immune response. The specific site on the antigen recognized by the antibody is an **epitope** (or antigenic determinant). Antigens may have multiple epitopes that each bind the antibody or TCR.

Other substances frequently encountered when discussing acquired immunity, in particular with respect to the role of biomaterials in the immune response, are haptens and adjuvants. A **hapten** is a low molecular weight substance that combines with a larger molecule (such as a protein) to produce a much greater immune response than to either the hapten or carrier alone. Upon second exposure, some antibodies may react against the hapten even without the presence of the carrier molecule. This is important in the immune response to metallic implants, as discussed later in the chapter. An **adjuvant** is a substance that non-specifically enhances the immune response to antigens, possibly by increasing their uptake by phagocytic cells or prolonging the time the antigen remains in the body.

12.2 Antigen Presentation and Lymphocyte Maturation

12.2.1 Major Histocompatibility Complex (MHC) Molecules

12.2.1.1 MHC Class I The first step in the acquired immune response is recognition of the antigen. To be recognized, in many cases, the antigen must be displayed together with a **major histocompatibility complex** (MHC) *Class I* or *Class II* molecule. The MHC is a genetic complex with multiple genes that encode for Class I and II molecules. As shown in Fig. 12.1, **Class I** molecules are transmembrane glycoproteins that are found on almost all nucleated cells in conjunction with a smaller protein, β2-macroglobulin. An MHC Class I molecule is composed of two noncovalently associated chains (α and β). The distal end of the α chain forms a cleft to interact with the antigen, although it is not

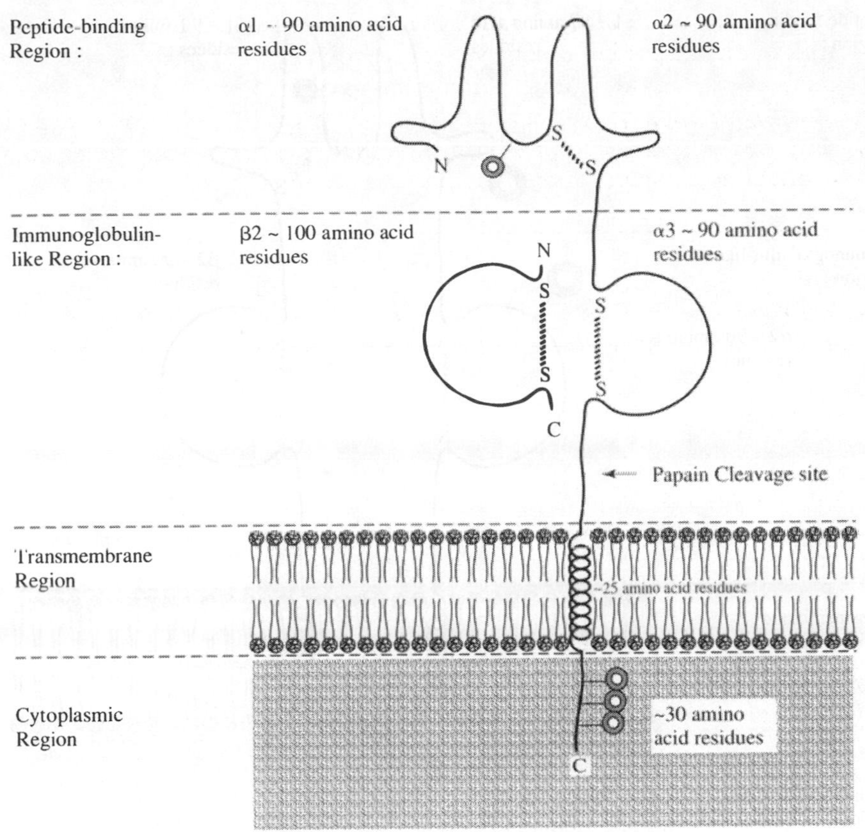

Figure 12.1
Schematic of major histocompatibility complex Class I molecule. Class I molecules are transmembrane glycoproteins that are found on almost all nucleated cells in conjunction with a smaller protein, β2-macroglobulin. A MHC Class I molecule is composed of two non-covalently associated chains (α and β). The cleft between the α_1 and α_2 portions interacts with the antigen, though this is not as specific as the binding sites for antibodies and T cell receptors. (Adapted with permission from [3].)

as specific as the binding sites for antibodies and T cell receptors. MHC Class I molecules are recognized by a subset of T cells (T cytotoxic or T_c cells).

12.2.1.2 MHC Class II MHC Class II molecules are also transmembrane glycoproteins having α and β chains (Fig. 12.2). In this case, the distal ends of both chains form the antigen-binding cleft, which has similar affinity for the antigen as MHC Class I molecules. As depicted in Fig. 12.3, MHC Class II molecules are recognized by a different subset of T cells (T helper or T_h cells) than Class I molecules. Also in contrast to Class I molecules, Class II molecules are only found on **antigen-presenting cells (APCs)**. APCs express MHC Class II molecules on their membranes and are able to deliver the co-stimulatory signal necessary for activation of T_h cells (see below for a more in-depth discussion of T cell activation). They include macrophages (a major point of interaction between the innate and acquired immune system), B lymphocytes, and dendritic cells.

12.2.1.3 MHC Molecule Variation and Tissue Typing It has been found that genes in three regions (**loci**) code for MHC Class I molecules, and genes in three different loci code for MHC Class II molecules. Because an individual inherits genes from both parents for each locus, each person has multiple types of MHC molecules present on the surface of his or her cells. However, MHC molecules not corresponding to any within the body (**non-self** molecules) are recognized and produce a primarily cell-based immune response. This is a main cause of organ rejection in transplant recipients. To counteract this, tissue typing is performed to determine how similar the MHC molecules are between the host and donor. The more similar the MHC molecules, the lower the chance of donor tissue rejection.

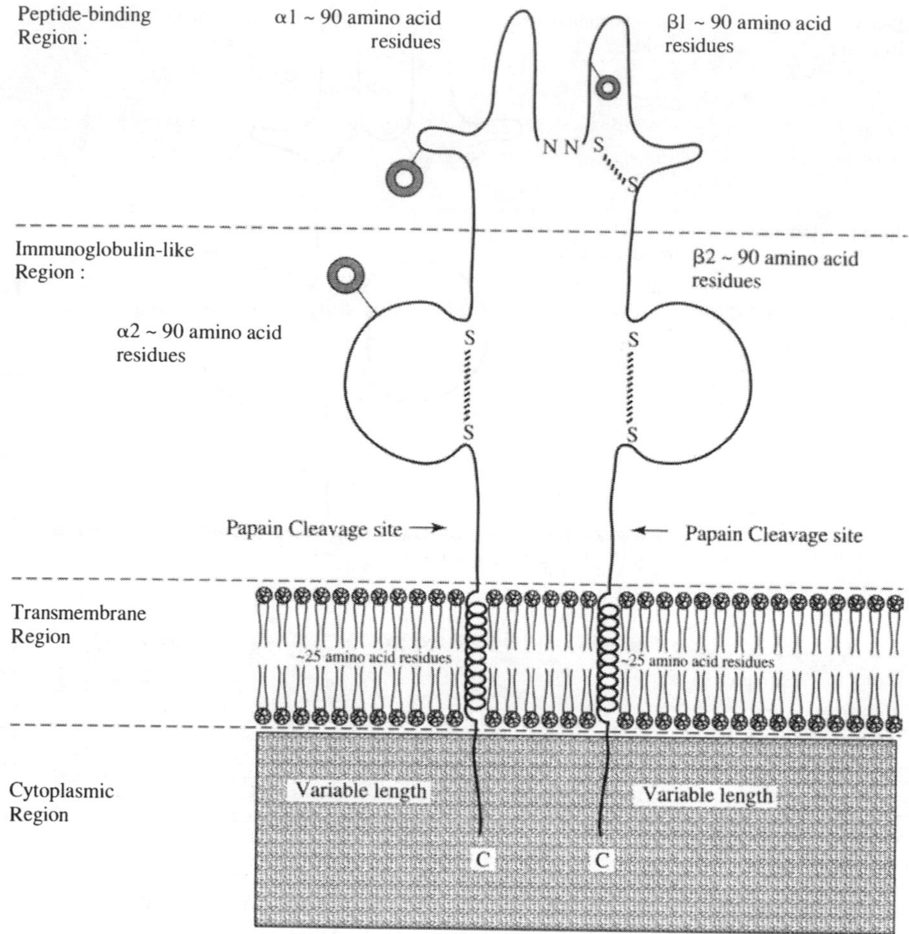

Figure 12.2
Schematic of a major histocompatibility complex Class II molecule. Class II molecules are transmembrane glycoproteins having α and β chains and are found only on antigen-presenting cells. The distal ends of both chains form the antigen-binding cleft, which has similar affinity for the antigen as MHC Class I molecules. (Adapted with permission from [3].)

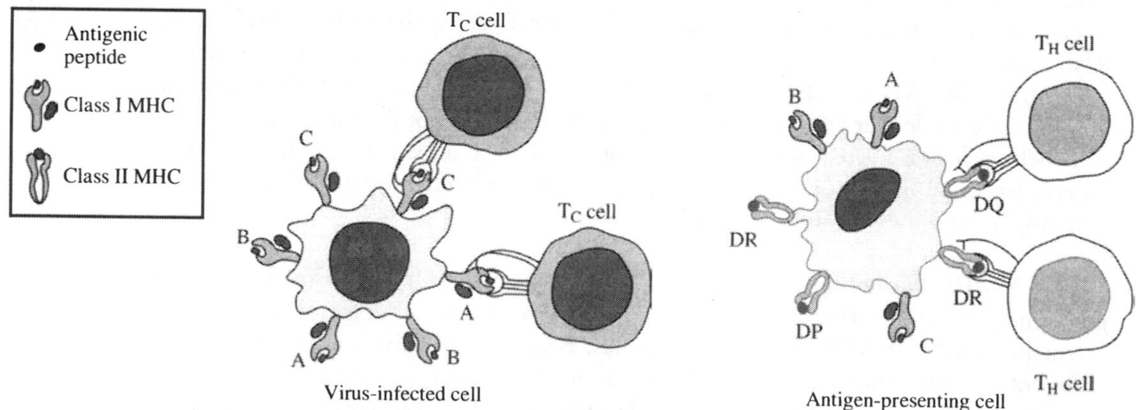

Figure 12.3
Recognition of MHC molecules by T cells. MHC Class I molecules are encoded by A, B, and C loci in humans and are recognized by T cytotoxic cells (T_c cells). MHC Class II molecules are encoded by DP, DQ, and DR loci in humans and are recognized by a different subset of T cells (T_h cells). Class II molecules are only found on antigen-presenting cells (APCs). (Adapted with permission from [2].)

EXAMPLE PROBLEM 12.1

A common treatment for bone defects is the introduction of bone grafts from either a donor site within the same patient (autograft) or a cadaver (allograft). In the case of an autograft, the bone is usually implanted with minimal processing following harvest. However, cadaver bone is generally subjected to stringent processing before implantation. One typical goal of the processing is to decellularize the bone graft. From an immunological point of view, why would removal of the cells from the allograft bone prior to implantation be important?

Solution: Rejection of grafts is generally mediated through a cellular immune response to MHC molecules present on the graft cells that are recognized as antigens by the host. Tissue typing should be performed to ensure similarity of MHC molecules between the donor and the recipient prior to implantation, if a graft is to contain cells. Otherwise, dissimilar MHC molecules present on the cells of the graft may be recognized as foreign by the host immune cells and induce a cellular immune response that can lead to graft rejection and ultimate failure of the treatment. ■

12.2.1.4 Intracellular Complexation with MHC Molecules Before extracellular presentation by MHC Class I or Class II molecules, antigens must first be processed intracellularly, where they complex with the appropriate MHC molecule, as depicted in Fig. 12.4. **Endogenous antigens**, or those resident within a host cell, such as viral proteins or proteins produced in cancerous cells, are first degraded into peptide fragments in the cytoplasm. At this point, they are free to bind to MHC Class I molecules in the rough endoplasmic reticulum. The antigen-MHC Class I complex is then transported to the cell membrane.

Exogenous antigens are produced outside the host cell and enter through phagocytosis [Fig. 12.4 (b)]. They are degraded into peptide fragments during endocytosis

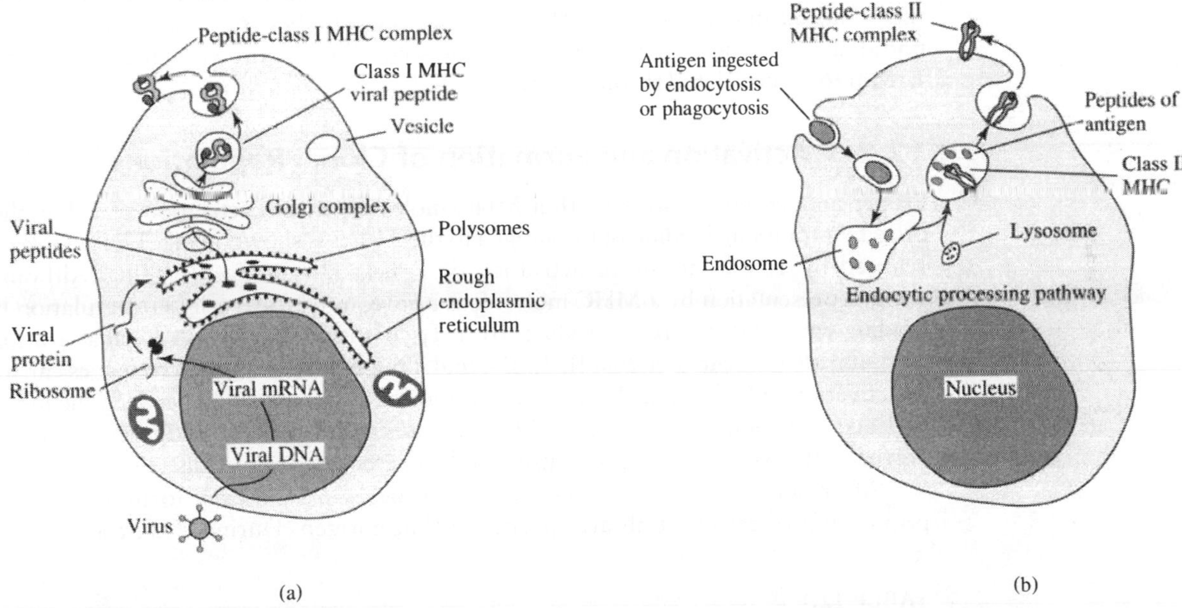

Figure 12.4
Intracellular processing of antigens. (a) Endogenous antigens, such as proteins produced in cancerous cells or viral proteins, are first degraded into peptide fragments in the cytoplasm. At this point, they are free to bind to MHC Class I molecules in the rough endoplasmic reticulum. The antigen-MHC Class I complex is then transported to the cell membrane. (b) Exogenous antigens are produced outside the host cell and enter through phagocytosis. They are degraded during endocytosis and the fragments bind to MHC Class II molecules in the endocytotic vesicles. The antigen-MHC Class II complex is then transported to the cell membrane. (Adapted with permission from [2].)

and the fragments bind to MHC Class II molecules in the endocytotic vesicles. The antigen-MHC Class II complex is then transported to the cell membrane. Exogenous antigens are the type more commonly formed as a direct result of biomaterial implantation, whereas endogenous antigens may be produced after alteration of a native cell due to toxic or carcinogenic properties of the biomaterial (see Chapter 14 for a more complete discussion of malignant transformations).

12.2.2 Maturation of Lymphocytes

There are two main types of lymphocytes that respond to antigens to produce the acquired immune response: B cells and T cells. B cells are mediators of humoral immunity and produce highly specific antibodies. T cells (T_c and T_h) are involved in cellular immunity and also produce proteins with high specificity, the T cell receptors (TCRs). Unlike antibodies, which can be released into the surrounding environment, TCRs remain bound to the cell membrane. A single lymphocyte possesses on the order of 10,000 antibodies/TCRs on its surface, all of which bind to the same antigen. However, each cell is reactive toward a different antigen, as determined by the rearrangement during cellular development of genes that encode for the antibody/TCR. The formation of antibodies and TCRs are examples of how the acquired immune system achieves its high specificity, while gene rearrangement in each cell provides immunologic diversity.

B cells are formed and processed in bone marrow, and further maturation occurs in the peripheral lymphoid tissues (lymph nodes and spleen). In contrast, T cells are formed in the bone marrow and mature in the thymus. After each cell expresses its specific antibody/TCR, it is exposed to "self" antigens during processing. Those cells that bind these antigens undergo apoptosis (up to 90% of cells generated), which prevents the production of cells that react against the body's own tissues. This process produces the self/nonself recognition that is critical to the proper function of the acquired immune system. After maturation, lymphocytes migrate to the lymphoid tissues, where they may remain for some time or directly enter the bloodstream to be circulated throughout the body.

12.2.3 Activation and Formation of Clonal Populations

Proper antigen presentation (with a MHC molecule) causes activation of T lymphocytes by promoting binding of the antigen to the TCR. As shown in Fig. 12.5, cytokines released by T_h cells aid in the activation of T_c cells after antigen binding. Although antigen presentation by a MHC molecule is not required for B cells, costimulation by binding with and/or secreted products from T_h cells is needed for full B cell activation. It should also be reiterated that IL-1, IL-6 and TNF-α secreted by macrophages can aid in activation of both B and T cells, thus promoting communication between the innate and acquired immune responses. Table 12.1 summarizes some of the cytokines involved in the wound healing response and their respective target cells.

After activation, the lymphocyte undergoes rapid mitosis, forming a clonal population of cells that all are specific to that antigen. During this process, both

TABLE 12.1

Cytokines in the Wound Healing Response

Cytokine Source	Cytokine Target	Specific Cytokines in this Response
Inflammatory Cells	Inflammatory Cells	IL-1, IL-8, MIP, TNF-α, TGF-β
Inflammatory Cells	Lymphocytes	IL-1, IL-6, TNF-α
Lymphocytes	Lymphocytes	IL-2, IL-4, IL-5, IL-6, TGF-β
Lymphocytes	Inflammatory Cells	IL-8, MIP, TGF-β

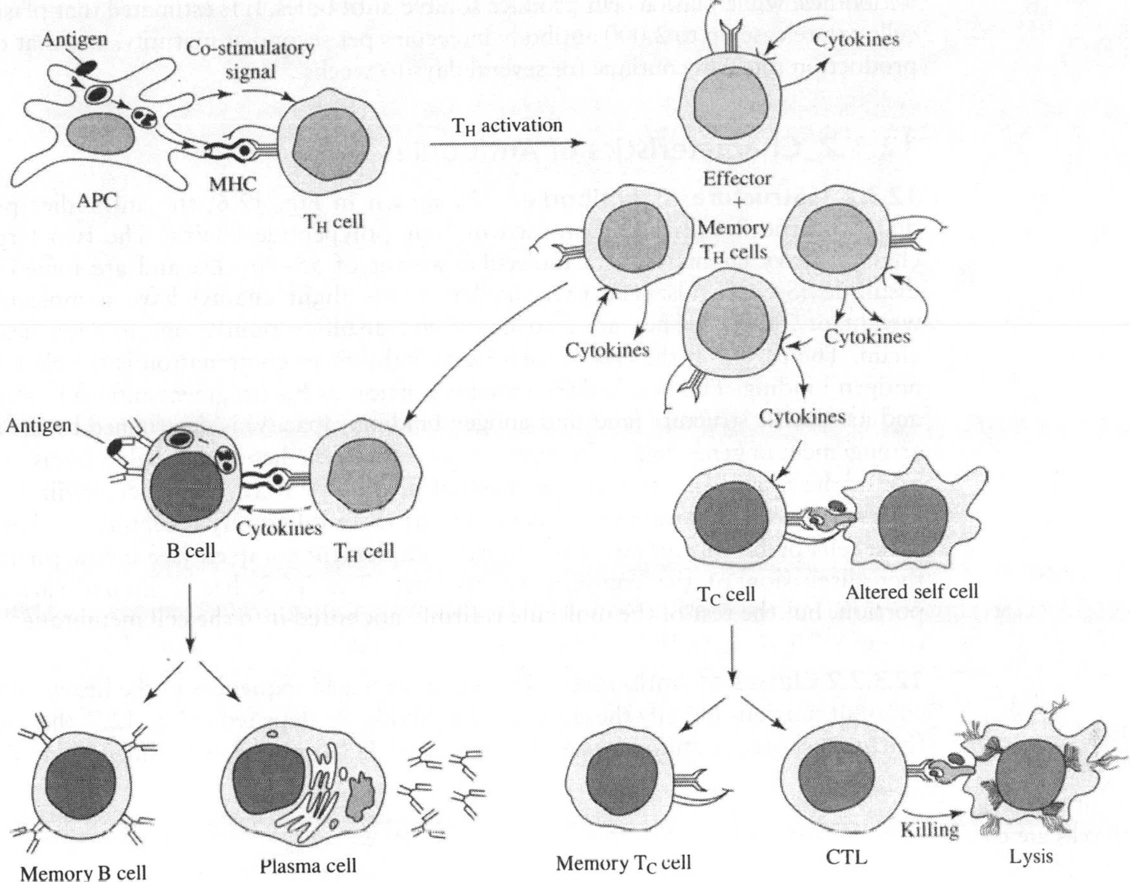

Figure 12.5
Interactions between T_h and other cell types in development of the immune response. Proper antigen presentation (with a Class II MHC molecule) causes activation of T_h lymphocytes by promoting binding of the antigen to the T cell receptor. T_c cells and B cells can also bind to the antigen, depending on the properties of the antigen and how it is presented. Cytokines released by T_h cells aid in the activation of T_c cells after antigen binding. Similarly, co-stimulation by binding with and/or secreted products from T_h cells is needed for full B cell activation after binding to the antigen. After activation, B and T_c cells undergo rapid mitosis, forming a clonal population of cells all specific to that antigen. During this process, both effector cells (cytotoxic T lymphocytes (CTLs) or plasma cells) and memory cells are created. (Adapted with permission from [2].)

effector cells and **memory cells** are created. Memory cells have longer lifetimes (up to years) than effector cells, but maintain their specificity for the given antigen. The existence of these cells causes a more rapid and heightened response if the body is exposed to the same antigen for a second time. It is through the production of both memory B and T cells that the acquired immune system's characteristic memory is achieved.

12.3 B Cells and Antibodies

12.3.1 Types of B Cells

As mentioned above, unlike T cells, B cells do not require antigen presentation by MHC molecules for activation. Once activated by both antigen binding and a stimulatory signal provided by T_h cells, they proliferate to form memory B cells and effector cells called **plasma cells** (Fig. 12.5). Memory cells express membrane-bound antibodies, while plasma cells produce soluble antibodies. It is estimated that plasma cells can release up to 2,000 antibody molecules per second at maturity, and that this production rate can continue for several days to weeks.

12.3.2 Characteristics of Antibodies

12.3.2.1 Structure of Antibodies As shown in Fig. 12.6, the antibodies produced by the B cells are composed of four polypeptide chains. The two larger chains (**heavy chains**) have a molecular weight of 55–70 kDa and are joined by disulfide (S–S) bonds. The two smaller chains (**light chains**) have a molecular weight of 24 kDa. They are also linked via disulfide bonds, one to each heavy chain. The region at the end of each heavy/light chain combination is the cleft for antigen binding. This is called the **variable portion** or $\mathbf{F_{ab}}$ (fragment antigen binding) and its specific structure (and thus antigen-binding capacity) is determined by the rearrangement of genes coding for amino acids in both the heavy and light chains. The rest of the molecule is termed the **constant portion** or $\mathbf{F_c}$ (fragment crystallizable). This section is responsible for recognition of the antibody by receptors in phagocytic cells or by certain molecules of the complement complex (see below for further discussion of the complement cascade). The TCR has a similar variable portion, but the rest of the molecule is firmly anchored into the cell membrane.

12.3.2.2 Classes of Antibodies Distinct amino acid sequences in the heavy-chain constant portions identify the **class** of the antibody. As depicted in Fig. 12.7, there are five main classes of antibodies, each named with Ig to abbreviate "immunoglobulin"

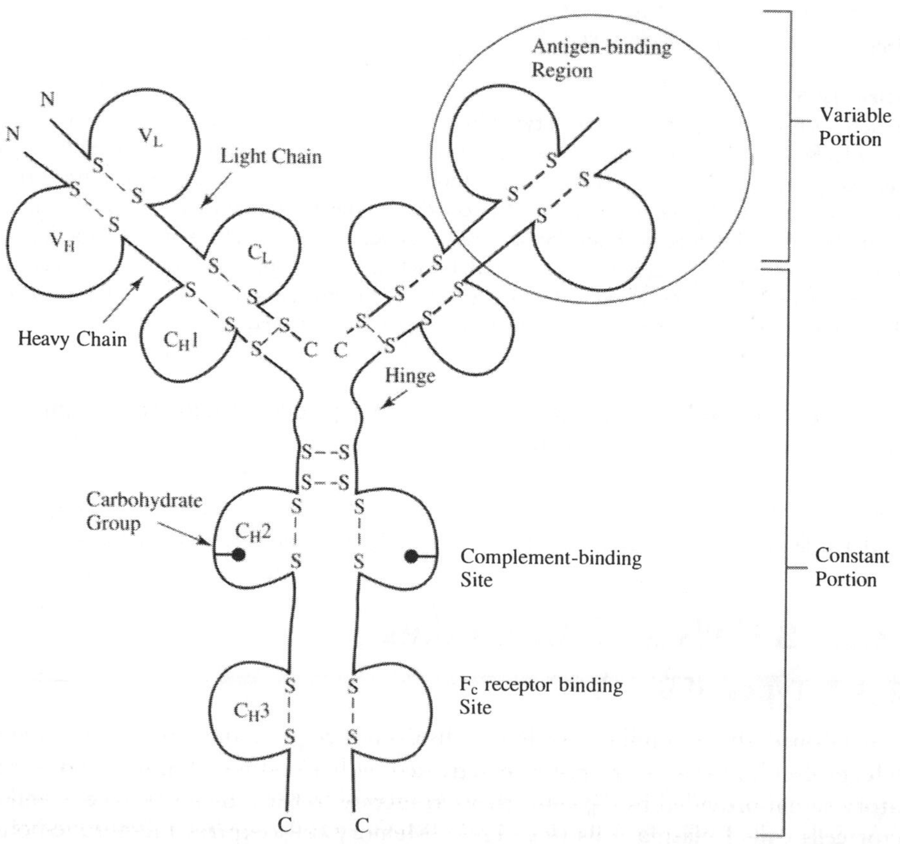

Figure 12.6
The structure of antibodies produced by B cells are composed of four polypeptide chains. The two larger chains (heavy chains) have a molecular weight of 55–70 kDa and are joined by disulfide (S–S) bonds. The two smaller chains (light chains) have a molecular weight of 24 kDa and are also linked via disulfide bonds, one to each heavy chain. The region at the end of each heavy/light chain combination is the cleft for antigen binding. This is called the variable portion and its specific structure (and thus antigen-binding capacity) is determined by the rearrangement of genes coding for amino acids in both the heavy and light chains. The rest of the molecule is termed the constant portion and is responsible for recognition of the antibody by receptors in phagocytic cells or by certain molecules of the complement complex. (Adapted with permission from [3].)

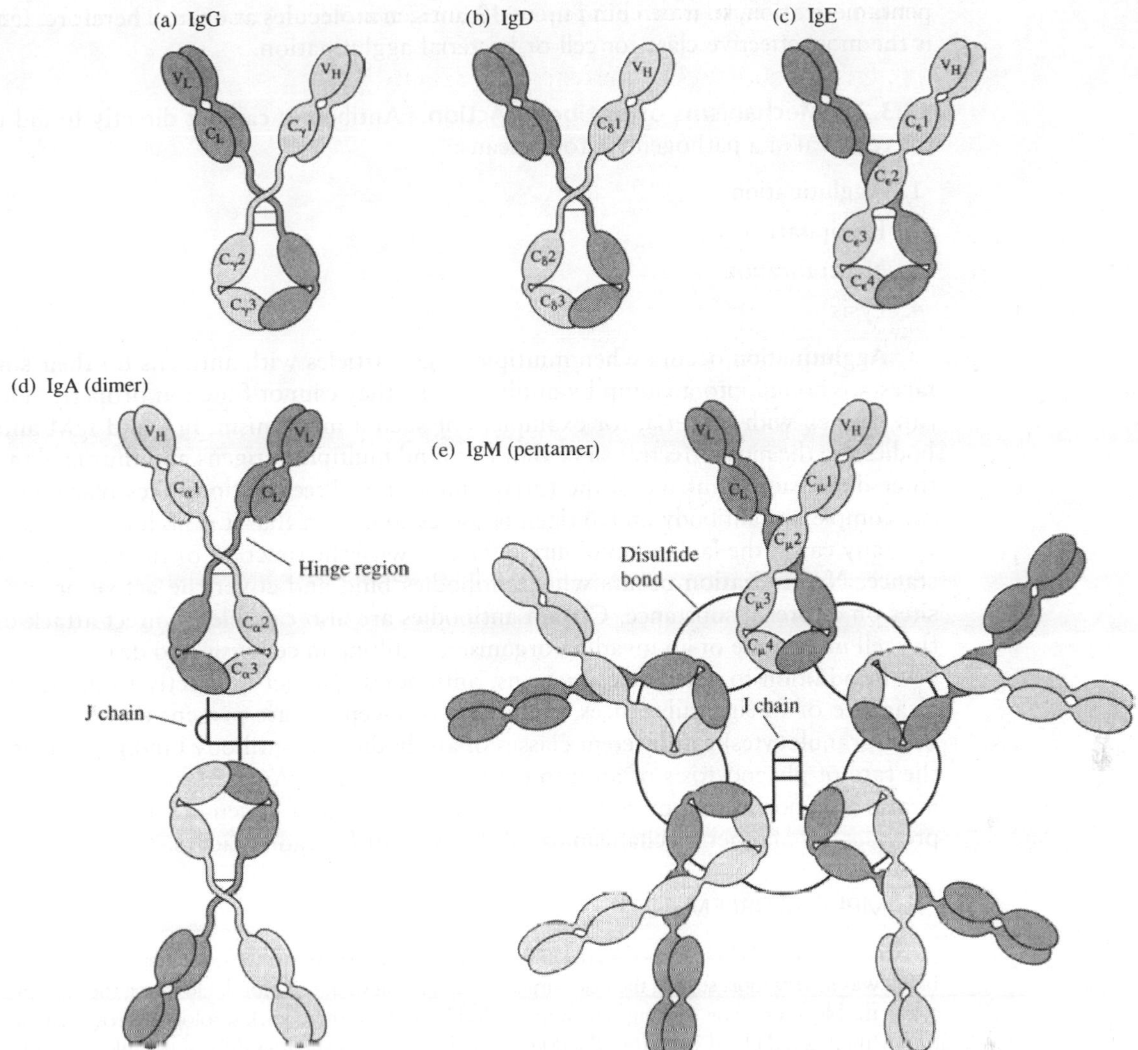

Figure 12.7
There are five main classes of antibodies, each named with Ig to signify "immunoglobulin" and then a capital letter indicating the class. (a–c) IgG, IgD, and IgE all possess the same general structure and have the capability to bind two antigen molecules simultaneously (one on each arm). (d) IgA has a similar structure to the other classes, but includes a J (joining) chain, which allows for dimerization. The dimer can then bind four antigen molecules at once. (e) IgM is characterized by the same general structure as the other antibody types, but its J chain allows for pentamerization, so it can bind up to 10 antigen molecules at once. (Adapted with permission from [2].)

and then a capital letter indicating the class. IgG, IgD and IgE all possess the same general structure for a generic antibody as described previously and have the capability to bind two antigen molecules simultaneously (one on each arm). IgG is the most prevalent antibody class, and composes about 75% of the antibodies in humans. The fraction of antibodies of the IgE type is much lower, but this class plays an important role in the allergic reaction, as discussed later. IgA has a similar structure to the other classes, but includes a J (joining) chain, which allows for dimerization. The dimer can then bind four antigen molecules at once, which can be important in *agglutination* reactions, as described below. IgM is characterized by the same general structure as the other antibody types, but its J chain allows for pentamerization, so it can bind up to 10 antigen molecules at once. Therefore, IgM is the most effective class for cell or bacterial agglutination.

12.3.2.3 Mechanisms of Antibody Action

Antibodies can act directly to aid in the removal of a pathogen via four means:

1. Agglutination
2. Precipitation
3. Neutralization
4. Lysis

Agglutination occurs when multiple large particles with antigens on their surfaces are bound into a clump by antibodies, so they cannot function properly. This can happen with bacteria, for example. For such a mechanism, IgA and IgM antibodies are the most effective since they can bind multiple antigens and thus facilitate three-dimensional linkage of the foreign molecules. **Precipitation** takes place when the complex of antibody and antigen becomes so large it that it is no longer soluble. In many cases, the lack of solubility interferes with the function of the foreign substance. **Neutralization** occurs when antibodies bind and cover the active or toxic sites on a foreign substance. Certain antibodies are also capable of direct attack on the cell membrane of an invading organism, resulting in cell **lysis** and death.

In addition to these direct actions, antibodies also act indirectly to aid in the clearance of foreign substances. A number of receptors are present on phagocytic cells (granulocytes) for different classes of antibodies, so antibody binding increases the rate of phagocytosis of antigen-containing particles. Antigen–antibody binding is also a major means of complement system activation (discussed below), which provides yet another mechanism to rid the body of foreign invaders.

EXAMPLE PROBLEM 12.2

A soldier in a battlefield sustained a critical injury and required a prompt blood transfusion. Although blood was in very short supply, the field surgeon found a unit of donor blood. However, the label indicating the blood type was missing. The surgeon decided to perform a quick serological cross-matching test by mixing red blood cells from the donor blood unit with a small sample of the injured soldier's serum. Through microscopic observation, the surgeon noted that small clumps of red blood cells were forming. Assuming that the clumping was not being caused by the clotting process, why might this clumping occur? Which antibody classes would most likely be involved? Should the donor blood unit be used in this patient, or should an alternate donor be found? Why or why not?

Solution: The clumping could be the result of agglutination of the red blood cells from the donor. Such agglutination would indicate that the serum of the injured soldier contained antibodies against proteins present on the surfaces of the donor red blood cells. As IgA and IgM are capable of forming dimers and pentimers, respectively, they would be the most effective antibody classes for agglutination. The donor blood unit should not be used in this patient, as it appears that the patient possesses antibodies against the donor blood. In the event that the donor blood was used, an immune response would ensue that would hinder the recovery of the patient. ■

12.4 T Cells

12.4.1 Types of T Cells

As indicated above, T cells require antigen presentation via a MHC complex to become activated. There are two main types of T cells: the helper T cell (T_h) and the cytotoxic T cell (T_c). T_h cells usually possess the surface glycoprotein **CD 4** and recognize antigens presented on MHC Class II molecules. In contrast, T_c cells generally possess the surface marker CD 8 and interact with antigens presented on MHC Class I molecules.

12.4.2 Helper T Cells (T_h)

T_h cells fulfill a key role in the acquired immune response—it is these cells that are destroyed in acquired immune deficiency syndrome (AIDS), with devastating effects. T_h cells become activated in response to antigen-MHC Class II complexes in combination with a co-stimulatory signal supplied by an APC. This co-stimulatory signal is usually the presence of B7-1 or B7-2 glycoproteins on the surface of the APC that can interact with specific receptors on the T_h cell (Fig. 12.8).

Once activated, these cells form a clonal population including effector and memory T_h cells (Fig. 12.5). Effector cells then secrete cytokines with a variety of actions (Table 12.1), including:

1. Stimulation of B cell growth and differentiation (result of IL-4, IL-5 and IL-6, among others).
2. Stimulation of T_c cell proliferation (see below) (result of IL-2 among others).
3. Further stimulation of T_h cell activation (result of IL-2 among others).
4. Promotion of chemotaxis and activation of macrophages (result of MIP, IL-8 among others). This is another example of how the acquired and innate immune systems work together to rid the body of foreign substances.

Activated T_h cells may also act directly by binding to B cells to stimulate the humoral response.

12.4.3 Cytotoxic T Cells (T_c)

As mentioned above, cytokines from T_h also act on T_c cells to encourage their activation and expansion into clonal populations including T_c memory cells and T_c effector cells called **cytotoxic T lymphocytes (CTLs)**. CTLs secrete perforins, which lyse cells by using mechanisms that are similar to the membrane attack complex of the complement system (discussed in the next section). The receptors on the surface of a CTL

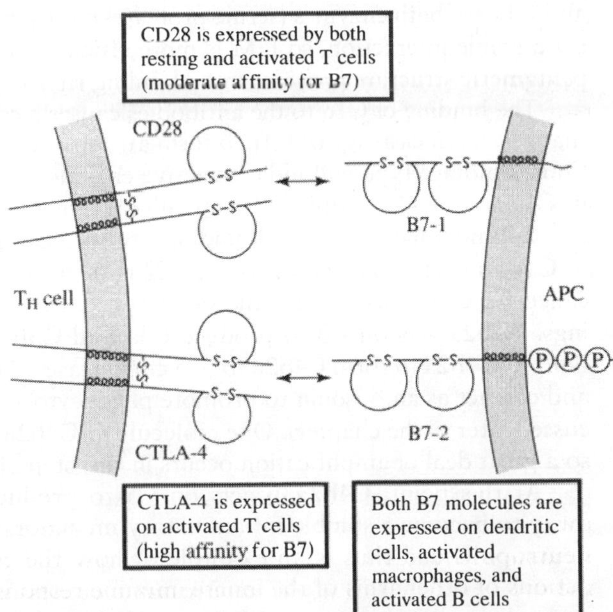

Figure 12.8
Activation of T_h cells. These cells become activated in response to antigen-MHC Class II complexes in combination with a co-stimulatory signal supplied by an antigen-presenting cell (APC). This co-stimulatory signal is usually the presence of B7-1 or B7-2 glycoproteins on the surface of the APC that can interact with specific receptors on the T_h cell. (Adapted with permission from [2] and [4].)

can disengage the antigen on a lysed cell and move to another cell, so they are very efficient at removing "altered self" cells. They are important for prevention of viral infection and cancer, and are the main mediators of graft/transplant rejection if MHC molecules are not sufficiently similar between donor and host. However, T_c cells generally play less of a role than T_h cells in potential acquired immune responses to biomaterials.

12.5 The Complement System

The complement system is actually a part of innate immunity, but it is discussed in this chapter since it is highly interrelated with the acquired immune response. The **complement system** is composed of over 20 plasma proteins involved in a cascade that ultimately causes the elimination of foreign elements. Like the blood coagulation cascade discussed in the next chapter, there is much amplification in this process, resulting in a swift and decisive response. There are two means of complement activation, the **classical pathway** and **alternative pathway**, which converge to cause formation of the membrane attack complex to lyse foreign cells.

12.5.1 Classical Pathway

The main steps in complement activation via the **classical pathway** are depicted in Fig. 12.9. Although many biomaterials activate the complement cascade via the alternative pathway (discussed below), there is evidence that, in some cases, the classical pathway may be involved.

The classical pathway begins with the binding of an antibody (IgG or IgM class) to an antigen on a suitable target (such as a bacterial cell or biomaterial). The attachment of the antibody to the target induces a conformational change in the F_c portion that exposes the binding site for the complement protein C1. This is one important example of how the complement system interacts with the acquired immune response.

C1 is actually a complex of C1q and two molecules each of C1r and C1s (Fig. 12.10). C1q is composed of 18 polypeptide chains forming six arms, each of which can bind to the F_c portion of an antibody through its globular "heads." C1r and C1s are both enzymes (serine proteases). C1q must attach to at least two F_c sites for a stable interaction, so IgM is more efficient in complement activation since its pentameric structure provides more binding sites in close proximity.

The binding of C1q to the antibodies causes a conformational change in the C1r that results in cleavage of C1r to form an active enzyme, **C1r**. (In the following sections, boldface type will indicate active enzymes.) **C1r** then cleaves C1s to activate it. **C1s** acts on C4, forming C4a (smaller fragment) and C4b (larger fragment).

C4b now has an exposed binding site, and can attach to the target surface near to **C1s** and act as a receptor for C2. C2 is then cleaved by **C1s** to form **C4b2a** (also called C3 convertase), while the smaller fragment, C2b, diffuses into the surroundings. **C4b2a** acts on C3 to produce C3a and C3b. The larger fragment, C3b, can bind to **C4b2a** to form **C4b2a3b** (C5 convertase). Alternatively, it may diffuse away and can act as an opsonin to promote phagocytosis of foreign materials (this is discussed later in the chapter). One molecule of **C4b2a** can cleave many C3 molecules, so a great deal of amplification occurs in this step of the cascade.

At this point, **C4b2a3b** acts on C5 to produce C5a and C5b. C5a diffuses away to become a soluble inflammatory mediator. C5a is a chemotactic agent for neutrophils and thus is an example of how the complement system aids in the actions of other arms of the innate immune response. The other product, C5b, remains bound to the target surface and initiates formation of the membrane attack complex (described later in this chapter.)

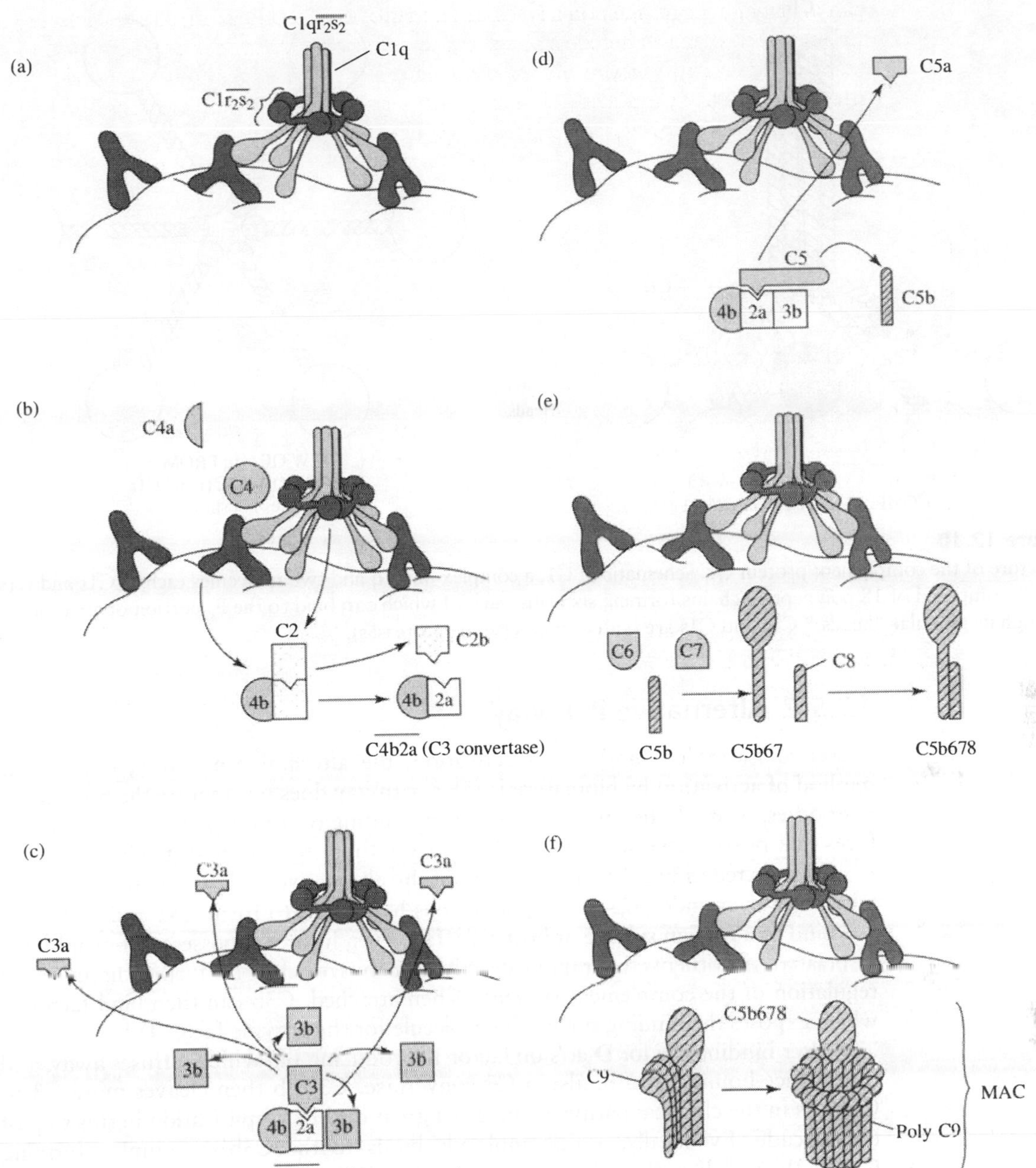

Figure 12.9
Main steps in complement activation via the classical pathway. (a–f) The classical pathway begins with the binding of an antibody (IgG or IgM class) to an antigen on a suitable target (such as a bacterial cell or biomaterial) (a). The attachment of the antibody to the target induces a conformational change, which causes a cascade of chemical reactions starting with the cleavage of C4 (b) and resulting in the formation of the membrane attack complex (MAC), which form pores with diameters of 70–100Å in the membrane (f). These pores allow continuous leakage of ions and small molecules out of the cell, so osmotic stability is impossible to maintain and the cell lyses. (Adapted with permission from [2].)

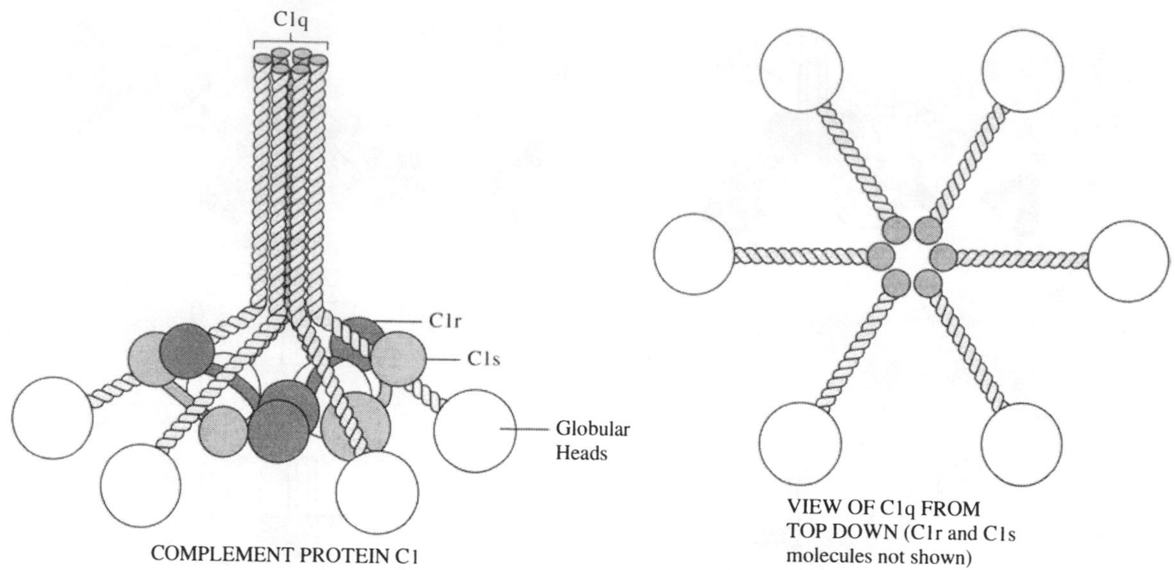

Figure 12.10
Structure of the complement protein C1. Schematic of C1, a complex of C1q and two molecules each of C1r and C1s. C1q is composed of 18 polypeptide chains forming six arms, each of which can bind to the F_c portion of an antibody through its globular "heads." C1r and C1s are both enzymes (serine proteases).

12.5.2 Alternative Pathway

A second means of complement activation, the **alternative pathway**, is the main method of activation by biomaterials. This pathway does not require the presence of antibodies. Instead, the cascade results from binding of complement proteins on surfaces that possess characteristics different from those found on host cells.

As depicted in Fig. 12.11, the origin of the alternative pathway is the serum protein C3, which undergoes slow spontaneous hydrolysis to form C3a and C3b. C3b can bind to a foreign surface or host cells. However, host cells possess cell-membrane-associated constituents that rapidly deactivate C3b (see below for further discussion of regulation of the complement system). When attached, C3b can then bind factor B, which exposes the binding site on this molecule for the enzyme **factor D.**[1]

After binding, **factor D** acts on factor B, producing Ba, which diffuses away, and the surface-bound **C3bBb**, also a C3 convertase. **C3bBb** then cleaves more C3 to C3b. As in the classical pathway, there is a great deal of amplification in this step of the cascade. Eventually, a C3b molecule binds to the **C3bBb** complex forming **C3bBb3b**, which is the C5 convertase of the alternative pathway. **C3bBb3b** then cleaves C5 to form C5b as in the classical pathway, thus initiating the formation of the membrane attack complex.

12.5.3 Membrane Attack Complex

Both the classical and alternative pathway result in the creation of C5b on the foreign surface. As depicted in Fig. 12.9, C5b provides a binding site for C6. C7 then binds to C5b6 and the complex undergoes a conformational transition that exposes hydrophobic regions for interaction with the phospholipid bilayer on the target cell. After the further

[1]Interestingly, there is evidence that the (fully intact) C3 molecule adsorbed to a biomaterial surface can also bind factor B, thus providing another means of alternative pathway activation, which is less easily controlled by the regulatory proteins discussed in the following sections.

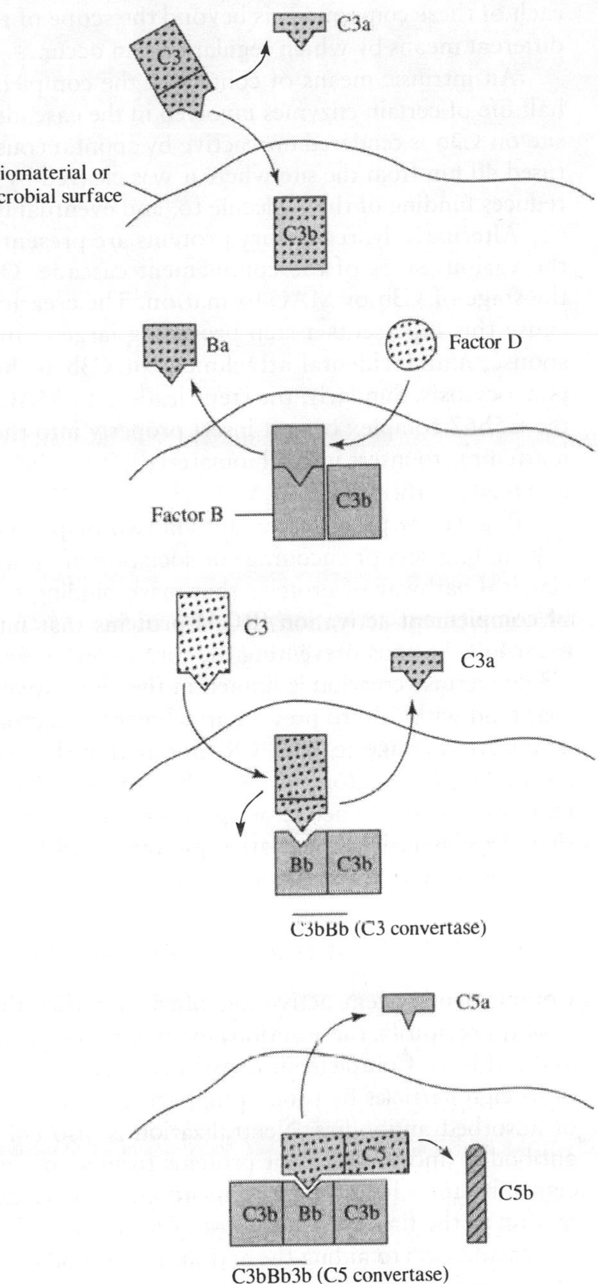

Figure 12.11 Complement activation via the alternative pathway. Serum protein C3 undergoes slow spontaneous hydrolysis to C3a and C3b, which commences a cascade that ends in the formation of **C3bBb3b**. **C3bBb3b** then cleaves C5 to form C5b as in the classical pathway, thus initiating the formation of the membrane attack complex (see Fig. 12.9). (Adapted with permission from [2].)

binding of C8, C5b678 inserts itself into the cell membrane, forming a small pore (diameter 10Å). The final step in the complement cascade is the binding and polymerization of C9 by C5b678. The C5b678 complex surrounded by the poly-C9 structure is termed the **membrane attack complex** (MAC) and it can form pores with diameters of 70–100Å. These pores allow continuous leakage of ions and small molecules out of the cell, so osmotic stability is impossible to maintain and the cell lyses.

12.5.4 Regulation of the Complement System

A plethora of molecules are involved in regulation of the complement cascade in order to confine its effects to a localized area and prevent host cells from being lysed by mechanisms intended to kill only foreign pathogens. A detailed discussion of each of these compounds is beyond the scope of this text. Instead, we will focus on different means by which regulation can occur.

An intrinsic means of control of the complement system is found in the short half life of certain enzymes involved in the cascade. For example, the target-binding site on C3b is rendered unreactive by spontaneous hydrolysis by the time it has diffused 40 nm from the site where it was cleaved by either of the C3 convertases. This reduces binding of the molecule to, and eventual lysis of, nearby host cells.

Alternatively, regulatory proteins are present to limit the actions that occur at the various steps of the complement cascade. Of these, many function at either the stage of C3b or MAC formation. The creation of C3b is tightly regulated because this represents a step providing large amplification of the complement response, and accidental attachment of C3b to host cells can cause their lysis or phagocytosis. Similarly, the steps leading to MAC formation are limited because if the C5b67 complex cannot insert properly into the target (such as may occur when it attempts to insert into a biomaterial), it can be released, attach to bystander cells, and mediate their lysis.

Regulatory proteins can act via two major mechanisms: they can compete for key binding sites or encourage dissociation of molecular complexes. Examples in the classical pathway of proteins that mask binding sites include a number of **regulator of complement activation (RCA) proteins** that bind with C4b to block its attachment to C2a, thus preventing the formation of the C3 convertase. In the same vein, C3 convertase creation is limited in the alternative pathway by other RCA proteins that bind with C3b to prevent attachment to factor B. Other regulatory proteins act at the MAC stage to bind C8, eliminating the assembly of the poly-C9 complex. Examples of regulatory proteins that affect molecular complexes include RCA proteins such as **decay-accelerating factor (DAF)**, which binds to C3 convertase in either the classical or alternative pathway and forces dissociation of the enzymatic component from the cell-bound component.

12.5.5 Effects of the Complement System

Complement system activation often amplifies the actions of antibodies. As discussed previously, these actions include agglutination, precipitation, neutralization, and cell lysis. Complement constituents, for example C3b, aid in the agglutination of foreign particles by promoting particle binding even with relatively low amounts of adsorbed antibodies. Neutralization is also enhanced when the combination of antibodies and complement proteins form a coating over the toxic sites of the foreign substance. In addition, as mentioned above, cell lysis is mediated via MAC formation as the final step in the complement cascade.

In addition to aiding the actions of antibodies, complement activation can stimulate another arm of innate immunity, the inflammatory response. In particular, C3a, C4a, and C5a bind to mast cells and basophils to induce the release of histamine and other agents from these cells (see the following section for further discussion). These molecules also cause smooth muscle cell contraction and an increase in vascular permeability, characteristic changes associated with inflammation (see Chapter 10). In addition, C3a, C5a, and the C5b67 complex promote chemotaxis of monocytes and neutrophils towards the site around the foreign agent. C3 has also been implicated in macrophage adhesion to poly(urethane) biomaterials.

Complement proteins act in concert with the inflammatory response in additional ways to encourage phagocytosis. In this case, the complement protein (mainly C3b) acts as an **opsonin**, and the foreign object is said to be **opsonized**. This process occurs when the C3b that is attached to the foreign surface binds to specific receptors on macrophages and neutrophils to facilitate uptake of the opsonized particle.

12.6 Undesired Immune Responses to Biomaterials

The previous sections of this chapter have explained the general response of the immune system to foreign surfaces derived either from nonself cells or proteins, or biomaterials. The acquired immune response is important to clear the body of pathogens; however, it can also have unwanted effects such as donor organ rejection, autoimmune disease, or allergies. Some of these undesired effects relating to biomaterials are discussed in this section.

12.6.1 Innate vs. Acquired Responses to Biomaterials

It is important to note that biomaterials themselves are rarely "rejected" like donor tissue. Since this phenomenon occurs primarily in response to foreign MHC molecules on cell surfaces, unless the biomaterials are carriers for foreign cells (as may be the case for some tissue engineering strategies), complete activation of the acquired immune system resulting in destruction of the implant is unlikely. This pertains even to naturally derived materials, since such materials often undergo treatments like freezing or gluteraldehyde fixation to reduce their antigenic character prior to implantation. Although the natural material may still possess sufficient foreign epitopes to activate the acquired immune system to some extent, this usually does not cause immediate destruction or resorption of the material.

Rather, the "immunocompatibility" of a biomaterial, particularly a synthetic biomaterial, often has more to do with its interaction with the nonspecific (innate) branch of the immune system. For example, complement activation by a biomaterial can lead to a continuing accumulation of inflammatory cells around the implant. While this is not "rejection," it can represent device failure in that the presence of inflammatory cells and/or a fibrous capsule may prevent integration of the implant with the surrounding tissue.

12.6.2 Hypersensitivity

However, sometimes another sort of undesired immune response mediated by the acquired immune system occurs, even with synthetic biomaterials. This is called the **hypersensitivity reaction** or **allergic reaction** and is defined as an unusual, excessive, or uncontrolled immune reaction. Allergies can be classified into four main groups (types I–IV), depending on the biological mechanism that causes the response.

12.6.2.1 Type I: IgE Mediated Type I hypersensitivity is caused by plasma cells (effector B cells) that secrete IgE molecules specific for the allergen (Fig. 12.12). The IgE molecules then bind to receptors on basophils and mast cells, resulting in sensitization of these cells. A second exposure to the antigen from the allergen causes crosslinking of these antibodies that are now membrane bound. This crosslinking provides a signal to induce degranulation of mast cells and the release of soluble mediators (e.g., histamine). These mediators then cause a number of localized and systemic effects, including vasodilation and smooth muscle cell contraction. Depending on its extent, this reaction can be fatal (e.g., allergy to peanuts or bee stings).

Type I reactions are the typical "allergic" response to environmental factors, such as ragweed pollen (known as "hay fever"). Documented cases of type I hypersensitivity to biomaterials are rare. However, it may be that an IgE-mediated response to metallic components could be generated if the patient was previously exposed to these compounds in the workplace, for example. Similarly, latex in latex examination gloves may produce a type I reaction in sensitized individuals. However, reports of type I hypersensitivity to silicone, as found in breast implants, remain controversial.

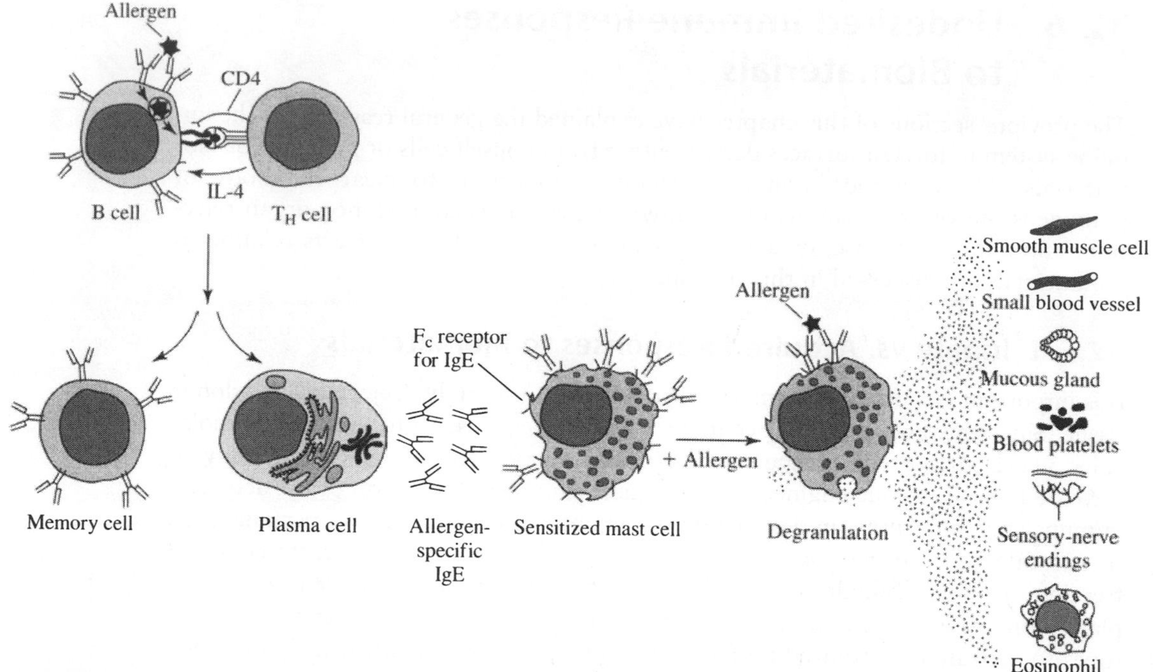

Figure 12.12

Type I hypersensitivity response. Type I hypersensitivity is caused by plasma cells (effector B cells) that secrete IgE molecules specific for the allergen. The IgE molecules bind to receptors on basophils and mast cells, resulting in sensitization of these cells. A second exposure to the antigen from the allergen causes crosslinking of these membrane-bound antibodies. This crosslinking provides a signal to induce degranulation of mast cells and the release of soluble mediators (e.g. histamine). These mediators cause a number of localized and systemic effects, including smooth muscle cell contraction and vasodilation. (Adapted with permission from [2].)

12.6.2.2 Type II: Antibody Mediated In type II reactions, generated antibodies work alone or in connection with the complement to destroy cells or platelets presenting a foreign antigen on their surface. A typical example of a type II reaction occurs when host cells respond to a mismatched blood type during blood transfusion. There are few documented cases of type II hypersensitivity to biomaterials.

12.6.2.3 Type III: Immune Complex Mediated Symptoms of type III reactions may appear days to weeks after original exposure to the antigen because, in this type of hypersensitivity, both antigen and antibody must be present in the tissue or circulation at the same time. When this occurs, a large number of immune complexes (antigen–antibody complexes) are precipitated within a localized area, or, if the antigen is present in the blood, systemically in blood vessel walls. The binding of the antigen and antibody encourages activation of the complement system, with the subsequent migration of phagocytic cells to the area. Much of the tissue damage in type III reactions results from the release of enzymes and other active substances by the recruited inflammatory cells. Type III reactions are the mechanism of action of autoimmune diseases such as lupus. This type of reaction may be a concern for biomaterial systems that are slowly degrading or involve slow drug release, but, in general, it is not a major cause of biomaterial hypersensitivity.

12.6.2.4 Type IV: T Cell Mediated Like type I reactions, type IV hypersensitivity reactions usually involve more than one exposure to the allergen. This response is also called **delayed-type hypersensitivity** since the symptoms can appear 24–72

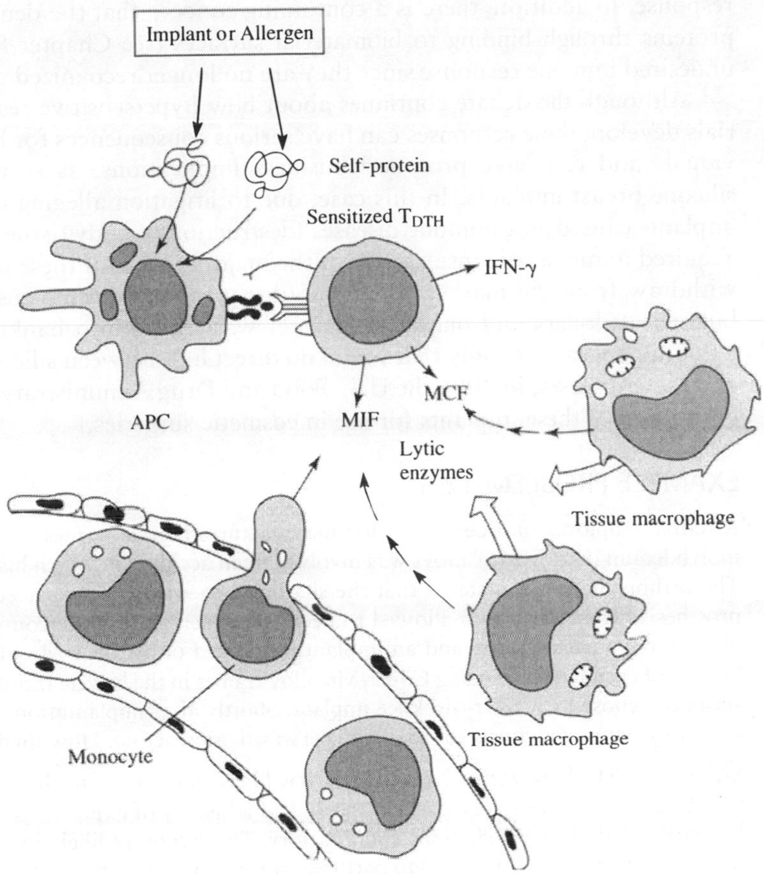

Figure 12.13 Diagram of a type IV hypersensitivity reaction. Specialized cells, T_{DTH} cells, are the main cause of the reaction. Upon first exposure to the antigen presented on an APC, T_h cells become sensitized and mature into T_{DTH} cells. Further exposure causes the activation of the T_{DTH} cells and secretion of cytokines to attract macrophages to the region. After their accumulation (one to three days later), release of lytic agents by the inflammatory cells results in local tissue damage and clinical symptoms. (Adapted with permission from [2].)

hours after the second contact with the allergen (antigen). This type of hypersensitivity is responsible for contact dermatitis.

As depicted in Fig. 12.13, unlike the previous types of hypersensitivity, antibodies are not involved in the type IV response. Instead, the action of specialized cells, T_{DTH} cells (usually formed from T_h cells) is the main cause of the reaction. Upon first exposure to the antigen presented on an APC, T_h cells become sensitized and mature into T_{DTH} cells. Further exposure causes the activation of the T_{DTH} cells and secretion of cytokines to attract macrophages to the region. After their accumulation (one to three days later), release of lytic agents by the inflammatory cells results in local tissue damage and clinical symptoms.

Reports of dermatitis or oral lesions after insertion of oral implants containing chromium, cobalt or nickel indicate that Type IV reactions could be a concern for biomaterial use. Similarly, deep tissue reactions of this type have also been seen with metallic, silicone and acrylic implants, indicating that this response is not confined to metallic biomaterials alone.

12.6.2.5 Hypersensitivity and the Classes of Biomaterials Hypersensitivity reactions to biomaterials have been most extensively studied for metals. However, it is thought that released products must act as haptens, requiring complexation with a native protein before immune system activation, due to the low molecular weight of the ions involved.

Very little study of hypersensitivity to ceramic materials has been performed, and evidence of type IV responses to polymers remain controversial. Chemical additives used in the manufacture of latex gloves may cause this type of hypersensitive response. In addition, there is a continuing concern that the denaturation of native proteins through binding to biomaterial surfaces (see Chapter 8) may result in an undesired immune response since they are no longer recognized as "self."

Although the debate continues about how hypersensitive reactions to biomaterials develop, these responses can have serious consequences for hypersensitive individuals and can have profound business implications, as seen with the sale of silicone breast implants. In this case, due to litigation alleging that silicone breast implants caused autoimmune diseases (destruction of body tissues due to unchecked acquired immune response), many of the major makers of these implants decided to withdraw from the market in 1992. Subsequent settlements cost these companies billions of dollars and one manufacturer was forced into bankruptcy. (As an epilogue, after years of study that found no direct link between silicone breast implants and these diseases, in 2006 the U.S. Food and Drug Administration approved a new generation of these implants for use in cosmetic surgeries.)

EXAMPLE PROBLEM 12.3

A retired employee of a company that manufactures bicycle frames from cobalt-chromium-molybdenum (Co-Cr-Mo) alloys was involved in an accident in which his knee was shattered. The orthopedic surgeon stated that the shattered knee must be replaced with an implanted prosthesis. The patient was allowed to decide between an implant composed of a titanium-aluminum-vanadium alloy and an implant composed of a Co-Cr-Mo alloy. Considering his history of cutting and grinding Co-Cr-Mo alloy frames in the bicycle factory, the patient enthusiastically chose the Co-Cr-Mo knee implant. Shortly after implantation, however, the patient exhibited symptoms consistent with a hypersensitivity reaction. How might this be explained?

Solution: The hypersensitivity reaction was likely in response to the implantation of a Co-Cr-Mo knee prosthesis. The patient clearly had a history of exposure to Co-Cr-Mo alloys in his work producing bicycle frames in a factory. This exposure likely included tactile contact, as well as inhalation of Co-Cr-Mo particles. It is possible that his body responded to the Co-Cr-Mo material as an antigen. The primary exposure to the material during his factory work led to the production of memory cells and release of IgE molecules specific for the material. The IgE molecules bound to receptors on mast cells and basophils, thereby sensitizing these cells. Upon the secondary exposure presented by the implantation of the knee prosthesis, the membrane-bound IgE antibodies on sensitized cells crosslinked, resulting in the release of histamine and other soluble mediators. Thus, a hypersensitivity reaction was initiated. ■

12.7 Techniques: Assays for Immune Response

Because of the strong interaction between the immune and inflammatory response, many of the *in vitro* and *in vivo* techniques employed to determine possible immune responses to biomaterials are the same as those outlined in Chapters 10 and 11 for inflammation. In fact, given the interplay between the innate and acquired immune responses, it is prudent to include both inflammatory cells and lymphocytes in *in vitro* tests for a more complete screening of the biocompatibility of a new material. As for other assays, it is expected that *in vitro* activation of lymphocytes in response to a particular substance is a predictor that this material may not be immunocompatible *in vivo*. A number of ASTM standards exist for immunotoxicity testing both *in vitro* (includes ASTM F1905, F1906, F1984, F2065) and *in vivo* (includes ASTM F720, F2147, F2148).

12.7.1 *In Vitro* Assays

As with the inflammatory response, cells involved in the immune response can be isolated from the blood and then cultured in the presence of the biomaterial before determining their state of activation. Both T and B cells are commonly tested for one or more of the same markers of activation as granulocytes:

1. Cell adhesion and spreading
2. Cell death
3. Cell migration
4. Cytokine release
5. Cell surface marker expression
6. Cell proliferation

The first five markers are identical to those for inflammatory cells. In addition, because cell expansion and the formation of clonal populations is important to lymphocyte function, assays for cell proliferation are also used as indicators of activation. Such assays are called **lymphocyte transformation tests (LTTs)** and are often performed by radiolabeling or fluorescent-labeling cellular DNA and monitoring the change in its amount over time. A large increase in DNA synthesis indicates that the lymphocytes are actively proliferating.

Many of the methods used to assay for the other parameters listed above have been discussed in Chapters 9 and 10 and are also used for lymphocytes. In contrast to macrophages and neutrophils, however, when a lymphocyte recognizes a target that binds to its antibody or TCR, it loses its ability to migrate. Therefore, although both the movements of individual and populations of lymphocytes have been tracked following procedures described previously, in this case smaller migration values are taken as an indicator of activation. This is referred to as a **lymphocyte migration inhibition assay**. Additionally, while ELISAs and FACS sorting are employed to determine the type and amount of released cytokines and cell-surface markers, respectively (see Chapter 10 for detailed discussion of these methods), the exact cytokines and cell surface markers targeted are different for lymphocytes than those examined for granulocyte activation.

12.7.2 *In Vivo* Assays

In vivo, an unresolved immune response has characteristics similar to chronic inflammation, but includes the presence of lymphocytes as well as inflammatory cells. Therefore, the techniques used to examine the *in vivo* immune response to implanted materials are very similar to those outlined in Chapter 11. Contrary to the case for inflammation, there is no ISO guidance for immune assessment. However, experimental design must address concerns like those for *in vivo* inflammatory tests, such as the choice of animal, choice of implant site, length of study, dose and administration of biomaterial, and inclusion of proper controls. To date, the most common means of assessment after implantation in an animal model is histology/immunohistochemistry, with an emphasis on visualizing the amount of lymphocytes present around the material.

It is also possible to monitor the immune response over the course of implantation without euthanizing the animal. Blood samples can be taken from the animal and tested for the presence of antibodies (usually IgG) against certain epiptopes derived from the implanted biomaterial. The presence of such antibodies suggests that the material is immunogenic and may result eventually in deleterious effects to the device or patient. This procedure can also be used for human patients, particularly if it is believed that a hypersensitivity has developed to an implant.

Another common hypersensitivity test in humans is to place possible antigens from the biomaterial on/under the skin and look for localized inflammation (**skin testing**). If redness or swelling is apparent near the site of application of the antigen, then it is an indication that the patient may be hypersensitive to the implanted material. Similar procedures are used to determine allergic reactions to environmental factors (such as pollen and dander).

EXAMPLE PROBLEM 12.4

Severe combined immunodeficiency (SCID) is a genetic disorder that results in a lack of B and T lymphocytes. People with SCID have severely compromised immune systems. Mice with SCID are capable of receiving transplanted tissue with a negligible risk of rejection. Consequently, they are useful as animal models for the evaluation of the biological activity of transplanted cells and/or tissues for therapeutic purposes. For instance, SCID mice can be used to evaluate the ability of marrow stromal cells to generate bone in an ectopic site *in vivo*. Would SCID mice be useful models for the evaluation of the immune response to a biomaterial? Why or why not?

Solution: SCID mice would not be a useful model for the evaluation of the immune response to an implanted biomaterial, as the immune system of SCID mice is severely compromised. The lack of an immune response to an implanted biomaterial in a SCID mouse would not be a reliable indicator of the potential immune response to this material in an individual with a fully functional immune system. ■

Summary

- The two types of acquired immunity are humoral, which is based on the actions of antibodies against foreign substances, and cellular, which utilizes specialized lymphocytes primarily to detect and neutralize altered cells of one's own body.
- A hapten is a low molecular weight substance that combines with a larger molecule to produce a much greater immune response than either entity would have alone. An adjuvant is a substance that non-specifically enhances the immune response to antigens.
- The acquired immune response is activated by the binding of an antigen to an antibody or a T cell receptor (TCR), through specific recognition of an epitope on the antigen. Antigen recognition generally occurs through presentation of the antigen with an MHC Class I or Class II molecule. MHC Class I molecules are present on nearly all nucleated cells and are recognized by T_c cells. MHC Class II molecules are only found on antigen-presenting cells (APCs) and are recognized by T_h cells. Antigens must be processed within the cell, where they complex with the appropriate MHC molecule before extracellular presentation.
- The two primary types of lymphocytes that respond to antigens to produce the acquired immune response are B cells, which are mediators of humoral immunity that produce highly specific antibodies that can either be released into the environment or remain bound to the cell membrane, and T cells, which are involved in cellular immunity and produce high specificity TCRs that remain bound to the cell membrane.
- B cells are formed and processed in the bone marrow and are further matured in the peripheral lymphoid tissues, whereas T cells are processed in the thymus. After maturation, the B cells and T cells migrate to the lymphoid tissues, where they may either remain for some time or enter directly into the blood stream to be circulated throughout the body.
- Antibodies are composed of two heavy and two light polypeptide chains, linked through disulfide bonds. The region at the end of each heavy/light chain combination is the cleft for antigen binding, called the variable portion (F_{ab}). The

remainder of the antigen is called the constant portion (F_c) and is responsible for recognition by the receptors in phagocytic cells or by certain molecules in the complement complex.

- Antibodies can assist in the removal of pathogens through agglutination (IgA and IgM are most effective at this), precipitation, neutralization, or lysis. Additionally, antibody binding can increase the rate of phagocytosis of antigen-containing particles and is a major mechanism for activating the complement system.
- Presentation of an antigen/MHC complex causes activation of T lymphocytes by promoting binding of the antigen to the TCR. Upon activation T_h cells release cytokines that aid in the activation of T_c cells. T_h cells also bind with and release cytokines to fully activate B cells. Following activation, each lymphocyte undergoes rapid division to form a clonal population of cells specific for its respective antigen. Both effector and memory cells are produced in this process. Effector B cells are called plasma cells, and secrete soluble antibodies. Effector T cells are cytotoxic T lymphocytes (CTLs), which can secrete perforins to lyse cells.
- Two means of complement activation (classical and alternative pathways) converge to result in the formation of the membrane attack complex to lyse foreign cells. The classical pathway is initiated with the binding of an antibody to an antigen on a suitable target. This results in a conformational change in the F_c region of the antibody that initiates a cascade of events that culminates in the production of C5b, which remains bound to the target surface and initiates formation of the membrane attack complex. The alternative pathway begins with the binding of a complement protein C3 to the foreign entity and ends ultimately in the formation of C5b. The membrane attack complex forms large pores in the membrane of the target cell that result in its lysis.
- Regulation of the complement cascade occurs through a number of means, including the short half life of many of the enzymes involved in the cascade and the action of regulatory proteins that occur at various stages of the cascade.
- Activation of the complement system allows for an amplification of the actions of antibodies. Additionally, complement activation can result in the stimulation of the inflammatory response through the action of C3a, C4a and C5a. Factors in the complement cascade can act in concert with inflammatory cells to encourage phagocytosis of targeted entities.
- Allergic responses can be divided into four general categories. Type I responses are mediated by IgE antibodies produced by plasma cells against a particular allergen. Type II responses are generated when antibodies work alone or in connection with the complement to destroy cells presenting a foreign antigen. Type III responses occur when a large number of antigen-antibody complexes are precipitated within a localized area or if the antigen is present systemically in the blood, in which cases the complement is activated and results in the recruitment and action of inflammatory cells. Type IV reactions are delayed-type hypersensitivity responses that do not involve the action of antibodies, but instead involve the sensitization and activation of T_{DTH} cells that recruit the action of macrophages.
- Techniques for *in vitro* determination of possible immune responses to biomaterials are very comparable to those for determining the inflammatory response to a material. Alternatively, the possibility of an immune response may be assessed *in vivo* with animal models.

Problems

12.1 A degradable scaffold material for bone tissue engineering is implanted into the body. Describe how the implantation could result in both exogenous and endogenous antigen presentation by the surrounding cells. What type of T cells are activated in each of these scenarios?

12.2 If a patient has lost his or her spleen, which type of acquired immunity is most affected?

12.3 (a) Describe the four ways that antibodies act in removing pathogens. (b) Explain how the complement proteins aid in these actions. (c) What immune system mechanism can be used to rapidly produce large amounts of antibodies if needed?

12.4 During an *in vivo* study to determine the efficacy of a new catheter design, you notice that a fibrous capsule has formed around the implant after eight weeks. Monitoring of the animal's blood via ELISA showed an initial spike in levels of C3 convertase, followed by a decrease in levels of this protein complex after week 1. Describe, in detail, a possible molecular/cellular mechanism for the formation of the fibrous capsule observed in this study.

12.5 What type of hypersensitivity reaction would be most likely observed following implantation of a synthetic, degradable polymer? What type of reaction would be expected with a long-term silicone implant, such as an artificial finger joint?

12.6 What are the main differences between the *in vitro* techniques to assess the inflammatory response and the immune response to a biomaterial?

12.7 What *in vivo* techniques can be used to determine the immune response to a biomaterial?

References

1. Anderson, J.M. and J.J. Langone. "Issues and Perspectives on the Biocompatibility and Immunotoxicity Evaluation of Implanted Controlled Release Systems," *Journal of Controlled Release*, vol. 57, pp. 107–113, 1999.
2. Kuby, J. *Immunology*, 3rd ed. New York: W.H. Freeman, 1997.
3. Silver, F.H. and D.L. Christiansen. *Biomaterials Science and Biocompatibility*. New York: Springer, 1999.
4. Linsley, P.S. and J.A. Ledbetter. "The Role of the CD28 Receptor During T Cell Responses to Antigen," *Annual Reviews in Immunology*, vol. 11, pp. 191–212, 1993.

Additional Reading

http://www.fda.gov/cdrh/breastimplants/consumerinfo.html

Black, J. *Biological Performance of Materials: Fundamentals of Biocompatibility*, 4th ed. New York: CRC Press, 2005.

Dee, K.C., D.A. Puleo, and R. Bizios. *An Introduction to Tissue-Biomaterial Interactions*. Hoboken: Wiley-Liss, 2002.

Granchi, D., G. Ciapetti, L. Savarino, E. Cenni, A. Pizzoferrato, N. Baldini, and A. Giunti. "Effects of Bone Cement Extracts on the Cell-Mediated Immune Response," *Biomaterials*, vol. 23, pp. 1033–1041, 2002.

Groth, T., K. Klosz, E.J. Campbell, R.R. New, B. Hall, and H. Goering. "Protein Adsorption, Lymphocyte Adhesion and Platelet Adhesion/Activation on Polyurethane Ureas Is Related to Hard Segment Content and Composition." *Journal of Biomaterials Science Polymer Edition*, vol. 6, pp. 497–510, 1994.

Guyton, A.C. and J.E. Hall. *Textbook of Medical Physiology*, 11th ed. Philadelphia: W.B. Saunders, 2006.

Hallab, N., J.J. Jacobs, and J. Black. "Hypersensitivity to Metallic Biomaterials: A Review of Leukocyte Migration Inhibition Assays," *Biomaterials*, vol. 21, pp. 1301–1314, 2000.

Hallab, N.J., K. Mikecz, and J.J. Jacobs. "A Triple Assay Technique for the Evaluation of Metal-Induced,

Delayed-Type Hypersensitivity Responses in Patients with or Receiving Total Joint Arthroplasty," *Journal of Biomedical Materials Research*, vol. 53, pp. 480–489, 2000.

Harris, G. "FDA Panel Backs Implants from One Maker." In *New York Times*, April 14, 2005.

Hensten-Pettersen, A. and N. Jacobsen. "Systemic Toxicity and Hypersensitivity." In *Biomaterials Science: An Introduction to Materials in Medicine*, B.D. Ratner, A.S. Hoffman, F.J. Schoen, and J.E. Lemons, Eds., 2nd ed. San Diego: Elsevier Academic Press, pp. 328–332, 2004.

Johnson, R.J. "Immunology and the Complement System." In *Biomaterials Science: An Introduction to Materials in Medicine*, B.D. Ratner, A.S. Hoffman, F.J. Schoen, and J.E. Lemons, Eds., 1st ed. San Diego: Elsevier Academic Press, pp. 173–188, 1996.

Matzelle, M.M. and J.E. Babensee. "Humoral Immune Responses to Model Antigen Co-Delivered with Biomaterials Used in Tissue Engineering," *Biomaterials*, vol. 25, pp. 295–304, 2004.

Mayesh, J.P. and M.F. Scranton. "Legal Aspects of Biomaterials." In *Biomaterials Science: An Introduction to Materials in Medicine*, B.D. Ratner, A.S. Hoffman, F.J. Schoen, and J.E. Lemons, Eds., 2nd ed. San Diego: Elsevier Academic Pres, pp. 797–804, 2004.

McNally, A.K. and J.M. Anderson. "Complement C3 Participation in Monocyte Adhesion to Different Surfaces," *Proceedings of the National Academy of Sciences*, vol. 91, pp. 10119–10123, 1994.

Merritt, K. "Systemic Toxicity and Hypersensitivity." In *Biomaterials Science: An Introduction to Materials in Medicine*, B.D. Ratner, A.S. Hoffman, F.J. Schoen, and J.E. Lemons, Eds., 1st ed. San Diego: Elsevier Academic Press, pp. 188–193, 1996.

Mitchell, R.N. "Innate and Adaptive Immunity: The Immune Respinse to Foreign Materials." In *Biomaterials Science: An Introduction to Materials in Medicine*, B.D. Ratner, A.S. Hoffman, F.J. Schoen, and J.E. Lemons, Eds., 2nd ed. San Diego: Elsevier Academic Press, pp. 304–318, 2004.

Palmer, E.M., B.A. Beilfuss, T. Nagai, R.T. Semnani, S.F. Badylak, and G.A. van Seventer. "Human Helper T Cell Activation and Differentiation Is Suppressed by Porcine Small Intestinal Submucosa," *Tissue Engineering*, vol. 8, pp. 893–900, 2002.

Rosales-Cortes, M., J. Peregrina-Sandoval, J. Banuelos-Pineda, R. Sarabia-Estrada, C.C. Gomez-Rodiles, E. Albarran-Rodriguez, G.P. Zaitseva, and M.L. Pita-Lopez. "Immunological Study of a Chitosan Prosthesis in the Sciatic Nerve Regeneration of the Axotomized Dog," *Journal of Biomaterials Applications*, vol. 18, pp. 15–23, 2003.

Thomas, P., S. Barnstorf, B. Summer, G. Willmann, and B. Przybilla. "Immuno-Allergological Properties of Aluminum Oxide (Al2O3) Ceramics and Nickel Sulfate in Humans," *Biomaterials*, vol. 24, pp. 959–966, 2003.

CHAPTER 13

Biomaterials and Thrombosis

Main Objective

To understand the steps involved in, and results of, the blood coagulation cascade stimulated by biomaterial implantation.

Specific Objectives

1. To understand the functions of platelets, including how platelets are activated and the results of this activation.
2. To compare and contrast the intrinsic and extrinsic pathways for blood coagulation and understand how these interact with the inflammatory response.
3. To understand the steps of the final common blood coagulation pathway and fibrin polymerization.
4. To understand approaches to limiting clot formation.
5. To understand the pro- and anticoagulant properties of the vascular endothelium.
6. To understand the concepts behind and possible limitations to the *in vitro*, *in vivo* and *ex vivo* tests presented.

13.1 Introduction: Overview of Hemostasis

Blood–biomaterials interactions are extremely important since almost all biomaterials are implanted in vascularized tissues and contact with blood occurs frequently, particularly during the implantation procedure. However, as reviewed in Chapters 7 and 8, it is important to remember that the body actually responds to the protein coat of the biomaterial in many cases, so controlling protein adsorption is a key method of altering blood coagulation caused by the implant.

After injury, **hemostatic** mechanisms in the body have been designed to arrest bleeding. These involve vascular constriction in the area of the insult, the formation of a platelet plug, and blood coagulation (**thrombosis**). The combination of these responses decreases regional blood flow and temporarily closes the hole in the vessel, thus preventing further blood loss from the area. Both proteinaceous and nonproteinaceous components of the blood (such as platelets), as well the endothelial lining of the blood vessels, play a large role in hemostasis. We begin with a discussion of the importance of platelets in the coagulation process.

13.2 Role of Platelets

13.2.1 Platelet Characteristics and Functions

Platelets are nonnucleated fragments of megakaryocytes with a diameter of 3–4 μm. Because they do not possess nuclei, platelets cannot proliferate and have a half-life in the body of only 8–12 days. Platelets perform two main hemostatic functions: they initially reduce bleeding through the creation of a platelet plug and then further stabilize this plug through activation of the blood coagulation cascade.

Although they are only cell fragments, platelets contain mitochondria for energy production, as well as portions of the ER and Golgi apparatus for packaging of secretory products. These products are usually chemical mediators to be released upon platelet activation and are stored in intracellular granules before secretion.

Several types of platelet intracellular granules can be distinguished. The **α granules** contain platelet-specific proteins (platelet factors) and β-thromboglobulin as well as various plasma proteins including fibrinogen and the coagulation-cascade proteins Factor V and Factor XIII. **Dense granules** carry adenosine diphosphate (ADP), calcium ions, and serotonin, while **lysosomal granules** contain hydrolytic enzymes.

13.2.2 Platelet Activation

13.2.2.1 Means of Activation Platelets can become activated via a variety of stimuli, including exposure to soluble factors or interaction with ECM and/or cells of injured vessel walls. In particular, collagen and von Willebrand factor (vWF) are potent platelet activators, and platelets may respond to these and other proteins either from damaged tissue or adsorbed on biomaterial surfaces. In all cases, interaction of these extracellular stimuli with receptors on the cell membrane is the first step in platelet activation.

13.2.2.2 Sequelae of Activation Once stimulated, platelets undergo a number of changes. Briefly, while unactivated platelets have a disc-like morphology, activated platelets swell and take on an irregular form, extending pseudopodia in various directions. Also at this time, contraction of cytoskeletal proteins results in release of storage granule contents. As a result of these changes, platelets express several new functionalities. Activated platelets are observed to adhere to ECM proteins, aggregate, secrete various bioactive factors for further platelet stimulation, and exhibit coagulatory activity. Each of these characteristics is discussed in more detail below.

Platelet adhesion near the injured area (or onto a biomaterial) is mediated through interactions between appropriate ligands from collagen, vWF, fibrinogen, fibronectin, and glycoprotein or integrin receptors on the platelet surface. As the platelets begin to adhere to the target area, they release their granule contents, including large amounts of adenosine diphosphate (ADP). Synthesis and release of **thrombin** (see Table 13.1) and thromboxane A_2 is also upregulated.

These soluble chemical mediators act on neighboring platelets to activate them and attract them to the growing aggregate. In particular, thrombin catalyzes the production of more thrombin and stimulates ADP and thromboxane A_2 release.

Also as a result of these soluble factors, platelets in the region of the aggregate begin to express the activated glycoprotein (GP) receptor **GP IIb/IIIa** on their surfaces. This receptor can then bind plasma proteins to increase platelet aggregation. Specifically, *fibrinogen* plays an important role in this process because it possesses two receptor binding sites, allowing for platelet–platelet bridging. Overall, these steps result in the formation of a platelet plug, although at this stage it is fairly fragile.

TABLE 13.1

Different Actions of Thrombin

Positive Effects on Coagulation	Negative Effects on Coagulation
Catalyzes production of more thrombin by platelets	
Stimulates release of granule contents by platelets (particularly ADP and thromboxane A_2)	Thrombomodulin–thrombin complex on endothelial cell membrane activates protein C, which can then inactivate Factors V and VIII
Cleaves fibrinogen to fibrin	
Activates Factor V	
Activates Factor XIII which crosslinks fibrin	

In order to stabilize the plug, platelets also promote localized blood coagulation. In particular, when stimulated, alterations in the platelet phospholipid membrane allow the expression of certain receptors that accelerate Factor X activation (Factor X is a key protein in the blood coagulation cascade; see below). Platelet membranes also form a catalytic environment for conversion of prothrombin to thrombin (see later discussion).

13.3 Coagulation Cascade

Blood coagulation can occur via two main mechanisms, called the **intrinsic** and **extrinsic** pathways. Like complement activation, both cascades end in a common pathway, in this case causing the conversion of fibrinogen to fibrin, the main constituent of the blood clot. The proteins involved in these pathways are designated with the word "Factor" and a Roman numeral, although many of them have alternate names. A list of factors and their common names is found in Table 13.2. Except for

TABLE 13.2

Coagulation Factors and their Common Names

Clotting Factor	Synonyms
Fibrinogen	Factor I
Prothrombin	Factor II
Tissue factor	Factor III, tissue thromboplastin
Calcium	Factor IV
Factor V	Proaccelerin, labile factor, Ac-globulin (Ac-G)
Factor VII	Serum prothrombin conversion accelerator (SPCA), proconvertin, stable factor
Factor VIII	Antihemophilic factor (AHF), antihemophilic globulin (AHG), antihemophilic factor A
Factor IX	Plasma thromboplastin component (PTC), Christmas factor, antihemophilic factor B
Factor X	Stuart factor, Stuart-Prower factor
Factor XI	Plasma thromboplastin antecedent (PTA), antihemophilic factor C
Factor XII	Hageman factor
Factor XIII	Fibrin-stabilizing factor
Prekallikrein	Fletcher factor
High-molecular weight kininogen	Fitzgerald factor, HMWK

(Adapted with permission from [1].)

the commencement of the intrinsic pathway, calcium is required for almost all reactions in the cascade, which is why substances that bind calcium (**calcium chelators**) are very effective anticoagulants.

13.3.1 Intrinsic Pathway

The intrinsic pathway is initiated by trauma to blood itself or exposure of blood to exposed ECM molecules in a damaged vessel wall. Clotting initiates in one to six minutes via this mechanism. Although in many classical hematology texts and much of the biomaterials literature, this pathway is treated as an equal alternative to the extrinsic pathway (described below), recent texts have placed more emphasis on the extrinsic pathway as the main means of clot formation. The role of the intrinsic pathway remains unclear, particularly in the case of coagulation near biomaterials, where the blood interacts with a foreign surface. If the surface is negatively charged, a requirement for the initiation of this cascade, the intrinsic pathway may remain an important means of coagulation.

As mentioned above, the intrinsic pathway begins with adsorption of one of the coagulation **contact proteins,** Factor XII, to a negatively charged surface (Fig. 13.1). This surface can be naturally occurring, such as with glycosylated ECM molecules, or can be an anionic biomaterial. The act of adsorption causes conversion of Factor

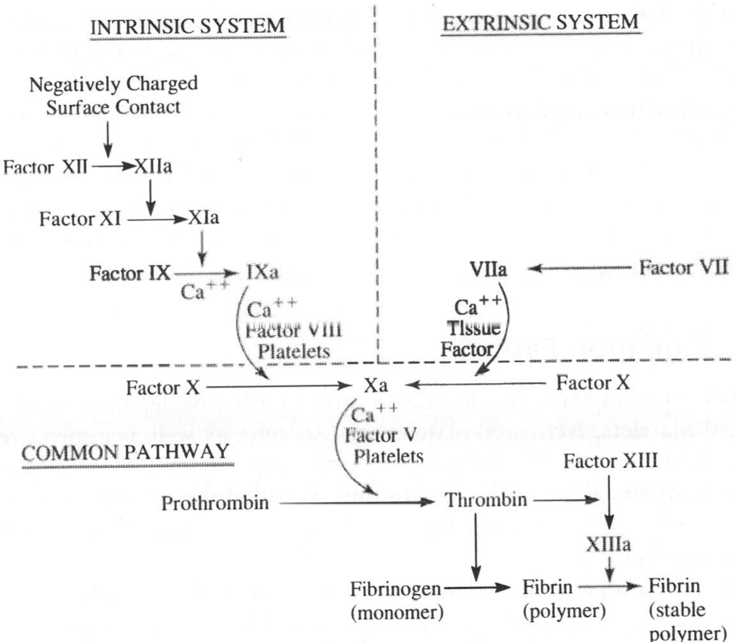

Figure 13.1
Diagram of the intrinsic and extrinsic pathways of blood coagulation. The intrinsic pathway is initiated by trauma to blood itself or exposure of blood to exposed ECM molecules in a damaged vessel wall. The intrinsic pathway begins with adsorption of one of the coagulation contact proteins, Factor XII, to a negatively charged surface. The extrinsic pathway is initiated by the release of tissue factor (TF), which binds with Factor VII on the surface of a phospholipid membrane. Both cascades converge on the common pathway, which begins with the conversion of Factor X to **Xa**. Factor V and stimulated platelets then react with Factor **Xa**, and thrombin is formed. Thrombin is responsible for the polymerization of fibrin monomers, and the presence of Factor **XIIIa** helps stabilize and crosslink the fibrin to strengthen the thrombus. (Adapted with permission from [2].)

XII to the activated **XIIa** (as in Chapter 12, active enzymes in the cascade will be designated by boldface type.) **XIIa** converts *prekallikrein* to **kallikrein** and Factor XI to **XIa**. This is accomplished because both prekallikrein and Factor XI bind to a cofactor, high molecular weight kininogen (HMWK), which anchors them to the charged surface and promotes interaction with Factor **XIIa**.

As an example of positive feedback within the cascade, the newly formed **kallikrein** converts Factor XII to more **XIIa. Kallikrein** also acts to cleave HMWK to release bradykinin, an inflammatory mediator (see Chapter 10). This provides an important point of crossover between thrombosis and the inflammatory response.

The coagulation pathway continues through the other major substrate of **XIIa**, Factor XI. As shown in Fig. 13.1, after activation, **XIa** converts Factor IX to **IXa**. In the final step, the initiation of the common pathway (see below), Factor **IXa** and Factor VIII associate on a phospholipid (usually platelet) membrane to convert Factor X to **Xa**. The function of Factor VIII is to accelerate the activation of Factor X, which occurs very slowly without this cofactor or the presence of the phospholipid membrane.

13.3.2 Extrinsic Pathway

An alternative mechanism of blood coagulation, the extrinsic pathway, is initiated by the release of tissue factor (TF) (Fig. 13.1). Clotting can commence via this pathway within 15 seconds. TF is a membrane-associated protein composed of a single polypeptide chain that acts as a cofactor in the extrinsic pathway, similar to HMWK in the intrinsic pathway. TF synthesis by macrophages and endothelial cells can be induced by IL-1 and TNF-α (see Chapter 10); by this means, inflammatory mediators can stimulate coagulation.

After its release, TF binds with Factor VII on the surface of a phospholipid membrane. Factor VII can then become activated to **VIIa** through cleavage by a number of proteases found in the blood. In the final part of the cascade, the TF/**VIIa** complex on the cell membrane converts Factor X to **Xa**, initiating the common pathway (see below).

13.3.3 Common Pathway

Like other steps in the cascade, the common pathway depends on the actions of stimulated platelets. Activated platelets can secrete, as well as express receptors for Factor V. When attached to the platelet membrane, Factor V is a receptor for Factor Xa. This complex, along with calcium ions, is called the **prothrombin activator.** Of these components, it is actually Factor **Xa** that converts prothrombin to the active enzyme **thrombin**.

Thrombin is an extremely important substance in the coagulation cascade, with both pro- and anticoagulant activities (see Table 13.1). Its main procoagulant role is to cleave fibrinogen found in the platelet granules or from blood plasma. This cleavage results in the creation of fibrin monomer and fibrinopeptides A and B. The peptides are chemotactic for neutrophils, and thus, are another point at which thrombosis and the inflammatory response overlap.

The fibrin monomers can then polymerize to form long fibrin fibers[1] (Fig. 13.2). These fibers are the basis of the blood clot, but at this point, they are held together by hydrogen bonding, so the structure is fairly weak. However, **thrombin** has two

[1]The combination of thrombin and fibrinogen has been explored as an injectable biomaterial. If they are taken from the patient into whom they will be reimplanted, there is no concern of an immune reaction.

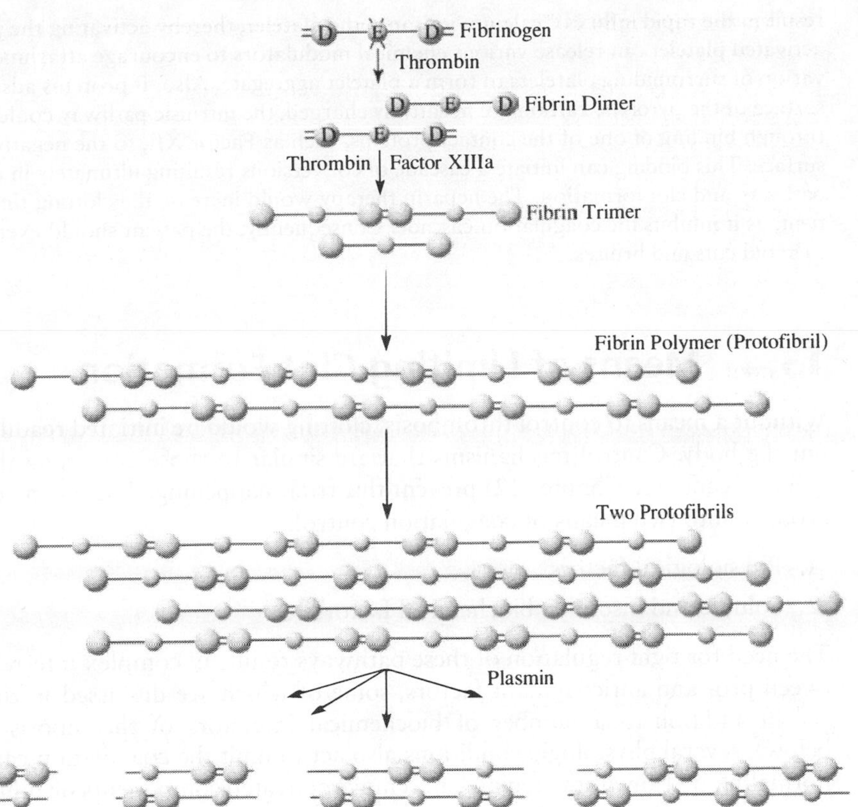

Figure 13.2
Process of fibrin polymerization. Crosslinking is initiated by the presence of Factor XIIIa, causing clot formation. After the wound has healed, activated plasmin then cleaves the fibrin to dissolve the thrombus. (Adapted with permission from [3].)

additional substrates: Factors V and XIII. Factor V, when converted to **Va**, accelerates the conversion of prothrombin to thrombin in a positive feedback mechanism designed to speed clotting. The other substrate, Factor XIII (**XIIIa**) acts in the presence of calcium to covalently crosslink fibrin chains (Fig. 13.2), which provides mechanical integrity to the clot (**thrombus**). This meshwork of fibrin encasing platelets, adhesive proteins, and other bioactive factors is considered the mature thrombus. Within the clot, the fibrin acts to bridge plasma proteins and the platelet interior and prevents further bleeding by attaching to the blood vessel ECM though adhesive proteins such as fibronectin.

EXAMPLE PROBLEM 13.1

A patient requires a replacement mitral heart valve. The cardiothoracic surgeon has determined that a tilting-disk pyrolytic carbon mechanical heart valve prosthesis will be the optimal choice for the patient. To reduce the risk of implant-related thrombosis, the patient will receive therapy with an anticoagulant drug such as heparin for the lifetime of the implant. Describe a mechanism by which clot formation might be initiated by the implant. Will heparin therapy increase or decrease the clotting time of the patient?

Solution: Clot formation could be initiated by a number of mechanisms. For example, flow conditions or surface properties associated with the implant could contribute to the damage and rupture of cells, resulting in the release of tissue factor. The extrinsic pathway could then be triggered with tissue factor binding Factor VII on the surface of a phospholipid membrane. The binding would initiate further steps that result in the conversion of Factor X to **Xa**, thereby beginning the common pathway. Alternatively, vWF may adsorb on the biomaterial surface and bind to receptors on the platelet surface. The binding of vWF to the receptors would result in the rapid influx of calcium ions into the platelet, thereby activating the platelet. The activated platelet can release various chemical modulators to encourage attachment and activation of surrounding platelets to form a platelet aggregate. Also, if proteins adsorbed to the surface of the pyrolytic carbon are negatively charged, the intrinsic pathway could be initiated through binding of one of the contact proteins, such as Factor XII, to the negatively charged surface. This binding can initiate a cascade of conversions resulting ultimately in the common pathway and clot formation. The heparin therapy would increase the clotting time of the patient, as it inhibits the coagulation cascade. Consequently, the patient should exercise caution to avoid cuts and bruises. ■

13.4 Means of Limiting Clot Formation

Without a means to control thrombosis, clotting would be initiated readily throughout the body. Control mechanisms that are similar to those governing the complement cascade (see Chapter 12) prevent this from happening. These can generally be grouped into two means of coagulation control:

1. Physiological factors
2. Soluble and insoluble biochemical factors

The need for tight regulation of these pathways results in complex interrelations between pro- and anticoagulant factors, some of which are discussed in this section.

In addition to a number of biochemical inhibitors of thrombosis (discussed below), several physiologic conditions also act to limit the coagulation cascade. The normal blood flow in the region can remove activated components or dilute them to an extent that they are not a concern in initiating systemic coagulation. Additionally, many reactions require or are catalyzed by a surface, such as the initial reactions of the intrinsic pathway, conversion of Factor X to **Xa** by either pathway, and cleavage of prothrombin to form thrombin. Without the presence of this membrane surface (usually supplied by activated platelets or platelet fragments), the cascade cannot proceed, thus limiting thrombosis to the traumatized region.

As an alternative means to control clotting, soluble agents may bind coagulation factors and inhibit their actions. An important example of this is the **heparin/antithrombin III (AT III) complex**. Heparin, a molecular cousin of the GAG heparan sulfate discussed in Chapter 9, is a highly negatively charged polysaccharide possessing anticoagulant properties that is secreted by basophils. It is found in small quantities in human blood and has been given to patients in soluble form as an anticoagulant since the 1930s. When heparin is conjugated with AT III, it increases AT III's effectiveness. AT III acts to inhibit thrombin by forming a tight complex and thus preventing the exposure of thrombin's catalytic site. AT III can also inhibit the actions of a number of other coagulation enzymes.

As discussed in Chapter 7, surface modification of cardiovascular biomaterials with heparin has been extensively explored due to the anticoagulant properties described above. Non-covalent modifications involving electrostatic interactions, as well as covalent coupling of the heparin to the material surface using methods like those described in Chapter 7, are possible. The advantage of covalent coupling is that it prevents protein exchange and thus allows the heparin to remain on the material for a longer period of time. Regardless of the method of immobilization, like with other biologically active molecules, heparin's native conformation must be maintained on the biomaterial surface in order to interact efficiently with AT III.

Alpha$_2$-macroglobulin is another soluble agent that acts as a secondary inhibitor for several important enzymes, including thrombin and plasmin (see below for discussion of the role of plasmin). The α_2-macroglobulin molecule has a quaternary structure that is arranged to "entrap" the target enzyme in a cage. Once bound in this manner, it is much more difficult for the enzyme to form a complex with its substrate, and its actions are effectively inhibited.

Although it is not soluble, the protein **thrombomodulin**, found on the endothelial surface of the blood vessel walls, plays a large role in the control of coagulation. Thrombomodulin is attached to the endothelial cell membrane and can bind and sequester thrombin in this location, thus preventing further cleavage of fibrinogen to fibrin. The thrombomodulin–thrombin complex can then activate **protein C**, which, in turn, inactivates Factors V and VIII, thus providing further feedback to limit the extent of thrombosis.

After the thrombus has been formed and the damaged area repaired, clot dissolution is required to restore normal blood flow to the region. This process occurs primarily via **fibrinolysis**, or cleavage of the fibrin fibers in a controlled manner. During the coagulation process, **plasminogen**, a plasma protein, is trapped in the thrombus. At some point after clot maturation (the timing of this event is not well understood), endothelial cells begin to release **tissue plasminogen activator (TPA)**, which converts plasminogen to **plasmin**. Activated plasmin then cleaves the fibrin to dissolve the thrombus, as shown in Fig. 13.2. To balance this, another molecule found in the blood, **α_2-plasmin inhibitor,** inhibits plasmin from acting on fibrin. Therefore, the relative amounts and locations of plasminogen, TPA, and α_2-plasmin inhibitor determine the rate of thrombus dissolution.

13.5 Role of the Endothelium

As mentioned in Chapter 10, blood vessels are complex tissues with several layers (Fig. 13.3). The interior wall (**endothelium**) is a heterogeneous surface, formed and maintained by the endothelial cells. A number of molecules exist on the surface, including mucopolysaccharides/GAGs, such as heparan sulfate (see Chapter 9), that are adsorbed to the endothelial cells and interact with carbohydrate moieties already on the surface to form a **glycocalyx**. This coating imparts smoothness to the walls of the vessel, unlike the comparatively rough surface of many biomaterials. Integrins and other receptors for attachment of cells and adhesive proteins can also be found on the endothelial surface.

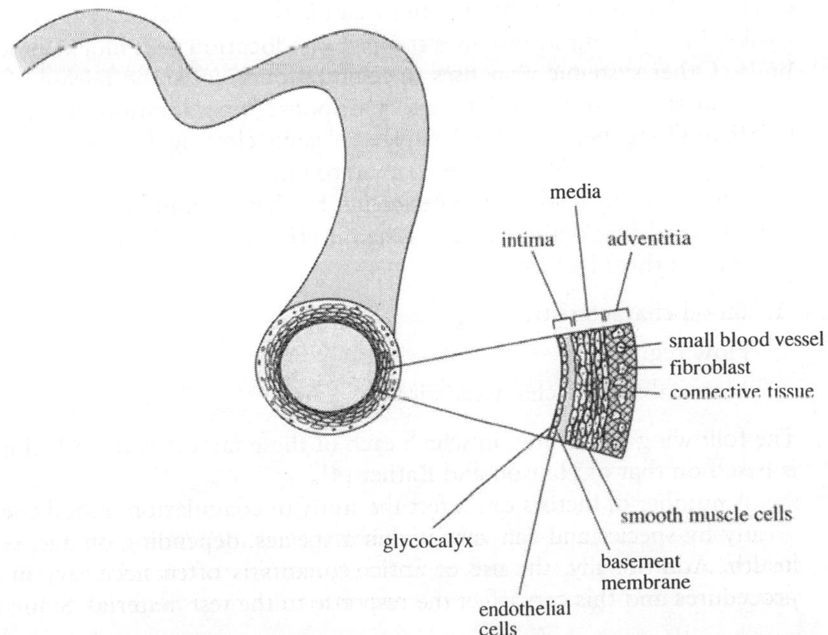

Figure 13.3
Structure of a blood vessel found in the human body. There are three main layers: the intima (endothelium), the media, and the adventitia. The innermost layer is composed of endothelial cells, the middle layer is populated by smooth muscle cells, and the outer layer has connective tissue and smaller blood vessels.

In its native state, the endothelium has a number of anticoagulative properties. The presence of heparan sulfate (like soluble heparin) may aid AT III in inhibiting thrombin. As discussed previously, thrombomodulin on the endothelial surface binds thrombin, and this complex then activates Protein C, which inhibits selected coagulation factors. Endothelial cells also secrete soluble chemical mediators, such as **prostaglandin I_2 (PGI_2)**, which prevents platelet aggregation, and TPA, which activates plasmin to promote thrombus lysis.

However, the overall composition of the endothelium at a given time is very important to determining whether or not coagulation is likely to occur. After injury, the protective glycocalyx is compromised, and the exposure of endothelial ECM molecules to reactive plasma proteins is a main mechanism of coagulation initiation (via the intrinsic pathway). Additionally, in response to certain stimuli (including cytokines IL-1 and TNF-α), the intact endothelial surface can become more coagulatory in nature. Because these cytokines are often products of granulocytes, this marks another means by which acute inflammation can promote coagulation. Examples of changes to the endothelium are a decrease in the amount of thrombomodulin at the surface and release of TF to promote coagulation through the extrinsic pathway. At this point, endothelial cells may also secrete vWF to mediate platelet aggregation.

13.6 Tests for Hemocompatibility

Another part of general biocompatibility testing is examination of hemocompatibility. Five categories of evaluation have been defined, including thrombosis, coagulation, platelets, hematology, and immunology (complement and leukocyte activation). *In vitro* and *in vivo* tests for immunological concerns were discussed in the previous chapter, so this section will focus on experiments to assess the other parameters.

13.6.1 General Testing Concerns

When designing hemocompatibility tests, one should consider both local and systemic effects. For example, localized blood clotting could negatively affect device function. Systemic results of device-mediated coagulation include thrombus **embolization**, in which pieces of the clot break off and are carried elsewhere in the circulatory system. In the most serious cases, this can lead to complications such as stroke if the thrombus becomes trapped in a location that blocks blood flow to the brain. Other systemic responses to coagulation involve the release of soluble products that stimulate the inflammatory response. Implantation of a coagulatory surface over long periods could deplete plasma clotting factors and platelets, thus reducing the patient's ability to respond to injury.

Also when considering experiments for hemocompatibility, it is important to keep in mind that both local and systemic effects from blood contacting devices can result from three factors:

1. Blood characteristics
2. Flow regime
3. Material surface characteristics

The following discussion, in which each of these factors is described in more detail, is based on that of Hanson and Ratner [4].

A number of factors can affect the study of coagulation. Blood chemistry differs greatly by species and can vary within a species, depending on age, sex, or state of health. Additionally, the use of anticoagulants is often necessary in experimental procedures and this can affect the response to the test material. Similarly, the act of pumping blood over a material can cause lysis of blood cells, which can also impact coagulation properties.

Blood flow parameters are also important to hemocompatibility studies since they can provide a limiting step for the transport of platelets and plasma proteins to the surface of the material. In addition, it has been found that under low flow rates (such as that found in the veins), thrombus formation often occurs on polymeric materials since synthetic substrates do not release or possess attached anticoagulant factors like those found on the endothelium.

As discussed in previous chapters, a number of material surface characteristics affect plasma protein adsorption and thus hemocompatibility. Some of these are surface physicochemical properties, such as charge, hydrophobicity, and steric concerns. However, interaction with blood components depends not only on the material, but on how the material is used in the final device design. Therefore, surface topography and device geometry are important factors in determining the overall hemocompatibility of the implant.

13.6.2 *In Vitro* Assessment

Like other types of biocompatibility testing, hemocompatibility can be assessed both *in vitro* and *in vivo*. For *in vitro* experiments, the interaction time is important: Short-term testing, such as examining platelet adhesion, may not be predictive of overall blood–material compatibility. However, the total length of *in vitro* experiments is often limited due to the fact that blood coagulation will occur over time, even in the presence of an anticoagulant.

In vitro testing can be either **static** or **dynamic**. In static coagulation experiments, the test material is exposed to freshly drawn whole blood (with or without an anticoagulant) and then the time for thrombus formation in reference to a control material (usually glass) is recorded. Dynamic tests measure similar parameters, but involve a variety of closed-loop flow systems with controlled flow regimes.

For these protocols, in addition to clotting time, it is also possible to measure further parameters to address other aspects of the ISO standards. Quantifiable parameters may include, but are not limited to the following:

1. Coagulation time
2. Amount of adhered platelets
3. Mass of adherent thrombus
4. Amount of platelet granule release (this requires specific assays for chemical mediators found in platelet granules, such as platelet factor-4 and β-thromboglobulin)

However, it is possible to misinterpret the results of any of these experiments. For example, if no adherent platelets are observed, this could mean that platelets did not aggregate on the surface, or that they did and were already "embolized" to another part of the system. Similarly, no apparent thrombus could mean that it has been sheared off the surface and transported to another area. If no soluble granule products are detected, it may be that the platelets were not stimulated, or perhaps mediators were released, but the volume of the system was large enough to dilute them to undetectable concentrations. These alternatives must be considered when interpreting data from *in vitro* hemocompatibility experiments.

Several additional concerns with *in vitro* experimentation can complicate data analysis. A major limitation is that the use of anticoagulants affects the recorded coagulation time. Also, control materials must be tested at the same time and with the same blood as the experimental material, since (as discussed above) there can be significant differences in blood composition. Overall, it is thought that *in vitro* hemocompatibility experiments have limited value for prediction of *in vivo* responses, but their low cost encourages their use for initial screening of new biomaterials.

13.6.3 *In Vivo* Assessment

While *in vivo* assessment provides more information about hemocompatibility of materials than *in vitro* testing, it is still not completely predictive due to differences in the coagulation proteins between animal species and humans. In designing appropriate *in vivo* experiments, similar concerns exist as those discussed in previous chapters, including:

1. Choice of animal
2. Length of study and choice of time points
3. Inclusion of proper control materials

Sample assessment is similar to that found *in vitro*, and may include histology at the end of the experiment to determine the extent of thrombus formation around the implant. Additionally, further information may be obtained if biochemical assays are performed on blood samples at various time points to examine the rate of depletion of key plasma coagulation factors.

However, in addition to differences in blood composition between animals and humans, other concerns about direct *in vivo* testing have been raised. One of these is that it is difficult to control or measure blood flow conditions in animal models. Also, variations in tissue trauma during implantation can affect the results of the experiments. In order to overcome some of these concerns, biomaterial testing using shunts has been developed.

In these experiments, which are usually considered ***ex vivo*** instead of *in vivo*, the material in tubular form is placed as an extension in a shunt that connects an artery to a vein or artery to an artery in a living animal (Fig. 13.4). The advantages to such a system are that the blood flow near the sample can be easily controlled and measured, native (non-anticoagulated) blood may be used, and the shunt can remain in place for up to several months, so long-term responses can be examined. However, a disadvantage to shunt-based systems is that this model does not replicate an implantation procedure, so the response from the trauma of surgery cannot be evaluated. Therefore, while shunts provide a more controlled experimental environment, the usefulness of this type of testing depends on the final application of the biomaterial.

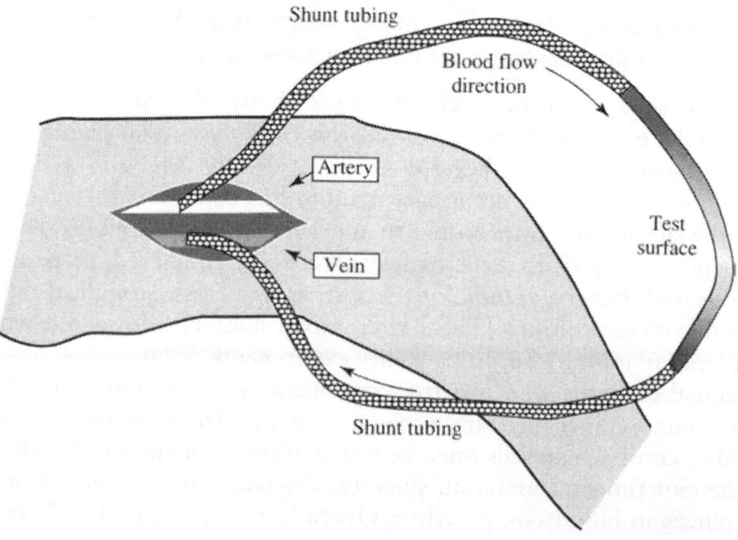

Figure 13.4
Ex vivo testing setup for a vascular material. The material (test surface) in tubular form is placed as an extension in a shunt that connects to the circulatory system of a living animal. (Adapted with permission from [4].)

EXAMPLE PROBLEM 13.2

A researcher has developed a vascular graft from a novel polymeric material and plans to evaluate the hemocompatibility of the implant in a canine model over the course of six weeks. However, it is known in the scientific literature that canines endothelialize vascular grafts spontaneously, while humans do not [5]. Should the canine model be used to evaluate the graft implant, or should another model be sought? Would endothelialization of a vascular graft be beneficial? Why?

Solution: The canine model should not be used in this case, as it does not appropriately approximate the human response to the vascular graft. The formation of an endothelial cell coating on the blood contacting surface of a vascular graft could result in the formation of a glycocalyx to impart smoothness to the walls of the graft. Further, endothelial cells present a number of anticoagulant properties that could reduce the risk of a thrombus formation response to the implant. Thus, endothelialization of the graft would be a substantial promoter of hemocompatibility. The spontaneous endothelialization of vascular grafts in canine models would result in more significant hemocompatibility of the graft than would be observed in humans, in which spontaneous endothelialization of vascular grafts does not occur. ■

Summary

- Platelets are nonnucleated fragments of megakaryocytes. They release soluble factors to initiate the formation of a platelet plug to stop bleeding and activate the blood coagulation cascade, which further stabilizes the plug.
- Platelets can become activated through a variety of means, including exposure to soluble factors or interaction with ECM components. Activated platelets transition to an irregular form and extend pseudopodia in various directions. Granule contents, including ADP and thrombin, are then released as a result of cytoskeletal protein contraction.
- The intrinsic blood coagulation pathway is initiated by trauma to the blood itself or to exposed ECM molecules in a damaged vessel wall. Factor XII can then adsorb to the negatively charged surface, resulting in a conversion to **XIIa**. The cascade continues until the common pathway is initiated with conversion of Factor X to **Xa**.
- The extrinsic pathway is initiated through the release of tissue factor from macrophages and endothelial cells, which can be induced through the inflammatory mediators IL-1 and TNF-α. A cascade ensues, resulting ultimately in the initiation of the common pathway through conversion of Factor X to **Xa**.
- In the common pathway, Factor V attached to the platelet membrane serves as a receptor for **Xa**. This complex, along with calcium ions, is called the prothrombin activator and allows Factor **Xa** to cleave prothrombin to form thrombin.
- Thrombin cleaves fibrinogen to form fibrin monomers. These monomers can then polymerize to form long fibrin fibers that form the foundation of the blood clot. Also, thrombin activates Factor XIII, which works to covalently crosslink fibrin chains to stabilize the clot. Clot dissolution occurs primarily by fibrinolysis, a result of the action of plasmin.
- Control of coagulation can generally be achieved through physiological factors or soluble and insoluble biochemical factors. Blood flow can regionally remove and/or dilute activated components of the coagulation cascade to inhibit coagulation. Also, limitations in the presence of surfaces (such as activated platelet membranes) to catalyze several of the steps of the coagulation cascade can result in limitation of coagulation. Soluble agents can bind coagulation factors to inhibit their actions.

- The endothelium in its native state presents anticoagulative properties through the presence and action of entities such as heparin sulfate, PGI_2, and TPA. However, disruption of the glycocalyx by injury results in exposure of the endothelial ECM molecules to the reactive plasma proteins to initiate coagulation through the intrinsic pathway. Also, the stimuli provided by cytokines such as IL-1 and TNF-α released by cells of acute inflammation can result in the endothelium becoming increasingly pro-coagulatory in nature.
- The examination of the general biocompatibility of a material should, in many cases, include assessment of the hemocompatibility of the material. Both local and systemic effects from blood-contacting materials can result from three factors: blood characteristics, flow parameters, and material surface characteristics.
- *In vitro* testing can be either static or dynamic and can include quantification of the coagulation time, number of adhered platelets, mass of adherent thrombus, and amount of platelet granule release.
- *In vivo* assessment of the hemocompatibility of materials provides more complete information than *in vitro* analyses. An alternative approach to assess hemocompatibility is *ex vivo* examination of a tubular material as a shunt. Although shunts allow for greater control of the experimental conditions, they do not replicate the implantation procedure.

Problems

13.1 A primary step for blood coagulation resulting from the contact of blood with a biomaterial is protein adsorption to the biomaterial surface. Name some proteins that can initiate coagulation.

13.2 Describe the main differences between platelets and other mammalian cells.

13.3 What changes occur within a platelet when it is activated? What differences can be observed in its morphology following activation? Which of the following two micrographs shows activated platelets? (Figures adapted with permission from [6].)

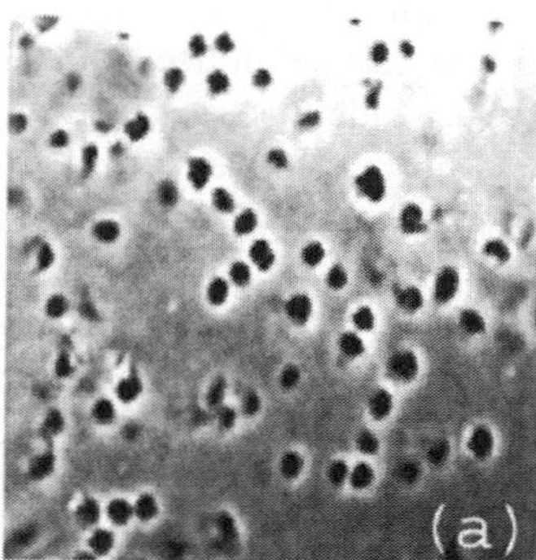

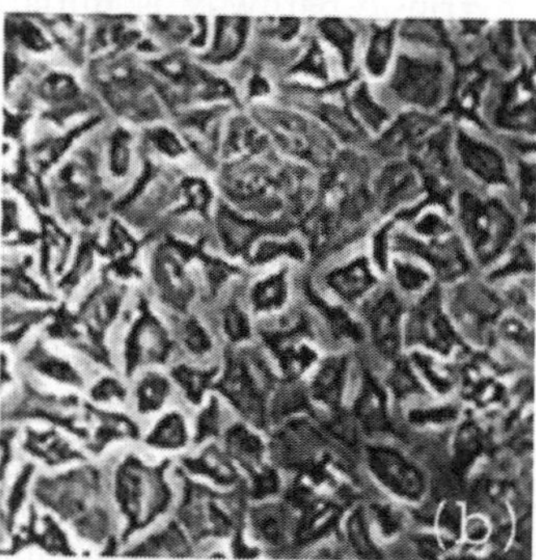

13.4 Do you expect blood coagulation to occur following injury of the endothelium of a blood vessel?

13.5 An experimental cardiovascular biomaterial with a positive surface charge was implanted in an animal model. Histological analysis of harvested implants revealed that coagulation occurred shortly after implantation.

(a) Which of the two pathways of the coagulation cascade is most likely responsible for this result?

(b) How would the coagulation time differ between this and the remaining pathway?

13.6 There are many examples of positive feedback mechanisms within the coagulation cascade to accelerate the coagulation process. What factors prevent coagulation throughout the body?

13.7 Would you expect the surface roughness of an implanted cardiovascular biomaterial to affect blood coagulation?

13.8 You are considering a new material for use in a vascular graft. Preliminary studies involving subcutaneous implantation of the material in the form of a disc in a rat model are promising. Subsequent *in vivo* studies with a larger animal model using a vascular graft configuration tested in an *ex vivo* setup similar to that shown in Fig. 13.4 indicate that the material is not hemocompatible. What is the reason for the different biological response observed in the larger animal model?

13.9 You are responsible for testing the hemocompatibility of a new poly(ethylene)-based material. You perform an experiment in which you incubate your material with platelets suspended in a mixture of blood plasma proteins containing different amounts of either fibrinogen (Fg) or vWF under either static or flow conditions. Using surface analysis techniques, you confirm that with increasing amounts of Fg or vWF in the plasma solution, you observe greater adsorption of each protein on the surface of the sample in both static and flow conditions. You then use the LDH assay to determine the number of adherent platelets in each case (results are shown below). (Figure (a) is adapted for educational purposes from [7], with a maintenance of the observed trends. Data appearing in (b) are purely hypothetical and for illustrative purposes only.)

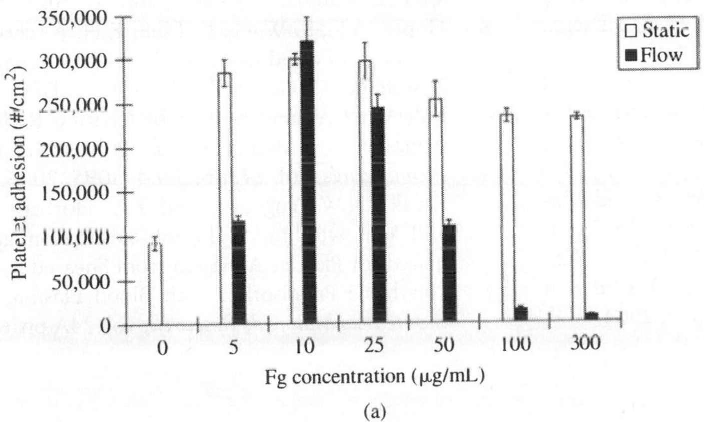

(a)

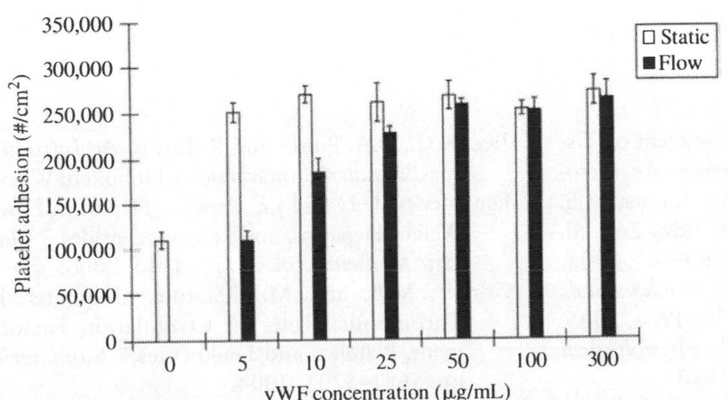

(b)

(a) How does the LDH assay work? Explain why this assay is a good choice to determine platelet adhesion in this experiment.

(b) Why are you particularly interested in the proteins Fg and vWF? Explain in terms of the role of these proteins in blood coagulation.

(c) Your company would like to use this material for a vascular graft application for small diameter blood vessels. You are asked to modify the material so that it releases an agent that deactivates (nullifies the effects of) either adsorbed Fg or adsorbed vWF. Based on the data presented, for this application, which protein is more important to deactivate and why?

(d) Your company has decided to turn its attention towards treating aneurysms (localized, mechanically compromised bulges in blood vessels). One treatment is to encourage clotting within the aneurysm so that blood flow is diverted to nearby vessels instead of stressing the aneurysm. A colleague suggests that a good way to use your material for this application would be to modify its surface to enhance Fg adsorption. Using the data you have already collected, do you agree? Why or why not?

References

1. Guyton, A.C. and J.E. Hall. *Textbook of Medical Physiology*, 9th ed. Philadelphia: W.B. Saunders, 1996.
2. Hanson, S.R. "Blood Coagulation and Blood-Material Interactions." In *Biomaterials Science: An Introduction to Materials in Medicine*, B.D. Ratner, A.S. Hoffman, F.J. Schoen, and J.E. Lemons, Eds., 2nd ed. San Diego: Elsevier Academic Press, pp. 332–338, 2004.
3. Colman, R.W., J. Hirsh, V.J. Marder, A.W. Clowes, and J.N. George. *Hemostasis and Thrombosis: Basic Principles and Clinical Practice*. Philadelphia: Lippincott, Williams, and Wilkins, 2001.
4. Hanson, S.R. and B.D. Ratner. "Evaluation of Blood-Materials Interactions." In *Biomaterials Science: An Introduction to Materials in Medicine*, B.D. Ratner, A.S. Hoffman, F.J. Schoen, and J.E. Lemons, Eds., 2nd ed. San Diego: Elsevier Academic Press, pp. 367–379, 2004.
5. Dixit, P., D. Hern-Anderson, J. Ranieri, and C.E. Schmidt. "Vascular Graft Endothelialization: Comparative Analysis of Canine and Human Endothelial Cell Migration on Natural Biomaterials," *Journal of Biomedical Materials Research*, vol. 56, pp. 545–555, 2001.
6. Gupta, A.S., S. Wang, E. Link, E.H. Anderson, C. Hofmann, J. Lewandowski, K. Kottke-Marchant, and R.E. Marchant. "Glycocalyx-Mimetic Dextran-Modified Poly(Vinyl Amine) Surfactant Coating Reduces Platelet Adhesion on Medical-Grade Polycarbonate Surface," *Biomaterials*, vol. 27, pp. 3084–3095, 2006.
7. Kwak, D.,W. Yuguang, and T.A. Horbett. "Fibrinogen and Von willebrand's Factor Adsorption are both Required for Platelet Adhesion from Sheared Suspensions to Polythlene Preadsorbec with Blood Plasma," *Journal of Biomedical Materials Research,* vol. 74A pp. 69–83, 2005.

Additional Reading

Anderson, J.M. and F.J. Schoen. "*In Vivo* Assesment of Tissue Compatibility." In *Biomaterials Science: An Introduction to Materials in Medicine,* B.D. Ratner, A.S. Hoffman, F.J. Schoen, and J.E. Lemons, Eds., 2nd ed. San Diego: Elsevier Academic Press, pp. 360–367, 2004.

Black, J. *Biological Performance of Materials: Fundamentals of Biocompatibility*, 4th ed. New York: CRC Press, 2005.

Bruck, S.D. *Properties of Biomaterials in the Physiological Environment*. Boca Raton: CRC Press, 1980.

Dee, K.C., D.A. Puleo, and R. Bizios. *An Introduction to Tissue-Biomaterial Interactions*. Hoboken: Wiley-Liss, 2002.

Dinwoodey, D.L. and J.E. Ansell. "Heparins, Low-Molecular-Weight Heparins, and Pentasaccharides," *Clinics in Geriatric Medicine*, vol. 22, pp. 1–15, 2006.

Gorbet, M.B. and M.V. Sefton. "Biomaterial-Associated Thrombosis: Roles of Coagulation Factors, Complement, Platelets and Leukocytes," *Biomaterials*, vol. 25, pp. 5681–5703, 2004.

Hanson, S.R. and B.D. Ratner. "Evaluation of Blood-Materials Interactions." In *Biomaterials Science: An Introduction to Materials in Medicine*, B.D. Ratner, A.S. Hoffman, F.J. Schoen, and J.E. Lemons, Eds., 2nd ed. San Diego: Elsevier Academic Press, pp. 367–379, 2004.

Horbett, T.A. "Principles Underlying the Role of Adsorbed Plasma Proteins in Blood Interactions with Foreign Materials," *Cardiovascular Pathology*, vol. 2, pp. 137S–148S, 1993.

Lafleur, M.A., M.M. Handsley, and D.R. Edwards. "Metalloproteinases and Their Inhibitors in Angiogenesis," *Expert Reviews in Molecular Medicine*, vol. 5, pp. 1–39, 2003.

Sefton, M.V. and C.H. Gemmell. "Nonthrombogenic Treatments and Strategies." In *Biomaterials Science: An Introduction to Materials in Medicine*, B.D. Ratner, A.S. Hoffman, F.J. Schoen, and J.E. Lemons, Eds., 2nd ed. San Diego: Elsevier Academic Press, pp. 456–470, 2004.

Silver, F.H. and D.L. Christiansen. *Biomaterials Science and Biocompatibility*. New York: Springer, 1999.

CHAPTER 14 Infection, Tumorigenesis and Calcification of Biomaterials

Main Objective

To understand the steps involved in, and results of, three potentially deleterious responses to implanted biomaterials: infection, tumorigenesis, and pathologic calcification.

Specific Objectives

1. To understand characteristics of implant-associated infection and common pathogens involved in these infections.
2. To understand the steps involved in implant infection.
3. To understand the characteristics of the bacterial surface and means to examine these surface properties.
4. To understand how bacterial surface properties, biomaterial surface properties, and media type contribute to specific and nonspecific bacterial adhesion.
5. To distinguish among classes of carcinogens and explain basic steps in tumor development.
6. To compare and contrast chemical and foreign body tumorigenesis.
7. To understand the causes and contributing factors for foreign body tumorigenesis.
8. To understand mechanisms of pathologic calcification and how this can affect properties of biomaterials.
9. To understand the concepts behind and possible limitations to the *in vitro* and *in vivo* models presented for examination of infection, tumorigenesis and pathologic calcification.

14.1 Introduction: Overview of Other Potential Problems with Biomaterial Implantation

Previous chapters have described possible negative responses stemming from the innate and acquired immune responses or the coagulation pathways after biomaterials implantation. However, there are several other serious complications that can occur due to the presence of a biomaterial in the body. These include device-related *infection*, *tumorigenesis* by the implant, and *pathologic calcification*. In each of these pathological responses, the presence of the biomaterial affects normal body function and may necessitate removal of the implant. Therefore, preventing these reactions is the subject of much current biomaterials research.

14.2 Infection

Infection can occur on or surrounding any type of implant, including artificial organs, synthetic blood vessels, joint replacements, intravenous catheters, and urologic devices. A number of characteristics of implant-associated infection have been identified that distinguish it from other types of infection, regardless of the area of the body afflicted:

1. Presence of biomaterial and/or damaged underlying ECM
2. Bacterial colonization of tissue
3. Resistance to host defense mechanisms and antibiotic therapy
4. Presence of characteristic bacteria types (see below)
5. Transformation of relatively innocuous bacterial species into virulent organisms by the presence of a biomaterial
6. Presence of multiple bacteria species
7. Persistence of infection until removal of the substratum
8. Absence of integration of the biomaterial with the host
9. Presence of cell damage or necrosis

14.2.1 Common Pathogens and Categories of Infection

One characteristic of implant-associated infections is the relatively small number of pathogens usually present in the afflicted area. In addition, many of these are commonly found on or in the human body and do not produce infection prior to biomaterial implantation. The organisms most often responsible for biomaterial-related infection are the gram-positive bacteria (see later sections of this chapter for explanation of this term) *Staphylococcus aureus* and *Staphylococcus epidermidis*, the gram-negative bacteria *Enterobacteriaceae* and *Pseudomonas aeriginosa*, and fungi such as *Candida* spp.[1]

The presence of these pathogens can result in infection immediately upon implantation or at some later time. Thus, three categories of implant-associated infections have been defined, depending on the time of onset and the location in the body. A **superficial immediate infection** occurs if there is growth of microorganisms on the skin in association with an implant (e.g. growth under burn dressings). These infections, which develop soon after the implantation procedure, are usually caused by skin-dwelling bacteria such as *Staphylococcus aureus* and *Staphylococcus epidermidis*. A **deep immediate infection** is one is which there is the presence of an infection at the implant site soon after surgery. Like the previous type, this is often a result of the proliferation of skin-dwelling bacteria that were transported to the implant site during the procedure. In contrast, a **late infection** may occur months to years after the implantation surgery. The cause of this type of infection remains unclear, although it is thought to be a consequence of the seeding of bloodborne pathogens originating in another site (e.g. tooth infection).

[1]The designation spp. after a genus refers to more than one unnamed species.

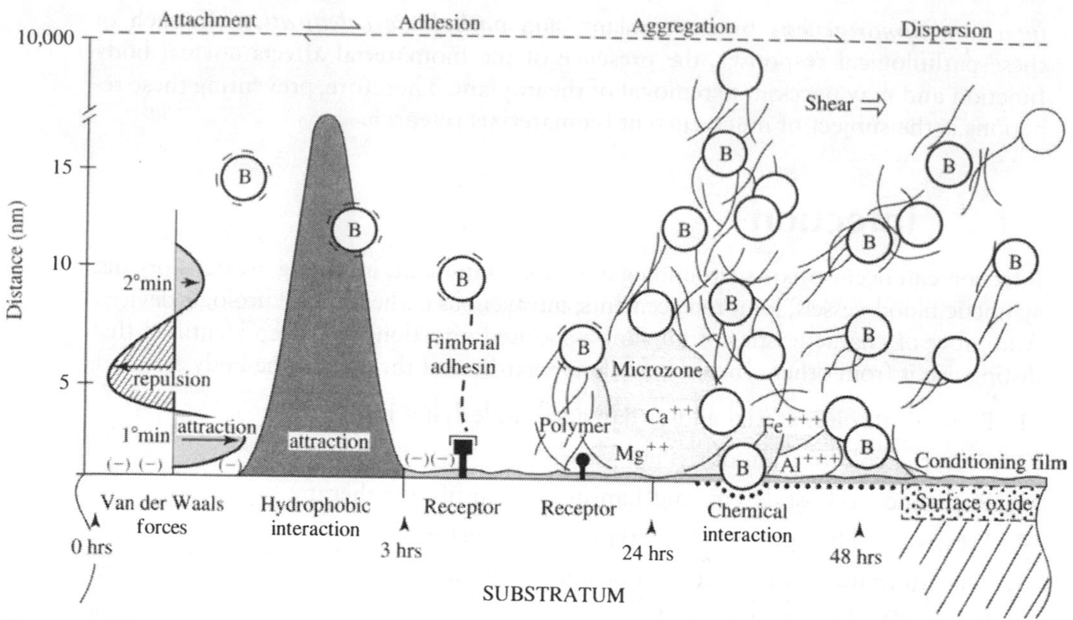

Figure 14.1
The four stages of infection. The first stage, bacterial (indicated by B) attachment to the surface, is reversible and is based on nonspecific interactions between the pathogen and the surface. In the second stage, adhesion, the microorganism becomes irreversibly bound to the biomaterial due to a combination of nonspecific and specific receptor–ligand interactions. The third stage, aggregation, occurs when the bacteria have firmly adhered to the substrate and begin to divide and form colonies. In the final stage, dispersion, shear forces from trauma, normal implant motion, or flowing blood may cause a portion of the bacterial colony to detach and move to other areas of the body. (Adapted with permission from [1].)

14.2.2 Steps to Infection

A number of steps must occur in order for bacterial attachment to a biomaterial to progress to a clinical infection. As summarized in Fig. 14.1, four distinct stages have been identified.[2] First, **bacterial attachment** to the surface is *reversible* and is based on nonspecific interactions between the pathogen and the surface. Therefore, the surface characteristics of bacteria and the substrate play a large role in this step.

In the next stage, **adhesion,** the microorganism becomes irreversibly (permanently) bound to the biomaterial due to a combination of nonspecific and specific receptor–ligand interactions between the pathogen and the surface (discussed further below). The strength of this interaction is time dependent and requires a matter of hours to develop.

After the bacteria have firmly adhered to the substrate, they begin to divide and form colonies. In this stage, termed **aggregation,** the pathogens often exude an extracellular polysaccharide slime (**biofilm**). This biofilm protects the microorganisms from phagocytosis by neutrophils or tissue macrophages and provides a favorable environment for bacterial growth. Biofilm formation may occur as early as one day after bacterial attachment.

In the final stage, **dispersion,** shear forces from normal implant motion, trauma, or flowing blood may carry a portion of the bacterial colony to other areas of the

---

[2]Although in this and subsequent sections, we will focus on bacterial interactions with biomedical implants, the principles are similar for other microorganisms, such as fungi.

body. This can occur as soon as two days after initial bacterial attachment. The result is spreading of the infection locally, or, in some cases, a secondary infection at a disparate location.

Since it is increasingly difficult to control the infection after the formation of a biofilm layer, many of the approaches to reducing implant-related infections have focused on preventing bacteria from firmly adhering to biomaterials. After implantation of a device, the reactions that occur can be considered a "race for the surface" between soluble proteins, surrounding cells, and potential pathogens. The outcome of this race determines whether or not infection develops and is highly affected by what proteins are initially adsorbed and how they interact with both mammalian cells and bacteria. For example, if a particular biomaterial surface supports attachment of cells that have mechanisms for preventing bacterial attachment to their membranes, infection may be reduced in these implants.

14.2.3 Characteristics of the Bacterial Surface, the Biomaterial Surface, and the Media

As mentioned above, the ideal biomaterial surface would be simultaneously bacteria resistant and cell friendly, both of which are directly related to the type of proteins that adsorb to the material. A wide variety of surface modification technologies have been employed in order to prepare biomaterial surfaces with the physicochemical properties to encourage cell adhesion while repelling bacteria. However, as with other protein adsorption processes described in Chapters 8–13, one must understand how the characteristics of the bacterial surface, the biomaterial surface, and the media interact in order to modify the biomaterial so it will discourage microbe binding in a biological milieu. All three aspects of bacterial adhesion are described in more detail in this section.

14.2.3.1 Bacterial Surface Properties: Gram-Positive vs. Gram-Negative Bacteria Two major classes of bacteria can be distinguished: *gram positive* and *gram negative*. As illustrated in Fig. 14.2, **gram-positive** species have a single bilayered phospholipid membrane and a thick cell wall composed of peptidoglycan (the chemical structure of this molecule is shown in Fig. 14.3). Several macromolecules are associated with this cell wall, including polysaccharides, teichoic and teichuronic acids, and proteins. Some of these may act as mediators for specific binding to the ECM or biomaterials.

In contrast, **gram-negative** bacteria possess two phospholipid membranes: the cell membrane and an outer membrane. In these species, the peptidoglycan layer is thinner and located between the two membranes, as shown in Fig. 14.2. Like gram-positive bacteria, gram-negative bacteria contain macromolecules that extend from their outer membranes to interact with the environment. In addition, they often demonstrate **fimbriae** or **pili** (surface appendages up to 1 μm long resembling small filaments). Gram-negative bacteria may also possess flagella, which are longer and used for locomotion. Any of these appendages may play an additional role in adhesion to tissue and biomaterial surfaces.

14.2.3.2 Bacterial Surface Properties: Cell Capsule and Biofilm Certain species of both gram-positive and gram-negative bacteria have an outer layer composed of polysaccharides called the **cell capsule**. These molecules are firmly attached to the cell wall and, thus, are distinguished from the slime that is also found near the exterior of many bacterial species. The polysaccharides produced as a part of the **slime** (or **biofilm**) coating are released into the surroundings, and therefore are not directly attached to the bacterial surface.

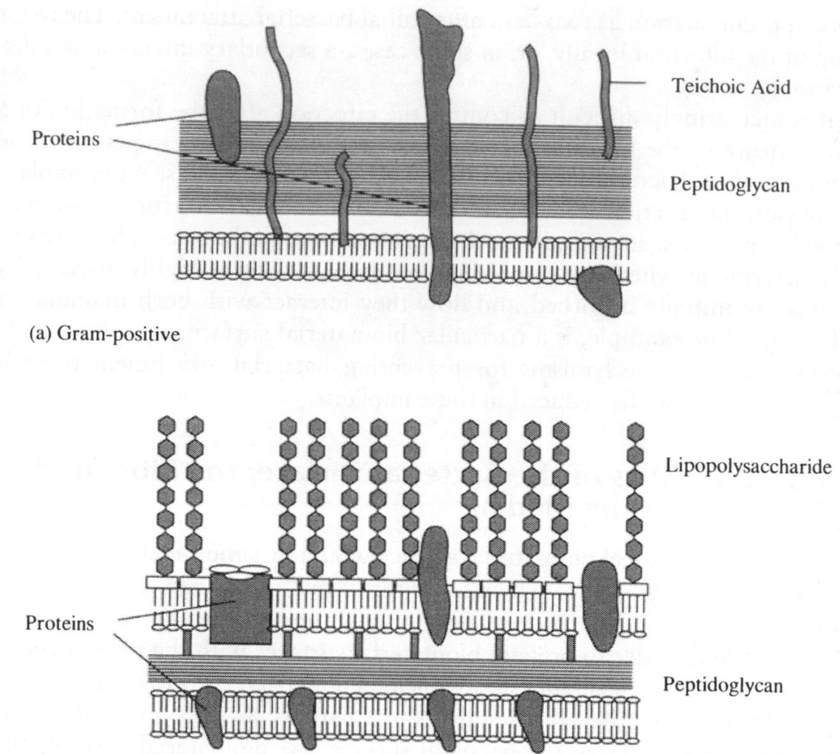

Figure 14.2
The two major classes of bacteria: gram-positive (a) and gram-negative (b). Gram-positive species have a single bilayered phospholipid membrane and a thick cell wall composed of peptidoglycan. Polysaccharides, teichoic and teichuronic acids, and proteins are among the macromolecules associated with this cell wall. Gram-negative bacteria possess two phospholipid membranes: the cell membrane and an outer membrane. In these species, the peptidoglycan layer is thinner and located between the two membranes. Like gram-positive bacteria, gram-negative bacteria contain macromolecules that extend from their outer membranes to interact with the environment. (Adapted with permission from [2] and [3].)

As discussed above, exudation of slime allows for the formation of a specialized microenvironment (a microzone) that allows the bacteria to trap ions important to their survival and protects them from the body's natural defenses. Several types of bacteria can be housed under a single biofilm coating. As depicted in Fig. 14.4, once encased in slime, bacterial colonies no longer remain attached to the surface, but are fixed to the biofilm, which takes on a mushroom-like appearance.

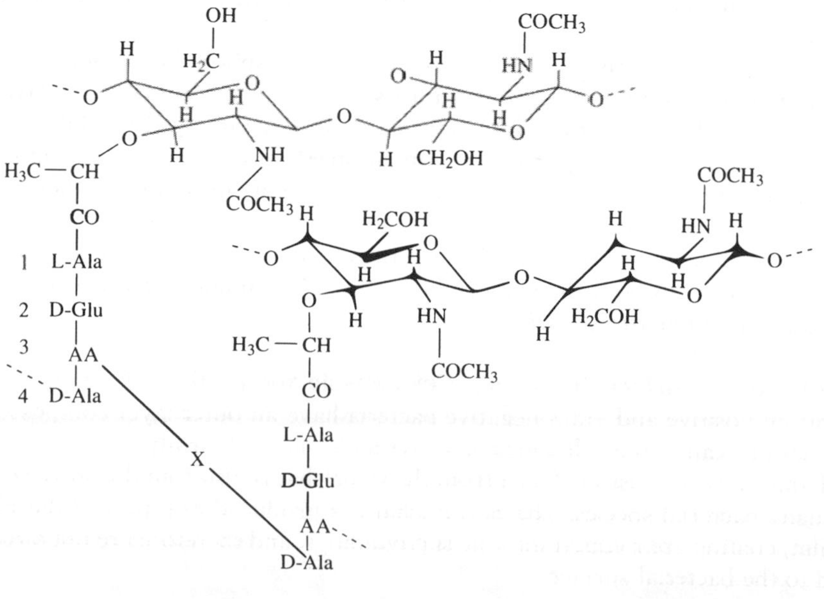

Figure 14.3
Chemical structure of peptidoglycan. The dotted lines indicate that additional repeat units of the depicted polymer are attached at these points. X represents a peptide crosslinker in this figure, and AA represents a diamino acid, such as that participating in the crosslink at position 3. (Adapted with permission from [4].)

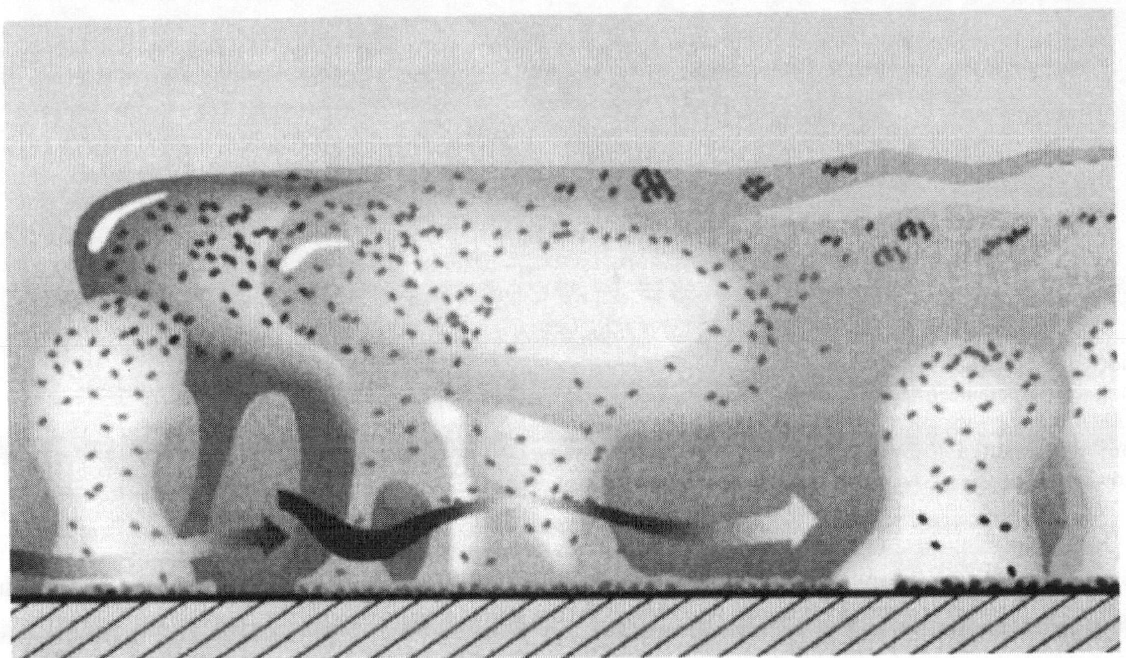

Figure 14.4
Schematic of a biofilm coating. Note that in a biofilm, the bacterial colonies (black spots) no longer remain attached to the surface, but are contained within the polysaccharide "slime." The arrow indicates the flow of water through open water channels in the biofilm. (Reprinted with permission from [5].)

The production of slime reduces the body's ability to kill adherent bacteria for several reasons. The biofilm forms a physical barrier to phagocytic cells, and certain components are thought to inhibit T and B cell formation, antibody production and bacterial opsonization, thus greatly decreasing the efficiency of both the innate and acquired immune responses. In addition, the presence of slime can impart antibiotic resistance. It has been found that the concentration of oral antibiotics required to kill biofilm bacteria is 100 times greater than the concentration needed to kill their planktonic counterparts. This may be partially due to the formation of a diffusional barrier for active agents. However, this effect may also be caused by phenotypic changes that render biofilm bacteria more resistant to oral antibiotics, many of which were developed to kill free-floating pathogens.

It should also be noted when designing experiments that bacterial surface properties may change depending on growth conditions. In fact, many laboratory-grown bacteria can have significantly different phenotypes than the wild strains from which they were derived. The bacterial surface properties of most importance in adhesion to biomaterials are surface hydrophobicity and charge, as well as the presence of any molecules, such as those mentioned above, that can promote specific interactions with the substrate. Means of bacterial surface characterization are discussed in the following techniques section.

14.2.3.3 Biomaterial Surface Properties The same material surface properties that govern protein adsorption (see Chapter 7) also affect bacterial adhesion because components of the adsorbed protein layer may form specific interactions with bacterial cell membrane constituents. Important biomaterial properties include surface hydrophobicity and charge as well as physical properties such as steric concerns and surface roughness.

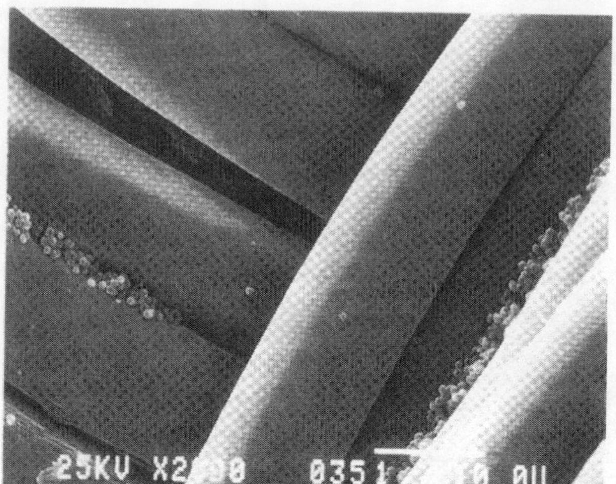

Figure 14.5
Scanning electron micrograph depicting bacteria entrapped between fibers of woven Dacron™. (Reprinted with permission from [6].)

As with cell attachment, bacteria may be prevented from adhering to surfaces due to steric repulsion from bulky hydrophilic groups. In contrast, grooves or valleys may trap bacteria and encourage the formation of colonies on the substrate, as shown in Fig. 14.5, which depicts bacteria entrapped between fibers of woven Dacron™. All of the surface characterization techniques described in Chapter 7 can be used to determine surface properties of biomaterials pertinent to bacterial adhesion. These include contact angle for hydrophobicity, ESCA, ATR-FTIR, and SIMS for chemical analysis, and SEM and AFM for topographical evaluation.

14.2.3.4 Media Properties As mentioned above, the proteins deposited on the biomaterial surface can play a significant role in bacterial adhesion. In addition to biomaterial surface properties, the nature of this coating is affected by the type of proteins found in the media surrounding the material. Additionally, the media characteristics are important because both protein adsorption and bacterial adhesion are governed by thermodynamic parameters. For either event to occur spontaneously, the overall change in the Gibbs free energy (ΔG) for the reaction must be negative. As discussed in Chapter 8, ΔG is partially dependent on the chemical properties of the media (solvent), such as the presence of ions that shield electrostatic repulsion between like-charged surfaces.

14.2.4 Specific and Non-Specific Interactions Involved in Bacterial Adhesion

Much like cell attachment, bacterial adhesion to biomedical implants can be caused by both nonspecific and specific interactions. As explained in Chapter 9, nonspecific binding can be modeled using DLVO theory (based on work from Derjaguin, Landau, Verway and Overbeek). Figure 14.6 depicts the free energy of interaction, $G(z)$, between a particle (the bacterium) and the surface, as determined by DLVO theory, as a function of separation distance (z). As the bacterium approaches the surface, there is a drop in potential energy (the secondary minimum), representing a balance between long-range electrostatic interactions (repulsive) and long-range van der Waals interactions (attractive). If the random (Brownian) motion of the bacterium is sufficient to overcome the potential energy barrier and reach the primary minimum (not shown in the figure), the pathogen can become firmly adherent to the surface.

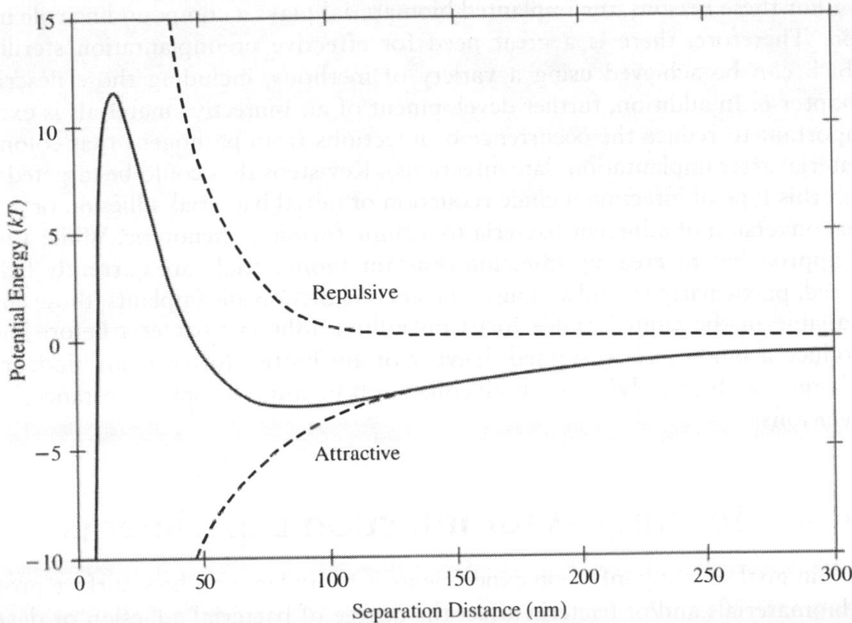

Figure 14.6
Dependence of the free energy of interaction between the bacterium and the biomaterial surface as a function of separation distance according to DLVO theory for bacterial adhesion. As the bacterium approaches the surface, there is a drop in potential energy (the secondary minimum), representing a balance between long-range electrostatic interactions (repulsive) and long-range van der Waals interactions (attractive). At this point, the bacterium is loosely (reversibly) bound to the surface. If the bacterium can overcome the potential energy barrier seen on the extreme left, it can reach the primary minimum (not shown) and become irreversibly bound. (Adapted with permission from [2].)

As discussed for cell attachment, DLVO theory is a highly idealized and simplified model. In reality, the complex nature of the bacterial cell membrane makes it probable that specific interactions between the membrane and the substrate also take place. In this case, receptors and ligands can extend into the media to promote binding and overcome the energy barrier depicted in the DLVO model. Many bacteria are known to have receptors for a variety of ECM components. These receptors are collectively called **microbial surface components recognizing adhesive matrix molecules (MSCRAMMs)**. For example, *Staphylococcus aureus* employs MSCRAMMs to bind to the ECM molecules fibronectin, vitronectin, and von Willebrand factor.

14.2.5 Summary of Implant-Associated Infections

Infections of biomedical implants are unique in that they are usually caused by transformation of relatively innocuous bacterial species into virulent organisms by the presence of a biomaterial. Several steps are required for this transformation, which is aided by the existence of the biomaterial and/or damaged underlying ECM as a surface for attachment of bacteria. The adherent bacteria then become resistant to host defense mechanisms and antibiotics for a number of reasons. The bacteria begin to form slime, which provides both a physical and a chemical barrier to the innate and acquired immune system and to the actions of antibiotics. In addition, the constant presence of the biomaterial may "exhaust" the granulocytes' ability to kill or phagocytose the pathogen.

For these reasons, the implanted biomaterial plays a compounding role in infection. Therefore, there is a great need for effective preimplantation sterilization, which can be achieved using a variety of methods, including those described in Chapter 6. In addition, further development of anti-infective materials is extremely important to reduce the occurrence of infections from pathogens that colonize the material after implantation (late infections). Key steps that could be targeted to prevent this type of infection include reduction of initial bacterial adhesion or arresting the conversion of adherent bacteria to a slime-forming phenotype. While a number of approaches to creating infection-resistant biomaterials are currently being explored, particularly for indwelling catheters and orthopedic implants, those currently available in the United States focus on killing adherent bacteria before they can produce a biofilm via sustained delivery of antibiotics (often from biodegradable polymers such as poly(lactic-co-glycolic acid) or antimicrobial substances such as silver ions.

14.3 Techniques for Infection Experiments

A main goal of many infection experiments is to understand how surface properties of biomaterials and/or bacteria affect the degree of bacterial adhesion or developed infection. Thus, a variety of techniques are required to relate measured parameters to overall infection potential. These include methods to characterize the biomaterial and bacterial surfaces and to quantify bacterial adhesion *in vitro* and the degree of infection *in vivo*. Biomaterial surface characterization was discussed in Chapter 7, and the other techniques are reviewed here.

14.3.1 Characterizing Bacterial Surfaces

As mentioned above, the bacterial surface properties of most importance to nonspecific binding are hydrophobicity and charge, and characterization methods for these parameters are discussed in this section. It may also be possible to use immunostaining or ELISA techniques (see Chapters 8 and 9) to examine bacteria for the presence of surface receptors that participate in specific binding to the substrate.

14.3.1.1 Surface Hydrophobicity As with biomaterial surfaces, bacterial hydrophobicity can be quantified using contact angle measurements as described in Chapter 7. Similar calculations can be completed to estimate the surface tension for a particular bacterial strain. In this case, the test surface is a material completely covered by bacteria. However, care must be taken in this procedure since contact angles can be difficult to measure and interactions between the test liquid (water) and the bacteria may change with time due to desorption of bacterial surface molecules into the water.

Another technique to assess bacterial hydrophobicity is called **microbial adherence to hydrocarbons (MATH)**. In this method, a test tube is filled with a mixture of two liquid phases: water and a hydrophobic hydrocarbon-based solvent. The bacteria are then added, and migration of bacteria from the water to the hydrocarbon phase is recorded. A more hydrophobic strain will show greater movement to the hydrocarbon phase because it is thermodynamically more stable for the bacteria to be suspended in a hydrophobic milieu. This is tracked by monitoring the turbidity (cloudiness) of the aqueous phase over time using optical density measurements. While this method is relatively simple and quick to perform, it is difficult to quantify and is therefore best suited to characterizing bacteria as generally "hydrophobic" or "hydrophilic."

A more quantitative assessment of the degree of bacterial hydrophobicity can be obtained through the use of **hydrophobic interaction chromatography (HIC)**. This is a type of affinity chromatography, as described in Chapter 8. In this case, the equipment may not be as extensive as that described for HPLC (see Chapter 2), but the technique is similar to any other reversed phase liquid chromatography. For HIC, bacteria suspended in an aqueous phase are passed through a column containing a hydrophobic packing material. The amount of bacteria remaining in the aqueous phase after exiting the column is measured, indicating the number of bacteria that were retained in the packing matrix. The fraction retained increases with greater strain hydrophobicity. As with other types of liquid chromatography, small changes in the chemistry of the packing material or composition of the aqueous phase reveal subtle differences in hydrophobicity between strains.

14.3.1.2 Surface Charge Another key bacterial surface characteristic, charge, can be assessed using variations on common techniques. For example, surface charge can be measured via an **electrophoretic mobility test.** In this method, microbes are introduced into an electrophoresis gel like that described in Chapter 8, using a buffer of known ionic strength. The velocity of migration in a known electric field is then determined and related to the surface charge through calculations based on the Helmholtz-Smoluchowski equation, the specifics of which are beyond the scope of this text.

Alternatively, bacterial surface charge may be quantified via **electrostatic interaction chromatography** (EIC). EIC is actually a type of liquid chromatography known as ion exchange chromatography. This technique is generally similar to HIC, except that the packing material is either cationic or anionic. Depending on the type of packing material and the amount of bacteria retained in each case, both the degree and nature of the surface charge (positive or negative) can be determined.

EXAMPLE PROBLEM 14.1

A biomaterials laboratory has had a persistent problem with a particular strain of bacteria adhering to an experimental biomaterial. The experimental material is inherently highly hydrophobic and uncharged. The researchers are considering chemical modification of the biomaterial surface through plasma treatment. The hydrophobicity of the bacteria in question was assessed with the microbial adherence to hydrocarbons assay. It was found that the optical density of the hydrocarbon phase was significantly greater than that of the aqueous phase. Assuming that the adhesion is controlled by nonspecific interactions, will surface modification of the experimental biomaterial with plasma treatment likely decrease the adhesion of the particular bacterial strain? Why or why not?

Solution: The nonspecific binding of bacteria to a biomaterial surface is highly influenced by the charge and hydrophobicity of both the bacteria and the biomaterial surface. It is stated that the material is uncharged, so the nonspecific binding of bacteria to the biomaterial surface in this case will be dominated by hydrophobicity. It is given that the material is highly hydrophobic and that the researchers are considering surface modification through plasma treatment. This technique will increase the hydrophilicity of the biomaterial. If the bacterial strain is hydrophobic, then this modification will discourage bacterial adhesion based on hydrophobic interactions. However, if the bacterial strain is hydrophilic, then this modification will encourage bacterial adhesion based on hydrophobic interactions. The microbial adherence to hydrocarbons assay results show that the optical density of the hydrocarbon phase is greater than that of the aqueous phase. Thus, more bacteria migrated to the hydrocarbon phase than the aqueous phase, suggesting that the bacteria are hydrophobic. Consequently, plasma treatment of the biomaterial surface will likely decrease the adhesion of the bacterial strain. ■

14.3.2 *In Vitro* and *In Vivo* Models of Infection

Like other tests for biocompatibility, both *in vitro* and *in vivo* experiments to assess a biomaterial's proclivity to infection can be performed. *Ex vivo* assays using shunts, like those described in Chapter 13 for hemocompatibility testing, are also common. An overview of these techniques is provided in this section.

14.3.2.1 *In Vitro* Bacterial Adhesion *In vitro* infection testing focuses on quantification of bacterial adhesion to biomaterials under static or well-defined flow conditions. The basic experimental design is similar to that described in Chapter 9 for cell attachment assays and begins with the introduction of the bacteria in the media surrounding the test material. The microbes are allowed to attach over a set period of time and then a well-controlled washing step is performed. Adherent bacteria are usually quantified by microscopic visualization of the surface and manual counting of the number of bacteria per image. The microbes can be stained with colored or fluorescent dyes to aid in quantification. In some cases, image analysis software may be employed to automate the counting procedure.

Inclusion of control materials for the given application is important when using this method to evaluate bacterial adhesion to novel biomaterials. In this way, it can be determined whether or not a new biomaterial discourages bacterial adhesion when compared with a material currently used for the target device.

14.3.2.2 *Ex Vivo* and *In Vivo* Infection Models *Ex vivo* models of infection involve the use of shunts, much like those described for hemocompatibility testing (see Chapter 13). In this case, the pathogen of interest is inoculated near the biomaterial, and bacterial adhesion (and subsequent developments) in the presence of flowing blood is followed over the course of several hours. These assays are most useful for examining infections of blood-contacting devices. They provide the advantage that the flow environment is similar to that seen *in vivo*; however, the use of shunts is more expensive than *in vitro* testing and therefore may not be cost-effective if screening a large number of samples.

In vivo models of infection use both small animals (rodents) and larger animals. Rodents are most often employed to screen new biomaterials (e.g. novel anti-infectives) rather than to test entire devices. The cage implant system described in Chapter 11 for *in vivo* assessment of inflammation may also be used in infection testing to examine how an "infected material" responds to soluble antibiotic therapies. In contrast, a complete device may be implanted in larger animal models. In these experiments, bacteria may be introduced via direct placement at the implant site or though injection into the bloodstream to mimic different sources of infection. As discussed in Chapter 11, the type of animal and implantation location chosen depends on the final use for the device.

For both *ex vivo* or *in vivo* experiments, assessment methods are similar and usually include histology and SEM of explants at various time points, using techniques described in Chapter 11. Additionally, the animal's blood may be tested over the course of the experiment for leukocyte and lymphocyte counts. As explained in earlier chapters, both of these cell types will be stimulated by the presence of certain molecules on the bacterial surface and, thus, a larger number of these cells would be expected if a severe infection is present.

Alternatively, the amount of bacterial cell wall antibodies found in the blood at different times may be quantified via ELISA techniques (see Chapter 8) to determine the extent of infection over time. In addition to antibody-based methods, the Limulus Amebocyte Lysate (LAL) assay, a colorimetric assay like that discussed in Chapter 8, has been developed to detect the presence of certain molecules (lipopolysaccharides, LPS) found in the outer membrane of gram-negative bacteria. LPS molecules have the potential to bind with receptors found on monocytes/macrophages and neutrophils to stimulate the inflammatory response. Thus, this assay is particularly important because, even after bacterial death, the presence of these molecules around the material could negatively affect the biocompatibility of the implant.

14.4 Tumorigenesis

14.4.1 Definitions and Steps of Tumorigenesis

Another potential problem with biomaterial implantation having serious consequences is the formation of tumors (**tumorigenesis**). Before beginning a detailed discussion of this phenomenon, a number of terms should be defined. **Neoplasia** refers to excessive and uncontrolled cell proliferation. This cell division is not related to the physiologic requirements of tissue and is not arrested by removal of the stimulus that caused it, so it can be separated from all other types of normal cell proliferation during development or wound healing. This new growth is called a **neoplasm** or a **tumor** and is composed of proliferating neoplastic cells and surrounding connective tissue and blood vessels.

Benign tumors do not invade adjacent tissues or spread to distant sites. However, **malignant tumors** do invade surrounding tissues and gain entry into lymph and blood vessels, so they can be transported to distant sites (this is called tumor **metastasis**). Malignant tumors usually contain cells that are less differentiated than normal tissue cells.

A **carcinogen** is a stimulus that causes malignant transformation, thought to occur due to mutations in the DNA of normal cells (**mutagenesis**). There are several classes of carcinogens, and their roles in cancer formation have not yet been fully elucidated. A **complete carcinogen** causes malignant transformation by itself, while a **procarcinogen** is not a carcinogen in its native form, but can be converted to one by metabolic processes found *in vivo*. A **cocarcinogen** possesses little or no inherent mutagenic potential, but enhances the activity of pro- or complete carcinogens.

Even in the presence of carcinogens, malignant transformation is often a result of an accumulation of genetic damage and is therefore a multistep process. The complexity of these events and their timing provides an additional challenge in relating biomaterial properties to carcinogenic potential. Three basic stages of tumorigenesis have been identified:

1. Initiation
2. Latency
3. Promotion

The primary cellular transformation occurs in the **initiation** phase. This can be followed by a **latency** period whose length varies by species. For humans, this may be on the order of 15–20 years. No tumor formation is visible during this period. At some point (the exact timing is not understood), the **promotion** stage is entered. This is the phase where obvious tumor development and growth can be observed.

14.4.2 Chemical vs. Foreign Body Carcinogenesis

Two main routes of malignant transformation can be encountered: chemical carcinogenesis and foreign body carcinogenesis. **Chemical carcinogenesis** is possible near biomaterials since tumors may be caused by substances that have leached from the implant. Similarly, transformations in organs distant from the device may occur if the carcinogen is transported away from the implant site. Known chemical carcinogens are usually hydrocarbon-based molecules. The role of metals is more controversial and there is no strong evidence of ceramics as chemical carcinogens.

The concept of **foreign body carcinogenesis** was developed based on data from implantation of various materials in rodents. In many experiments, a solid material with no chemical carcinogenic activity was observed to cause tumor formation, and the ability of the material to induce malignant transformation increased with the size of the implant. Materials exhibiting a resolved inflammatory response (fibrous encapsulation) were usually more able to cause tumorigenesis. The exact cause of foreign-body carcinogenesis remains unclear, but chemical and electrical conditions near the tissue–implant interface differ from those found in regular tissue, so alterations in the local environment may be one factor (see below for further discussion of potential causes).

14.4.3 Timeline for Foreign Body Tumorigenesis

14.4.3.1 Foreign Body Tumorigenesis with Large Implants Like other types of tumor formation, foreign body tumorigenesis involves several steps. The process begins during the foreign body reaction to an implanted material, which is described in more detail in Chapter 11. During this time, cellular proliferation associated with creation of a fibrous capsule is common. Preneoplastic cells may be present at this point, but transformation has not yet occurred. A cell type implicated in foreign body tumorigenesis is the pericyte, which is associated with the microvasculature formed during this stage.

After the fibrous capsule is fully generated, the inflammatory response becomes quiescent. However, there is continued contact of the preneoplastic cells with the implanted material. During this phase, malignant transformation may occur, followed by a latent period. At a later time, there is final maturation of preneoplastic cells, resulting in tumor growth.

Certain aspects relating to the mechanism of foreign body tumorigenesis have been observed in *in vivo* experiments. It is thought that the transformation event occurs early in implantation and is not directly caused by the foreign body (material). Additionally, the final steps leading to tumor growth can only occur if the malignant cells are in a relatively protected, quiet environment such as the fibrous capsule. This is not permitted in implants with continued macrophage activity (unresolved inflammation). Among the possible causes of foreign-body carcinogenesis are the following [7]:

1. Bulk chemical properties of the implant
2. Physicochemical surface properties of the implant
3. Viral contamination of the implant
4. Interruption of cellular communication due to the presence of the implant
5. Local tissue damage leading to insufficient nutrient exchange
6. Disturbed cellular growth around the implant

14.4.3.2 Foreign Body Tumorigenesis with Small Fibers The previous discussion of foreign body tumorigenesis has focused on implants where the material was much larger than the size of a cell. However, it should be noted that small fibers (less than 1 μm in diameter and more than 8 μm in length) have been implicated in certain cancers, regardless of chemical composition. This was first discovered in humans who had inhaled asbestos fibers and subsequently developed a type of cancer known as mesothelioma. The proposed mechanism of malignant transformation in these cases is that the small fibers can penetrate the cell membrane and cause direct mechanical damage to the nucleus, resulting in genetic alterations in the cell.

14.4.4 Summary of Biomaterial-Related Tumorigenesis

Tumorigenesis results from a complex series of events, most likely involving genetic mutation, that are not at present fully understood (Fig. 14.7). Tumor formation can be caused by the presence of a biomedical implant, which may lead to disruption of cell–cell communication or physical damage to surrounding cells, or by chemicals leached from the device. There is a relatively low incidence of implant-related tumorigenesis in humans. This may be because the solubility of many implant materials (like metals) is low in physiologic fluids, so the concentration may stay below threshold values for initiation of malignant transformation in humans.

If transformation does occur, it also remains unclear what controls the time line of tumor formation and the length of the latent phase between mutagenesis and tumor growth. No solid correlation between biomedical implants and tumor formation has been found, but the latent period creates difficulties in directly correlating the presence of biomaterials with tumorigenesis.

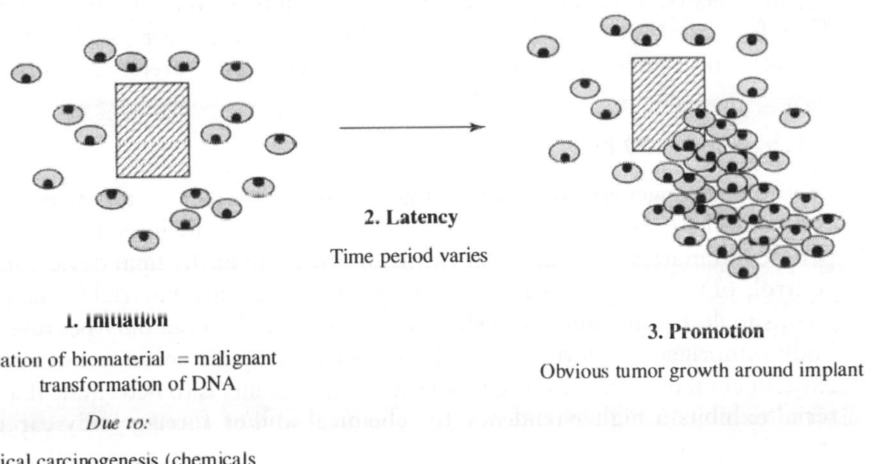

Figure 14.7
Steps of tumorigenesis, which results from a complex series of events, most likely involving genetic mutation, that are not at present fully understood. Tumor formation can be initiated by the presence of a biomedical implant, which may lead to disruption of cell–cell communication or physical damage to surrounding cells, or by chemicals leached from the device. It also remains unclear what controls the time line of tumor formation and the length of the latent phase between initiation and promotion (tumor growth). No solid correlation between biomedical implants and tumor formation has been found, but the latent period creates difficulties in directly correlating the presence of biomaterials with tumorigenesis.

14.5 Techniques for Tumorigenesis Experiments

Of the implant-associated pathologies described in this chapter, tumorigenesis testing is the best regulated by organizations such as ISO and ASTM. ISO standards require assays for carcinogenesis, although they may be combined with tests for other long-term sequelae, such as chronic toxicity. ISO regulations are most concerned with *in vivo* testing, but, due to generally low incidence of implant-related tumors in humans, this is only necessary when other sources (initial trials or *in vitro* testing) indicate a potential for tumor formation.

14.5.1 *In Vitro* Models

In vitro assays for tumorigenesis are actually tests for mutagenic potential, since all carcinogens are mutagens. (The reverse is not necessarily true.) A commonly used method of predicting mutagenic potential is the Ames test. This technique employs a mutant bacteria line that requires the amino acid histidine for growth. The bacteria are cultured with the sample material and an enzyme preparation in histidine-free media, so only the bacteria able to mutate to a non-histidine-dependent phenotype will be able to survive and proliferate. The number of surviving colonies are then quantified to provide an indicator of the mutagenic potential of the sample. Although this method is quick and inexpensive, it may have limited sensitivity to mutagenic agents, particularly when they are administered at low concentrations. Therefore, the Ames test should be conducted using proper positive and negative controls and should be considered only as a preliminary screening mechanism.

14.5.2 *In Vivo* Models

In vivo carcinogenesis assessment is generally undertaken as a part of general biocompatibility testing, as suggested by ISO and ASTM guidelines. In this case, the experimental material is usually fabricated in the form of the final device. In addition, controls of the same shape made from a noncarcinogenic material [often poly(ethylene)] should be implanted to distinguish responses observed only because of foreign body tumorigenesis (foreign-body based tumors should occur to both control and experimental materials). The goal of these experiments is to determine if a novel material exhibits a higher tendency for chemical and/or foreign body carcinogenesis than the control.

As discussed previously, the exact animal type and implantation location for these procedures depend on the final intended device function. In order to expedite assessment, particularly for pharmaceutical applications, recently the Food and Drug Administration has considered replacement of long-term rodent carcinogenicity studies with six-month studies in a transgenic mouse (RasH2) that was designed to be sensitive to a number of human carcinogens. Regardless of the animal model or duration of the study, at various time points during the experiment, the tissue around the implant should be excised and evaluated using general histological techniques and/or SEM (see Chapter 11) to detect tumor growth.

EXAMPLE PROBLEM 14.2

A research lab has developed a dental implant composed exclusively of a well known and characterized biomaterial. The biomaterial has been studied extensively in various *in vivo* models to evaluate the chemical carcinogenicity of the material. The results consistently indicate that the biomaterial is not a chemical carcinogen. To the surprise of the research lab, however, it was found during the *in vivo* evaluation of the dental implants that tumors were forming in the mandibles of the recipient animals. Is this dental implant an example of a chemical or a foreign body carcinogen? Would nondental implants composed of this material be expected to form a tumor? Is the material a mutagen?

Solution: The dental implant is an example of a foreign body carcinogen, as the implant material was known not to be a chemical carcinogen, yet resulted in tumor formation in the dental implant application. The size and shape of the implant, the implantation site, and the procedure could influence the tumorigenicity of the implant. Thus, although the implant resulted in tumor formation in the dental site, other implants of different sizes and shapes composed of this material might not necessarily result in tumor formation in other implantation sites. The implant is a mutagen, as it resulted in carcinogenesis in this case, and all carcinogens are mutagens. ■

14.6 Pathologic Calcification

14.6.1 Introduction to Pathologic Calcification

In addition to infection or tumor formation around a biomedical implant, an additional pathology that may occur to disrupt device function is pathologic calcification. **Pathologic calcification**, or undesired formation of nodules of calcium phosphate within or on the surface of an implanted material, has affected the operation of such devices as cardiac valves, cardiac assist devices (blood pumps), urinary prostheses, and soft contact lenses. Often ECM-derived materials are associated with this pathology, but calcification (or mineralization) of synthetic polymers is also a large concern. Although calcification can be desired in conjunction with some biomaterials applications, such as in bone tissue engineering to produce mineralized bone matrix, calcification can be undesirable in other applications, such as in artificial heart valves, which require flexibility for function. In this text, the term mineralization will denote the deposition of inorganic material in a tissue, whereas calcification will denote a subset of mineralization in which calcium is the major specific inorganic material deposited in the tissue.

The presence of mineral deposits can be considered deleterious to device function in some applications because they can have a large impact on the mechanical properties of biomaterials. As discussed in Chapter 4, ceramics, like the calcium phosphate materials that are deposited in pathologic calcification, are quite brittle. Therefore, pathologic calcification of natural or synthetic polymers can lead to premature fracture, particularly in devices that perform continued movement, such as pumps or heart valves.

The extent of pathologic calcification in a given system is dependent on the structure and chemistry of the biomaterial, as expected, but also on host metabolic factors and on the mechanical environment of the implant. The role of mechanical factors has not been fully elucidated, but the state of mineral metabolism in the host has a large effect on calcium deposition. For example, pathologic calcification occurs more quickly in younger patients, possibly because the metabolism of children with rapidly growing bones favors mineralization.

14.6.2 Mechanism of Pathologic Calcification

Pathologic calcification is found with either synthetic or naturally based materials, but natural materials treated with gluteraldehyde or formaldehyde are extremely susceptible. In many cases, these natural materials are not composed of individual ECM components, such as collagen, but are those in which the entire ECM is intact, and the material has been exposed to the agents listed above to preserve them and render them less immunogenic. A common example of an implant that often undergoes calcification in humans is the porcine heart valve.

Initiation of calcium deposits on these pretreated natural materials is thought to occur on dead cells or cell membrane fragments. As mentioned in Chapter 9, cell membranes contain proteins with attached phosphate groups that may act as nucleation sites to form calcium phosphate crystals. In addition, the enzyme alkaline phosphatase is linked to the membrane and is thought to have a role in promoting calcification in bone. Nonviable cells also do not possess the transport mechanisms (such as cell membrane pumps) to control the intracellular calcium concentration, leading to a potential increase in calcium ions near the phosphorous-containing proteins on the cell membrane. Fixing agents, such as gluteraldehyde, may promote these interactions by crosslinking and stabilizing the cell-surface proteins. Localized mechanical forces can increase the probability of calcification in an area, possibly due to an increase in regional cell death.

Later in the process, collagen, a major component of most natural biomaterials, can act as a template for the growth of mineral crystals, similar to what occurs in normal bone formation. As with calcification in bone, there are also a number of negatively charged, noncollagenous proteins that are associated with pathologic calcification and may act to direct or regulate crystal formation.

14.6.3 Summary and Techniques to Reduce Pathologic Calcification

Pathologic calcification of biomedical implants depends on the host metabolism, surface and bulk properties of the biomaterial chosen, and the mechanical environment of the device. Calcium phosphate deposition occurs first near cell membrane fragments and later in the collagen-rich ECM of naturally derived implants. It is thought that crystal formation in pathologic calcification follows a similar mechanism as that observed for normal bone formation.

One way to reduce the occurrence of this pathology is to target calcium phosphate crystal initiation. This is due to the fact that, once nucleated, crystal growth continues quickly because the blood and bodily fluids are nearly saturated in Ca and P ions. Several means to reduce unwanted calcification have been explored. These include localized release of inhibitors of calcium-phosphate crystal formation, such as trivalent metal ions (Fe^{3+} or Al^{3+}), which are thought to compete with calcium for complexation with free phosphate groups. Other treatments studied involve soaking naturally derived implants in ethanol or surfactants such as sodium dodecyl sulfate to remove the phosphate-containing cell membrane proteins that attract calcium ions to nucleate crystal formation.

14.7 Techniques for Pathologic Calcification Experiments

Both *in vitro* and *in vivo* models of pathologic calcification have been developed, although *in vivo* studies provide more information and, thus, are more commonly used. A review of various experimental systems is provided in this section.

14.7.1 *In Vitro* Models of Calcification

In *in vitro* studies of calcium deposition, materials or entire devices can be placed in a bath containing media approximating the chemical composition of a particular *in vivo* location (e.g., urine or blood). In alternate experimental configurations, the liquid may be either static or continuously circulating, and the implant may be in motion (such as flexion) or remain immobile during the course of the experiment. At appropriate time points, the sample is removed and analyzed for degree of calcification using the techniques described in subsequent sections. While these methods do not completely re-create the *in vivo* environment, like other *in vitro* experiments, they can be useful for initial screening of new biomaterials.

14.7.2 *In Vivo* Models of Calcification

Two types of *in vivo* experiments can be performed to assess the pathologic calcification of a biomaterial: subcutaneous implantation and insertion of the final device directly at the target location. In **subcutaneous** experiments, the material to be tested is placed under the skin, usually in mice or rats, although rabbit models are sometimes used. The advantage of such a procedure is that a smaller animal can be used and an extensive surgery is not required for implantation. In addition, similar types of calcium deposits are seen as those that would normally be found at the device site, but mineralization occurs at a more rapid rate, thus decreasing the overall time needed for the study. While subcutaneous assays may be used for preliminary or secondary testing of new biomaterials, it should be noted that this model does not fully recreate the dynamic environment found at the site of device function.

Another option for *in vivo* experiments is the placement of a prototype of the final device at the site where it would be found in human patients. This usually requires a large animal model such as a cow or sheep, particularly with cardiovascular implants. Other disadvantages include that the implantation procedure can be lengthy and complex (involving cardiopulmonary bypass) and thus operative costs may be high. However, this model is often used as a final test of a new device design or material because it best represents the environment that such a device would encounter in human patients.

14.7.3 Sample Assessment

Specimens from both *in vitro* and *in vivo* experiments can be evaluated for degree of calcium deposition in a similar manner. Entire samples may be subjected to biochemical assays to determine calcium content via color change after reaction with the appropriate reagent. As described in more detail in Chapter 8, the color change is quantified on a microplate reader equipped with a spectrophotometer and compared with a standard curve to determine the amount of calcium present in the sample.

Alternatively, the sample may be sectioned as per standard histological techniques (see Chapters 9 and 11) and stained for calcium content to examine the location of the calcification. Explants can also be analyzed via SEM or TEM to visualize the specimen, as well as to quantify Ca and P content using the EDXA X-ray attachment described in Chapter 7. X-ray diffraction experiments (see Chapter 2) on a ground portion of the sample may provide additional useful information about the structure of the crystals formed.

For assessment that does not require explantation of *in vivo* specimens, radiographs (traditional X-rays) can be used to monitor calcification within samples from both *in vitro* and *in vivo* experiments (Fig. 14.8). Radiography is a nondestructive technique that can be used with living animals and is based on principles similar to those of X-ray diffraction. However, in radiographic imaging, elements with high atomic numbers (such as calcium phosphates) in essence absorb the X-rays as they travel through the sample and do not allow them to reach the detector, usually a radiographic film. This leaves a white area on the film directly under the calcified material. The size and location of these white (radiopaque) areas can reveal changes in

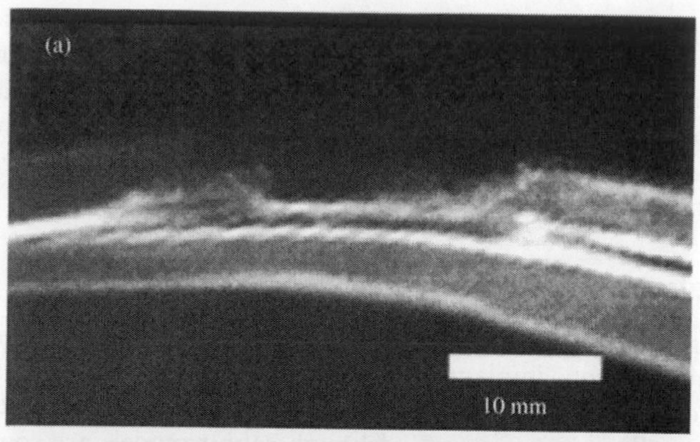

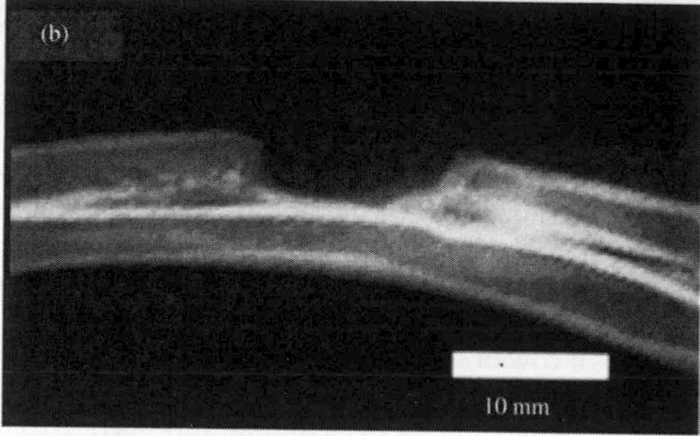

Figure 14.8
Radiographic imaging of a healing defect in the radius (long bone in forearm) of a rabbit. A tissue engineering scaffold was placed in the defect, and radiographs were used to determine the extent of bone formation that occurred at the defect site. The bone from the rabbit in (a) exhibits some degree of repair whereas the bone from a different rabbit in (b) shows minimal repair. Although in this case calcified matrix deposition was desired, similar methods can be also be used to determine the extent of pathologic calcification in a tissue. (Reprinted with permission from [8].)

calcification over time within the same sample. However, conventional radiography only yields two-dimensional representations of three-dimensional samples and often presents limited spatial resolution.

Microcomputed tomography (μCT) is an alternative nondestructive method to evaluate calcification in a sample using X-rays (Fig. 14.9). In this case, a fine-beam X-ray source exposes the sample to X-rays. The X-rays projecting through the sample are detected by a two-dimensional detector array. The sample is then rotated and another projection is rendered, and the process is repeated until two-dimensional projections

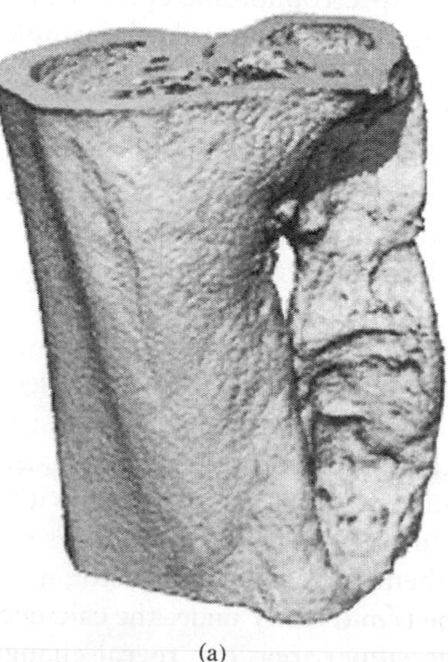
(a)

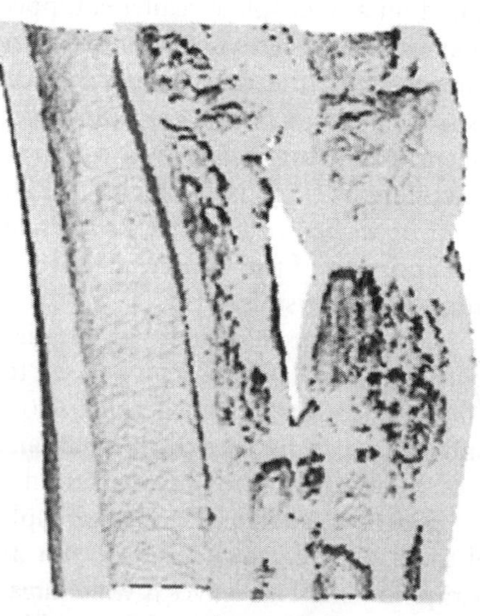
(b)

Figure 14.9
Microcomputed tomography imaging of engineered bone tissue following the implantation of a scaffold in a bone defect in the radius of a rabbit. (a) shows an exterior view and (b) shows a cross-section of the repaired region. Because this imaging modality creates a three-dimensional image, it can be used for quantification of calcified matrix production in a certain volume. (Reprinted with permission from [8].)

have been collected for the entire specimen. A computer processes these projections into images of two-dimensional cross-sections of the sample, which can be combined to reconstruct the three-dimensional internal and external architecture of the sample. The spatial resolution of this technique is of the order of micrometers. It is important to note that a suitable difference must exist in the X-ray attenuation coefficient between the calcified material and the other materials (such as surrounding soft tissue and/or implant material) in order to differentiate them by this and other radiographic techniques.

EXAMPLE PROBLEM 14.3

A company plans to evaluate a new heart valve prosthesis fabricated with crosslinked porcine pericardium in an *in vitro* model. The company is specifically interested in assessing whether the tissue in the heart valve prosthesis will calcify with time. The researcher in charge of the project has decided to place the prosthesis in a pulsatile flow circuit with porcine blood being perfused through the system to simulate physiologic conditions. However, to prevent coagulation of the blood in the system, the researcher wants to supplement the porcine blood with large amounts of ethylenediaminetetraacetic acid (EDTA), a chelating agent for calcium ions. How might EDTA serve to inhibit coagulation? Could the EDTA affect the validity of the calcification study? How? Should the EDTA be used in this system?

Solution: Recalling from Chapter 13 that calcium ions play a crucial role in the coagulation cascade, EDTA will work to inhibit coagulation by sequestering the calcium ions in the blood, limiting their availability to promote coagulation. Additionally, as the EDTA sequesters the calcium in solution, it could reduce the concentration of calcium present during the *in vitro* assays to levels significantly below the values that would normally be found in blood *in vivo*. Thus, if calcification is found not to occur in this *in vitro* analysis, it could be an artifact of the chelation of calcium and might not reflect what would normally happen *in vivo*. It follows that the EDTA should not be used in this system. It would be more suitable to use an anticoagulant that does not sequester calcium as an alternative to EDTA. ■

Summary

- Implant-associated infections have a number of related characteristics. The pathogens most commonly connected with implant-associated infection are the gram-positive bacteria *Staphylococcus aureus* and *Staphylococcus epidermidis*, the gram-negative bacteria *Enterobacteriaceae* and *Pseudomonas aeriginosa*, and fungi such as *Candida*. These pathogens can result in different categories of infections, including superficial immediate infection, deep immediate infection, and late infection.
- Four distinct stages are involved in the development of implant-associated infection. First, preliminary reversible bacterial attachment to the surface occurs through nonspecific interactions (attachment). Second, the preliminary attachment becomes permanent as specific receptor-ligand interactions develop and nonspecific interactions remain (adhesion). Third, the bacteria divide after firmly attaching to the surface, causing the development of a biofilm (aggregation). Fourth, the bacteria travel from the colony to other areas of the body (dispersion).
- The biofilm produced by bacteria assists in trapping ions important to bacterial survival, offers protection against the natural defenses of the body, and can impart antibiotic resistance.
- The two major classes of bacteria are gram-positive and gram-negative species. Gram-positive species have a single bilayered phospholipid membrane and a

thick cell wall composed of peptidoglycan. Gram-negative species have two phospholipid membranes (cell membrane and outer membrane), with the peptidoglycan layer between them.

- The bacterial surface properties of most importance to adhesion to biomaterial surfaces are surface hydrophobicity and charge. The surface hydrophobicity of bacteria can be assessed by contact angle measurements, the microbial adherence to hydrocarbons (MATH) technique, or through hydrophobic interaction chromatography (HIC). Bacterial surface charge can be assessed through electrophoretic mobility tests or electrostatic interaction chromatography (EIC).
- Bacterial adhesion to a biomaterial can be strongly influenced by the layer of proteins adsorbed to the material surface; thus, material properties can influence protein adsorption and bacterial attachment. Further, the protein and/or ion content of the media can affect the composition of the protein layer adsorbed to a material and consequently the attachment of bacteria.
- A carcinogen is a stimulus that results in malignant transformation of cells. A complete carcinogen causes malignant transformation by itself, while a procarcinogen is not a carcinogen in its native form, but can be converted to one by metabolic processes found *in vivo*. A cocarcinogen possesses little or no inherent mutagenic potential, but enhances the activity of pro- or complete carcinogens.
- The three basic stages of tumorigenesis are initiation, latency, and promotion. The initiation phase involves the primary cellular transformation. It is followed by a period of no visible tumor formation called latency. The point at which tumor development and growth can be observed marks the onset of the promotion phase.
- There are two primary routes of malignant transformation: chemical carcinogenesis and foreign body carcinogenesis. Chemical carcinogenesis involves exposure to chemicals that are known to be carcinogens. Foreign body carcinogenesis occurs when materials with no known chemical carcinogenic activity are observed to cause tumor development.
- Possible contributing factors to foreign body carcinogenesis include bulk chemical properties of the implant, physicochemical surface properties of the implant, viral contamination of the implant, interruption of cellular communication due to the presence of the implant, local tissue damage leading to insufficient nutrient exchange, and disturbed cellular growth around the implant. Foreign body tumorigenesis has also been observed with small fibers (less than 1 μm in diameter and more than 8 μm in length).
- Undesired calcification is termed pathologic calcification, and it can be deleterious to device function as it imparts stiffness and brittleness to the material. Pathologic calcification of biomedical implants depends on the host metabolism, surface and bulk properties of the biomaterial chosen, and the mechanical environment of the device. Naturally based ECM materials are especially susceptible to pathologic calcification.
- *In vitro*, *in vivo*, and *ex vivo* experiments can be performed to assess a biomaterial's proclivity to infection and, in most cases, they are very similar to the ones employed in other biocompatibility assays.
- *In vitro* assays for tumorigenesis are actually tests to assess the mutagenic potential of a material and/or its leachable products. *In vivo* carcinogenesis assessment is generally undertaken as part of general biocompatibility testing in accordance with the guidelines of standards organizations.

- The potential for a material to be calcified can be assessed preliminarily through *in vitro* studies employing media that approximate the physiological environment that the device would face in its intended application. *In vivo* models of calcification generally provide more complete information and can be conducted either subcutaneously or at the site of intended final application.

Problems

14.1 You perform an *in vivo* study and discover during the first time point after implantation that there are *Staphylococcus aureus* bacteria at the external surface of the incision site. Does their presence indicate an infection?

14.2 Is implant sterilization sufficient to prevent infection following implantation? Why or why not?

14.3 You implant a sample material subcutaneously in the back of a rabbit model in an effort to evaluate the tissue response. After 24 hours, you notice the presence of an infection in one of the hind legs. Is this infection due to the presence of the implanted material?

14.4 Would the occurrence of tumorigenesis be more or less likely to occur with an implant that is encased in a fibrous capsule (compared with an integrated implant)? Why or why not?

14.5 Preliminary *in vitro* testing shows that treating a porcine heart valve with a surfactant before implantation reduces calcification. You decide to design and run an *in vivo* experiment to verify these results. What would you do?

14.6 The following graph shows the results from a study in which the adhesion of *Staphylococcus epidermidis* to two different material surfaces was examined. In this study the "adhesive coefficient" is defined as the percent of the bacteria transported to the biomaterial surface that were retained per unit surface area. The surfaces consisted of either poly(ethylene) that was coated with plasma proteins or poly(ethylene) with adherent platelets. Shear stress was applied to the samples to determine how well the bacteria attached to the experimental surfaces. What do these results indicate? How would you apply this information if you were to design a cardiovascular implant? (Figure adapted with permission from [9].)

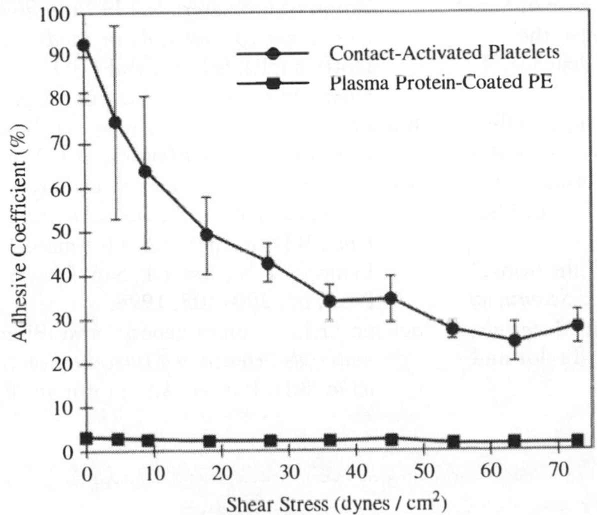

References

1. Gristina, A.G. "Biomaterial-Centered Infection: Microbial Adhesion versus Tissue Integration," *Science*, vol. 237, pp. 1588–1595, 1987.
2. Dickinson, R.B., A.G. Ruta, and S.E. Truesdail. "Physiochemical Basis of Bacterial Adhesion to Biomaterial Surfaces." In *Antimicrobial/Anti-Infective Materials: Principles, Applications, and Devices*, S.P. Sawan and G. Manivannan, Eds. Lancaster: Technomic Publishing, pp. 67–93, 2000.
3 Madigan, M.E., Martinko, J.M., and J. Parker. *Brock Biology of Microorganisms*, 9th ed. Upper Saddle River: Prentice Hall, 2000.
4. Hancock, I. and I. Poxton. *Bacterial Cell Surface Techniques.* New York: John Wiley and Sons, 1988.
5. Costerton, B., G. Cook, M. Shirtliff, P. Stoodley, and M. Pasmore. "Biofilms, Biomaterials, and Device-Related Infections." In *Biomaterials Science: An Introduction to Materials in Medicine*, B.D. Ratner, A.S. Hoffman, F.J. Schoen, and J.E. Lemons, Eds., 2nd ed. San Diego: Elsevier Academic Press, pp. 345–354, 2004.
6. Wang, I.W., J.M. Anderson, M.R. Jacobs, and R.E. Marchant. "Adhesion of *Staphylococcus epidermidis* to Biomedical Polymers: Contributions of Surface Thermodynamics and Hemodynamic Shear Conditions," *Journal of Biomedical Materials Research*, vol. 29, pp. 485–493, 1995.
7. Black, J. *Biological Performance of Materials: Fundamentals of Biocompatibility*, 4th ed. New York: CRC Press, 2005.
8. Hedberg, E.L., H.C. Kroese-Deutman, C.K. Shih, J.J. Lemoine, M.A. Liebschner, M.J. Miller, A.W. Yasko, R.S. Crowther, D.H. Carney, A.G. Mikos, and J.A. Jansen. "Methods: A Comparative Analysis of Radiography, Microcomputed Tomography, and Histology for Bone Tissue Engineering," *Tissue Engineering*, vol. 11, pp. 1356–1367, 2005.
9. Wang, I.W., J.M. Anderson, and R.E. Marchant. "Platelet-Mediated Adhesion of *Staphylococcus epidermidis* to Hydrophobic NHLBI Reference Polyethylene," *Journal of Biomedical Materials Research*, vol. 27, pp. 1119–1128, 1993.

Additional Reading

Anderson, J.M. "Mechanisms of Inflammation and Infection with Implanted Devices," Cardiovascular Pathology, vol. 2, pp. 33S–41S, 1993.

Anderson, J.M. and F.J. Schoen. "*In Vivo* Assesment of Tissue Compatibility." In *Biomaterials Science: An Introduction to Materials in Medicine*, B.D. Ratner, A.S. Hoffman, F.J. Schoen, and J.E. Lemons, Eds., 2nd ed. San Diego: Elsevier Academic Press, pp. 360–367, 2004.

Appelmelk, B. and W. Lynn. "Chapter 2: The Cause of Sepsis: Bacterial Cell Components That Trigger the Cytokine Cascade." In *Septic Shock*, J.-F. Dhainaut, L. Thijs, and G. Park, Eds. London: WB Sanders, 2000.

Gristina, A.G. and P.T. Naylor. "Implant-Associated Infection." In *Biomaterials Science: An Introduction to Materials in Medicine*, B.D. Ratner, A.S. Hoffman, F.J. Schoen, and J.E. Lemons, Eds., 1st ed. San Diego: Elsevier Academic Press, pp. 205–214, 1996.

Higashi, J.M. and R.E. Marchant. "Implant Infections." In *Handbook of Biomaterials Evaluation: Scientific, Technical, and Clinical Testing of Implant Materials*, A.F. von Recum, Ed., 2nd ed. Philadelphia: Taylor and Francis, pp. 493–506, 1999.

Levy, R.J., F.J. Schoen, H.C. Anderson, H. Harasaki, T.H. Koch, W. Brown, J.B. Lian, R. Cumming, and J.B. Gavin. "Cardiovascular Implant Calcification: A Survey and Update," *Biomaterials*, vol. 12, pp. 707–714, 1991.

Morton, D., C.L. Alden, A.J. Roth, and T. Usui. "The Tg Rash2 Mouse in Cancer Hazard Identification," *Toxicologic Pathology*, vol. 30, pp. 139–146, 2002.

Pathak, Y., F.J. Schoen, and R.J. Levy. "Pathological Calcification of Biomaterials." In *Biomaterials Science: An Introduction to Materials in Medicine*, B.D. Ratner, A.S. Hoffman, F.J. Schoen, and J.E. Lemons, Eds., 1st ed. San Diego: Elsevier Academic Press, pp. 272–281, 1996.

Ratner, B.D. "Characterization of Biomaterial Surfaces," *Cardiovascular Pathology*, vol. 2, pp. 87S–100S, 1993.

Schoen, F.J. "Tumorigenesis and Biomaterials." In *Biomaterials Science: An Introduction to Materials in Medicine*, B.D. Ratner, A.S. Hoffman, F.J. Schoen, and J.E. Lemons, Eds., 1st ed. San Diego: Elsevier Academic Press, pp. 200–205, 1996.

Schoen, F.J., "Tumorigenesis and Biomaterials." In *Biomaterials Science: An Introduction to Materials in Medicine*, B.D. Ratner, A.S. Hoffman, F.J. Schoen, and J.E.

Lemons, Eds., 2nd ed. San Diego: Elsevier Academic Press, pp. 338–345, 2004.

Schoen, F.J. and R.J. Levy. "Pathological Calcification of Biomaterials." In *Biomaterials Science: An Introduction to Materials in Medicine*, B.D. Ratner, A.S. Hoffman, F.J. Schoen, and J.E. Lemons, Eds., 2nd ed. San Diego: Elsevier Academic Press, pp. 439–453, 2004.

Smith, A.W. "Biofilms and Antibiotic Therapy: Is There a Role for Combating Bacterial Resistance by the Use of Novel Drug Delivery Systems?" *Advanced Drug Delivery Reviews*, vol. 57, pp. 1539–1550, 2005.

Von Recum, A.F. *Handbook of Biomaterials Evaluation: Scientific, Technical, and Clinical Testing of Implant Materials.* Philadelphia: Taylor and Francis, 1999.

Zhang, X. "Anti-Infective Coatings Reduce Device-Related Infections." In *Antimicrobial/Anti-Infective Materials: Principles, Applications, and Devices*, S.P. Sawan and G. Manivannan, Eds. Lancaster: Technomic Publishing, pp. 149–180, 2000.

APPENDIX I

List of Abbreviations and Symbols

List of Abbreviations (alphabetical)

3DP	Three-dimensional printing
A	Adenine
ADP	Adenosine diphosphate
AFM	Atomic force microscopy
AIDS	Acquired immune deficiency syndrome
amu	Atomic mass unit
APC	Antigen-presenting cell
APF	Atomic packing factor
ASTM	American Society for Testing and Materials
AT III	Antithrombin III
ATP	Adenosine triphosphate
ATR-FTIR	Attenuated total reflectance-Fourier-transform infrared
BCC	Body-centered cubic
C	Cytosine
CAD	Computer-aided design
CAMs	Cell adhesion molecules
CS	Chondroitin sulfate
CTL	Cytotoxic T lymphocyte
CVD	Chemical vapor deposition
DLVO	Derjaguin, Landau, Verway, and Overbeek
DMA	Dynamic mechanical analysis
DNA	Deoxyribonucleic acid
DS	Dermatan sulfate
DSC	Differential scanning calorimetry
dsDNA	Double-stranded DNA
ECM	Extracellular matrix
EDXA	Energy-dispersive X-ray analysis
EIC	Electrostatic interaction chromatography
ELISA	Enzyme-linked immunosorbent assay
emf	Electromotive force
ER	Endoplasmic reticulum
ESCA	Electron spectroscopy for chemical analysis
F_{ab}	Fragment antigen-binding
F_c	Fragment crystallizable
FACS	Fluorescence-activated cell sorter
FBGC	Foreign body giant cell
FCC	Face-centered cubic
FT-IR	Fourier-transform-infrared
G	Guanine
GAGs	Glycosaminoglycans
GFC	Gel filtration chromatography
GP	Glycoprotein
GPC	Gel permeation chromatography
HA	Hyaluronic acid
HCP	Hexagonal close-packed
HIC	Hydrophobic interaction chromatography
HIP	Hot isostatic pressing
HMWK	High molecular weight kininogen
HPLC	High-performance liquid chromatography
Ig	Immunoglobulin
IR	Infrared
IL-1	Interleukin-1
IL-1ra	IL-1 receptor agonist
IL-6	Interleukin-6
IL-8	Interleukin-8
ISO	International Organization for Standardization
KS	Keratan sulfate
LB-film	Langmuir-Blodgett-film
LDH	Lactate dehydrogenase
LTT	Lymphocyte transformation test
MAC	Membrane attack complex
MATH	Microbial adherence to hydrocarbons
MHC	Major histocompatibility complex
MIP-1a	Macrophage inflammatory protein-1a
MIP-1b	Macrophage inflammatory protein-1b
MMP	Matrix metalloproteinase
mRNA	Messenger RNA
MSCRAMM	Microbial surface components recognizing adhesive matrix molecules
MWNT	Multiwalled nanotube
NMR	Nuclear magnetic resonance
PCR	Polymerase chain reaction
PGI_2	Prostaglandin I_2

PI	Polydispersity index
P/M	Powder metallurgy
PVD	Physical vapor deposition
RNA	Ribonucleic acid
rRNA	Ribosomal RNA
RT-PCR	Reverse transcription-polymerase chain reaction
SAL	Sterility assurance level
SAM	Self-assembled monolayer
SDS	Sodium dodecyl sulfate
SDS-PAGE	SDS-poly(acrylamide)gel electrophoresis
SEC	Size exclusion chromatography
SEM	Scanning electron microscopy
SFF	Solid freeform fabrication
SIMS	Secondary ion mass spectrometry
SLS	Selective laser sintering
SMAs	Surface-modifying additives
SPM	Scanning probe microscopy
ssDNA	Single-stranded DNA
SWNT	Single-walled nanotube
T	Thymine
T_c	Cytotoxic T cell
T_h	Helper T cell
TCR	T cell receptor
TEM	Transmission electron microscopy
TF	Tissue factor
TGA	Thermogravimetric analysis
TGF-β	Transforming growth factor-β
TIMP	Tissue inhibitor of metalloproteinase
TNF-α	Tumor necrosis factor-α
TPA	Tissue plasminogen activator
tRNA	Transfer RNA
U	Uracil
UV-VIS	Ultraviolet and visible light spectroscopy
vWF	von Willebrand factor
XPS	X-ray photoelectron spectroscopy
μCT	Microcomputed tomography

List of Symbols (alphabetical)

Symbol	Definition	Chapter
A	Absorbance	2
A	Amplitude	2
A	Cross-sectional area	2
a	Length of a crack on the surface or half the length of an internal crack	4
A_0	Original cross-sectional area	4
A_f	Cross-sectional area at fracture	4
A_{in}	Instantaneous area	4
a, b, c	Unit cell edge lengths	2
b	Burger's vector	3
b, d	Specimen dimensions	4
C	Molar concentration of a compound	2
C	Concentration of a protein	8
C	Concentration of a chemical signal	9
C	Concentration of a receptor-ligand complex	9
D	Diffusivity	2, 8
E	Energy	1
E	Modulus of elasticity (Young's modulus)	4
E_1^0, E_2^0	Measured potential of materials 1 and 2	5
E_A	Attractive energy	1
E_b	Binding energy	7
E_k	Kinetic energy	7
E_R	Repulsive energy	1
E_{total}	Total energy	1
F	Force	1, 4
F	Faraday's constant	5
F_A	Attractive force between two atoms	1
F_C	Coulombic force	1
F_f	Load at fracture	4
F_R	Repulsive force between two atoms	1
F_{total}	Total force between two atoms	1
G	Shear modulus	4
G	Gibbs free energy	8, 14
h	Planck's constant	2, 7
h	Distance between plates	9
H	Enthalpy	8
J	Diffusion flux	2
k	Boltzmann's constant	2
k	Kinetic rate constant of crystal growth	3
k_0	Proportionality constant	1
k_f	Kinetic rate constant of complex formation	9
k_r	Kinetic rate constant of complex dissociation	9
l	Thickness of a sample through which light is passed	2
L	Distance between supports	4
L	Concentration of a free ligand	9
l_0	Length of sample before loading (gauge length)	4
l_f	Length at fracture	4
l_i	Sample length at any point during a testing procedure (instantaneous length)	4
M	Mass (or number of atoms)	2
M	Molecule	2
M	Flux of cells	9
M^*	Molecule excited to a new state	2
M_i	Average molecular weight for a chosen molecular weight range	2
$\overline{M}_n$	Number-average molecular weight	2
$\overline{M}_w$	Weight-average molecular weight	2
N	Total number of atomic sites	2
N	Cell number	9
n	Number characteristic of the mechanism of crystal nucleation and growth	3
N_f	Fatigue life	4
N_i	Number of chains with molecular weight M_i	2

Symbol	Definition	Chapter
N_i	Number of cycles required for crack initiation	4
N_{in}	Number of interstitials	2
N_p	Number of cycles for propagation of a crack to critical size for failure	4
N_v	Number of vacancies	2
$N_{v,an}$	Number of anion vacancies	2
$N_{v,cat}$	Number of cation vacancies	2
p	Persistence time	9
q	Charge of a single electron	1
Q	Activation energy for diffusion	2
Q	Volumetric flow rate	8, 9
Q_v	Activation energy for formation of a vacancy	2
Q_{vi}	Activation energy for formation of a vacancy and an interstitial	2
Q_{vp}	Activation energy for formation of a cation/anion vacancy pair	2
r	Separation distance between ions 1 and 2	1
r	Atomic radius	2
r	Distance coordinate	8
R	Gas constant	2, 5
R	Radius of cylinder	8
R	Concentration of the free receptor	9
r_0	Separation distance between two atoms where equilibrium is reached	1
r_a	Radius of an anion	2
r_c	Radius of a cation	2
s	Translocation speed	9
S	Entropy	8
t	Time	2
T	Absolute temperature	2, 5, 8
T	Torque force	4
T_c	Crystallization temperature	3
T_g	Glass transition temperature	3, 4
T_m	Melting temperature	3, 4
t_r	Time to rupture	4
V	Velocity	8
w	Width	9
x	Distance coordinate	9
$X(t)$	Degree of crystallinity of a polymer at time t	3
y	Distance coordinate	8
Z	Atomic number	1
Z_1, Z_2	Valance of ions 1 and 2	1
%EL	% elongation	4
%AR	% area reduction	4
α, β, γ	Angles between axes of unit cell	2
γ	Shear strain	4
γ	Surface tension (surface free energy)	7
$\dot{\gamma}$	Rate of applied (shear) strain, or rate of deformation	3, 4

Symbol	Definition	Chapter
γ_c	Critical surface tension	7
γ_{LV}	Liquid-vapor surface tension	7
γ_{SL}	Solid-liquid surface tension	7
γ_{SV}	Solid-vapor surface tension	7
ΔE^0	Electrochemical potential	5
ΔG	Gibbs free energy change	14
ΔG_{ads}	Change in G for the entire adsorption process	8
ΔG_{prot}	Change in G for a protein during an adsorption process	8
ΔG_{sol}	Change in G for a solvent during an adsorption process	8
ΔG_{surf}	Change in G for a surface during an adsorption process	8
ϵ	Molar absorption coefficient for a compound at a given wavelength	2
ε	Engineering strain	4
$\dot{\varepsilon}$	Creep rate	4
ε_a	Strain along loading axis	4
ε_t	Transverse strain	4
ε_t	True strain	4
ε_{yp}	Yield point strain	4
η	Viscosity	3, 4
θ	Contact angle	7
λ	Wavelength	2
λ	Angle between slip direction and direction of applied force	4
μ	Viscosity	8, 9
ν	Poisson's ratio	4
ν	Frequency	2, 7
ρ_a	Density of polymer in amorphous form	3
ρ_c	Density of polymer in crystalline form	3
ρ_s	Density of polymer sample	3
ρ_t	Radius of curvature of a crack tip	4
σ	Engineering stress	4
σ	Random motility coefficient	9
σ_0	Overall applied stress	4
σ_f	Fracture strength	4
σ_m	Maximum stress at a crack tip	4
σ_{mr}	Modulus of rupture	4
σ_t	True stress	4
σ_{uts}	Ultimate tensile strength	4
σ_y	Yield strength	4
τ	Shear stress	3, 4, 9
τ_{crss}	Critical resolved shear stress	4
τ_r	Resolved shear stress	4
ϕ	Angle between normal to the slip plane and direction of force	4
χ	Chemotactic coefficient	9
$\perp$	Edge dislocation	3
$\circlearrowleft$	Screw dislocation	3

Index

D

E

Q